# PEDIATRIC STEM CELL TRANSPLANTATION

*Edited by*

## PAULETTE MEHTA, MD

Professor of Internal Medicine and Pediatrics
Director of Hematology/Oncology
Central Arkansas Veterans Healthcare System
Little Rock, Arkansas

**JONES AND BARTLETT PUBLISHERS**
*Sudbury, Massachusetts*
BOSTON　　TORONTO　　LONDON　　SINGAPORE

*World Headquarters*
Jones and Bartlett Publishers
40 Tall Pine Drive
Sudbury, MA 01776
978-443-5000
info@jbpub.com
www.jbpub.com

Jones and Bartlett Publishers Canada
2406 Nikanna Road
Mississauga, ON L5C 2W6
CANADA

Jones and Bartlett Publishers International
Barb House, Barb Mews
London W6 7PA
UK

**Library of Congress Cataloging-in-Publication Data**

Pediatric stem cell transplantation / edited by Paulette Mehta.
    p. ; cm.
   Includes bibliographical references and index.
   ISBN 0-7637-1855-6
      1. Bone marrow–Transplantation. 2. Hematopoietic stem cells–Transplantation. 3. Transplatation of organs, tissues, etc. in children. I. Mehta, Paulette.
   [DNLM: 1. Bone Marrow Transplantation–Child. 2. Stem Cell Transplantation–Child. WH 380 P371 2003]
   RD123.5.P436 2003
   617.4'4–dc21

                                 2003047423

Executive Publisher: Christopher Davis
Production Manager: Amy Rose
Associate Production Editor: Renée Sekerak
Editorial Assistant: Elizabeth Peterson
Manufacturing Buyer: Therese Bräuer
Design and Composition: Studio Montage
Cover Design: Kristin E. Ohlin
Printing and Binding: Malloy Incorporated
Cover Printing: Malloy Incorporated

Printed in the United States of America
07 06 05 04 03   10 9 8 7 6 5 4 3 2 1

# TABLE OF CONTENTS

**CHAPTER VI**    **Pediatric Stem Cell Transplantation: Ethical Concerns** . . . . . . . . . . 91

*Puneet Cheema and Paulette Mehta*

**CHAPTER VII**    **Psychosocial Adjustment After Stem Cell Transplantation** . . . . . . . . . 99

*Allen C. Sherman, Stephanie Simonton, and Umaira Latif*

**CHAPTER XI**

## High Dose Chemotherapy and Stem Cell Rescue for Treatment of Brain Tumors

**CHAPTER XII**

## Acute Lymphoblastic Leukemia

# PREFACE

This book grew from my experiences as a pediatric hematologist-oncologist-stem cell transplanter at the University of Florida from 1977 to 2000. I joined the pediatric hematology/oncology faculty before the transplant unit opened in 1980, and helped to recruit its first director, Dr. Samuel Gross. Under his leadership, the bone marrow transplant program was born and started growing. Later, the leadership moved to Dr. John Wingard, who is currently the director of the combined pediatric-adult bone marrow transplant unit. During my time on the faculty (including 7 years as its Medical Director), I watched the unit open, blossom, and give rise to miracles undreamed of at the time it began. In effect, my bone marrow transplant unit was, and is, a microcosm of the universe of hematology/oncology-stem cell transplantation, which has grown from infancy to maturity in just a few years.

These pages contain the story of these few years of momentous change in pediatric stem cell transplantation. Some of the giants who paved the field, including Dr. Robert Good, have contributed chapters describing their early work. Other contributing authors pioneered treatments for graft-versus-host disease, for bacterial, viral, and fungal infections associated with transplantation, and/or made major strides in developing conditioning regimens for different diseases. Some of the authors "dared to dream the impossible" of using unrelated and/or mismatched stem cells, or of using stem cells derived from places in the body other than the bone marrow itself, which was once thought to be the only source of hematopoietic stem cells. Now other sources–peripheral blood, umbilical cord blood, and even fat cells–are being used or being considered for stem cell engineering and transplantation. Other authors of this book have been instrumental in developing the banks that made transplantation available to children of minority groups, who previously lacked available donors. The widening sources of bone marrow stem cells now make stem cell transplantation, once reserved for a small elite of children, a possibility for all children.

Many of the authors in this book are members of the collaborative groups through which my colleagues and I made our connections and started our trials. These collaborative groups include the Children's Oncology Group (COG, wedded from the Pediatric Hematology/Oncology and the Children's Cancer Group in 2000) and the Pediatric Bone Marrow Transplantation Consortium. I owe special thanks to these groups for nurturing the careers of myself and others, and in so doing, inspiring so many projects and landmark discoveries in stem cell transplantation.

I am grateful to all of the authors of this book, who spent endless hours recording years of work in a few pages. All were incredibly cooperative, forthcoming, and kind. I also thank the editors at Jones and Bartlett Publishers, especially Chris Davis. We made contact several years before the idea of this book took hold, and he kept its vision alive even as I switched universities, programs, and career paths. Thanks also to Renée Sekerak, Elizabeth Peterson, and the other editors at Jones and Bartlett for urging me onwards to finish just one more chapter, edit one more passage, or suggest one more author.

A final note is a sad one. Shortly after the finalization of most of this book's chapters, the world learned of Dr. Robert Good's untimely and unfortunate passing. Dr. Good was a giant in our field, inarguably the father of modern immunology. In 1968, he became the first physician ever to successfully complete a transplant on a patient with severe immuno-deficiency, using allogeneic stem cells. This patient is alive and well—the longest survivor of stem cell transplantation.

Dr. Good's move to Florida in 1985 enriched both the state itself and his many Florida colleagues, including me. I am humbled by the thought that one of the great pioneers of stem cell transplantation and of immunology, Dr. Robert Good, completed the last great chapter of his life by summarizing his life's achievements in a chapter for this book.

As we are entering the new millennium, stem cell transplantation still offers untold opportunities for the engineering and delivery of cells and for the healing and cure of disease. We can predict new sources of stem cells, new ways to engineer new genes into old cells, new ways to harness graft-versus-host disease, and new ways to avoid or treat complications. We can predict ever-increasing numbers of patients saved and ever-increasing diseases eradicated by stem cell transplantation. One day we will look back and realize that we have only just begun, and truly the best is yet to come.

To my mother and father, now departed, whose memories
   continue to inspire every day's work,

To my husband with whom I have shared my entire adult life,
   for his patience and support,

To my beautiful children Asha and Jason who make every day worthwhile
   and who are my most sacred gifts from and to the world,

To all the many families who trusted me with the care of their children,
   to the dignity of those who survived,
   and the memory of those who fell,

To my teachers, peers, friends, and students who created the web
   that makes all of life meaningful....

**TO LIFE!**

   – *Paulette Mehta, MD*

**Paulette Mehta, MD**
Director of Hematology/Oncology
Central Arkansas Veterans Healthcare System
Professor of Internal Medicine and Pediatrics
University of Arkansas for Medical Sciences
Little Rock, Arkansas

**Elias Anaissie, MD**
Professor of Medicine
University of Arkansas for Medical Sciences
Little Rock, Arkansas

**Miriam A. Botwinick, MS, MEd, RD**
Senior Pediatric Nutritionist
Division of Pediatric Hematology/Oncology
Stem Cell Transplantation Program
Schneider Children's Hospital
North Shore-Long Island Jewish Health System
New Hyde Park, New York

**Paul A. Carpenter, MD**
Division of Clinical Research
Fred Hutchinson Cancer Research Center
University of Washington
Department of Pediatrics
Seattle, Washington

**Suneetha Challagundla, MD**
University of Arkansas for Medical Sciences
Central Arkansas Veterans Healthcare System
Little Rock, Arkansas

**Puneet Cheema, MD**
Department of Oncology
Ministry Medical Group
Rhinelander, Wisconsin

**Seth J. Corey, MD**
Division of Hematology/Oncology
Children's Hospital of Pittsburgh
Pittsburgh, Pennsylvania

## Jonathan Finlay, ChB, MB

Director of the Steven D. Hassenfeld Center for Children With Cancer and Other
   Blood Disorders
NYU Medical Center
New York, New York

## Vicki L. Fisher, RN, MSN, CPNP

Program Manager of the Pediatric and Adult Blood and Marrow Transplant Program
Rainbow Babies and Children's Hospital
University Hospitals of Cleveland
Ireland Cancer Center
Case Western Reserve University School of Medicine
Cleveland, Ohio

## Sharon Gardner, MD

The Steven D. Hassenfeld Center for Children With Cancer and Other Blood Disorders
NYU Medical Center
New York, New York

## Robert A. Good, PhD, MD, DSc

Director of Children's Research Institute
Physician in Chief
All Children's Hospital
Distinguished Research Professor
University of South Florida
Tampa, Florida
Deceased: June 13, 2003

## Dennis P. M. Hughes, MD, PhD

Lecturer, Pediatric Hematology/Oncology
University of Michigan Medical Center
Ann Arbor, Michigan

## Michael Joyce, MD, PhD

Director of Pediatric HSCT
Nemours Children's Clinic
Associate Professor of Pediatrics
Mayo Medical School
Jacksonville, Florida

## Morris Kletzel, MD, FAAP

Division Head of Hematology/Oncology and Stem Cell Transplant
Director of the Stem Cell Transplant Program
Children's Memorial Hospital
Northwestern University Feinberg School of Medicine
Chicago, Illinois

**Lakshmanan Krishnamurti, MD**
Director of the Hemoglobinopathy Program
Division of Hematology/Oncology/BMT
Children's Hospital of Pittsburgh
Assistant Professor of Pediatrics
Pittsburgh, Pennsylvania

**Umaira Latif, M.Sc.**
Research Coordinator of Behavioral Medicine
University of Arkansas for Medical Sciences
Arkansas Cancer Research Center
Little Rock, Arkansas

**Choon Kee Lee, MD**
Associate Professor of Medicine
University of Arkansas for Medical Sciences
Myeloma Institute for Research and Therapy
Central Arkansas Veterans Administration Healthcare System
Little Rock, Arkansas

**John Levine, MD**
Clinical Associate Professor of Pediatrics
University of Michigan
Blood and Marrow Stem Cell Transplantation Program
Ann Arbor, Michigan

**Jeffrey Michael Lipton, MD, PhD**
Cornell University Hospital
Schneider Children's Hospital
New Hyde Park, New York

**Bertram H. Lubin, MD**
President of Children's Hospital Oakland Research Institute
Director of Sibling Donor Cord Blood Program
Adjunct Clinical Professor of Pediatrics
University of California San Francisco
San Francisco, California

**Robert B. Marcus Jr., MD**
Professor of Radiation Oncology and Pediatrics
Department of Radiation Oncology
Emory University
Atlanta, Georgia

**Joan Morris, MD**
Associate Professor of Pediatrics
Medical Director of Pediatric Stem Cell Transplantation
Loma Linda University Medical Center
Loma Linda, California

**Naomi Moskowitz, MD**
Pediatric Hematology/Oncology Fellow
The Steven D. Hassenfeld Center for Children With Cancer and Other Blood Disorders
NYU Medical Center
New York, New York

**Michael L. Nieder, MD**
Director of the Pediatric Blood and Marrow Transplant Program
Rainbow Babies and Children's Hospital
Associate Professor and Vice Chairman of Pediatrics
Case Western Reserve University School of Medicine
Cleveland, Ohio

**Charles Peters, MD**
Associate Professor of Pediatrics
Hematology/Oncology, Blood and Marrow Transplant
University of Minnesota
Minneapolis, Minnesota

**William Reed, MD**
Assistant Medical Director of Research
Blood Centers of the Pacific, Irwin Center
Associate Clinical Professor of Laboratory Medicine
University of California San Francisco
Medical Director of the Human Islet Cell and Cellular Transplantation Laboratory
San Francisco, California

**Indira Sahdev, MD**
Head of Stem Cell Transplant Program
Schneider Children's Hospital
North Shore-Long Island Jewish Health System
Division of Pediatric Hematology/Oncology
Stem Cell Transplantation Program
New Hyde Park, New York

**Jean E. Sanders, MD**
Fred Hutchinson Cancer Research Center
Professor of Pediatrics
University of Washington
Director of Pediatric Transplantation, FHCRC
Seattle, Washington

**Eric Sandler, MD**
Chief of Pediatric Hematology/Oncology
Nemours Children's Clinic
Associate Professor of Pediatrics
Mayo Medical School
Jacksonville, Florida

**Peter Shaw, MD**
Division of Hematology/Oncology
Children's Hospital of Pittsburgh
Pittsburgh, Pennsylvania

**Allen C. Sherman, PhD**
Director of Behavioral Medicine
Associate Professor of Otolaryngology
University of Arkansas for Medical Sciences
Arkansas Cancer Research Center
Little Rock, Arkansas

**Stephanie Simonton, PhD**
Director of the Program Development of Behavioral Medicine
Associate Professor of Otolaryngology
University of Arkansas for Medical Sciences
Arkansas Cancer Research Center
Little Rock, Arkansas

**Ann Steele, PhD, PMIAC, CLDir**
Department of Pathology and Laboratory Medicine
All Children's Hospital
St. Petersburg, Florida

**Tazim Verjee**
Division of Allergy and Immunology
Department of Pediatrics
University of South Florida/All Children's Hospital
St. Petersburg, Florida

**Adrianna Vlachos, MD**
Cornell University Hospital
Schneider Children's Hospital
New Hyde Park, New York

**Donna A. Wall, MD**
Director of Pediatric Blood and Marrow Transplant Program
Texas Transplantation Institute
San Antonio, Texas

**John R. Wingard, MD**
Price Eminent Scholar and Professor of Medicine
Director of Blood and Marrow Transplant Program
Associate Director of Clinical and Translational Research
University of Florida Shands Cancer Center
Division of Hematology/Oncology
Gainesville, Florida

# PART *I*

# SCIENTIFIC BASIS OF CELL TRANSPLANTATION IN CHILDREN

# CHAPTER I

# The Scientific Basis Of Pediatric Bone Marrow Transplantation

PAULETTE MEHTA

The evolution of bone marrow transplantation springs from advances in many fields including immunology, transfusion medicine, infectious diseases, and supportive care (▼ Table 1.1). Bone marrow transplantation was first tried as early as 1959 when two patients were reported by Thomas et al. to have been treated with high dose radiation therapy followed by subsequent marrow grafting.[1] The patients survived the immediate treatment, but died shortly thereafter. It was not until the 1970s, after years of basic animal experimentation, that serious attempts at bone marrow transplantation would again be attempted.[2-8] During this hiatus, animal models were developed to test the basic concepts in transplantation medicine, and to experiment with different forms of conditioning, different modes of administration of stem cells, and different preventive and therapeutic regimens for complications after bone marrow transplantation. Initially, mice were used as models of disease; however, these animals did not live long enough to evaluate short- or long-term consequences after bone marrow transplantation. Thus, subsequent experiments were carried out using a dog model; these experiments allowed for identification of the DLA [analogous to the human lymphocyte antigen (HLA) system], the role of DLA/HLA matching, and the consequences, prevention, and treatment of graft-versus-host disease (GVHD). These topics dominated the area of clinical bone marrow transplantation for the next several decades.

| TABLE 1.1 | Developments in Supportive Care Making the Development of Bone Marrow Transplantation Possible |
|-----------|------------------------------------------------------------------------------------------------|
| Central catheter | |
| Hyperalimentation | |
| Specific anti-emetics | |
| Growth factors | |
| HLA typing | |
| Virtual banks for unrelated matches | |
| Banks for umbilical cord | |

# DEVELOPMENTS IN OTHER FIELDS THAT ENHANCED BONE MARROW TRANSPLANTATION

## Immunology

The concepts of self and non-self and of tolerance[10-13] suggested that transplantation of mature cells could not be grafted to another subject without it being recognized as non-self and therefore rejected, except under two conditions. First, the antigen could be mistaken for "self" if the antigen was presented early in life or early in reestablishing immunity after transplant (as in microchimerism, see later in this chapter). Second, the antigen could be accepted as "self" if the immune system was sufficiently suppressed with radiation and/or chemotherapy to mistake the antigen as "self". Much of the developments in this area arose from the work of Good et al., as described in Chapter X.

## Transfusion Medicine

Major advances in transfusion medicine took place, especially after World War II. These advances related to collection of blood component therapy, development of pheresis and apheresis equipment, use of ABO and Rh blood groups, HLA typing and matching, and isolation of stem cells. Developments in transfusion support and other systems were required, since conditioning prior to infusion of stem cells results in intense and prolonged myelosuppression.

The time of aplasia lasting until engraftment is fraught with an intense need for fractionated blood products. In particular, platelets and red blood cells are given frequently and other components as needed. Blood must be irradiated to prevent graft-versus-host disease, often must be leuko-depleted and/or cytomegalovirus (CMV) screened for CMV negative blood in order to prevent CMV infections, and products often must be matched by HLA type in order to prevent, or lessen, alloimmunization and/or reactions from alloimmunization if it has already occurred.

Also, stem cells are collected using the standard storage bags and filter devices developed for other blood products. Stem cell collection from peripheral blood requires similar equipment as for apheresis of blood products, albeit for days on end until a sufficient number of CD34+ cells could be collected.

## Infectious Diseases

During the time of aplasia, patients are at risk for overwhelming infection from bacterial, viral, fungal, and other types of infections. Much of the mortality of the early days of bone marrow transplantation was averted in subsequent years as antiviral, antibiotics, antifungals, and other agents developed, and as methods for early detection of small amounts of viral load improved. Drs. Anaissie and Wingard were pioneers in much of this work, as described by them in Chapter X.

The advent of bone marrow transplantation saw a change in predominantly gram-negative to gram-positive bacterial organisms, mostly related to the implantation of catheters and to prolonged mucositis beginning at the time of neutropenia, leading to increased staphylococcal and streptococcal infections, respectively. Although white blood cell infusions were successfully used, especially for gram-negative infections early on, leukocyte infusions have lost favor in recent years because of their short half-life and because of the ease and efficacy with which granulocyte colony stimulating factors can hasten engraftment. Also, the switch from bone marrow to peripheral blood stem cell collections (see later in this chapter) has enabled much faster engraftment and thereby greatly reduced infectious disease complications.

Viral infections were at one time the bane of bone marrow transplantation. These were due to activation of latent viruses at the time of immunosuppression, or due to primary virus infections acquired from blood products. Viral disease dissemination has become much less of a problem with early and prolonged use of acyclovir in herpes simplex virus positive (HSV+) patients, and occasionally with gancyclovir for CMV positive patients. The incidence of CMV infections has drastically declined due to the use of filters to deplete leukocytes in which the virus resides and/or screening for CMV in all blood products and restriction of blood products to only CMV negative for CMV negative bone marrow transplant patients. The widespread use of the varicella vaccine has also greatly reduced the risk of acquiring varicella in the community. Nevertheless, patients exposed to varicella who have lost their antibody resistance should be treated with zoster immune globulin or zoster immune plasma to avoid serious complications of the disease.

The area of antifungal drug development is now rapidly expanding. Conventional amphotericin is now available in liposomal forms, allowing for reduced renal toxicity. Also, new classes of antifungal drugs have become available; these developments are described in detail in Chapter X.

## Supportive Care

Many developments in supportive care needed to be in place before bone marrow transplantation could be possible. Many of these advances became available as a result of renal transplantation, which preceded bone marrow transplantation by several years. These advances included development of an indwelling central catheter with two, three, or more lumens. The Hickman and Broviac varieties of catheters remain the standards-of-care not only for transplant patients, but also for others who require long-term intensive care. Since renal transplantation preceded bone marrow transplantation, some of these advances were already being developed. Development of extremely effective, safe, and non-sedating antiemetics made the use of high dose chemotherapy more palatable and tolerable for patients. Granulocyte growth factors facilitated engraftment after infusion of stem cells, greatly decreasing the period of aplasia and thereby reducing infections.

## EVOLVING PARADIGMS

The scientific evolution of bone marrow transplantation also can be seen as evolving paradigms (▼ Table 1.2). Initially, bone marrow transplantation was considered a way of simply replacing a damaged or failed organ, the bone marrow. During this early time, bone marrow failure was of national interest because the atomic bomb testing injury to the bone marrow was shown to be immediate and life threatening.[14–16] Sadly, this risk has again become the focus of national concern.[17,18] Subsequently, bone marrow transplantation was considered to be a way of replacing bone marrow damaged through other insults, in

| TABLE 1.2 | Evolving Paradigms for Understanding the Role of Bone Marrow Transplantation |
| --- | --- |

- Bone marrow transplant can be used to replace bone marrow damaged by radiation or other injury
- Bone marrow transplantation can be used to replace bone marrow damaged by viruses, chemicals, etc., as in aplastic anemia
- Bone marrow transplant can be used to replace bone marrow lymphocyte failure, as in severe combined immunodeficiencies
- Bone marrow transplant can be used to replace failure of bone marrow preemptively if lethal injury can be predicted (as when using high dose chemotherapy for hematologic or non-hematologic malignancy, i.e., to rescue bone marrow from chemotherapy-induced injury)
- To induce graft-versus-leukemia effect
- To induce graft-versus-solid tumor effect

particular, infections, toxins, and other undefinable factors. Accordingly, bone marrow transplantation was tried, successfully, in patients with aplastic anemia.[19,20] Patients who had fewer than 100 transfusions prior to transplant, who were young (i.e., < 20 years of age), who were fortunate enough to have a matched sibling, and who were in good general health did well with this procedure. It remains the treatment of choice today as well for newly diagnosed patients who have an HLA-matched sibling donor.

Bone marrow failure also can present as immunodeficiency, since the bone marrow is the source of undifferentiated lymphocytes that later will acquire their T and B cell differentiating factors as they traverse through lymph nodes, spleen, and other reticular tissue. Thus, bone marrow transplantation was considered and used successfully as a method of restoring immunity to patients who had severe combined immunodeficiency (SCID).[21,22] Unlike bone marrow transplantation in other settings, the natural immunodeficiency of these patients is sufficient to preclude the need for any further radiation or chemotherapy conditioning to further reduce immunity.

Later, the concept of bone marrow transplantation for anticipatory bone marrow failure was adopted and embraced. Thus, it was recognized that certain therapies had dose limiting toxicities that were mostly restricted to the bone marrow. These drugs could be escalated in extremely high doses, if bone marrow cells were rescued by removing them prior to chemotherapy attack and then re-infusing after the attack. Such an approach allowed for autologous transplants for hematologic and non-hematologic malignancies. A variation on this theme would be rescuing the bone marrow cells destroyed by chemotherapy and/or radiation with stem cells from another donor, i.e., allogeneic bone marrow transplantation. This also was used for hematologic as well as non-hematologic malignancies.

Surprisingly, patients undergoing allogeneic bone marrow transplantation had very low rates of relapsed disease compared to patients receiving autologous bone marrow transplantation. However, overall survival was not affected, because the gain from better remission was offset by the losses from graft-versus-host disease (GVHD), a serious complication of allogeneic but not autologous bone marrow transplantation.[23,24] This finding was replicated in other studies,[25–27] and has led to a newer, more modern paradigm of bone marrow transplantation, that is, that bone marrow transplantation is immunologically active, and that this activity may be as, or more, important than the high dose chemotherapy used as conditioning prior to the transplant.

Analysis of patients who survived toxicity of allogeneic bone marrow transplantation showed that the presence of GVHD correlated to a longer and better remission. Patients who did not develop GVHD, either because of T cell depletion of marrow cells, syngeneic donors, excessive preventive therapy, or other reasons, had a higher relapse rate than patients who developed GVHD. Chronic GVHD was associated with a low relapse rate after transplantation for patients with acute non-lymphocytic leukemia in relapse or for patients with chronic myelogenous leukemia in blast crisis. Also, aggressive treatment of chronic GVHD often led to re-emergence of the underlying malignancy.

## THE NEW PARADIGM: BONE MARROW TRANSPLANTATION IS A FORM OF IMMUNOTHERAPY

The revelation that bone marrow transplantation (BMT) acts as immunotherapy gave rise to new developments in BMT not previously available.[24,28–30]

First, if BMT acts as immunotherapy, then a myeloablative regimen may not be necessary. Since the myeloablative condition is presumably not the key element to cure, a less-than-ablative dose regimen may be less toxic with little impingement on remission rates. Indeed, if bone marrow transplantation is working through an immunologic rather than cytotoxic pathway, then it may no longer be "necessary to kill to cure".[29,30]

A second consequence of this observation is that mixed chimeras can exist indefinitely, each donor type developing tolerance for the other. Mixed donor chimerism is now accepted as adequate for non-malignant tumors, and mixed donor chimerism is accepted as a platform from which to deliver subsequent doses of donor lymphocytes to acquire full donor chimerism eventually in the case of malignant conditions. The use of slow, chronic treatment with repeated doses of donor lymphocytes allows for much greater tolerance to treatment, and also for much lower risks of severe acute GVHD.

The third consequence of this reinterpretation of the use of bone marrow transplantation was the use of donor lymphocyte infusions (DLI) as follow-up therapy for patients who relapse after bone marrow transplantation. For DLI, the administration of the donor lymphocytes (CD3 cells predominantly) can be used for treatment of relapsed chronic myelogenous leukemia (CML) after bone marrow transplantation. It also is being used experimentally to induce chimerism from the donor in graded, staggered measures[31] so as to avoid overwhelming acute GVHD at the onset. The use of graded DLI to convert to donor chimerism gradually appears promising in several diseases and offers an interesting aspect to bone marrow transplantation (▼ Table 1.3).

### GVHD Treatment Conundrum

These developments of graft-versus-leukemia effects has led to a conundrum of treatment for chronic GVHD.[32] Whether one should treat chronic GVHD (and thereby risk re-emergence of the malignant clone) or not treat (and thereby limit the patient's functional capacity) has been a very difficult, and still not yet resolved, issue in transplantation medicine.

| TABLE 1.3 | Relative Efficacy of Donor Lymphocyte Infusions in Different Malignancies |
|---|---|
| CML+++ | |
| AML++ | |
| MM+++ | |
| HD− ? | |
| NHL, Intermediate Grade+ | |
| NHL, Low Grade++ | |
| NHL, High Grade+ | |
| EBV Lymphoproliferative Disease+++ | |

Symbols: +++ = very effective; ++ = effective; + = may be effective; ? = unknown efficacy. Abbreviations: CML = cell/chronic myelogenous leukemia; AML = acute myelogenous leukemia; MM = multiple myeloma; HD = Hodgkin's Disease; NHL = non-Hodgkin lymphoma; EBV = Epstein-Barr virus.

## Stem Cells Obtained From Sources Other Than Bone Marrow Are Increased

Bone marrow transplantation has become a misnomer, since stem cells can come from many different sources including bone marrow, adult peripheral blood, umbilical cord blood, and adipose tissue. Peripheral blood stem cell has become the major source of stem cells and is usually preferred over bone marrow as a source of stem cells because of the far greater yield.

## UMBILICAL CORD BLOOD TRANSPLANTATION

A more recently explored source of stem cells is in umbilical cord blood, first described by Broxmeier[33,34] and first used by Gluckman, Rocha, and Chevret.[34] Not only is the umbilical cord and the placenta at birth a rich source of immature blood cells, but these cells also have abundant proliferative capability, and are less immunologically reactive, giving rise to less GVHD than would be expected for the degree of mismatch, thus allowing for greater mismatching than would be otherwise permissible.

In patients with leukemia, the relapse rate is similar to that of conventional bone marrow transplantation, and the overall similarity with unrelated cord blood transplantation is not significantly different from bone marrow transplantation. Therefore, even with less GVHD, graft-versus-leukemia (GVL) still occurs, even in adults.

### Umbilical Cord Blood Banks

The development of national central blood banks funded by the National Institutes of Health (NIH) gave great impetus to this resource by collecting cord blood from newborns from large cities, from large numbers of patients of diverse ethnic backgrounds, thus for the first time making stem cells available for the white population and the minority populations alike. This organization, named COBLT (cord blood transplant), overviews quality control studies and protocols.[35] The NIH funded three banks, six transplant centers, and a medical coordinating center. Other umbilical cord blood banks have also developed. Dr. Donna Wall oversaw the establishment and development of the umbilical cord blood bank in St. Louis and describes her experience in Chapter XIX. Similarly in Europe, Eurocord has developed to evaluate results from umbilical cord blood transplant. A recent report from Eurocord showed that related bone marrow transplantation was similar for cord or for adult blood stem cell donors, but that the former was associated with delayed engraftment and that early bone marrow transplant complications consequently were greater.[34]

A unique model of an umbilical cord blood center for patients with hematologic disorders has been developed at the University of California in Oakland, California. Lubin and his collaborators at this center have developed an NIH-sponsored program whereby siblings of patients with hematologic disorders (e.g., sickle cell disease, thalassemia, etc.) can have their cord blood stem cells saved so as to be used subsequently for their sibling's transplant if the transplant becomes necessary. He describes his experience in Chapter VIII.

## FUTURE DIRECTIONS

The uses of stem cell transplantation are rapidly expanding into new applications (▼ Table 1.4). One important area for current and new research is the field of gene therapy, in which genes can be transferred into hematopoietic cells for different activities.[36–40] For example, genes can be included to reduce sensitivity of myeloid cells to chemotherapy, thereby allowing chemotherapy to progress more safely. Donor T cells can be transduced to become sensitive to otherwise nontoxic prodrugs. Neoplastic cells also can be modified to enhance their immunogenicity using genes that encode immune stimulatory cytokines or cell surface proteins (e.g., transferring cdl54, the ligand for CD40+ to make cells more immunogenic). Subsequent therapy with CD40+ containing cell vaccines would then home specifically and selectively to those leukemia cells transduced to carry the ligand for the CD40+ antigen.

Also, the GVL effect that has been identified and shown to be so successful in warding off leukemia may be targeted to exploit immunological reactions against solid organs malignancy.[29,41–43] The single best example of this is the graft-versus-tumor effect of renal cell carcinoma.

An exciting new concept is that hematopoietic stem cells have plasticity; they can dedifferentiate into more primitive cells, transdifferentiate into specialized cells of other organs, and redifferentiate into differentiated cells similar to the cells with which they

---

**TABLE 1.4    Potential Future Uses for Stem Cell Transplantation**

- Facilitate gene therapy
- Harness graft-versus-solid tumor
- Microchimerism to induce tolerance to solid organ transplantation
- Repair and remodeling of other tissue after injury and scarring (cardiac, renal, liver, CNS)

maintain contiguity.[44–49] For example, we recently found that patients undergoing autologous bone marrow transplantation may have improved cardiac condition, possibly because of healing from stem cells homing to the heart and transdifferentiating into myocardiocytes.

Another interesting concept of bone marrow transplantation is microchimerism, a state in which the immune system gains tolerance for solid organ transplantation through transfer of solid organ and the same donor's bone marrow cells.[50,51] Thus, for many years now, renal transplantation physicians have experimented with grafts of bone marrow stem cells from the same source as the renal donor.[41,50,52] In a recent study, Ciancio et al. reported the six-year clinical effects of donor marrow infusions in renal transplant patients.[41] This study included 63 cadaver renal transplant recipients who were given one or two donor bone marrow cell infusions, at two different doses ($7.01 \times 1$-87/kg on days 4 and 11; or $3.5 \times 109$-8/kg $\times 1$ on day 4). Both received similar immunosuppressive regimens (OKT3 induction, with tacrolimus, mycophenolate mofetil, and methylprednisolone). The rate of biopsy-confirmed chronic rejection was significantly lower in the group that received donor bone marrow cells compared to the control group (3% vs. 18%). There were significantly fewer patients who had ongoing deterioration in kidney function among those who received donor bone marrow cells compared to those who did not (2 vs. 40). Chimerism tripled from the time of infusion over a four year period of time, and there was no chimerism in the control group. Thus, donor bone marrow cell infusions induce immunologic tolerance in renal transplant recipients.

Presently, there is also intense research in this field of expanding stem cells; if stem cells could be expanded in vitro, then greater numbers of cells obtained could allow for many more recipients for cord blood stem cells.

# REFERENCES

1. Thomas ED, Cannon JH, Lochte HL Jr et al. Supralethal whole body irradiation and isologous marrow transplantation in man. J Clin Invest 1959;38:1709–1716.
2. Fibbe WE, Noort WA, Schipper F et al. Ex vivo expansion and engraftment potential of cord blood-derived CD34 + cells in NOD/SCID mice. Ann N Y Acad Sci 2001;938:9–17.
3. Michejda M, Peters SM, Bacher J et al. Intrauterine xenotransplantation of bone marrow stem cells in non-human primates. Transplantation 1992;54:759–762.
4. Roodman GD, Vandeberg JL, Kuehl TJ. In utero bone marrow transplantation of fetal baboons with mismatched adult marrow: initial observations. Bone Marrow Transplant 1988;3:141–147.
5. Storb R, Raff RF, Appelbaum FR et al. What radiation dose for DLA-identical canine marrow grafts? Blood 1988;72:1300–1304.
6. Storb R, Thomas ED. Graft-versus-host disease in dog and man: the Seattle experience. Immunol Rev 1985;88:215–238.
7. Storb R, Weiden PL, Deeg HJ et al. Marrow graft studies in dogs. Hamatol Bluttransfus 1980;25:43–52.
8. Turner CW, Archer DR, Wong et al. In utero transplantation of human fetal haemopoietic cells in NOD/SCID mice. Br J Haematol 1998;103:326–334.
9. Testa NG, Hendry JH, Molineux G. Long-term bone marrow damage in experimental systems and in patients after radiation or chemotherapy. Anticancer Res 1985;5:101–110.
10. Brent L, Brooks CG, Medawar PB et al. Transplantation tolerance. Br Med Bull 1976;32:101–106.
11. Gunn A, Medawar P. Studies on the induction of transplantation tolerance at low zones of dosage. Br J Surg 1971;58:858–864.
12. Medawar PB. The Nobel Lectures in Immunology. The Nobel Prize for Physiology or Medicine, 1960. Immunological tolerance. Scand J Immunol 1991;33:337–344.
13. Medawar PB. Tolerance reconsidered—a critical survey. Transplant Proc 1973;5:7–9.
14. Dritschilo A, Sherman DS. Radiation and chemical injury in the bone marrow. Environ Health Perspect 1981;39:59–64.
15. Lvovsky E, Baze WB, Hilmas DE et al. Radiation damage and the interferon system. Tex Rep Biol Med 1977;35:388–393.
16. Stewart AM. Delayed effects of A-bomb radiation: a review of recent mortality rates and risk estimates for five-year survivors. J Epidemiol Community Health 1982;36:80–86.
17. Waeckerle JF, Seamans S, Whiteside M et al. Task Force of Health Care and Emergency Services Professionals on Preparedness for Nuclear, Biological, and Chemical Incidents. Ann Emerg Med 2001;37:587–601.
18. Mettler FA Jr, Voelz GL. Major radiation exposure—what to expect and how to respond. N Engl J Med 2002;346:1554–1561.
19. Camitta BM, Storb R, Thomas ED. Aplastic anemia (first of two parts): pathogenesis, diagnosis, treatment, and prognosis. N Engl J Med 1982;306:645–652.
20. Camitta BM, Storb R, Thomas ED. Aplastic anemia (second of two parts): pathogenesis, diagnosis, treatment, and prognosis. N Engl J Med 1982;306:712–718.
21. Kane L, Gennery AR, Cooks BN et al. Neonatal bone marrow transplantation for severe combined immunodeficiency. Arch Dis Child Fetal Neonatal Ed 2001;85:F110–F113.
22. Kapoor N, Cooks G, Kohn DB et al. Hematopoietic stem cell transplantation for primary lymphoid immunodeficiencies. Semin Hematol 1998;35:346–353.
23. Hansen JA, Anasetti C, Beatty PG et al. Allogeneic marrow transplantation: the Seattle experience. Clin Transpl 1989:105–114.
24. Sullivan KM, Fefer A, Witherspoon R et al. Graft-versus-leukemia in man: relationship of acute and chronic graft-versus-host disease to relapse of acute leukemia following allogeneic bone marrow transplantation. Prog Clin Biol Res 1987;244:391–399.
25. Anasetti C, Beatty PG, Storb R et al. Effect of HLA incompatibility on graft-versus-host disease, relapse, and survival after marrow transplantation for patients with leukemia or lymphoma. Hum Immunol 1990;29:79–91.
26. Weiden PL, Flournoy N, Thomas ED et al. Antileukemic effect of graft-versus-host disease in human recipients of allogeneic-marrow grafts. N Engl J Med 1979;300:1068–1073.
27. Weiden PL, Sullivan KM, Flounoy N et al. Antileukemic effect of chronic graft-versus-host disease: contribution to improved survival after allogeneic marrow transplantation. N Engl J Med 1981;304:1529–1533.
28. Champlin R, Khouri I, Kornblau S et al. Allogeneic hematopoietic transplantation as adoptive immunotherapy. Induction of graft-versus-malignancy as primary therapy. Hematol Oncol Clin North Am 1999;13:1041–1957, vii-viii.
29. Childs R, Barrett J. Nonmyeloablative stem cell transplantation for solid tumors: Expanding the application of allogeneic immunotherapy. Semin Hematol 2002;39:63–71.

30. Prigozhina TB, Gurevitch O, Morecki S et al. Nonmyeloablative allogeneic bone marrow transplantation as immunotherapy for hematologic malignancies and metastatic solid tumors in preclinical models. Exp Hematol 2002;30:89–96.
31. Slavin S, Morecki S, Weiss L et al. Donor lymphocyte infusion: the use of alloreactive and tumor-reactive lymphocytes for immunotherapy of malignant and nonmalignant diseases in conjunction with allogeneic stem cell transplantation. J Hematother Stem Cell Res 2002;11:265–276.
32. Wingard J. The conundrum of chronic graft-versus-host disease. Blood Marrow Transplant Rev 2002;12:1–54.
33. Broxmeyer HE. Cord blood as an alternative source for stem and progenitor cell transplantation. Curr Opin Pediatr 1995;7:47–55.
34. Gluckman E, Rocha V, Chevret S. Results of unrelated umbilical cord blood hematopoietic stem cell transplants. Transfus Clin Biol 2001;8:146–154.
35. Fraser JK, Cairo MS, Wagner EL et al. Cord Blood Transplantation Study (COBLT): cord blood bank standard operating procedures. J Hematother 1998;7:521–561.
36. Locatelli F, Burgio GR. Transplant of hematopoietic stem cells in childhood: where we are and where we are going. Haematologica 1998;83:550–563.
37. Lutzko C, Omori F, Abrams-Ogg AC et al. Gene therapy for canine alpha-L-iduronidase deficiency: in utero adoptive transfer of genetically corrected hematopoietic progenitors results in engraftment but not amelioration of disease. Hum Gene Ther 1999;10:1521–1532.
38. Porada CD, Tran N, Eglitis M et al. In utero gene therapy: transfer and long-term expression of the bacterial neo(r) gene in sheep after direct injection of retroviral vectors into preimmune fetuses. Hum Gene Ther 1998;9:1571–1585.
39. Thomas ED. Marrow transplantation and gene transfer as therapy for hematopoietic diseases. Cold Spring Harb Symp Quant Biol 1986;51 Pt 2:1009–1012.
40. Wierda WG, Kipps TJ. Gene therapy of hematologic malignancies. Semin Oncol 2000;27:502–511.
41. Ciancio G, Miller J, Garcia-Morales RO, Singh BK et al. Six-year clinical effect of donor bone marrow infusions in renal transplant patients. Transplantation 2001;71:827–835.
42. Rini BI, Zimmerman T, Stadler WM et al. Allogeneic stem-cell transplantation of renal cell cancer after nonmyeloablative chemotherapy: feasibility, engraftment, and clinical results. J Clin Oncol 2002;20:2017–2024.
43. Rini BI, Zimmerman TM, Gajewski TF et al. Allogeneic peripheral blood stem cell transplantation for metastatic renal cell carcinoma. J Urol 2001;165:1208–1209.
44. Burt RK, Traynor AE, Oyama Y et al. Plasticity of hematopoietic stem cells: enough to induce tolerance and repair tissue? Arthritis Rheum 2002;46:855–858.
45. Condorelli G, Borello U, De Angelis L et al. Cardiomyocytes induce endothelial cells to transdifferentiate into cardiac muscle: implications for myocardium regeneration. Proc Natl Acad Sci USA 2001;98:10733–10738.
46. Goodell MA, Jackson KA, Majka SM et al. Stem cell plasticity in muscle and bone marrow. Ann N Y Acad Sci 2001;938:208–218; discussion 218–220.
47. Mertelsmann R. Plasticity of bone marrow-derived stem cells. J Hematother Stem Cell Res 2000;9:957–960.
48. Orkin SH. Diversification of haematopoietic stem cells to specific lineages. Nat Rev Genet 2000;1:57–64.
49. Zhao LR, Duan WM, Reyes M et al. Human bone marrow stem cells exhibit neural phenotypes and ameliorate neurological deficits after grafting into the ischemic brain of rats. Exp Neurol 2002;174:11–20.
50. Burke GW, Ciancio G, Garcia-Morales R et al. Evidence for microchimerism in peripheral blood, bone marrow, and skin following donor bone marrow/kidney-pancreas transplantation at 3 years. Transplant Proc 1998;30:1555.
51. Hayward A, Ambruso D, Battaglia F et al. Microchimerism and tolerance following intrauterine transplantation and transfusion for alpha-thalassemia-1. Fetal Diagn Ther 1998;13:8–14.
52. Ciancio G, Garcia-Morales R, Mathew J et al. Donor bone marrow infusions are tolerogenic in human renal transplantation. Transplant Proc 2001;33:1295–1296.

# CHAPTER II

# Clinical and Research Background of Stem Cell Transplantation

ROBERT A. GOOD, ANN STEELE, AND TAZIM VERJEE

This chapter describes my lifelong dedication and contributions to the field of immunology through my medical and scientific triumphs. The historical perspective of immune deficiencies as rare diseases must be considered in the context of the reality that the clinical understanding and new pathways to therapy provided by these discoveries has had a major consequence on clinical medicine and revolutionized our current understanding of the complexity of the immune system.

Herein, I describe milestones. With my studies of X-linked agammaglobulinemia, we bisected immunologically the microbial universe, the universe of viruses, the immunologic universe, and the universe of lymphoid systems as could be done in no other way. My research achievements include the discovery of function of thymus, and definition of the two distinct, major cellular components of the immunity systems. My contribution to understanding function of plasma cells, defining and understanding T cells and B cells, and the inestimable insights gained from the study of "Experiments of Nature" are now scientific tenets. Attempts to harness learning into a curative format, where I coined the term "cellular engineering", underscored the achievement of the very first successful bone marrow transplantation (BMT) in the world to cure a fatal genetic disease, XLSCID, and a fatal acquired disease, aplastic anemia, that complicated the initial successful transplant. This transplant catalyzed a rapid and subsequent multi-targeted application of cellular engineering. The treatment modality was extended to other primary immunodeficiencies and all forms of SCID. The thrust of research expanded to include the evolution of BMT across multimajor and multiminor barriers, thereby extending curative potential to the unmatched recipient. BMTs interfaced us squarely with our limited knowledge regarding the precarious process of immune reconstitution. Ongoing refinement and understanding of transplantation dynamics catalyzed the advent of the hematopoietic stem cell (HSC) transplant, begged definition of the, as yet, undefined, pleuripotency of the mesenchymal stem cell (MSC), and necessitated its assessment in conjunction with its hematopoietic counterpart as a possible valuable new transplantation therapy.

My life's work has been both fulfilling and rewarding. In addition to the study of our patients, who have taken us often to the laboratory with critical questions where we have been able to seek answers which we then could return to the bedside as useful new approaches to diagnosis and clinical treatment, our other great teacher of immunology has been the many different short-lived inbred strains of laboratory mice. These lowly animals have allowed us to generate an extremely hopeful new perspective. We are only at the very beginning of an era which will involve cellular engineering to include the potential for gene correction. Many of us consider these advances to be reflections of the end of the beginning for cellular engineering—however, it is just the end of a beginning and not the beginning of the end in immunology!

I have been richly accompanied on my life's journey by more than 200 outstanding students, each of whom has specialized in analyses and development of cellular and humoral immunology and in genetics and molecular biology of primary and secondary immunodeficiency diseases. Over 100 of these young associates have now become professors, department chairmen, deans, or leaders of research worldwide, again promising renewed beginning and growth.

The future of immunology promises further striking revelations; I embrace its challenge!

The diversified array of cells that defend the body against microbial and viral invaders arises from precursors that first appear about nine weeks after conception. From that point onward, the cells of the immune system commence a repeated cycle of development. The stem cells on which the immune system depends can both reproduce themselves and also give rise to specialized cell lineages: B cells, macrophages, killer T cells, helper T cells, cytotoxic T cells, and myeloid cells.

Immune cells are highly mobile but identifiable entities in terms of the markers they express. These characteristics are not only crucial to function, but also confer an advantage that enables isolation of immune or hematopoietic cells in relatively pure form at every stage of differentiation. Experiments thus can determine the properties of these cells in a non-confounded format.

Such information serves those attempting to understand cellular development and differentiation, a process that starts with a fertilized egg and culminates in the consummate complexity of an adult organism. More importantly, this knowledge enables the treatment of diseases subsequent to a failure of fetal immune cells to develop normally or, alternatively, in response to a deviation from normal patterns of development and growth coincident to age.

In the early 1960s, three monumental discoveries reshaped current thought, research, and clinical approaches involving hematopoiesis and immunology. First, Till and McCulloch[1] demonstrated that bone marrow contained clonogenic precursors capable of self-renewal and multilineage differentiation into colonies within splenic tissues known as colony-forming units-spleen, or CFU-S.[2-4] This provided the first evidence of hematopoietic stem cells (HSCs) as an entity. Next, the thymus was shown to be indispensable for the development of a subset of lymphocytes now known to be T cells, and, finally, the thymus was identified as necessary for the development of cell-mediated immunity.[5-7]

Peterson, Cooper, and Good[8] likened Bruton's agammaglobulinemia to chickens that were bursectomized and irradiated in the neonatal period and, after its description, the DiGeorge syndrome with its defective thymus development and failure of T cell development to the neonatally thymectomized mice, rats, chickens, and hamsters. Severe combined immunodeficiency disease (SCID) we likened to irradiated newly hatched chickens[9-11] that had been subjected to both thymectomy and extirpation of the bursa of Fabricius. We called the latter "severe dual system immunodeficiency." The fact that it was necessary to use irradiated chickens in these experiments when the thymus and/or bursa of Fabricius was extirpated required further clarification.[4] Cooper,[12] a first year fellow, and also van Alten,[12,13] an embryologist who was taking a sabbatical with Dr. Good, showed that essentially the same results could be obtained with thymectomy or bursectomy without irradiation when these operations were performed within the maturing egg. We had clearly defined thymus-dependent lymphoid systems and a bursa-dependent lymphoid system.[14] The central lymphoid organ for each system was the thymus for cell-mediated immunities and the bursa of Fabricius for humoral immunity, antibody production, B cells, germinal centers, and the antibody-secreting plasma cells. This set the stage for the two-component system.[10,15]

## THE TWO-COMPONENT LYMPHOID SYSTEM

The bursa of Fabricius plays a role parallel to that of bone marrow in humans. In 1965, Peterson, with Cooper and Good[14] showed that either removal of the thymus from x-irradiated, newly hatched chickens, or removal of the bursa of Fabricius from similarly sub-lethally-irradiated newly hatched chickens, or removal of both thymus and bursa from such newly hatched chickens each produced very different resultant immunodeficiencies. Removal of the thymus early in life prevented the development of lymphocytes in the blood and in the dense aggregates of lymphocytes in the white pulp of chicken spleen, leaving the germinal center and plasma cell development impressively intact. According to the new view of lymphoid development, cell-mediated immunities and certain small lymphocytes were dependent on the thymus, while antibody production, germinal center formation, other lymphocyte and plasma cell formation depended on the bursa of Fabricius. These studies and further experimental results enabled us to simultaneously formulate our rather revolutionary two-component concept of immunity.[14,16–19]

To reiterate, we found that thymus was related to the development of a population of small lymphocytes, which we called thymus-dependent cells or T cells.[2] The bursa of Fabricius in chickens on the other hand was shown to be responsible for development of a second system of cells, the B cells responsible for antibody-producing plasma cells and germinal centers in lymph nodes, tonsil, and spleen.[14,17,18] The two lymphoid systems were promptly shown to be maximally interactive both with one another and with other hematopoietic cells, e.g., in the germinal centers and bone marrow.[20–23]

Back in the clinic, these parallel observations provided complementary evidence for the existence of two lymphoid lineages. For example, in some infants the thymus developed normally, but the bone marrow malfunctioned. The classic example of this is X-linked agammaglobulinemia–Bruton's disease. Afflicted children have lymphocytes in their peripheral tissues, but suffer a congenital deficiency of plasma cells and plasma cell precursors. Conversely, infants born without a thymus, as in DiGeorge syndrome (DGS), but with normal bone marrow produce plasma cells but only a small number of T lymphocytes.

To summarize, the discovery of the central role played by the thymus in the development of the immune system in rodents,[2,3,24] chickens,[9,17,25–29] rabbits,[2,30,31] mice,[2,3,31] and hamsters,[32,33] and the new insight gained of the role of the bursa of Fabricius increased the clinical experimental, phylogenetic, and clinical evidence for a two-component concept of the lymphoid system,[14,16,25,34] which led us to postulate that a lymphoid stem cell population exists that is induced to differentiate along two distinct and separate cell lines related to two separate central immune functions.[14] This suggests that two separate channels might be available for the cellular engineering necessary to correct the immunological deficiencies that can make survival impossible.

# CORRECTION OF DIGEORGE SYNDROME BY THYMUS TRANSPLANTATION

No sooner had Cooper et al., Perey et al.,[14,16,24,34,35] and Warner et al.[9,29] presented their findings differentiating the separate origins of two distinct lymphoid systems, than DiGeorge[36] described the complex set of developmental anomalies that provide the human counterpart of animal experiments suggesting a separate central lymphoid organ controls the maturation of cellular immune functions.

DiGeorge syndrome (DGS) was first considered a rare disorder attributable to failure to develop the thymus and other derivatives of the third and fourth pharyngeal pouches, which explains the association of hypoparathyroidism, malformations of the aortic arch, and facial abnormalities. This disease was recognized and first described by Angelo DiGeorge, a Philadelphia endocrinologist.[36,37] This "experiment of nature" became a major subject of investigation for geneticists and immunologists. DiGeorge recognized that survival of these athymic patients was limited by overwhelming susceptibility to infection due to failure to develop thymus-dependent immunity, which is characterized by failure to develop a T cell-dependent immune function.

Having defined DGS immunologically as selective deficiency of T cell development due to failure of differentiation of thymus, it seemed likely that this abnormality should be correctable by thymus transplant. Cleveland's group attempted embryonic thymus transplantation.[38] Soon thereafter August and his co-workers,[39] and then Biggar, Stutman, and Good[40] appeared to have achieved correction of immunological function in children by transplantation of an embryonic thymus. In two patients, HLA-identical BMT may have restored T cell function by adoptive transfer of mature T cells;[41,42] immune reconstitution was reported also after transplantation of peripheral blood mononuclear cells in one patient.[43]

Several approaches have been implemented in the treatment of immunodeficiency associated with DGS. Some published trials of postnatal thymus transplantation were unsuccessful.[44–46] However, Markert et al.[47] treated five infants (age one to four months) with complete DGS by transplantation of cultured postnatal human thymus tissue. Two of the patients survived with impressive restoration of immune function; three patients died from infection or abnormalities unrelated to transplantation. Markert's work taught us that transplanting pieces of human thymus, indeed, can rescue children with DGS through reconstruction of their thymus-dependent immunological function. It is a medical and scientific triumph that transplantations of fetal or postneonatal thymus fragments can lead to T cell neogenesis, and the achievement of T cell immune-competence.[45–47] Although complete DiGeorge syndrome is rare, it represents a unique opportunity to observe how scientific studies spanning over four decades of research on mice can translate into effective treatment in humans.

# X-LINKED AGAMMAGLOBULINEMIA

Originally described by Col. Ogden C. Bruton in 1952,[48,49] X-linked agammaglobulinemia (XLA) is caused by an arrest of B cell development. Frequently recognized as a prototype of primary immunodeficiency,[50] XLA was the first human immune disorder for which an underlying defect was clearly identified. It is difficult to overemphasize the importance of Bruton's observation, which established beyond any reasonable doubt the crucial role of gammaglobulins in immune defense.[48,49]

Bruton's initial report[48] described a single patient for whom life was one severe life-threatening bacterial infection after another. Following his description of the association of immunodeficiency with agammaglobulinemia in a single patient, Janeways's group in Boston,[51] Gitlin et al.,[52] and our group in Minneapolis[53–55] launched studies on a substantial series of patients with agammaglobulinemia. Good et al. encountered a small group with an X-linked agammaglobulinemia who demonstrated extreme deficiency of gammaglobulins. The patients lacked plasma cells, made no antibodies, and lacked germinal centers in their hematopoietic and lymphoid tissues, but possessed circulating lymphocytes and all the same cellular immunities as normal children. Most of these agammaglobulinemic patients exhibited perfectly normal delayed and contact allergies; they usually rejected skin allografts with vigor,[56] and particularly were shown to exhibit second set graft rejections and viral immunities. Their lymph nodes showed very characteristic morphology.[57] The far-cortical areas where B lymphocytes abound and where germinal centers usually appear were strikingly underpopulated, as were the medullary cords of lymph nodes in which plasma cells are usually present following antigenic stimulation. Later, when studies were made of the thymus, this organ was found to have unusual features in children who had agammaglobulinemia associated with the extreme antibody deficiency syndrome and this rare disease was shown to be genetically X-linked. Life for these children was a succession of threatening episodes of infection caused by high-grade encapsulated bacteria such as, *Streptococcus pneumoniae, Hemophilus influenzae,* meningococci, or other encapsulated pyogenic pathogens such as *Pseudonomas aeruginosa.* However, the agammaglobulinemic patients who could not produce antibodies had quite normal adaptive immune responses that enabled them to resist recurrences of childhood exanthems, e.g., measles, German measles, chicken pox, and vaccinia, and they resisted bacille Calmette-Guérin (BCG) quite normally. XLA, therefore, was one of the first, if not the first, primary immunodeficiency to be well described in humans.[48,49] In addition, much has been learned not only about XLA, but also about how the immunity systems work and how the different cellular components of the immunity systems work together to subserve the bodily defenses. This information was derived from cellular, immunopathologic, immunologic, and immunogenetic analyses of other immunodeficiencies and from experiments in animals, especially mice and chickens.[2,9,17,31]

# THYMOMA-AGAMMAGLOBULINEMIA SYNDROME

Another contribution of our clinical and pathologic studies was obtained through studies of a farmer from Western Minnesota.[53,55,58–61] This man had both cellular and humoral immunodeficiencies and antibody-based immunodeficiency. These complex immunodeficiencies were associated with a huge thymic tumor of the mediastinum, which proved to be a stromal epithelioma of the thymus made up largely of "spindle-shaped" stromal thymic epithelial cells.[58] He had agammaglobulinemia, a markedly deficient ability to produce antibodies and also significant deficits of the cell-mediated immunities. Surgical removal of the huge tumor did not correct the apparent immunodeficiencies. The epithelioma, which was benign, was found histologically to occupy almost all of the thymic gland. However, the association of this thymic abnormality with the profound and broadly based immunodeficiency provoked us to question what role the thymus plays in development or maintenance of bodily defenses or, even better, the role of the thymus in immunologic development. This patient thus caused us to launch extensive analyses of the role of the thymus in immunity and as such the revolution of modern immunology.

In view of the preceding, the cellular basis of immunodeficiencies seemed to have been so greatly clarified that Good et al. began to plan strategies to correct, by cellular engineering,[8,19,20,53,55,57,62] some primary immunodeficiencies of humans.

# FIRST BONE MARROW TRANSPLANTATION TO CORRECT SCID

In the midst of the excitement generated by these insights into the cellular development of the immunity systems and the putative cellular developmental pathogenesis of many of the primary immunodeficiency diseases,[10,15] we believed that enough had been learned to focus our efforts on developing a form of cellular engineering that might provide a cure for some of our patients with primary immunodeficiency diseases. Our interpretation, based on these critical immunologic and morphologic analyses, and our analyses of the two major immunologic systems of mice and chickens and of immunodeficient humans[14,35] indicated that hematopoietic stem cells ultimately must give rise to both of these two major cellular components of immunity. Based on the anomalies in XLA, DGS, and SCID, we concluded that it might be possible to correct an immunodeficiency disorder associated with severe combined immunodeficiency disease (SCID) by bone marrow transplant (BMT) from a human leukocyte antigen (HLA)-matched sibling donor.

We followed evidence that in experimental animals BMT from a major histocompatibility (MHC)-matched donor could correct the hematopoietic and immunologic abnormalities produced by lethal doses of total body x-irradiation.[63] Main and Prehn[64] showed that when they achieved successful allogeneic BMT in mice, long-lasting immunologic tolerance of the donor was produced in the recipient's mice. In these experiments, x-irradiation was given in large doses to destroy all hematopoietic and lymphopoietic cells and their precursors in the recipient. Then, donor marrow, syngeneic or allogeneic, that contained hematopoietic and lymphopoietic stem cells could be given to fully reconstitute all blood cell and lymphoid tissue and cellular deficits produced by lethal total body irradiation. In such a model system, the hematopoietic and lymphoid cells that developed were all derived from donor stem cells of the MHC-matched sibling donor.

In June of 1968,[15,65] we encountered our first potential BMT recipient. This baby was a four-month-old child with the otherwise uniformly lethal immunodeficiency SCID. This infant came from a family in which 11 male relatives had died from XLSCID. He had already suffered three or four bouts of pneumonia and most certainly would have succumbed to one lethal infection soon thereafter. Although he was not perfectly matched at the MHC with his sister, who was the best donor available, nonetheless we went ahead and performed a bone marrow transplant to the child with severe combined immunodeficiency. Our attempt to cure the XLSCID turned out to be the very first successful bone marrow transplant in the world.[65–67] The infant's XLSCID was impressively and quite fully corrected. However, because of an A locus mismatch, he developed a severe graft-versus-host reaction (GVHR) that also led to aplastic anemia. Instead of attempting to eliminate the bone marrow graft as colleagues suggested, we took steps to apply a second successful BMT to cure severe aplastic anemia, again, also for the very first time.[68–71] This second transplant with his sister's donor cells resulted in full immunologic, lymphoid, and hematopoietic reconstitution. Twice he was exposed to chicken pox but failed to develop the disease because his sister, whose marrow cells had been used to correct his immunodeficiency, already was immune to this disease; his red blood cell type switched from his genetic A entirely to his sister's blood group 0. Today, at 35 years of age, he remains robustly healthy (▼ Figure 2.1).[15,72–75] Subsequently, BMT has been applied as a frequent cure of many different diseases. These include all other known forms of SCID, other primary immunodeficiencies, high risk leukemias, non-Hodgkin's lymphomas, inborn errors of metabolism, genetic abnormalities of red blood cell and leukocyte development, thalassemias, sickle cell anemia, and other diseases such as collagen, vascular diseases and, perhaps, certain other cancers.

The work of our laboratory over the years has been based almost entirely upon efforts to interpret "nature's experiments," and virtually all of the questions we have asked originated in clinical relationships. Our studies began with a derivative analysis of the association between hypergammaglobulinemia and plasmacytosis made by Bing and Plum in 1937.[76] This association led Good's teacher of hematology, Fred Kolouch,[77] to become curious about the meaning of the many plasma cells in the lymphoid tissues that he observed in the bone marrow of a patient with subacute bacterial endocarditis. This observation led him to ask whether antigenic stimulation (vaccination) might not lead to plasma cell accumulations. Kolouch's observations led directly to the studies of Bjoerneboe and Gormsen[78] and these in turn to those of Fagraeus and Coons and co-workers.[79–81] Together, these studies established the function of the plasma cells as factories of gammaglobulin and antibody synthesis was established.

## TREATMENT OF DIABETES MELLITUS BY STEM CELL (WITH OR WITHOUT PANCREAS) TRANSPLANTATION

Insulin-dependent diabetes mellitus (IDDM) is mainly of juvenile-onset, non-obese, and ketosis-prone. In IDDM, as in non-obese diabetic (NOD) mice, deduction of insulin-producing beta cells of the pancreatic islets are progressively destroyed, insulin production is reduced, and the plasma insulin level becomes extremely low.[82] Exogenous insulin injection has prolonged the survival of diabetic patients and prevented systemic complications.[83] However, it is difficult to tightly control glucose homeostasis using insulin injections. Transplantation of isolated pancreas is a physiologic approach to the replacement of pancreatic endocrine functions and may be easily performed.

It is also well known that the portal venous administration of alloantigens can induce tolerance. Ikebukuro with Ikehara et al.[84] found that the administration of allogeneic cells via the portal vein (p.v.) induces donor-specific tolerance across MHC barriers[85] and that donor HSCs, which are trapped in the liver after p.v. injection, induce anergy to host CD8+

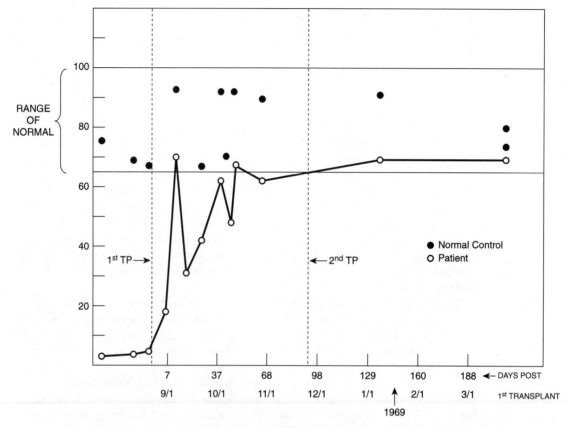

**FIGURE 2.1 (A)** Number of transformed blastoid cells after stimulation with PHA in lymphocyte cultures from the patient's peripheral blood before and after bone marrow transplantation. A gradual rise to low-normal levels promptly followed the first transplantation.

T cells owing to the absence of co-stimulatory signals.[86] With Ikehara, we also found that the injection of HSCs via the p.v. plus short-term administration of an immunosuppressant (cyclosporine, tacrolimus, or FK506) can sometimes induce persistent tolerance in the skin allografts in mice[87] and pigs.[88]

Successful transplantation of tissues, cells, and organs between fully MHC-mismatched donor and recipient combinations has been dependent on the use of immunosuppressive agents to control acute and chronic rejection. Immunosuppressants generally have some toxic effects that can result in significant morbidity and mortality. It has been recognized that the induction of donor-specific tolerance by bone marrow chimerism can eliminate the problem of allograft rejection.[89–93] Although bone marrow chimerism can successfully prevent even chronic graft rejection, the clinical application of the lethal conditioning approach to induce tolerance would be limited by the excessive toxicity associated with lethal conditioning. It has been reported that the transplantation of whole pancreas can

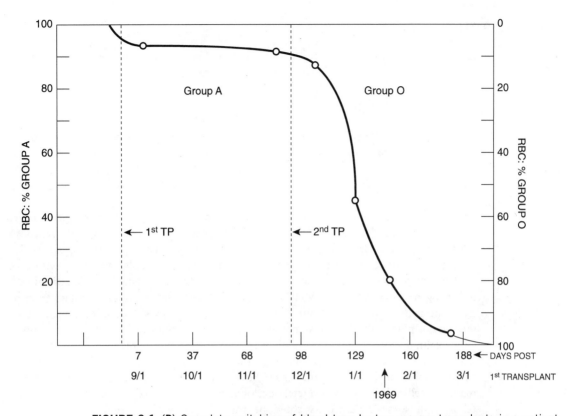

**FIGURE 2.1 (B)** Complete switching of blood type by two marrow transplants in a patient with XLSCID dual-system immunodeficiency. The second marrow transplant corrected the genetically determined dual system immunodeficiency. The second marrow transplant, leading to complete switching of blood type "A" to donor type "O" corrected an immunologically-based aregenerative pancytopenia, an acquired disease. This switching took place approximately 120 days after the onset of graft-versus-host disease.

maintain normal blood glucose levels and effectively control IDDM.[94] The transplantation of the endocrine tissue alone—isolated pancreatic islets (PIs)—is a more technically simple approach than the whole pancreatic transplantation. It also has been reported that the survival term of grafts in the transplantation of PIs is short owing to their antigenicity and their high sensitivity to graft rejection.[95]

The NOD mouse is a well-known animal model for IDDM. We previously showed that allogeneic BMT can prevent and treat insulitis in this model[82] and that allogeneic BMT plus fetal pancreas grafts can treat overt diabetes in NOD mice.[90] However, Ikehara et al. found that in (BALB/c + NOD) chimeric mice, NOD hematopoietic cells become dominant, which results in the recurrence of IDDM because the abnormal HSCs of autoimmune-prone mice are more resilient than normal hemopoietic stem cells (HSCs), as previously described.[96] These findings suggest that allogeneic BMT instead of mixed allogeneic BMT should be carried out in conjunction with organ transplantation.

# HEMATOPOIETIC STEM CELLS

Dependence on allogeneic marrow transplantation that employed only MHC-matched sibling donors placed a serious restriction on the development of BMT. Only 25% of those needing a marrow transplant have a matched sibling who can be used as a suitable donor. Recognizing this limitation, we continued to press the concept that cellular engineering by BMT can more generally be applied, and showed for the first time that non-sibling donors from the extended family[97–102] and even a donor in the general population might be employed as the basis for successful treatment of severe combined immunodeficiency or other disease by BMT.[103] Following von Boehmer's lead in pursuing our experimental research,[104] we then showed that if all T lymphocytes plus the immediate precursors of T cells were completely purged from bone marrow preparations of mice, bone marrow of mice could be transplanted across multimajor plus multiminor histocompatibility barriers without producing GVHR.[104–107] Such experimental marrow transplants regularly produced tolerance of donor and tolerance of recipient and permitted expression of impressive immunologic capacity that could reject third party allogeneic cells and tissues with cell-mediated responses of normal vigor. Although such mice transplanted with T-cell-purged, fully allogeneic marrow across MHC barriers[106–111] showed demonstrable immunodeficiencies, especially in primary immune responses, mice of many strains transplanted across multimajor plus multiminor histocompatibility barriers could survive well and remain in good health in conventional environments.[105–110] When donor and recipient mice were haploidentical at MHC, primary antibody production as well as all cell-mediated responses could be marshaled without problems.[111] Fetal or neonatal liver transplants, when free of mature T cells relatively early in fetal development, T-cell-purged marrow or even neonatal liver in some experiments could be transplanted without producing GVHR or GVHD.[112–114] To extend the latter findings from mice to humans, we[115] and later Jean Louis Touraine[116] performed fetal liver transplants from very immature donors that were regularly free of fully mature lymphocytes and could in a few instances restore immunologic function to children who had been born with SCID and who had no MHC-matched donor.[115,116] Occasionally these fetal liver transplants, as in inbred mice, restored impressive immunologic function and corrected most if not all of the immunodeficiency with which the children had been born.

At the same time, Reisner from Sharon's laboratory[117,118] had been using a nonimmunologic method of purging mouse marrow cells using plant lectins to aggregate cell populations, plus differential centrifugation of mouse marrow and spleen cells to remove all T cells. These preparations of MHC-mismatched marrow permitted bone marrow or bone marrow plus spleen cell transplantation in mice without inducing GVHD. Because the monoclonal antibodies available at the time did not permit in humans sufficient purging of T cells and T cell precursors that could develop into T cells that initiated GVH reactions, Reisner, then in our laboratory, changed the lectin-purging technique to one that employed initial aggregation with soybean agglutinin, followed by centrifugation and rosetting of T cells with sheep red blood cells (as a second lectin), followed by differential centrifugation, and was able to remove the T cells from human marrow sufficiently.[119] With this new technique, we found that parental marrow could be employed for successful initial treatment of SCID.[120] We also used this approach to prepare parental marrow for BMT in patients with leukemia if a matched sibling or perfectly matched relative was not available.

Both O'Reilly et al.[121,122] at Memorial Sloan Kettering Cancer Center and Buckley et al.[123] at Duke have used these relatively crude preparations of haploidentical marrow stem cells, purged of T cells and T cell precursors, to treat many patients who have SCID with frequent life-saving success. The success rate for marrow transplants to correct various forms of SCID with haploidentical donor marrow purged of T cells by the lectin technique under the very best conditions has been only slightly lower than the rates achieved with MHC-matched sibling donor marrow transplants.[121–123] The T cell reconstruction is slower when haploidentical T-cell-purged marrow is transplanted, as the development of B cells and antibody production may be delayed and therefore must be treated.

More recently, hematopoietic stem cell transplantation (HSCT) has been used successfully to cure many pediatric disorders. However, the immunologic alterations associated with transplantation result in profound immunodeficiencies in the transplant recipient, resulting in significant infectious morbidity and mortality.[124] The precarious process of immune reconstitution in the transplant recipient is neither instantaneous nor complete, but influenced by multiple factors such as GVHD, conditioning regimen, patient age, and underlying disease. Studies in pediatric HSCT have revealed unique attributes of immune recovery in pediatric transplant recipients.

Upon transplantation into lethally irradiated hosts with SCID, self-renewing HSCs migrate to lymphoid and hematopoietic organs and give rise to all lymphoid[125] and myeloid[126] cell lineages. The concept of specificity of HSCs and other tissue stem cells is now being challenged following reports that have documented a plasticity of these cells and their ability to transdifferentiate into cells of multiple lineages.[127]

# MESENCHYMAL STEM CELLS

In addition to HSC from which all the formed elements of blood originate, the bone marrow contains a second type of stem cell, mesenchymal (MSC), capable of giving rise to multiple mesenchymal cell lineages. The human MSC has recently been identified and characterized. Present technology enables the *ex vivo* expansion of human MSC without apparent loss of phenotype or function. Recent studies undertaken to determine the effects of MSC transplantation in relation to hematopoietic counterparts may prove to be a valuable new form of therapy.[128]

Stem cells for non-hematopoietic tissue until recently were referred to either as MSCs or as bone marrow stroma cells with comparatively little consistency.[129] It now has become possible to distinguish MSCs from bone marrow stroma cells on a molecular level. Moreover, MSCs can be induced to differentiate into bone marrow stroma cells.[130] Consequent to this finding, MSCs are now regarded as the less mature precursor cells. Nevertheless, it has not yet been conclusively determined whether there is a difference between MSCs and certain cell populations of the bone marrow stroma.

MSCs reside in the bone marrow and release a large number of growth factors. Therefore, it is to be expected that they have to settle in the bone marrow following systemic infusion and will contribute there to the growing medium for hematopoietic cell within this microenvironment.[129] Thus, the co-transplantation of MSCs would be a furth possible clinical application to support the immigration and growth of transplanted HS Studies conducted *in vitro* have shown that MSCs in long-term cultures contain hematopoietic precursor cells known as long-term culture initiating cells, and ca their growth to their close association with HSCs in the bone marrow, hematopoietic stroma or MSCs, which have been described as facilitators of HSC engraftment. Several reports also have suggested that MSCs can transdifferentiate into different cells of other tissues.

To reiterate, bone marrow stromal cells (BMSCs) are not derived directly from HSCs, but rather from pluripotential mesenchymal stem cells. These stromal cells support hematopoiesis and are now being replaced or used in humans based on our previous animal work.[131,132] Mesenchymal stem cells are multipotent and capable of differentiation into bone, cartilage, osteoblasts, stromal cells, and adipose tissue *in vitro* and *in vivo*.[28,133] These pluripotential cells may be important for effective HSC differentiation, which occurs in direct proximity to osteoblasts within the bone marrow cavity[134,135] and, presumably, by providing other regulators such as c-kit ligand and cytokines (IL-6, G-CSF, GM-CSF) to stimulate and enhance marrow cell proliferation.[136,137] At the single cell level, mesenchymal stem cells appear to differentiate into endothelial cells in addition to other mesodermal cells, e.g., skeletal myoblasts.[138] Initial evidence from experiments in our laboratory suggests that HSCs from healthy mice migrate to target organs and possibly differentiate into renal cells when transplanted into irradiated autoimmune-affected mice. Very recently (2003), Jones et al.[139] and Steele et al.[140] were able to identify donor chimerism consistent with mesangial cell differentiation within the autoimmune kidney of mice pre-conditioned with either sub-lethal (550 cGy) or lethal (950 cGy) levels of irradiation prior to transplantation using whole bone marrow injected via tail vein. Interestingly, the group pre-conditioned with the gentler preparatory regimen (550 cGy) appears to have a greater number of cells of donor origin within their glomeruli as opposed to the lethally-irradiated group. Gok et al. (2003, unpublished data) in our lab are currently studying intraperitoneal versus intravenous routes for mesenchymal stem cell transplantation. Preliminary evidence suggests that engraftment by either route is precluded in younger disease-free BXSB mice in comparison to older BXSB mice at disease onset.[139,140] Earlier studies (2000) by Ying et al.[141] and Terada et al.[142] speculated that stem cells may fuse with other tissue elements and become hyper diploid, thus taking on genes and the somatic characteristics of the cells among which the mesenchymal stem cells settle. The mechanics of transdifferentiation are still under intensive investigation.

Cahill et al.,[143] when in our laboratory, transplanted a patient with a rare, regularly fatal, metabolic bone disease, hypophosphatasia. This patient presented clinically with severe rickets; failure to thrive, severe bone pain, hypercalcemia/hypercalcinosis, kyphosis, and marked bowing of long bones. This "experiment of nature" has demonstrated an important role for alkaline phosphatase in the secondary mineralization of bone and the formation of secondary dentition. Our strategy was to replace the patient's osteoblasts with her father's osteoblasts, which were only a 4/6 HLA match. We elected to give her IV, cultured osteoblasts obtained from crushed iliac donor bone, as well as inserting bone intraperitoneally (IP). These two methods were based on animal work by Hisha et al.[144] and Ishida et al.[145] in Ikehara's laboratory in Japan, where they demonstrated the replacement of the recipient stroma using bone fragments placed under the kidney capsule. This process enhanced engraftment, immune recovery, and accelerated tolerance.

To reiterate, our patient was given IP bone marrow and bone fragments obtained from donor's iliac crest. Cultured osteoblasts also obtained from the iliac crest were given IV. ...s no evidence of engraftment of hematopoietic stem cells or increase in her circu- ...kaline phosphatase, but there was most impressive clinical and radiological evidence ...full mineralization of her bones had occurred. A bone biopsy of the patient's iliac crest

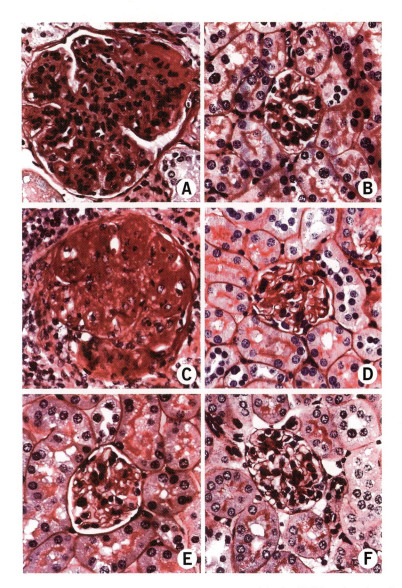

**COLOR PLATE 1** Prevention of lethal glomerulonephritis in BXSB mice by allogeneic (healthy) BMT + syngeneic (autoimmune) BMT into lethally irradiated BXSB mice. (**A**) Untreated BXSB mice. Note profound proliferative glomerulonephritis that characterizes mice of this autoimmune strain. (**B**) BALB/c (healthy) + BXSB → lethally irradiated BXSB mice. Glomerulonephritis is prevented by mixed BMT. (**C**) BXSB → BXSB mouse. The glomerulonephritis is fulminant PAS stain. (**D**) BALB/c + B6 → BXSB also prevented glomerulonephritis. (**E**) Normal glomerulus from BALB/c healthy mouse. (**F**) BALB/c → lethally irradiated BXSB mouse. This also prevented glomerulonephritis.

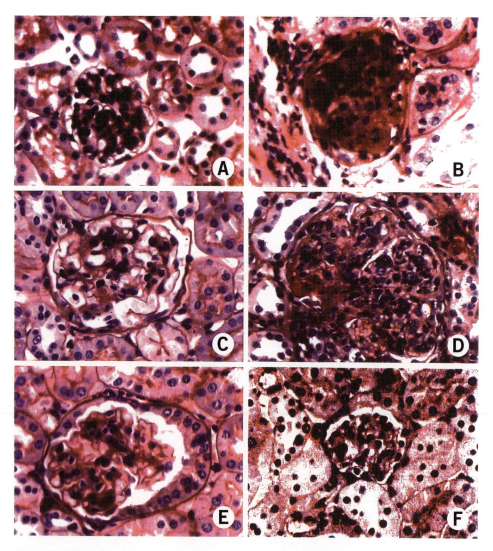

**COLOR PLATE 2** Treatment of lethal glomerulonephritis in BXSB mice by allogeneic (healthy) BMT + syngeneic (autoimmune) BMT → lethally irradiated BXSB mice. (**A, B**) Biopsies which show glomerulonephritis to already be expressed in BXSB mice at 16 weeks of age. (**C**) Treatment of BXSB mice by mixed allogeneic BALB/c (healthy) BMT + syngeneic (autoimmune) BMT → lethally irradiated BXSB mice normal glomerulus at autopsy of 50 weeks of age. (**D**) BXSB → (syngeneic) BXSB shows fulminating glomerulonephritis at 50 weeks of age. (**E**) BALB/c allogeneic (healthy) BMT → BXSB minimal glomerular lesion at 50 weeks of age. (**F**) Normal C57BL/6 glomerulus for comparison. Mixed BMT in BXSB mice can be effective on treatment as well as prevention of the fulminant glomerulonephritis of BXSB mice.

(Reprinted with permission from, Effective treatment of autoimmune disease and progressive renal disease by mixed bone marrow transplantation that establishes a stable mixed chimerism in BXSB recipient mice. Wang et al. Proc Natl Acad Sci USA 96:3012–3016, 1999, ©1999 by the National Academy of Sciences, U.S.A.)

revealed the presence of male donor cells by polymerase chain reaction amplification of male-specific sex-determining region (SRY) sequences. The success of this transplant seems real and suggests that there was a selective advantage of the donor's normal cells over the abnormal cells in sufficient quantities to assure proper mineralization.[143]

Cahill (2001; personal communication) aptly illuminates the dynamics underlying the preceding transplantation success. "It is believed that pluripotent cells whatever their origins have a selective advantage over the abnormal or damaged cell and thus will replace them in sufficient quantity to cure their disease.[146–148] The HSC also contain some pluripotent, probably mesenchymal stem cells, but in human studies there is no evidence that they can duplicate the effectiveness of stromal cells. In many cases of genetic diseases and malignancy in both human and animal models, it has been shown that the bone marrow stroma is also abnormal or damaged as are many of the HSCs and other tissue cells in the body. The bone marrow stroma may not be transplanted during the current practice of stem cell transplantation. The recipient's marrow stroma survives and is incompatible with the donor HSCs. More important, the stroma is made up of the pluripotent stem cell capable of differentiating into all tissues as well as the osteoblasts, one of the most important cells for hematopoiesis, lymphopoiesis as well as normal bone formation."

## STEM CELL PLASTICITY

Marrow stromal cells (SC) were initially isolated by a Russian scientist in 1968 who defined them as adherent, clonogeneic, non-phagocytic, and fibroblastic.[149]

Marrow stroma include reticular endothelial cells, macrophages, fibroblasts, osteoblasts, chondrocytes, adipocytes, tenocytes, neural precursors, and osteogenic precursor cells,[128] the complex orchestration of which provides growth factors, essential cell-to-cell interactions, and production of matrix proteins essential to maintenance, growth, and differentiation of HSC within specifically defined conditions comprising the marrow microenvironment. In fact, normal hematopoiesis is contingent upon intact and fully functional bone marrow stroma.

Within the stromal environment resides another type of stem cell, the non-hematopoietic mesenchymal stem cell (MSC). *In vitro* MSCs display a multiplicity in differentiation to adipocytes, chondrocytes, osteoblasts, tenocytes, hematopoietic supporting stroma, skeletal muscle, smooth muscle, carida muscle, astrocytes, oligodendrocytes, and neurons[150] along with appropriate molecular phenotypic verification markers and cellular morphological and metabolic identifiers.

MSCs demonstrate three criteria for stem cells definition: extensive proliferation, differentiation into multiple cell types, and engraftment *in vivo*. In keeping with the preceding, studies have shown that MSC cells infused into swine[151] demonstrate myogenic differentiation; MSC transplantation in the presence of HSCs and bony elements in a canine has shown pulmonary osteoblastic ossification with evidence of trilineage marrow engraftment;[152] the potential of MSCs to differentiate not only into mesodermal cells, but also adopt the fate of endodermal and ectodermal cell types was recognized by the ability of human MSCs grafted into ischemic rat brain to express markers for astrocytes, oligodendroglia, and neurons.[153] Compelling data demonstrating the expansive potential of these pluripotent cells have been derived from in utero xenographic transplantations wherein human MSCs engrafted fetal sheep and demonstrated specific differentiations in chondrocytes, adipocytes, myocytes, cardiomyocytes, bone marrow stromal cells, and thymic stroma.[154]

In a similar study of pleuripotency, a human MSC xenotransplantation into a damaged sheep fetus sustained cellular reconstitution of all damaged tissues (heart, lung, and muscle), which were replaced by human cells.[155]

It remains unresolved how, after BMT, despite an abnormal microenvironment or injury from chemotherapy and irradiation in the preparative regimen or from prior chemotherapy, there is no evidence of engraftment of donor stromal cells in human patients with non-malignant or malignant diseases.[156–160] Many studies indicate that the bone marrow stroma is damaged following BMT.[130] Accordingly, since the marrow stroma is critical for the maintenance of hematopoiesis, its ability to support hematopoiesis following stem cell transplantation (SCT) may be impaired. Animal models suggest that the transplantation of healthy stromal elements, including MSCs, may enhance the ability of the bone marrow microenvironment to support hematopoiesis after SCT. Present technology permits *ex vivo* expansion of human MSC without apparent loss of phenotype or function. Thus, recent studies have been undertaken that ultimately will determine effects of MSC transplantation with hematopoietic counterparts, which may prove to be a valuable form of cellular therapy.

Investigators have found an unprecedented level of apparent plasticity in bone marrow-derived stem cells that are CD34+ (MSC are CD34−) and are capable of developing into many different tissues and demonstrate functionality.[159] Most studies have shown that differentiation into cell types occurs almost exclusively in damaged organs.[159] Contribution of non-hepatic cells to liver and biliary epithelium has been seen in cirrhosis[60] and differentiation of marrow derived cells to skeletal muscle in the setting of muscular dystrophy.[161] An attempt to cure a B-glucoronidase deficient mouse model (Sly disease) using large quantities of IV bone marrow in mice without myeloablative therapy was unsuccessful, but with some amelioration of many of the disease symptoms, improvement in life span, and reduction of lysosomal storage. However, the authors were not able to demonstrate significant changes in the architecture of the bones and brain.[162] In several cases of carbonic anhydrase II deficiency (osteopetrosis and renal tubular acidosis), bone marrow transplant was performed with large doses of unmanipulated marrow that resulted in full donor chimerism and cure of their osteopetrosis. However, there was no effect on the renal tubular acidosis.[163]

From our laboratory, Cahill (personal communication, 2001) stated that "stem cells are those cells which, in addition to their ability to differentiate into more mature stages and into various lineages, possess the capability of renewing themselves without loss of potential. A location that is particularly rich in different types of stem cell is the bone marrow. In addition to the hematopoietic part of bone marrow, which contains the most thoroughly studied stem cells, bone marrow also contains stem cells for endothelial and mesenchymal tissue, such as bones, fatty tissue, and cartilage. More recently, precursor cells or possibly stem cells for liver and nerve cells have been identified. Their wide applicability for tissue regeneration, in transplantation medicine or for gene therapy has made mesenchymal stem cells a focus of research, in addition to the hematopoietic stem cells."

## MURINE MODELS FOR AUTOIMMUNE DISEASES

BMT has facilitated our understanding of the etiology of autoimmune disease and has enabled us to determine whether this approach may be of benefit to affected patients.[74,164] For over three decades it has been known that in many rodent models of spontaneously arising as well as antigen-induced autoimmune disease, disease pathogenesis can be blocked and often reversed by BMT.[164–166] Data from many animal studies demonstrate mixed results, possibly because some models donors are from MHC-mismatched non-susceptible (healthy) strains, while in others the donors are either MHC-congeneic or -syngeneic. Favorable outcomes in allogeneic transplants appear to be in those studies where there is a mismatch between donor and host at the MHC.[74,167]

The availability of several murine strains that develop system lupus erythematosus like autoimmune disease (SLE) has prompted better understanding of the fundamental nature of autoimmune diseases through study of the immunological abnormalities. Insights have catalyzed attempts at correction or cure of autoimmune diseases in these mice. MRL/MP-*lpr/lpr* (MRL/1) and BXSB strains, (NZB × NZW)F1, as well as NZB mice and also (NZW × BXSB)F1 hybrids spontaneously develop life-threatening autoimmune diseases. Such diseases are characterized by the development of many different autoantibodies, anti-double-stranded (ds)DNA, immune-complex glomerulonephritis, and rapid death from renal failure.[168,169] The (NZW × BXSB)F1 (W/BF1) mice are increasingly used as a murine model for the most severe systemic autoimmune disease,[170,171] which includes human SLE.[172,173] Mice of the (W/B)F1 model develop occlusive cardiovascular disease (CVD) related to anticardiolipin autoantibodies, pulmonary disease and glomerulonephritis that results from deposition of immune complexes in the small coronary vessels and in the glomeruli of affected animals.[174,175] Other models successfully prevented or treated by BMT include autoimmune-mediated lupus erythematosus in NZB, (NZB × NZW)F1 (B/W)F1, and (NZW × BXSB)F1.[174–176] The latter mice develop lupus-like diseases, including fulminating glomerulonephritis, pulmonary, coronary vascular disease with myocardial infarction, and autoimmune thrombocytopenia. Other informative murine models include BXSB mice[177,178] whose autoimmune-associated pulmonary, cardiac, renal, and humoral disease can be either prevented or cured by mixed syngeneic (autoimmune) plus allogeneic (normal healthy) BMT or, mixed syngeneic plus allogeneic peripheral blood HSCT. Both produce a stable mixed chimerism. NZB/Bin J female mice[179–182] demonstrate abnormalities in both lymphoid and non-lymphoid progenitor populations. Allogeneic BMT (NZB/Bin J into DBA/2cum) precipitated abnormalities in clonable lymphoid and myeloid cells within the normal murine recipient and so demonstrated that these abnormalities like other autoimmune phenomena are transferable with hematopoietic cell grafts.

In light of the preceding evidence, these experiments encouraged us to speculate that life-threatening human autoimmune diseases may be treated effectively using mixed BMT or mixed allogeneic-syngeneic HSCT. The latter may involve relatively gentle cellular engineering with incomplete myeloablation. Curative success may establish precedent for milder approaches to cellular engineering as treatment of life-threatening autoimmune diseases for which current therapies remain inadequate.

## ROLE OF PRIMITIVE, SELF-RENEWING HEMATOPOIETIC STEM CELLS TO TREAT AUTOIMMUNE-PRONE MICE

Our earlier insights into the cellular development of the immune systems, coupled with our increased understanding of the cellular developmental pathogenesis of many autoimmune diseases of mice enabled us to develop a frequently curative form of cellular engineering in both prevention and treatment of complex and severe murine autoimmunities.

Thus, the etiologic and pathogenic basis of many murine autoimmune diseases appears to reside in the primitive, self-renewing hematopoietic stem cells (HSC) population.[183] Replacement of this population in the recipient using healthy donor non-autoimmune allogeneic HSCT plus syngeneic autoimmune (diseased) HSCT creates stable mixed chimerism of healthy autoimmunity-free recipients. Preclinical studies in our experimental animals demonstrated that allogeneic BMT,[184] either alone or coupled with syngeneic BMT, or bone,[144] stromal cell,[145] or thymus transplantation[185] could both prevent and/or treat to cure organ-specific (diabetes in NOD mice[186,187] and thyroid autoimmune disease[188]) as well as systemic autoimmune diseases in mice, e.g., bone marrow plus bone chips plus fetal thymus in MRL/+ old female mice with pancreatitis and sialoadenitis, similar to Sjögren's-type autoimmune disease[185] of humans.

Mizutani et al.[174] under Good's directive used reciprocal haploidentical BMT to investigate whether CVD of male W/BF1 mice is transferable as a component of systemic autoimmunity based in abnormalities in hematopoietic marrow cells. Bone marrow or HSCT preparations from male W/BF1 mice transplanted to murine autoimmune-free strains produces thrombocytopenic purpura,[189] SLE, and lupus-type nephritis in normal healthy mice, and also produces coronary artery disease in recipients.[175,190] Moreover, transfer of splenic lymphoid cells from male to female W/BF1 mice accelerates the development of lupus nephritis and increases the incidence of CVD in the recipient females.[191] T cell-depleted (TCD) marrow from male W/BF1 mice was transplanted to autoimmune-free B6C3F1 mice and the recipients were monitored for subsequent development of autoantibodies to cardiolipin (aCL) and other autoantibodies, thrombocytopenia, lupus nephritis, and vasculo-occlusive and lethal CVD. Conversely, the reciprocal haploidentical transplantation of TCD marrow from autoimmune-free B6C3F1 mice to male W/BF1 mice showed that CVD of W/BF1 is regularly prevented and, also, possibly, successfully treated. Murine lupus-associated CVD is an aspect of systemic autoimmunity and as such is transferable to autoimmune-free mice by TCD BMT or HSCT. These findings suggest similarities in pathogenesis of human and murine lupus-associated CVD and also show that the W/BF1 male mouse may prove itself an ideal model for clarifying attempts to cure autoimmune-associated CVD.[174,175]

## ALLOGENEIC BMT CURED AUTOIMMUNE DISEASES IN MICE

Allogeneic, but not syngeneic, marrow transplants have proven to be effective treatments for genetically-based spontaneous models of autoimmune diseases.[131] Long-term effects of allogeneic BMT[192] across major histocompatibility complex barriers were studied and shown to be effective treatments for B/WF1, BXSB, MRL/*lpr*, and SCG/Kj (Kinjoh discovered this strain in Dr. Good's laboratory)[193] mice. In the BXSB or B/WF1 mice, allogeneic BMT could be used either as a prevention or as a cure of the autoimmunities and tissue injuries. In both instances, glomerular and pulmonary lesions could be either prevented or corrected to cure the disease. Serological abnormalities and immunologic functions were restored to normal. In the MRL/*lpr* mice, however, autoimmunities and renal disease initially improved after allogeneic BMT following TBI, but then recurred. The mice did not tolerate high doses of TBI and the recipient stem cells proved resistant to irradiation. For this reason, the severe autoimmunities and lupus-like disease of MRL/*lpr* mice was not cured by

BMT alone. If, however, the BMT was given along with bone or stromal cell transplantation, the MRL/*lpr* mice were cured permanently of their autoimmune lupus-like disease. The long-lasting cures obtained with BXSB mice treated by mixed BMT or mixed HSCT via stable mixed chimerism stand in striking contrast to the recurrent autoimmunity and renal damage apparent after BMT in attempts to cure MRL/*lpr* mice. However, by providing stromal cells the disease of MRL/*lpr* mice could be abrogated by BMT plus bone transplants.[141] Thus, our experiments support the work of Ikehara et al.,[192] who showed that in autoimmune-prone mice, this problem is negated using allogeneic BMT if bone marrow cells are completely depleted of T cells, if myeloablation and immunosuppression have been adequate, and if donor stromal cells (bone transplants) also are transplanted.[141] The preceding further supports more recent work by Kaufman, Ildstad, and co-workers,[194,195] who discovered that certain cells in bone marrow can act as facilitating cells. El-Badri et al.[196] showed that osteoblasts can act as facilitating cells for HSCT engraftment.

# EFFECT OF STEM CELL TRANSPLANTATION ON AUTOIMMUNE DISEASE IN MICE

Fully allogeneic BMT, after TBI and purging the marrow of destructive T cells, can prolong the span of life, inhibit the production of serum autoantibodies, and treat or prevent the development of autoimmune-associated histopathologic lesions in some autoimmune-prone strains of mice.

A most dramatic property of successful BMT within and across MHC barriers is that it regularly provides a high degree of specific immunologic tolerance that is either life-long or lasts as long as the transplanted marrow.[75] Main and Prehn[64] first recognized that immunologic tolerance-inducing capacity may be achieved by BMT even across MHC barriers. Tolerance in successful BMT is bidirectional toward both donor and recipient MHC.[106–108] Such immunologic tolerance induced by BMT is reminiscent of the life-long tolerance that is consequent of the hematopoietic precursor exchange accompanying the mutually tolerant state observed in synchorial fraternal twin cattle during embryonic life.[197,198] Another model of this form of tolerance is neonatal tolerance produced by injections of hematopoietic cells in late embryonic or neonatal mice. Life-long tolerance also was produced regularly by classic parabiosis in mice, especially those mice that first had been matched at the MHC.[199,200] Thus, recipients of successful BMT, whether prepared when donor and recipient are matched or whether they are mismatched at MHC, if prepared correctly, almost always exhibit fully stable long-lasting chimerism.

Such mice are tolerant of donor MHC determinants, tolerant of recipient MHC determinants, and fully responsive to third-party MHC determinants, as repeatedly shown by allograft rejection experiments or quantitation of proliferative responses of their lymphocytes to stimulation with allogeneic cells. Such fully tolerant bone marrow chimeric mice, although somewhat immunocompetent, develop deficiencies of both humoral and cell-mediated immune responses when the marrow transplant or HSCT bridges the MHC barrier.[107,108,201,202] The immunodeficiencies are especially apparent when primary antibody production responses to SRBC and ability to resist certain pathogens are considered.[203] Partial histocompatibility matching eliminates this immunologic deficiency, i.e., haploidentical bone marrow transplants of mice and humans do not exhibit recognizable immunodeficiencies.[111]

To eliminate these immunodeficiencies that exist in fully allogeneic chimeric mice and rats, Ildstad and Sachs[204] discovered that lethally irradiated animals transplanted simultaneously with mixed TCD marrow from both allogeneic (healthy) plus syngeneic (autoimmune) donors can fully reconstitute hematopoietic and immunologic function following supralethal TBI, and such animals do not express the type of immunological deficits observed after TBI plus transplantation of fully allogeneic bone marrow chimeras. El-Badri in Good's laboratory[205,206] has pursued this investigation as well,[188,200] and reported the induction and maintenance of specific bilateral immunologic tolerance using a mixed BMT model that crossed major plus multiminor histocompatibility barriers.[207] Thus, co-transplantation of syngeneic/autoimmune, together with allogeneic, bone marrow cells significantly improved survival and produced chimeras with normal looking thymus and peripheral lymphoid tissues that did not exhibit the immunological deficits observed in fully allogeneic BMT chimeras. Such stable mixed allogeneic chimerism was achieved, for the first time, crossing the entire major plus multiminor histocompatibility antigen barriers.[205-207]

Mixed BMT then were used to prevent (See Color Plate 1)[177] and later to treat (See Color Plate 2)[178] lethal manifestations of autoimmunity. Such mixed BMT or mixed HSCT required myeloablation and immunosuppression using lethal TBI. We found such allogeneic (healthy) plus syngeneic (autoimmune) BMT and HSCT, when applied in an effort to prevent the fulminant lupus or lupus-like glomerulonephritis, to be highly effective in suppressing development of SLE, including the otherwise lethal glomerulonephritis in the BXSB strain of lupus-prone mice. Accordingly, we found it possible to regularly prevent all manifestations of autoimmunity in the BXSB strain of mice.[177,178]

The key to successful prevention of genetically determined lethal autoimmune disease appeared to be consequent to establishment of a stable mixed chimerism with HSCs from healthy BALB/c donors plus HSCs or bone marrow also from the autoimmune-prone syngeneic BXSB recipients.[177] No facilitating cells were required for the combined BALB/c plus BXSB HSCT given preventatively. These mice receiving mixed allogeneic donor and syngeneic recipient HSCs at 8–10 weeks of age remained in good health, and tolerated the dual BMT that established mixed bone marrow chimerism without any apparent adverse consequences. Furthermore, they were capable of vigorous antibody production against a thymus T cell-dependent antigenic stimulation, e.g., SRBC. These mice were shown to exhibit significant advantage over mice that had been successfully allotransplanted across a multi-MHC barrier. Such mice given fully allogeneic BMT could not generate effective antibody responses nor defend against a variety of potential microbial pathogens.

Assured that the complex autoimmunity of BXSB mice can be prevented (See Color Plate 1)[177] by mixed allogeneic syngeneic BMT and mixed HSCT, we also attempted to determine whether such a complex autoimmune SLE-like disease can be cured (See Color Plate 2)[178] by cellular engineering that involves mixed BMT or mixed HSCT given with lethal total body irradiation.

For this experiment, we analyzed serum and biopsied the kidneys of 16-week-old BXSB mice, first to verify that both autoimmunities and renal disease were already quite fully expressed by this age. We then used mixed allogeneic-syngeneic BMT or mixed HSCT and showed that renal disease as well as complex autoimmunities were all corrected in BXSB mice by creating the stable allogeneic-syngeneic mixed chimerism.[178] Moreover, serum levels of anti-ds DNA autoantibodies in TCD marrow-recipient male BXSB mice at 50 weeks

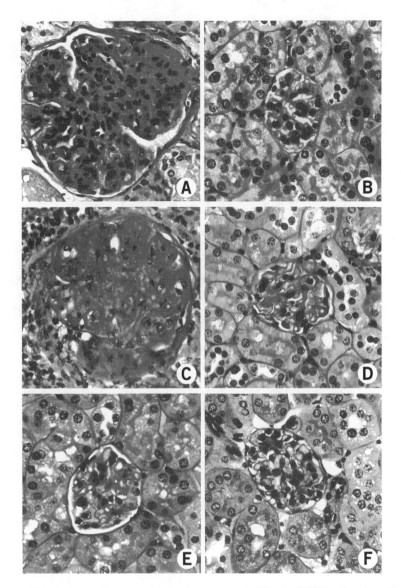

**COLOR PLATE 1** Prevention of lethal glomerulonephritis in BXSB mice by allogeneic (healthy) BMT + syngeneic (autoimmune) BMT into lethally irradiated BXSB mice. **(A)** Untreated BXSB mice. Note profound proliferative glomerulonephritis that characterizes mice of this autoimmune strain. **(B)** BALB/c (healthy) + BXSB → lethally irradiated BXSB mice. Glomerulonephritis is prevented by mixed BMT. **(C)** BXSB → BXSB mouse. The glomerulonephritis is fulminant PAS stain. **(D)** BALB/c + B6 → BXSB also prevented glomerulonephritis. **(E)** Normal glomerulus from BALB/c healthy mouse. **(F)** BALB/c → lethally irradiated BXSB mouse. This also prevented glomerulonephritis.

(Reprinted with permission from, Prevention of development of autoimmune disease in BXSB mice by mixed bone marrow transplantation. Wang et al. Proc Natl Acad Sci USA 94:12065–12069, 1997, ©1997 by the National Academy of Sciences, U.S.A.) (See Color insert within this chapter.)

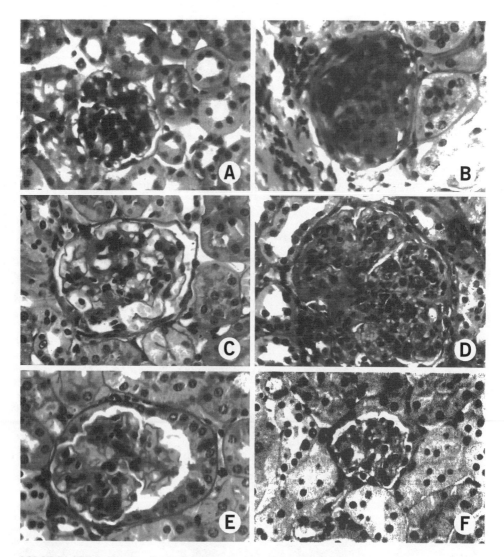

**COLOR PLATE 2** Treatment of lethal glomerulonephritis in BXSB mice by allogeneic (healthy) BMT + syngeneic (autoimmune) BMT → lethally irradiated BXSB mice. (**A, B**) Biopsies which show glomerulonephritis to already be expressed in BXSB mice at 16 weeks of age. (**C**) Treatment of BXSB mice by mixed allogeneic BALB/c (healthy) BMT + syngeneic (autoimmune) BMT → lethally irradiated BXSB mice normal glomerulus at autopsy of 50 weeks of age. (**D**) BXSB → (syngeneic) BXSB shows fulminating glomerulonephritis at 50 weeks of age. (**E**) BALB/c allogeneic (healthy) BMT → BXSB minimal glomerular lesion at 50 weeks of age. (**F**) Normal C57BL/6 glomerulus for comparison. Mixed BMT in BXSB mice can be effective on treatment as well as prevention of the fulminant glomerulonephritis of BXSB mice.

(Reprinted with permission from, Effective treatment of autoimmune disease and progressive renal disease by mixed bone marrow transplantation that establishes a stable mixed chimerism in BXSB recipient mice. Wang et al. Proc Natl Acad Sci USA 96:3012–3016, 1999, ©1999 by the National Academy of Sciences, U.S.A.) (See Color insert within this chapter.)

demonstrated a decrease in recipients transplanted with a mixed TCD marrow from both BALB/c and BXSB donors.

## TRANSPLANTATION OF HIGHLY PURIFIED HSCS

Purification and transplantation of HSCs from among the cells present in hematopoietic tissues such as bone marrow (BM) and fetal liver have been investigated.[208] Cell preparations enriched for HSCs have facilitated the study of the role of stem cells in prevention and treatment of immunologic and hematologic disease. Experimental evidence suggests that the etiopathogenesis of systemic and organ-specific autoimmune diseases originate from defects present within the HSCs. Several studies from our laboratory[170] and others[209-211] indicate that replacement of stem cells can dramatically modulate (prevent or cure) autoimmune disease. Purified peripheral blood stem cell transplantation (PBSC) in the absence of marrow T cells induces significantly less graft-versus-host disease than does the usual allogeneic BMT that may contain some mature T lymphocytes from peripheral blood. This provides a substantial advantage because GVHD compromises marrow transplantation and limits its use to lethal or highly morbid diseases, thus hampering the application of cellular engineering for less morbid, but still distressing diseases such as the autoimmunities of SLE. PBSC transplantation also was successfully achieved when the PBSC of allogeneic origin exceeded the syngeneic PBSC in the transplantation at a ratio of at least 5:1.[212]

Purified pluripotent HSCs used alone in SCT do not always engraft lethally irradiated fully allogeneic recipients.[194,196,208-211] Due to the success of mixed allogeneic/syngeneic mismatched BMT, a population of cells resident, but absent in the usual stem cell preparations, have been investigated as the facilitators of successful mismatched BMT. Several studies have been carried out to investigate this hypothesis and several kinds of apparent-facilitating cells have been described.[194,196]

Ogata et al.[213] showed that using highly purified marrow stem cells, only one to four cells were required to repopulate the entire hematopoietic cell lineage after total body irradiation. More recently, we employed the same HSC purification technique to investigate whether an increase in the number of well-defined highly purified HSCs used alone (without facilitating cells) can repopulate lethally irradiated, fully allogeneic recipient mice. We reported[208] the successful long-term engraftment of highly purified HSCs (without facilitators) in fully allogeneic recipient mice across the entire MHC transplantation barrier. $1 \times 10^5$ HSCs alone from 5-FU treated donors repopulated hematopoietic lineages of the fully allogeneic recipients. Interestingly, 1000 HSCs were sufficient to repopulate semi-allogeneic recipients, but $1 \times 10^4$ HSCs, also failed to reconstitute fully allogeneic recipients. Transplantation of primary marrow stromal cells or bones of the donor strain into recipient, together with $1 \times 10^4$ HSCs failed to reconstitute fully allogeneic recipients. Suppression of resistance of recipients by thymectomy or injections of granulocyte colony-stimulating factor (G-CSF) prior to HSCT enhanced the engraftment of allogeneic HSCs.[208]

Thus, successful engraftment across the entire MHC transplantation barrier, and cure of SLE may be achieved by transplanting allogeneic HSCs alone if a sufficient number of these cells are used.[171]

Accordingly, cell number is crucial to survival, engraftment, and cure of the autoimmune disease. An increase in the number of allogeneic stem cells was necessary to overcome the disadvantage of reintroducing the disease by including syngeneic bone marrow cells. Fully allogeneic chimeras overcome any possible disadvantages provided by the host cells and provide only healthy allogeneic cells. Sections of the kidneys from such transplanted mice showed striking improvement in the glomerular and pulmonary lesions.[171]

## AUTOIMMUNE DISEASE PATHOGENESIS AND STEM CELL FUNCTION

Due to the incidental causation of autoimmune diseases, it may be speculated that the pathogenesis of autoimmune disease involves stem cell function. Accordingly, stem cell research could provide a foundation for therapeutic advancement impacting a diverse array of degenerative disorders, as well as a new era of disease treatment, prevention, or cure.

The characterization of reliable stem cell markers is of immediate importance to HSCT. Progressive understanding of stem cell biology has resulted in the establishment of stem cell transplantation as a treatment for malignancies and other fatal disorders. Originally based on treatment for malignancy, stem cell transplantation preparative protocols must impact procedure-associated mortality by producing lower toxicity in gentler non-lethal myeloablative conditioning regimens[214] appropriate for use in treatment of autoimmunity in humans. For example, gentler non-lethal conditioning procedures may reduce the burden of host autoreactivity while permitting stem cells to repopulate the recipient with a re-regulated tolerant immune system.[215] Moreover, a complete understanding of the basic biology of hematopoiesis will accelerate progress toward the clinical goal of improved stem cell-based therapies.

Our approach to the management of autoimmune diseases using mixed allogeneic-syngeneic BMT to create stable mixed chimerism in experimental animals already may have a degree of consonance with observations pertaining to the ability of BMT or HSCT to prevent, treat, or cause autoimmune diseases in humans. Other studies have shown that after total myeloablative allogeneic BMT, several cases of rheumatoid arthritis (RA)[216] have been put into long-lasting remission when the RA occurred as a complicating factor to leukemia or aplastic anemia; remissions lasting as long as six years or more have been recorded.[217] Similarly, allogeneic BMT has induced regression of inflammatory bowel disease and psoriasis vulgaris,[218,219] providing increasing evidence that some autoimmune diseases may originate as stem cell disorders in humans as well as experimental animals, and that allogeneic HSCT may be used effectively in the treatment[220–222] of human diseases that are based on an autoimmune mechanism.

## NON-MYELOABLATION VERSUS FULL MYELOABLATION APPROACHES TO INTRODUCE THERAPEUTIC CONCEPTS

The efficacy of graft-versus-leukemia induction to treat relapses after allogeneic progenitor cell transplantation in a variety of hematologic malignancies suggests that it may be possible to use graft-versus-leukemia as a primary therapy for some malignancies without the need of full myeloablative therapy. Although a potentially lower level of inflammatory cytokines may be present after non-myeloablative therapies, fatal GVHD still occurs and remains a major obstacle to the use of isolated stem cell transplantation for treatment of autoimmune diseases. Giralt, Khouri, and Champlin[223] demonstrated that non-ablative chemotherapy using fludarabine combinations is sufficiently ablative and immunosuppressive to permit engraftment of allogeneic blood progenitor cells and also to reduce toxicity of the transplant procedure. Patients treated with fludarabine plus donor lymphoid infusion have a higher overall and complete response rate in addition to long disease-free survival advantage compared to other regimens over certain diseases.

One rationale of the non-myeloablative approach to cellular engineering is to establish a stable mixed chimerism that has already been shown capable of gradually increasing the donor phenotype by donor lymphocyte infusions (DLI) following stem cell transplantation.[224] We proposed studies aimed at addressing achievement of high levels of mixed, healthy allogeneic donor plus syngeneic recipient autoimmune donor phenotype by titrating the numbers of bone marrow cells transplanted. Stable mixed chimerism can be induced in total-myeloablative regimens by transplanting a mixture of MHC-mismatched allogeneic bone marrow cells from healthy autoimmune-free donors plus autoimmune-prone syngeneic bone marrow cells of the recipient.[178] In light of this, we will further analyze the use of incompletely myeloablative, fully MHC-matched allogeneic BMT or HSCT in averting disease progression in BXSB mice.

To reiterate, BXSB mice spontaneously develop a disease apparently more severe than most cases of human SLE. It can be prevented or cured by total myeloablative, allogeneic plus syngeneic BMT.[177, 178] By optimizing the pretransplant conditioning regimen comprising chemotherapy and low dose irradiation, we plan to produce stable mixed chimerism after non-myeloablative or incompletely myeloablative stem cell transplantation. However, we will study the survival and effect on lupus-like disease activity in the BXSB mice after allogeneic plus syngeneic mixed BMT to determine the level of stable mixed chimerism required regularly to achieve prolonged remission or cure of autoimmune disease. Our results should provide a framework and direction for future studies to determine whether stable mixed chimerism achieved by mixed HSCT or BMT can be employed to modify lupus-like disease activity and/or provide a cure for SLE in humans as well as in mice using non-myeloablative BMT of mixed allogeneic-syngeneic BMT given at the same time.

The current modalities for SLE treatment are limited in the presence of severe disease activity and they impose significant adverse effects on the host. Pediatric cases constitute about 15% to 17% of the total lupus population and the concerns related to damaging treatment are even greater for children than for adults. Aggressive treatment is usually indicated in children since clinically evident nephritis affects more than 75% of pediatric patients with lupus. In fact, the nephritis is not only more common, but often is more severe among children as compared to adults with SLE.[225,226] Clearly, there is a need for developing new approaches to control disease activity in SLE or other severe life-threatening autoimmune diseases. The production of stable mixed chimerism using simultaneous allogeneic (healthy) BMT plus syngeneic (autoimmune) BMT after either myeloablative technology or non-myeloablative technology remains an attractive approach.

# HEMATOPOIETIC STEM CELL TRANSDIFFERENTIATION IN VIVO

In more recent work, El-Badri and Steele et al.[227] attempted to study the contribution of transplantation of hematopoietic stem cells to restructuring of non-hematopoietic organs, particularly the kidneys, and their role in the correction and reversal of the autoimmune pathology. We report that HSCs from healthy, autoimmune-resistant mouse strains apparently have the capacity to transdifferentiate into renal tubular epithelial cells and, possibly, vascular endothelial cells when transplanted into autoimmune-prone mice. MHC matching between donor HSCs and host stroma was not essential for engraftment, repopulation, and reconstitution of both host hematopoietic and non-hematopoietic tissue. Migration of donor-phenotype cells to the autoimmune-injured glomerular tissues was accompanied by evidence of apoptosis and signs of decreased inflammation, decreased autoimmune deposits, and replacement of cells in the affected glomeruli and mesangium with cells from the healthy donor mice.[227]

Immunological tolerance has been successfully induced in liver and heart transplants by passenger leukocytes. In animal models, lymphocytes from the donor can induce tolerance when injected via the portal vein (87,228). Kushida et al.[229] have been able, in a sense, to reproduce this phenomenon by a BMT method consisting of fractionated irradiation, 5.5 Gy × 2, followed by intra-bone marrow (IBM) injection of whole bone marrow cells + (< 3%) of T cells, HSCs, and stromal cells from allogeneic normal C57BL/6 mice (5.5 Gy × 2 + IBM) directly into the recipient bone marrow cavity so that donor-derived hematopoietic cells, including stromal cells can effectively accumulate in the bone marrow. This is a first report that shows the effect of IBM-BMT on autoimmune diseases in MRL/*lpr* mice. There are a few reports in which bone marrow cells aspirated from the bone marrow cavity were used for serial BMT and gene therapy.[230] These investigators have shown that: (a) GVHD was not developed, even if T cells were not depleted from the bone marrow; (b) graft failure did not occur even if the dose of radiation as the conditioning for BMT was reduced to 5 Gy × 2; (c) hematopoietic recovery is rapid; and (d) the restoration of T cell function is complete, even in donor-recipient combinations across the MHC barriers. Because intraosseous infusion (IBM injection) is now an established method for administering fluids, drugs, and blood to critically ill patients, particularly infants, we believe that this IBM-BMT method also may be applicable to humans of other ages.[229]

The original curative allogeneic BMT[65–72] established precedent for use of this modality as treatment for an extensive array of otherwise fatal immunodeficient, or alternatively, genetically determined abnormalities of hematopoietic development. These pioneering efforts permeate our evolving understanding of inherent immune plasticity, and belie both directed construction and reconstruction of tissues damaged by autoimmunities using cellular engineering. The treatment and curative potential demonstrated by BMT and more recently stem cell transplantation should continue to impact disease definition and treatment.

# THE STEM CELL

## Progressive Conceptualization

The concept of stem cell, now nearing its hundredth year as one of the organizing principles of developmental biology, shows no sign of losing its youthful luster. At a time when the transfer of biological concepts to clinical practice drives much of science, the properties of stem cells in various tissues are attracting increasing interest. This attention is not restricted to the germ line and blood, the traditional domain of stem cells as defined by early 20th century studies on animal development, but has been extended to tissues not typically thought to turn over. As novel sites, properties, and functions have been identified for these cells, the definition of a stem cell has shifted repeatedly. Like some stem cells, this concept has expanded greatly and has displayed a remarkable degree of plasticity. The evidence for true plasticity of stem cell populations challenges the imagination and is difficult to accept. One recent explanation concerning observed apparent plasticity of some stem cells suggests that they may induce a spontaneous fusion with other cells, i.e., the stem cells settle over target cells and induce, or undergo, a fusion, the products of which serve as a combined source for all cellular components comprising the original stem and target cell. This concept might provide a mechanism that could explain apparent stem cell plasticity, for example, useful in restructuring damaged kidneys, lungs, and heart or other parenchymal tissues in instances where major plasticity has apparently been observed.

## Classical Concepts

Since the 19th century, histology and medicine recognized variance in the capacity of different tissues to regenerate and identified those capable of self-renewal over an organism's lifespan. Based on his studies of spermatogenesis, Regaud[231,232] first postulated the existence of a stem cell that by definition is the ultimate unit or entity of self-renewal in self-renewing tissues. Weidenreich, Dantschakof, and Maimow, a group of hematologists, concurrently proposed that all blood cells are derived from a common stem cell. The classic work of Ferrata and Pappenheim supported and extended these historical studies.[233,234] These observers recognized that a constant replenishment of cells via spermatogenesis or hematopoiesis throughout an organism's life span required a self-renewing ancestral cell. Accordingly, the concepts of stem cells and tissue self-renewal became closely linked.[235]

The discovery that clonogenic progenitors could give rise to progeny capable of complete reconstitute hematopoiesis coupled with the development of appropriate hematological assays[1] served to delineate the role of the stem cell. The preceding provided the basis for the most distinct transplantation of stem cell biology into medical treatment: BMT. Consequently, the stem cell's ability to reconstitute a dependent tissue during the life span of an organism was assimilated into the generic definition of a cell's "stemness."[236]

The "classical" basis for defining a stem cell's identity, namely, self-renewal and tissue reconstitution, is currently being challenged, redefined, expanded, and biologically evolving. Tissues previously identified as non-self-renewing (nervous tissue), slowly self-renewing (bone), or non-renewing but with a limited capacity to repair (skeletal muscle) are postulated to include stem cells. However, these examples remain unproven due to a lack of evidence for self-renewal *in vivo*. In most cases, progenitor cells demonstrate a disparity with endogenous stem cells, as their expansion is limited as is the amounts of the dependent tissues to be generated.[237]

Stem cells and their progeny display variable degrees of plasticity. As shown in the bone marrow stromal system, differentiated cells shift between osteoblastic cells, myelosupportive stroma, and adipocytes within the context of the bone marrow microenvironment.[237,238] Striking experimental observations indicate lineage plasticity within stem cells proper. For example, neural and muscle stem cells can give rise to blood, while marrow stroma-derived stem cells can generate neural tissue.[237,239] Some stem cells thus display a higher degree of plasticity upon removal from their normal microenvironment and take on the phenotype of cells indigenous to the new context in which they are placed. This increasingly familiar lack of cellular fidelity to a specific tissue or lineage violates classical expectations and provokes renewed thought concerning developmental pathways. Perhaps, however, demonstration of unanticipated plasticities no longer should be surprising after the recent and spectacular demonstration that a nucleus transplanted from a differentiated somatic tissue can contribute to all or many of the cells of a complete organism.

## Regeneration and Disease

The recognition that somatic stem cells can be isolated and are able to renew a particular tissue motivated immediate efforts to apply these cells in the clinic. BMT, albeit not successful in all circumstances, has become a mainstay in the treatment of many hematologic and some non-hematologic diseases and cancers.[240] Extensive skin lesions are now being treated with the use of autologous and even nonautologous grafts generated by the *ex vivo* expansion of epidermal cells.[241] The reconstruction of damaged articular cartilage has been attempted using *ex vivo* expanded chondrogenic cells.[242] More recently, it also has been suggested that skeletal tissue, muscle, and even nervous tissue can be regenerated from stem cell populations.[237,239] Potential applications extend beyond tissue regeneration into the realm of gene transfer and gene therapy. With the advance of molecular techniques, it is envisioned that stem cells could be engineered to replace or repair a defective gene. Because of their self-renewal and ability to regenerate a tissue, transgenic stem cells could provide a long lasting clinical benefit to a recipient. Although the precise techniques for accomplishing these goals are not yet in hand, our biotechnological imaginations have been tantalized with the possibility of recreating organs and correcting genetic diseases.

Similar to the Holy Grail, with its promise of eternal youth and renewal of life, stem cells have arguably achieved mythological status in our world with their potential to self-renewal and in regeneration of vital heart muscle, neurons, and blood cells. To understand and utilize the full potential of both embryonic and adult stem cells requires complete understanding of their biology. In passing this unique challenge to the 21st century scientific adventurer, the mythological Holy Grail may finally be poised to become reality.

## ACKNOWLEDGMENTS

The authors thank Dr. Peter Steele, Director, Special Anatomic Pathology, for his expert analysis, photomicrographic digital reproduction, and assistance. We also thank Dr. Joe Jones for his helpful suggestions in the preparation of this manuscript. The authors are supported by grants from USPHS-NIH Institute on Aging # AGO5628-15.

# REFERENCES

1. Till J, McCulloch EA. A direct measurement of the radiation sensitivity of normal mouse bone marrow cells. Radiat Res 1961;14:1419–1430.
2. Archer O, Pierce JC (introduced by Good RA). Role of thymus in development of the immune response (Abstr). Fed Proc 1961;20:26.
3. Miller JFAP. Immunological function of the thymus. Lancet 1961;2:748–749.
4. Martinez C, Kersey J, Papermaster B et al. Skin homograft survival in thymectomized mice. Proc Soc Exp Biol Med 1962;109:193–196.
5. Dalmasso AP, Martinez C, Good RA. Studies of immunologic characteristics of lymphoid cells from thymectomized mice. In: Good RA, Gabrielsen AE (eds). The Thymus in Immunobilogy: Structure, Function and Role in Disease. New York: Hoeber Harper, 1964:478–491.
6. Martinez C, Dalmasso AP, Good RA. Effect of thymectomy on development of immunological competence in mice. Ann NY Acad Sci 1964;113:933–946.
7. Martinez C, Dalmasso AP, Good RA. Homotransplantation of normal neoplastic tissue in thymectomized mice. In: Good RA, Gabrielsen AE (eds). The Thymus in Immunobilogy: Structure, Function, and Role in Disease. New York: Hoeber-Harper, 1964:465–477.
8. Peterson RDA, Cooper MD, Good RA. The pathogenesis of immunologic deficiency diseases. Am J Med 1965;38:579–604.
9. Warner NL, Szenberg A. Immunologic studies on hormonally bursectomized and surgically thymectomized chickens: Disassociation of immunologic responsiveness. In: Good RA, Gabrielsen AE (eds). The Thymus in Immunobiology: Structure, Function and Role in Disease. New York: Hoeber-Harper, 1964:395–413.
10. Good RA. Immunodeficiency in developmental perspective. The Harvey Lectures, Series 67. 1973;67:1–107.
11. Martinez C, Kersey J, Papermaster BW et al. Skin homograft survival in thymectomized mice. Proc Soc Exp Biol Med 1962;109:193–196.
12. Cooper MD, Cain WA, van Alten PJ et al. Development and function of the immunoglobulin producing system: I. Effect of bursectomy at different stages of development on germinal centers, plasma cells, immunoglobulins and antibody production. Int Arch Allergy Appl Immunol 1969;35:242–252.
13. van Alten PJ, Cain WA, Good RA et al. Gammaglobulin production and antibody synthesis in chickens bursectomized as embryos. Nature 1968;217:358–360.
14. Cooper MD, Peterson RDA, Good RA. Delineation of the thymic and bursal lymphoid systems in the chicken. Nature 1965;205:143–146.
15. Good RA. The Minnesota Scene: A crucial portal of entry to modern cellular immunology. In: Champlin RE, Gale RP (eds). The Immunological Revolution: Facts and Witnesses. Boca Raton: University Presses of Florida, 1993:105–168.
16. Cooper MD, Perey DY, Peterson RDA et al. The two-component concept of the lymphoid system. Birth Defects: Original Article Series. In: Bergsma D, Good RA (eds). Immunologic Deficiency Diseases in Man. New York: The National Foundation, 1968;IV:7–16.
17. Cooper MD, Peterson RDA, South MA et al. The functions of the thymus system and the bursa system in the chicken. J Exp Med 1966;123:75–102.
18. Good RA, Gabrielsen AE, Cooper MD et al. The role of the thymus and bursa of Fabricius in the development of effector mechanisms. Ann NY Acad Sci 1966;129:130–154.
19. Good RA, Peterson RDA, Perey DY et al. The immunological deficiency diseases of man: consideration of some questions asked by these patients with an attempt at classification. Birth Defects: Original Article Series. In: Bergsma D, Good RA (eds). Immunologic Deficiency Diseases in Man. New York: The National Foundation, 1968;IV:17–39.
20. Good RA, Martinez C, Gabrielsen AE. Clinical considerations of the thymus in immunobiology. In: Good RA, Gabrielsen AE (eds). The Thymus in Immunobiology: Structure, Function and Role in Disease. New York: Hoeber-Harper, 1964:3–48.
21. Chaperon EA, Claman HN. Effect of histocompatibility differences on the plaque-forming potential of transferred lymphoid cells (Abstr). Fed Proc 1967;26:640.
22. Mitchell GF. T cell modification of B cell responses to antigen in mice. In: Cooper MD, Warner NL (eds). Contemporary Topics in Immunobiology. New York: Plenum Press, 1974;3:97–116.
23. Chiller JM, Habicht GS, Weigle WO. Kinetic differences in unresponsiveness of thymus and bone marrow cells. Science 1971;171:813–815.
24. Jankovic BD, Isakovic K. Role of the thymus and the bursa of Fabricius in immune reactions in chickens. I. Changes in lymphoid tissues of chickens surgically thymectomized at hatching. Int Arch Allerg 1964;24:278–295.
25. Arnason BG, Jankovic BD, Waksman BH. The role of the thymus in immune reactions in rats. In: Good RA, Gabrielsen AE (eds). The Thymus in Immunobiology: Structure, Function and Role in Disease. New York: Hoeber Medical Division, 1964:492–503.

26. Aspinall RL, Meyer RK, Graetzer MA et al. Effect of thymectomy and bursectomy on the survival of skin homografts in chickens. J Immunol 1963;90:872–877.
27. Glick B, Chang TS, Jaap RG. The bursa of Fabricius and antibody production. Poultry Sci 1956;35:224–225.
28. Mueller AP, Wolfe HR, Meyer RK et al. Further studies on the role of the bursa of Fabricius in antibody production. J Immunol 1962;88:354–360.
29. Warner NL, Szenberg A, Burnet FM. The immunological role of different lymphoid organs in the chicken. I. Dissociation of immunological responsiveness. Aust J Exp Biol Med Sci 1962;40:373–387.
30. Archer OK, Pierce JC, Papermaster BW et al. Reduced antibody response in thymectomized rabbits. Nature 1962;191:191–192.
31. Good RA, Dalmasso AP, Martinez C et al. The role of the thymus in development of immunologic capacity in rabbits and mice. J Exp Med 1962;116:773–796.
32. Sherman JD, Adner MM, Costea N et al. The function of the thymus in the golden hamster (Abstr). Fed Proc 1963;22:599.
33. Hard RC, Martinez C, Good RA. Intestinal crypt lesions in neonatally antibody thymectomized hamsters. Nature 1964;204:455–457.
34. Perey DYE, Good RA. Experimental arrest and induction of lymphoid development in intestinal lymphoepithelial tissues of rabbits. Lab Invest 1968;18:15–26.
35. Cooper MD, Peterson RDA, Good RA. A new concept of the cellular basis of immunity (Abstr). J Pediatr 1965;67:907–908.
36. DiGeorge AM. Discussions on new concept of cellular basis of immunity (following presentation by Cooper, Peterson and Good). J Pediatr 1965;67:907–908.
37. DiGeorge AM. Congenital absence of the thymus and its immunologic consequences: concurrence with congenital hypoparathyroidism. In: Bergsma D, Good RA (eds). Immunologic Deficiency Diseases in Man. New York: The National Foundation, 1968:116–123.
38. Cleveland WW, Fogel BS, Brown WT, Kay HEM. Foetal thymus transplant in a case of DiGeorge syndrome. Lancet 1968;2:1211–1214.
39. August CS, Rosen FS, Miller RM et al. Implantation of a fetal thymus, restoring immunological competence in a patient with thymus aplasia (DiGeorge's syndrome). Lancet 1970;2:1210–1211.
40. Biggar WD, Stutman O, Good RA. Morphological and functional studies of fetal thymus transplants in mice. J Exp Med 1972;135:793–807.
41. Goldsobel AB, Haas A, Stiehm ER. Bone marrow transplantation in DiGeorge syndrome. J Pediatr 1987;111:40–44.
42. Borzy MS, Ridgway D, Noya FJ et al. Successful bone marrow transplantation with split lymphoid chimerism in DiGeorge syndrome. J Clin Immunol 1989;9:386–392.
43. Bowers DC, Lederman HM, Sicherer SH et al. Immune reconstitution of complete DiGeorge anomaly by transplantation of unmobilized blood mononuclear cells. Lancet 1998;352:1983–1984.
44. Reece ER, Gartner JG, Seemayer TA et al. Epstein-Barr virus in a malignant lymphoproliferative disorder of B cells occurring after thymic epithelial transplantation for combined immunodeficiency. Cancer Res 1981;41:4243–4247.
45. Dictor M, Fasth A, Olling S. Abnormal B cell proliferation associated with combined immunodeficiency, cytomegalovirus, and cultured thymus grafts. Am J Clin Pathol 1984;82:487–490.
46. Borzy MS, Hong R, Horowitz SD et al. Fatal lymphoma after transplantation of cultured thymus in children with combined immunodeficiency disease. N Engl J Med 1979;301:565–568.
47. Markert ML, Boeck A, Hale LP et al. Transplantation of the thymus tissue in complete DiGeorge syndrome. N Engl J Med 1999;341:1180–1189.
48. Bruton OC. Agammaglobulinemia. Pediatrics 1952;9:722–728.
49. Bruton OC, Apt L, Gitlin D et al. Absence of serum gammaglobulins. Am J Dis Child 1952;84:632–636.
50. Rosen FS, Cooper MD, Wedgwood RJP. The primary immunodeficiencies (first of two papers). N Engl J Med 1984;311:235–242.
51. Janeway CA, Apt L, Gitlin D. Agammaglobulinemia. Trans Assoc Am Physicians 1953;66:200–202.
52. Gitlin D, Hitzig WH, Janeway CA. Multiple serum protein deficiencies in congenital and acquired agammaglobulinemia. J Clin Invest 1956;35:1199–1204.
53. Good RA, Zak SJ. Disturbances in gamma globulin synthesis as "experiments of nature." Pediatrics 1956;18:109–149.
54. Good RA. Agammaglobulinemia: a provocative experiment of nature. Bull Univ Minn Hosp Minn Med Fdn 1954;26:1–19.
55. Good RA. Studies on agammaglobulinemia. II. Failure of plasma cell formation in the bone marrow and lymph nodes of patients with agammaglobulinemia. J Lab Clin Med 1955;46:167–181.
56. McKneally MF, Ph.D, Thesis. The influence of the thymus and appendix on the immune responses of x-irradiated newborn and adult rabbits. Minneapolis: University of Minnesota, 1970.
57. Good RA, Varco RL. A clinical and experimental study of agammaglobulinemia. Lancet 1955;75:245–271.

58. MacLean LD, Zak SJ, Varco RL et al. Thymic tumor and acquired agammaglobulinemia: A clinical and experimental study of the immune response. Surgery 1956;40:1010–1017.
59. Good RA. Absence of plasma cells from bone marrow and lymph nodes following antigenic stimulation in patients with agammaglobulinemia. Revue d'Hematol 1954;9:502–503.
60. Gabrielsen AE, Good RA. Thymoma. Ann Intern Med 1966;65:607–611.
61. Jeunet FS, Good RA. Thymoma, immunologic deficiencies and hematological abnormalities. In: Bergsma D, Good RA (eds). Immunologic Deficiency Diseases in Man. New York: The National Foundation, 1968;192–206.
62. Hoyer R, Cooper MD, Gabrielsen AE et al. Lymphophenic forms of congenital immunologic deficiency: clinical and pathologic patterns. In: Bergsma D, Good RA (eds). Immunologic Deficiency Diseases in Man (Birth Defects: Original Article Series). New York: The National Foundation, 1968;IV:91–103.
63. Lorenz ED, Uphoff TR, Reid TR et al. Modification of irradiation injury in mice and guinea pigs by bone marrow injections. J Natl Cancer Inst 1951;12:197–201.
64. Main JM, Prehn RT. Successful skin homografts after the administration of high dosage X irradiation and homologous bone marrow. J Natl Cancer Inst 1955;15:1023–1029.
65. Gatti RA, Meuwissen HF, Allen HD et al. Immunological reconstitution of sex-linked lymphophenic immunological deficiency. Lancet 1968;2:1366–1369.
66. Good RA. Immunologic reconstitution: the achievement and its meaning. Hosp Pract 1969;4:41–47.
67. Meuwissen HJ, Gatti RA, Terasaki PI et al. Treatment of lymphopenic hypogammaglobulinemia and bone marrow aplasia by transplantation of allogeneic marrow. N Engl J Med 1969;382:691–697.
68. Good RA, Meuwissen HF, Hong R et al. Successful marrow transplantation for correction of immunological deficit in lymphopenic agammaglobulinemia and treatment of immunologically induced pancytopenia. Exp Hematol 1969;19:4–10.
69. Good RA, Meuwissen HJ, Hong R et al. Bone marrow transplantation: correction of immune deficit in lymphopenic immunologic deficiency and correction of an immunologically induced pancytopenia. Trans Assoc Am Physicians 1969;82:278–284.
70. Gatti RA, Good RA. Follow-up of correction of severe dual system immunodeficiency with bone marrow transplantation. J Pediatr 1971;79:475–479.
71. Good RA. Bone marrow transplantation: cellular engineering to correct primary immunodeficiency, aregenerative anemia and pancytopenia. In: Bergsma D (ed). Good RA, Finstad J (scientific eds). Immunodeficiency in Man and Animals: Proceedings (Birth Defects: Original Article Series). Massachusettes: Sinauer Associates, Inc., 1975;XI:377–379.
72. Good RA. Progress toward a cellular engineering (Lasker Award Lecture). JAMA 1970;214:1289–1300.
73. Good RA, Finstad J (scientific eds). Immunodeficiency in Man and Animals: Proceedings (Birth Defects: Original Article Series). Massachusetts: Sinauer Associates, Inc., 1975;XI:377–379.
74. Good RA. Marrow transplantation and stem cell transplantation in 1996 (The developmental perspective. In: Ikehara S, Takaku F, Good RA (eds). Bone Marrow Transplantation: Basic and Clinical Studies. Proceedings of the International Symposium on Bone Marrow Transplantation, Tokyo: Springer-Verlag; 1996;277–301.
75. Good RA. Organization and development of the immune system: Relation to its reconstruction. In: Sackstein R, Janssen WE, Elfenbein GJ (eds). Bone Marrow Transplantation (Foundations for the 21st Century). New York: Academy of Sciences, Ann NY Acad Sci 1995;770:8–31.
76. Bing J, Plum P. Serum proteins in leucopenia. Acta Med Scand 1937;92:415–428.
77. Kolouch F, Good RA, Campbell B. The reticulo-endothelial origin of the bone marrow plasma cells in hypersensitive states. J Lab Clin Med 1947;32:749–755.
78. Bjoerneboe M, Gormsen H. Preliminary report in investigations on occurrence of plasma cells in experimental hyperglobulinemia in rabbits. Nordisk Medicin Hospitalstid 1941;9:891–894.
79. Fragraeus A. Antibody production in relation to the development of plasma cells: *in vivo* and *in vitro* experiments. Acta Med Scandinav 1948;(Suppl 204)130:3–122
80. Coons AH, Ledric EH, Connolly JM. Studies on antibody production. I. A method for the histochemical demonstration of specific antibody and its application to a study of the hyperimmune rabbit. J Exp Med 1955;102:49–60.
81. Coons AH, Ledric EH, Connolly JM. Studies on antibody production. II. The primary and secondary responses in the popliteal lymph node of the rabbit. J Exp Med 1955;102:61–72.
82. Ikehara S, Ohtsuki H, Good RA et al. Prevention of type I diabetes in non-obese diabetic mice by allogeneic bone marrow transplantation. Proc Natl Acad Sci USA 1985;82:7743–7747.
83. Castano L, Eisenbarth GS. Type I diabetes: a chronic autoimmune disease of human, mouse, and rat. Annu Rev Immunol 1990;8:647–679.
84. Ikebukuro K, Adachi Y, Yamada Y et al. Treatment of streptozotocin-induced diabetes mellitus by transplantation of islet cells plus bone marrow cells via portal vein in rats. Transplantation 2002;73:512–518.
85. Zhang Y, Yasumizu R, Sugiura K et al. Fate of allogeneic or syngeneic cells in intravenous or portal vein injection: possible explanation for the mechanism of tolerance induction by portal vein injection. Eur J Immunol 1994;24:1558–1565.

86. Sugiura K, Kato K, Hashimoto F et al. Induction of donor-specific T cell anergy by portal venous injection of allogeneic cells. Immunobiology 1997;197:460–477.

87. Morita H, Sugiura K, Inaba M et al. A new strategy for organ allografts without using immunosuppressants and irradiation. Proc Natl Acad Sci USA 1998;95:6947–6952.

88. Morita H, Nakamura N, Sugiura K et al. Acceptance of skin allografts in pigs by portal venous injection of donor bone marrow cells. Ann Surg 1999;23:114–119.

89. Nakamura T, Good RA, Yasumizu R et al. Successful liver allografts in mice by combination with allogeneic bone marrow transplantation. Proc Natl Acad Sci USA 1986;83:4529–4532.

90. Yasumizu R, Sugiura K, Iwai H et al. Treatment of type 1 diabetes mellitus in non-obese diabetic mice by transplantation of allogeneic bone marrow and pancreatic tissue. Proc Natl Acad Sci USA 1987;84: 6555–6557.

91. Iwai H, Yasumizu R, Sugiura K et al. Successful pancreatic allografts in combination with bone marrow transplantation in mice. Immunology 1987;62:457–462.

92. Exner BG, Fowler K, Ildstad ST. Tolerance induction for islet transplantation. Ann Transplant 1997;2:77–80.

93. Neipp M, Exner BG, Ildstad ST. A nonlethal conditioning approach to achieve engraftment of xenogenic rat bone marrow in mice and to induce donor-specific tolerance. Transplantation 1998;66:969–975.

94. Gruessner RW, Sutherland DE, Najarian JS et al. Solitary pancreas transplantation for nonuremic patients with labile insulin-dependent diabetes mellitus. Transplantation 1997;64:1572–1577.

95. Li H, ColsonYL, Ildstad ST. Mixed allogeneic chimerism achieved by lethal and nonlethal conditioning approaches induces donor-specific tolerance to simultaneous islet allografts. Transplantation 1995;6: 523–529.

96. Kawamura M, Hisha H, Li Y et al. Distinct qualitative differences between normal and abnormal hemopoietic stem cells in vivo and in vitro. Stem Cells 1997;15:56–62.

97. Kapoor N, Good RA. Bone marrow transplantation in 1985. In: Aiuti F, Rosen F, Cooper MD (eds). Recent Advances in Primary and Acquired Immunodeficiencies. New York: Raven Press, 1986;327–381.

98. Koch C, Herriksen K, Juhl F et al. Copenhagen Study Group of Immunodeficiencies. Bone-marrow transplantation from an HL-A non-identical but mixed-lymphocyte-culture identical donor. Lancet 1973;1: 1146–1150.

99. Hansen JA, O'Reilly RJ, Good RA et al. Relevance of major human histocompatibility determinants in clinical bone marrow transplantation. Transplant Proc 1976;8:581–589.

100. O'Reilly RJ, Pahwa R, Dupont B et al. Severe combined immuno-deficiency: transplantation approaches for patients lacking an HLA genotypically identical sibling. Transplant Proc 1978;10:187–199.

101. O'Reilly RJ, Pahwa R, Kirkpatrick D et al. Successful transplantation of marrow from an HLA-A, -B, -D-mismatched heterozygous sibling donor into an HLA-D-homozygous patient with aplastic anemia. Transplant Proc 1978;10:957–962.

102. O'Reilly RJ, Kapoor N, Pollack M et al. Reconstitution of immunologic function in a patient with severe combined immunodeficiency following transplantation of marrow from an HLA-A, B, C non-identical but MHC-compatible paternal donor. Transplant Proc 1979;11:1934–1937.

103. O'Reilly RJ, Dupont B, Pahwa S et al. Reconstitution in severe combined immunodeficiency by transplantation of marrow from an unrelated donor. N Engl J Med 1977;297:1311–1318.

104. Von Boehmer H, Spren J, Nabholj M. Tolerance to histocompatibility determinants in tetraparental bone marrow chimeras. J Exp Med 1975;141:322–334.

105. Onoé K, Fernandes G, Good RA. Humoral and cell-mediated immune responses in fully allogeneic bone marrow chimera in mice. J Exp Med 1980;151:115–132.

106. Krown SE, Coico R, Scheid M et al. Immune function in fully allogeneic mouse bone marrow chimeras. Clin Immunol Immunopathol 1981;19:268–283.

107. Coico R, Krown SE, Good RA et al. Helper cell factors restore antibody responses of allogeneic bone marrow chimeras: Evidence for ineffective cellular interactions. J Immunol 1982;128:1590–1593.

108. Onoé K, Good RA. Immune responses in fully allogeneic chimera. Proc Jpn Soc Immunol 1979;9:45–46.

109. Onoé K, Yasumizu R, Oh-ishi T et al. Restricted antibody formation to sheep erythrocytes of allogeneic bone marrow chimeras histoincompatible at the K end of the H-2 complex (Brief Definitive Report). J Exp Med 1981;153:1009–1014.

110. Onoé K, Yasumizu R, Noguchi M et al. Analyses of H-2 restriction specificity of helper T cells in fully allogeneic bone marrow chimera in mice. Immunobiology 1985;169:60–70.

111. Ishii E, Gengozian N, Good RA. Influence of dimethyl myleran on tolerance induction and immune function in major histocompatibility complex-haploidentical murine bone-marrow transplantation. Proc Natl Acad Sci USA 1991;88:8435–8439.

112. Yunis EJ, Fernandes G, Smith J et al. Long survival and immunologic reconstitution following transplantation with syngeneic or allogeneic fetal liver and neonatal spleen cells. Transplant Proc 1976;8:521–525.

113. Yunis EJ, Good RA, Smith J et al. Protection of lethally irradiated mice by spleen cells from neonatally thymectomized mice. Proc Natl Acad Sci USA 1974;71:2544–2548.

114. Tulunay O, Good RA, Yunis EJ. Protection of lethally irradiated mice with allogeneic fetal liver cells: influence of irradiation dose on immunologic reconstitution. Proc Natl Acad Sci USA 1975;72:4100–4104.

115. O'Reilly RJ, Pahwa R, Sorrell M et al. Transplantation of fetal liver and thymus in patients with severe combined immunodeficiencies. In: Doria G, Eshkol A (eds). The Immune System: Functions and Therapy of Dysfunction: Proceedings of the Seronon Symposia. New York: Academic Press, 1980;27:241–253.

116. Touraine JL. T lymphocyte maturation after bone marrow, fetal liver, or thymus transplantation in immunodeficiencies. Transplant Proc 1979;11:494–497.

117. Reisner Y, Sharon N: Cell fractionation by lectins. Trends Biochem 1980;5:29–31.

118. Reisner Y, Itzicovitch L, Meshorer A et al. Hemopoietic stem cell transplantation using mouse bone marrow and spleen cells fractionated by lectins. Proc Natl Acad Sci USA 1978;75:2933–2936.

119. Reisner Y, Kapoor N, Hodes MZ et al. Enrichment for CFU-C from murine and human bone marrow using soybean agglutinin. Blood 1982;59:360–363.

120. O'Reilly RJ, Kapoor N, Kirkpatrick D et al. Transplantation for severe combined immunodeficiency using histoincompatible parental marrow fractionated by soybean agglutinin and sheep red blood cells: Experience in six consecutive cases. Transplant Proc 1983;15:1431–1435.

121. O'Reilly RJ, Collins NH, Kernan N et al. Transplantation of marrow depleted of T cells by soybean lectin agglutination and E-rosette depletion: Major histocompatibility complex-related graft resistance in leukemic transplant recipients. Transplant Proc 1985;17:455–459.

122. O'Reilly RJ, Kernan NA, Cunningham I et al. Allogeneic transplants depleted of T cells by soybean lectin agglutination and E-rosette depletion. Bone Marrow Transplant 1988;3:3–6.

123. Buckley RH, Schiff SE, Sampson HA et al. Development of immunity in human severe primary T cell deficiency following haploidentical bone marrow stem cell transplantation. J Immunol 1986;136:2398–2407.

124. Auletta JJ, Fisher VL. Immune reconstitution in pediatric stem cell transplantation. Front Biosci 2001;6: G23–G32.

125. Kondo M, Weissman IL, Akashi K: Identification of clonogeneic common lymphoid progenitors in mouse bone marrow. Cell 1997;91:661–672.

126. Akashi K, Traver D, Miyamoto T et al. A clonogeneic common myeloid progenitor that gives rise to all myeloid lineages. Nature 2000;404:193–197.

127. Pittenger MF, Mackay AM, Beck SC et al. Multilineage potential of adult human mesenchymal stem cells. Science 1999;284:143–147.

128. Devine SM, Hoffman R. Role of mesenchymal stem cells in hematopoietic stem cell transplantation. Curr Opin Hematol 2000;7:358–363.

129. Kapp U, Hackanson B. Mesenchymal stem cells. Biomed Progr 2001;14:30–35.

130. Majumdar MK, Thiede MA, Mosca JD et al. Phenotypic and functional comparison of cultures of marrow-derived mesenchymal stem cells (MSCs) and stromal cells. J Cell Physiol 1998;176:57–66.

131. Ikehara S, Inaba M, Ishida S et al. Rationale for transplantation of both allogeneic bone marrow and stromal cells in the treatment of autoimmune diseases. In Champlin RE, Gale, RP (eds). New Strategies in Bone Marrow Transplantation, New York: Wiley-Liss, Inc., 1991:251–257.

132. Ikehara S. Pluripotent hematopoietic stem cells in mice and human. Exp Biol Med 2000;223:149–155.

133. Caplan AI. The mesengenic process. Clin Plast Surg 1994;21:429–435.

134. Taichman RS, Reilly MJ, Emerson SB. Human osteoblasts support human hematopoietic progenitor cells in vitro bone marrow cultures. Blood 1996;518–524.

135. Taichman RS, Emerson SB. The role of osteoblasts in the hematopoietic microenvironment. Stem Cells 1998;16:7–15.

136. Haynesworth SE, Baber MA, Caplan AI. Cytokine expression by human marrow-derived mesenchymal progenitor cells in vitro; effects of dexamethasone and IL-Ia. J Cell Physiol 1996;166:585–592.

137. Nota JA, Hanley MB, Kohn DB. Sustained human hematopoiesis in immunodeficient mice by cotransplantation of marrow stroma expressing human IL-3; analysis of gene transduction of long-lived progenitors. Blood 1994;83:3041–3051.

138. Reyes M, Lund T, Lenvik T et al. Purification and ex vivo expansion of postnatal human marrow mesodermal progenitor cells. Blood 2001;98:2615–2625.

139. Jones OY, Steele A, Marikar Y et al. Treatment of BXSB lupus mice with fully matched allogeneic bone marrow transplantation using nonmyeloablative conditioning (Abstr). Seattle, Washington, 2003: Pediatric Academic Societies' Annual Meeting. Ped Res 53.

140. Steele AM, Jones OY, Gok F et al. Rapid in-situ methodology for post-transplant detection of donor chimerism in paraffin-embedded recipient target tissue sections (Abstr). Tampa: Health Science Center Research Day, University of South Florida, 2003;USF Research Day Abstract Book.

141. Ying QL, Nichols J, Evans EP et al. Changing potency by spontaneous fusion. Nature 2002;416:545–548; 416:485–487 (comment).

142. Terada N, Hamazaki T, Oka M et al. Bone marrow cells adopt the phenotype of other cells by spontaneous cell fusion. Nature 2002;416:542–545; 416:485–487 (comment).

143. Cahill RA, Jones OY, Mueller T et al. Replacement of recipient stromal/mesenchymal cells (SC/MSCs) after bone marrow transplant using bone fragments and cultured osteoblast-like cells (Abstr #228). Blood 2002; 100:63a.
144. Hisha N, Nishino T, Kawamura M et al. Successful bone marrow transplantation by bone grafts in chimeric-resistant combination. Exp Hematol 1995;23:347–352.
145. Ishida T, Inaba M, Hisha H et al. Requirement of donor-derived stromal cells in the bone marrow for successful allogeneic bone marrow transplantation: complete prevention of recurrence of autoimmune diseases in MRL/lpr mice by transplantation of bone marrow plus bone (stromal cells) from the same donor. J Immunol 1994;3119–3127.
146. Almeida-Porada G, Fale AW et al. Cotransplantation of stroma cells in enhancement of engraftment and early expression of donor hematopoietic stem cells in utero. Exp Hematol 1999;27:1569–1575.
147. Simmons PJ, Przopiorka D, Thomas ED et al. Host origin of marrow stromal cells following allogeneic bone marrow transplantation. Nature 1987;328:429–432.
148. Perkins S, Fleischman RA. Hematopoietic microenvironment. Origin, lineage, and transplantability of the stromal cells in long-term bone marrow cultures from chimeric mice. J Clin Invest 1988;81:1072–1080.
149. Friedenstein AJ, Petrakova KV, Kurolesova AI et al. Heterotopic of bone marrow. Analysis of precursor cells for osteogenic and hematopoietic tissues. Transplantation 1968;6:230–247.
150. Minguell JJ, Erices A, Conget P. Mesenchymal stem cells. Soc Exp Biol Med 2001;226:507–520.
151. Shake JG, Gruber PJ, Baumgartner WA et al. Mesenchymal stem cell implantation in a swine myocardial infarct model: engraftment and functional effects. Ann Thorac Surg 2002;73:1919–1925.
152. Sale GE, Storb R. Bilateral diffuse pulmonary ectopic ossification after marrow allograft in a dog. Evidence for allotransplantation of hematopoietic and mesenchymal stem cells. Exp Hematol 1983;11:961–966.
153. Zhao LR, Duan WM, Reyes M et al. Human bone marrow stem cells exhibit neural phenotypes and ameliorate neurological deficits after grafting into the ischemic brain of rats. Exp Neurol 2002;174:11–20.
154. Liechty KW, MacKenzie TC, Shaaban AF et al. Human mesenchymal stem cells engraft and demonstrate site-specific differentiation after in utero transplantation in sheep. Nat Med 2000;6:1282–1286.
155. Koc ON, Peters C, Aubourg P et al. Bone marrow-derived mesenchymal stem cells remain host-derived despite successful hematopoietic engraftment after allogeneic transplantation in patients with lysosomal and peroxisomal storage diseases. Exp Hematol 1999;27:1675–1681.
156. Lazarus HM, Haynesworth SE, Gerson SL et al. Human bone marrow-derived mesenchymal (stromal) progenitor cells (MPCs) cannot be recovered from peripheral blood progenitor cell collections. J Hematother 1997;6:447–455.
157. Lazarus HM, Haynesworth SE, Gerson SL et al. Ex vivo expansion and subsequent infusion of human bone marrow-derived stromal progenitor cells (mesenchymal progenitor cells): Implications for therapeutic use. Bone Marrow Transplant 1995;16:557–564.
158. Gerson SL. Mesenchymal stem cells: No longer second class marrow citizens. Nat Med 1999;5:262–264.
159. Krause DS, Theise ND, Collector MI et al. Multi-organ, multi-lineage engraftment by a single bone marrow-derived stem cell. Cell 2001;105:369–377.
160. Thiese ND, Nimmakayalu M, Gardner R et al. Liver from bone marrow in humans. Hepatology 2000; 32:11–16.
161. Gussoni E, Pavlath GK, Miller RG et al. Specific T cell receptor gene rearrangements at the site of muscle degeneration in Duchenne muscular dystrophy. J Immunol 1994;153:4798–4805.
162. Soper BW, Lessard MD, Vogler CA et al. Nonablative neonatal marrow transplantation attenuates function and physical defects of beta-glucuronidase deficiency. Blood 2001;97:1498–1504.
163. McMahon C, Will A, Hu P et al. Bone marrow transplantation corrects osteopetrosis in the carbonic anhydrase II deficiency syndrome. Blood 2001;97:1947–1950.
164. van Bekkum DW. BMT in experimental autoimmune diseases. Bone Marrow Transplant 1993;11:183–187.
165. Ikehara S, Good RA, Nakamura T et al. Rationale for bone marrow transplantation in the treatment of autoimmune diseases. Proc Natl Acad Sci USA 1985;82:2483–2487.
166. Ikehara S, Yasumizu R, Inaba M et al. Long-term observations of autoimmune-prone mice treated for autoimmune disease by allogeneic bone marrow transplantation. Proc Natl Acad Sci USA 1989;86: 3306–3310.
167. Aguila HL, Akashi K, Domen J et al. From stem cells to lymphocytes: biology and transplantation. Immunol Rev 1997;157:13–40.
168. Burt RK, Marmont A, Schroeder J et al. Intense suppression for systemic lupus – the role of hematopoietic stem cells. J Clin Immunol 2000;20:31–37.
169. Yoshida S, Castles JJ, Gerswhin ME. The pathogenesis of autoimmunity in New Zealand mice. Semin Arthritis Rheum 1990;19:224–242.
170. Sardiña EE, Sugiura K, Ikehara S et al. Transplantation of WGA+ hematopoietic cells to prevent or induce systemic autoimmune disease. Proc Natl Acad Sci USA 1991;88:3218–3222.
171. El-Badri NS, Wang B-Y, Steele A et al. Successful prevention of autoimmune disease by transplantation of adequate number of fully allogeneic hematopoietic stem cells. Transplantation 2000;70:870–877.

172. Hang L, Izui S, Dixon F. (NZW × BXSB)F1 hybrid. A model of acute lupus and coronary vascular disease with myocardial infarction. J Exp Med 1981;154:216–221.
173. Berden J, Hang L, McConahey P et al. Analysis of vascular lesions in murine SLE. I: association with serologic abnormalities. J Immunol 1983;130:1699–1705.
174. Mizutani H, Engelman RW, Kinjoh K et al. Prevention and induction of occlusive coronary vascular disease in autoimmune (W/B)F1 mice by haploidentical bone marrow transplantation: possible role for anticardiolipin autoantibodies. Blood 1993;82:3091–3097.
175. Kirzner RP, Engelman RW, Mizutani H et al. Prevention of coronary vascular disease by transplantation of T cell depleted bone marrow and hematopoietic stem cell preparation in autoimmune-prone W/BF1 mice. Biol Blood Marrow Transplant 2000;6:13–22.
176. Oyaizu N, Yasumizu R, Miyama-Inaba M et al. (NZW × BXSB)F1 mouse, a new animal model of idiopathic thrombocytopenic purpura. J Exp Med 1988;167:2017–2022.
177. Wang B-Y, Cherry, El-Badri NS et al. Prevention of development of autoimmune disease in BXSB mice by mixed bone marrow transplantation. Proc Natl Acad Sci USA 1997;94:12065–12069.
178. Wang B-Y, Yamamoto Y, El-Badri-Dajani N et al. Treatment of autoimmune disease in BXSB mice by mixed bone marrow transplantation. Proc Natl Acad Sci USA 1999;3012–3016.
179. Jyonouchi H, Kincade PW, Good RA et al. Reciprocal transfer of abnormalities in clonable B lymphocytes and myeloid progenitors between NZB and DBA/2 mice. J Immunol 1981;127:1232–1238.
180. Kincade, PW, Lee G, Fernandes G et al. Abnormalities in clonable B lymphocytes and myeloid progenitors in autoimmune NZB mice. Proc Natl Acad Sci USA 1979;76:3464–3468.
181. Kotzin BL, Strober S. Reversal of NZB/NZW disease with total lymphoid irradiation. J Exp Med 1979;10:371–378.
182. Warner NL, Moore MAS. Defects in hematopoietic differentiation in NZB and NZC mice. J Exp Med 1971;134:313–334.
183. Ikehara S, Kawamura M, Takao F et al. Organ-specific and systemic autoimmune diseases originate from defects in hematopoietic stem cells. Proc Natl Acad Sci USA 1990;87:8341–8344.
184. Good RA, Ikehara S. Preclinical investigations which subserve efforts to employ bone marrow transplantation for rheumatoid or autoimmune diseases. J Rheumatol 1997;24(Suppl 48):5–12.
185. Hosaka N, Nose M, Kyogoku M et al. Thymus transplantation, a critical factor for correction of autoimmune disease in aging MRL/+ mice. Proc Natl Acad Sci USA 1996;93:8558–8562.
186. Yasumizu R, Sugiura K, Iwai H et al. Treatment of type 1 diabetes mellitus in non-obese diabetic mice by transplantation of allogeneic bone marrow and pancreatic tissue. Proc Natl Acad Sci USA 1987;84:6555–6557.
187. Ikehara S, Ohtsuki H, Good RA et al. Prevention of type I diabetes in nonobese diabetic mice by allogeneic bone marrow transplantation. Proc Natl Acad Sci USA 1985;82:7743–7747.
188. Wyatt DT, Lum L, Casper J et al. Autoimmune thyroiditis after bone marrow transplantation. Bone Marrow Transplant 1990;5:357–361.
189. Mizutani H, Furubayashi T, Kashiwagi H et al. Effects of splenectomy on immune thrombocytopenic purpura in (NZW × BXSB)F1 mice: Analyses of platelet kinetics and antiplatelet antibody production. Thromb Haemost 1992;67:563–566.
190. Mizutani H, Engelman RW, Kurata Y et al. Development and characterization of monoclonal antiplatelet autoantibodies from autoimmune thrombocytopenic purpura-prone (NZW × BXSB)F1 mice. Blood 1993;82:837–844.
191. Hang L, Stephen-Larson PM, Henry JP et al. Transfer of renovascular hypertension and coronary heart disease by lymphoid cells from SLE-prone mice. Am J Pathol 1984;115:42–46.
192. Ikehara S, Yasumizu R, Inaba M et al. Long-term observations of autoimmune-prone mice treated for autoimmune disease by allogeneic bone marrow transplantation. Proc Natl Acad Sci USA 1989;86:3306–3310.
193. Kinjoh K, Kyogoku M, Good RA. Genetic selection for crescent formation yields mouse strain with rapidly progressive glomerulonephritis and small vessel vasculitis. Proc Natl Acad Sci USA 1993;9:3413–3417.
194. Kaufman CL, Colson YL, Wren SM et al. Phenotypic characterization of a novel bone marrow-derived cell that facilitates engraftment of allogeneic bone marrow stem cells. Blood 1994;84:2436–2446.
195. Ildstad ST, Wren SM, Bluestone JA et al. Characterization of mixed allogeneic chimeras. Immunocompetence, in vitro reactivity and genetic specificity of tolerance. J Exp Med 1985;162:231–244.
196. El-Badri NS, Wang B-Y, Cherry et al. Osteoblasts promote engraftment of allogeneic hematopoietic stem cells. Exp Hematol 1998;26:110–116.
197. Owen RD. Immunogenetic consequences of vascular anastomoses between bovine twins. Science 1945;102:400–401.
198. Anderson D, Billingham RE, Lampkin GH et al. The use of skin grafting to distinguish between monozygotic and dizygotic twins in cattle. Heredity 1952;5:379–397.
199. Martinez C, Shapiro F, Kelman H et al. Tolerance of F1 hybrid skin homografts in the parent strain induced by parabiosis. Proc Soc Exp Biol Med 1960;103:266–269.

200. Martinez C, Shapiro F, Good RA. Essential duration of parabiosis and development of tolerance to skin homografts in mice. Proc Soc Exp Biol Med 1960;104:256–259.
201. Onoé K, Fernandes G, Shen FW et al. Sequential changes of thymocyte surface antigens with presence or absence of graft-vs-host reaction following allogeneic bone marrow transplantation. Cell Immunol 1982;68:207–219.
202. Onoé K, Yasumizu R, Geng L et al. Analyses of Ia restriction specificity of helper T cells in H-2 subregion compatible bone marrow chimera in mice. Immunobiology 1985;169:71–82.
203. Onoé K, Good RA, Yamamoto K. Anti-bacterial immunity to Listeria monocytogenes in allogeneic bone marrow chimera in mice. J Immunol 1986;136:4264–4269.
204. Ildstad ST, Sachs DH. Reconstitution with syngeneic plus allogeneic or xenogeneic bone marrow leads to specific acceptance of allografts or xenografts. Nature 1984;307:168–170.
205. El-Badri NS, Good RA. Lymphohemopoietic reconstitution and induction of immunological tolerance using WGA hemopoietic stem cell transplantation in a mixed chimerism model. Ph.D. Dissertation. Tampa: University of South Florida, 1992.
206. El-Badri NS, Good RA. Lymphohemopoietic reconstitution using wheat germ agglutinin-positive hemopoietic stem cell transplantation within but not across the major histocompatibility barriers. Proc Natl Acad Sci USA 1993;90:6681–6685.
207. El-Badri NS, Good RA: Induction of immunological tolerance in full major and multiminor histocompatibility-disparate mice using a mixed bone marrow transplantation model. Proc Soc Exp Biol 1994;205:67–74.
208. Wang B-Y, El-Badri NS, Cherry et al. Purified hematopoietic stem cells without facilitating cells can repopulate fully allogeneic recipients across entire major histocompatibility complex transplantation barrier in mice. Proc Natl Acad Sci USA 1997;94:14632–14636.
209. Ikehara S. Treatment of autoimmune diseases by hematopoietic stem cell transplantation. Exp Hematol 2001;29:661–669.
210. Wulffraat N, van Royen A, Bierings M et al. Autologous haemopoietic stem cell transplantation in four patients with refractory juvenile chronic arthritis. Lancet 1999;353:550–553.
211. Burt RK, Traynor AE, Cohen B et al. T cell depleted autologous hematopoietic stem cell transplantation for multiple sclerosis: report on the first three patients. Bone Marrow Transplant 1998;21:537–541.
212. Yamamoto Y, Wang B-Y, Fukuhara S et al. Mixed peripheral blood stem cell transplantation for autoimmune disease in BXSB/Mpj mice. Blood 2002;100:1886–1893.
213. Ogata H, Bradley WG, Inaba M et al. Long term repopulation of hematolymphoid cells with only a few hemopoietic stem cells in mice. Proc Natl Acad Sci USA 1995;92:5945–5949.
214. Prigozhina TB, Urevitch O, Zhu J et al. Permanent and specific transplantation tolerance induced by non-myeloablative treatment to a wide variety of allogeneic tissues: I. induction of tolerance by a short course of total lymphoid irradiation and selective elimination of the donor-specific host lymphocytes. Transplantation 1997;63:1394–1399.
215. Rao SS, Peters SO, Crittenden RB et al. Stem cell transplantation in the normal nonmyeloablated host: relationship between cell dose, schedule and engraftment. Exp Hematol 1997;25:114–121.
216. Lowenthal RM, Cohen ML, Atkinson K et al. Apparent cure of rheumatoid arthritis by bone marrow transplantation. J Rheumatol 1993;20:137–209.
217. Marmont AM. Immune ablation followed by allogeneic or autologous bone marrow transplantation: a new treatment for severe autoimmune diseases? Stem Cells 1994;12:125–135.
218. Nelson JL, Torrez R, Louie FM et al. Pre-existing autoimmune diseases in patients with long-term survival after allogeneic bone marrow transplantation. J Rheumatol 1997;24(Suppl):S23–S29.
219. Eedy DJ, Burrows D, Bridges JM et al. Clearance or severe psoriasis after allogeneic bone marrow transplantation. [comment] BMJ 1990;300:908.
220. Ikehara S. Autoimmune diseases as stem cell disorders: Normal stem cell transplant for their treatment (Review). Int J Mol Med 1998;1:5–16.
221. Sullivan KM, Furst DE. The evolving role of blood and marrow transplantation for the treatment of autoimmune diseases. J Rheumatol 1997;24(Suppl 48):1–4.
222. Burt RJM, Traynor AE. Hematopoietic stem cell transplantation. a new therapy for autoimmune disease. Stem Cells 1999;17:366–372.
223. Giralt S, Khouri I, Champlin R. Non-myeloablative "mini transplants" (Review). Cancer Treat Res 1999;101:97–108.
224. Slavin S. New strategies for bone marrow transplantation. Curr Opin Immunol 2000;12:542–551.
225. Meislin AG, Rothfield NF. Systemic lupus erythematosus in childhood: Analysis of 42 cases with comparative data on 200 adult cases followed concurrently. Pediatrics 1968;42:37–49.
226. Niaudet P. Treatment of lupus nephritis in children. Pediatr Nephrol 2000;14:158–166.
227. El-Badri-Dajani N, Shah B, Steele A et al. Migration and repopulation of hematopoietic stem cells in autoimmune glomerulonephritis (Abstr #2283.5). Blood 2001;98:546a.
228. Starzl TE, Demetris AJ, Murase N et al. Cell migration, chimerism, and graft acceptance (Review; see comments). Lancet 1992;339:1579–1582.

229. Kushida T, Inaba M, Hisha H et al. Intra-bone marrow injection of allogeneic bone marrow cells: a powerful new strategy for treatment of intractable autoimmune disease in MRL/lpr mice. Blood 2000;97:3292–3299.
230. Jin L, Zeng H, Chien S et al. In vivo selection using a cell-growth switch. Nat Genet 2000;26:64–66.
231. Regaud C. Etudes sur la structure des tubes seminferes et sur la spematogenese chezles mammiferes. Part I. Arch Anat Microsc Morphol Exp 1901;4:101–156.
232. Regaud C. Etudes sur la structure des tubes seminferes et sur la spermatogenese chez les mammiferes. Part 2. Arch Anat Microsc Morphol Exp 1901;4:231–280.
233. Baserga A, Zavagli G. Ferrata's stem cells: an historical review on hemocytoblasts and hemohistioblasts. Blood Cells 1981;7:537–545.
234. Pappenheim A. Prinzipien der neueren morphologischen Haematozytologie nach zytogenetischer Grundlage. Folia Haematol (Frankf) 1917;21:91.
235. Leblond CP. Classification of cell populations on the basis of their proliferative behaviour. Natl Cancer Inst Monogr 1964;14:119–150.
236. Robey PG. Stem cells near the century mark. J Clin Invest 2000;105:1489–1491.
237. Bianco P, Robey PG. Marrow stromal stem cells. J Clin Invest 2000;105:1663–1668.
238. Bianco P, Riminucci M, Kuznetsov S et al. Multipotential cells in the bone marrow stroma: regulation in the context of organ physiology. Crit Rev Eukaryot Gene Expr 1999;9:159–173.
239. Cossu G, Mavilio F. Myogenic stem cells for the therapy of primary myopathies: wishful thinking or therapeutic perspective? J Clin Invest 2000;105:1669–1674.
240. Treleaven J, Barrett J. Introduction to bone marrow transplantation. In: Treleaven J, Barrett J (eds). Bone Marrow Transplantation in Practice. New York: Churchill Livingstone, 1992;3–9.
241. Green H. Regeneration of the skin after grafting of epidermal cultures. Lab Invest 1989;60:583–584.
242. Brittberg M, Lindahl A, Nilsson A et al. Treatment of deep cartilage defects in the knee with autologous chondrocyte transplantation. N Engl J Med 1994;331:889–895.

# CHAPTER III

# Finding Histocompatible Donors for Allotransplantation

CHOON KEE LEE

Whether a patient survives stem cell transplantation largely depends on the degree of similarity of tissue antigens (human leukocyte antigen, HLA) between the patient and donor.[1-4] Of the T lymphocytes in both donor and recipient that recognize the differences in tissue antigens between them, cytotoxic CD8+ T cells recognize class I molecules and helper/suppressor CD4+ T cells recognize class II molecules on the cell surface. Since recognition is bi-directional between the donor and recipient, immunosuppressive therapy for the recipient is required to prevent rejection of the donor graft by the recipient's T lymphocytes. Of course, insufficient immunosuppressive therapy or transplantation of mismatched stem cells potentially result in rejection or mixed chimerism of hemopoietic stem cells from the donor. However, the most important clinical significance of tissue typing is to reduce the reaction of donor T lymphocytes to dissimilar host tissue antigens.

Reaction, i.e., graft-versus-host disease, can occur where there are host antigens that would be recognized. Some antigens (class I antigens) are present on all available cells, while others (class II antigens) are detected only on certain cells, such as B lymphocyte, macrophage, and dendritic cells. Furthermore, certain dissimilarities of tissue antigens are clinically more important. For example, mismatches in HLA Cw or DR antigens are associated with more serious graft-versus-host disease than mismatches in HLA A or B antigens. HLA antigens that are identified and known to be important for histocompatibility are named as major antigens, and the other antigens that are present but not yet identified are called minor antigens.[5,6]

A donor search among siblings usually results in the best possible chance for match, since there should be significant genetic similarity in HLA minor antigens if HLA major antigens are matched between a sibling pair. For patients who do not have matched sibling donors, alternate choices for stem cells are autologous stem cells, haploidentical stem cells from a parent, mismatched stem cells from a sibling, or matched or partially mismatched stem cells from an unrelated donor. Matched unrelated donor cells can be from an unrelated adult, or from umbilical cord blood cells.

Finding the right donor necessitates matching of HLA antigens or histocompatibility genes by serologic or molecular methodology. These antigens are present in all species and are known as major histocompatibility (MHC) genes. These gene products are known as H2 in the mouse, DLA in the dog, and HLA in humans. The designation of these antigens as human leukocyte antigens comes from the initial discovery in the 1960s of tissue antigens only in leukocytes, but not in red blood cells.

The HLA system contains several hundred class I and II genes, located on chromosome 6, which encode cell surface glycoprotein molecules and restrict the specific T cell responses.[3,4,7–10] Class I antigens are composed of three α subunits encoded by HLA A, B, C, E, F, and G genes, and one molecule of β2-microglobulin from chromosome 15. Both α and β subunits of class II antigens are encoded by DM, DO, DP, DR, and DQ genes that reside in the HLA-D region.

# ANTIGEN CLASSES

There are two types of genes for the major histocompatibility complex. Class I MHC genes code for cell surface glycoproteins that are present on almost all nucleated cells. These glycoproteins consist of three globular domains from a large α polypeptide chain and a β2-microglobulin, forming a tetrameric structure. The α3 and the β2 microglobulin are close to the cell membrane and are called the immunoglobulin constant domains. In contrast, the α1 and α2 domains are located farther away from the membrane and form a U-shaped groove into which a processed antigenic peptide sits and to which the T cell receptor binds. Processed antigens are intracellular proteins such as viral protein that is synthesized in the cells. The ends of α1 and α2 that are recognized by corresponding T cell receptors are called the "complementarity determining region," which are unique in each individual. The diversity of class I antigens comes from differences in α1 and α2 molecules. Of all of the class I antigens, HLA A, B, and C are most diverse and polymorphic. HLA E and G are oligomorphic and F is monomorphic. Therefore, in clinical practice, HLA E, F, and G are not investigated due to their relatively similar structure between donor and recipient.

Class II antigens are mostly confined to specific antigen presenting cells including dendritic cells, Langerhans' cells, macrophages, B lymphocytes, activated T lymphocytes, and endothelial cells. Unlike class I antigens, all four domains (α2β2) come from chromosome 6, without β2-microglobulin. The proximal domains close to the cell membrane (α2 and β2) are similar to members of the immunoglobulin superfamily, while the distal domains (α1 and β1) form an antigen binding groove to which a processed antigen can be found and to which T cell receptors attach. Processed antigens associated with class II molecules are exogenous molecules that are taken into the cells by endocytosis and broken down in the endosomes before merging with newly synthesized class II molecules.

The entire HLA region (p21) of the chromosome 6 is present as an allele, designated as the HLA haplotype, similar to any other pair of chromosomes. Thus, each person has one complete haplotype set from each parent. The genes encoding HLA class I and II antigens are co-dominantly expressed as cell surface molecules and transmitted by dominant inheritance. Therefore, each person has two different sets of expressed HLA molecules on the cell membrane, for example, HLA A 1, 2.

There are also class III antigens on chromosome 6, in close proximity to class I and II antigens, which are involved in many important functions of the body, such as adrenal 21 hydroxylase, serum complement components, tumor necrosis factors, and heat shock proteins. These molecules are not involved in the recognition between donor and recipient.

# POLYMORPHISM OF GENES

As described earlier, HLA A, B, and C of the class I antigens are polymorphic and E, while F and G are either oligo- or monomorphic. The differences are most commonly found in exon 2 and 3, which correspond to the α1 and α2 domains, respectively. In class II antigens, α1 and β1 domains from each exon 2 of α and β chain genes are the most polymorphic and α2 and β2 domains from the exon 3 are preserved. In HLA DQ and DP, there are a few non-functioning genes except α and β, called pseudogenes, which do not contribute to histo-incompatibility. α and β genes transcribe the A1 and B1 of each HLA DQ and DP, respectively. Therefore, histocompatibility information on DQ and DP antigens are mainly restricted to DQA1, DQB1, DPA1, and DPB1.

Unlike other class II antigens, polymorphism of HLA DR (D-related) antigens comes exclusively from β chain genes and the α chain is monomorphic. Furthermore, there are several motifs (DRB1 through DRB9) that constitute β chain genes, increasing the degree of polymorphism by different arrangements among the motifs. The usual arrangement of these motifs is DRB1 on the 5′ end, DRB9 on the 3′ end, and other DRB motifs in between. Of the nine DRB motifs, only DRB3, DRB4, and DRB5 are expressed genes. In one haplotype, there can be up to three DRB genes, but only one DRB gene can be expressed. Therefore, for clinical practice of DNA DR typing, DRB1 and at least one of DRB-3, -4, or -5 are reported.

# HLA TESTING

The HLA system was first described and classified by serologic differences, using a panel of standard HLA-specific sera that recognized certain antigenic determinants.[11–16] As the degree of difference in HLA antigens has been refined, earlier classifications were modified to incorporate new ones and change or delete existing classifications. One important theme of sequential changes in the scheme of HLA classification has been the designation of further refined or newly discovered antigenic determinants from a previous classified antigen. In this case, the previously classified antigens are called a broad antigen, and newly discovered differences (or different antigenic determinants) are referred to as splits. For example, the previously defined A10 is now classified as A25, A26, A34, or A66. By convention, broad antigens are described in parentheses, after a numeric designation of the most recent and refined serologic determinant to indicate the origin of the splits. In the case of A10, the splits are designated A25,[10] A26,[10] A34,[10] and A66.[10] In some instances, reaction patterns of monoclonal antibodies to HLA antigens may look similar even without a clear-cut split from a broad antigen, due to the comparable reactions to shared public epitopes of HLA antigens. This pattern of reaction is grouped in one category of cross reactive group (CREG), which may be clinically useful for a mismatched transplantation. For example, A11 is related to A1, A3, and A10 as a cross reactive group.

HLA antigens now can be analyzed at the DNA level by polymerase chain reaction and molecular DNA fingerprinting, achieving precise definitions of the HLA alleles for each of the HLA genes.[8,11,17] Polymerase chain reactions that utilize sequence specific oligonucleotide probes (PCR-SSOP) or allele specific oligonucleotide (PCR-ASO) are used for typing DRB and DQ.[11,14] The sequence-specific oligonucleotide probes are short complementary sequences for the first domain of heavy chains of hypervariable regions in exon 2. For DPB and class I antigens, PCR-restriction fragment length polymorphism (PCR-RFLP) is preferred, which measures the length of cleaved HLA genes by the restriction endonucleases.

## HLA TERMINOLOGY

The HLA terminology is designated by the World Health Organization Nomenclature Committee.[19] By convention, the first two digits following the HLA class represent serotype and the two additional digits after the serotype describe information on the DNA, which is assigned in the order in which DNA sequences were determined. Differences in the first four digits come from significant nucleotide substitutions, changing the amino acid sequence of the encoded protein. For example, of HLA A 2402, 24 is a serotype and 02 indicates the fact that it was found after the first identified DNA sequence 01.

Differences in silent, non-coding nucleotide substitution are presented as the fifth digit, and differences in introns or in the 5' and 3' untranslated regions of HLA DNA sequence as the sixth and seventh digits. In HLA A 2402102, 1 following 2402 indicates it is a non-coding substitution and 02 following 24021 represents the untranslated regions. Therefore, the first four digits of HLA are clinically important, whereas there may not be a significant reaction between the donor and patient based on the differences in the latter three digits.

The w in HLA Bw denotes 'workshop,' indicating that it is indistinct or not so clarified. However, w in HLA Cw is used so that it will not be confused with C of serum complements.

## FREQUENCY OF HLA HAPLOTYPES

Certain haplotypes are more commonly found among populations while others are very rare and difficult to find; the incidence of haplotypes can be ranked by population analyses.[19,20] This association of particular HLA antigens with others results from linkage disequilibrium inherently present in chromosomes.[21] The rank of haplotypes in general is dependent on ethnicity.[21–24] For example, the haplotypes of HLA A1, B8, DR3 are most common in the Caucasian American and Native American populations, while it ranks as second in African Americans and third in Hispanic Americans. In clinical practice, the chance of finding an unrelated donor can be predicted based on the rank of the patient's haplotypes. If the patient's haplotypes are one of the first ten most common types of a particular ethnic group, finding a matched unrelated donor is very likely. The ten most common haplotypes are described in ▶ Table 3.1.

## PROBABILITY OF FINDING AN HLA MATCHED DONOR

Currently, HLA A, B, Cw, and DR are the minimum number of antigens for histocompatibility typing. A and B antigens may be tested by serological methods, but DNA typing of antigens is preferred if available. In general, the first four digits of HLA antigen information (so-called low-resolution DNA typing) are required. If serologic methods are used, an algorithm for broad antigens is necessary as well as cross reactive groups to see if the reported numerical information of an HLA antigen corresponds to the one being searched. Otherwise a certain degree of mismatch can be accepted for transplantation. For example, HLA A28, 30 is not significantly different from A68, 31 since A28 and A68 are in the same category for a broad antigen specificity, and A30 and A31 are cross reactive to each other. Of course, these may not used for allotransplant if the protocol for transplantation requires

**TABLE 3.1**   Frequency of Haplotypes, Based on Ethnicity

### African American Haplotype

| Rank | A | B | DR |
|---|---|---|---|
| 1 | 30 | 42 | 3 |
| 2 | 1 | 8 | 3 |
| 3 | 3 | 7 | 2 |
| 4 | 2 | 44 | 4 |
| 5 | 33 | 53 | 8 |
| 6 | 2 | 7 | 2 |
| 7 | 28 | 58 | 12 |
| 8 | 2 | 45 | 6 |
| 9 | 30 | 42 | 8 |
| 10 | 34 | 44 | 2 |

### Caucasian Haplotype

| Rank | A | B | DR |
|---|---|---|---|
| 1 | 1 | 8 | 3 |
| 2 | 3 | 7 | 2 |
| 3 | 2 | 44 | 4 |
| 4 | 2 | 7 | 2 |
| 5 | 29 | 44 | 7 |
| 6 | 2 | 62 | 4 |
| 7 | 3 | 35 | 1 |
| 8 | 1 | 57 | 7 |
| 9 | 2 | 60 | 6 |
| 10 | 2 | 8 | 3 |

### Native American Haplotype

| Rank | A | B | DR |
|---|---|---|---|
| 1 | 1 | 8 | 3 |
| 2 | 3 | 7 | 2 |
| 3 | 2 | 44 | 4 |
| 4 | 2 | 7 | 2 |
| 5 | 29 | 44 | 7 |
| 6 | 2 | 62 | 4 |
| 7 | 1 | 57 | 7 |
| 8 | 3 | 35 | 1 |
| 9 | 2 | 60 | 6 |
| 10 | 24 | 51 | 4 |

### Hispanic Haplotype

| Rank | A | B | DR |
|---|---|---|---|
| 1 | 2 | 35 | 8 |
| 2 | 29 | 44 | 7 |
| 3 | 1 | 8 | 3 |
| 4 | 2 | 35 | 4 |
| 5 | 3 | 7 | 2 |
| 6 | 28 | 39 | 4 |
| 7 | 2 | 39 | 4 |
| 8 | 24 | 39 | 6 |
| 9 | 33 | 14 | 1 |
| 10 | 24 | 35 | 4 |

### Asian American Haplotype

| Rank | A | B | DR |
|---|---|---|---|
| 1 | 33 | 58 | 3 |
| 2 | 33 | 44 | 6 |
| 3 | 24 | 52 | 2 |
| 4 | 2 | 46 | 9 |
| 5 | 33 | 44 | 7 |
| 6 | 30 | 13 | 7 |
| 7 | 24 | 7 | 1 |
| 8 | 33 | 58 | 6 |
| 9 | 11 | 62 | 4 |
| 10 | 1 | 57 | 7 |

an exact serologic match or match at the DNA level. In contrast, HLA Cw and DR require DNA typing since any degree of mismatch in these antigens affects the incidence and intensity of graft-versus-host disease.

The chance of finding an HLA matched sibling depends on the number of available siblings. The likelihood of a match can be estimated by using the equation $[1 - (\frac{3}{4})n]$, where n is the number of siblings. Therefore, if there is one sibling, the chance of a match is 25%;

for two siblings 44%, three siblings 58%, and four siblings 68%. For an unrelated donor search, both ethnicity and haplotypes of the patient affect the chances of a match, as described earlier. One important search strategy among unrelated donors is to use data related to linkage disequilibrium of haplotypes. Therefore, at the outset for donor search, for either a sibling or unrelated donor, it is important to know the haplotypes of the patient. The information on haplotypes can be deduced easily by comparing the patient's haplotypes to those of the existing siblings. If it is difficult to identify the haplotypes, HLA typing of parents, children, or uncles/aunts may provide additional information.

# REFERENCES

1. Beatty PG, Clift RA, Mickelson EM et al. Marrow transplantation from related donors other than HLA-identical siblings. N Engl J Med 1985;313:765–771.
2. Petersdorf EW, Hansen JA, Martin PJ et al. Major-histocompatibility-complex class I alleles and antigens in hematopoietic-cell transplantation. N Engl J Med 2001;345:1794–1800.
3. Beatty PG, Anasetti C, Hansen JA et al. Marrow transplantation from unrelated donors for treatment of hematologic malignancies: effect of mismatching for one HLA locus. Blood 1993;81:249–253.
4. Sasazuki T, Juji T, Morishima Y et al. Effect of matching of class I HLA alleles on clinical outcome after transplantation of hematopoietic stem cells from an unrelated donor. Japan Marrow Donor Program. N Engl J Med 1998;339:1177–1185.
5. Goulmy E. Human minor histocompatibility antigens: New concepts for marrow transplantation and adoptive immunotherapy. Immunol Rev 1997;157:125–140.
6. Martin PJ. Increased disparity for minor histocompatibility antigens as a potential cause of increased GVHD risk in marrow transplantation from unrelated donors compared with related donors. Bone Marrow Transplant 1991;8:217–223.
7. Eiermann TH. HLA and bone marrow transplantation. Arch Immunol Ther Exp (Warsz) 1995;43:83–87.
8. Hansen JA, Choo SY, Geraghty DE et al. The HLA system in clinical marrow transplantation. Hematol Oncol Clin North Am 1990;4:507–515.
9. Howell WM, Navarrete C. The HLA system: An update and relevance to patient-donor matching strategies in clinical transplantation. Vox Sang 1996;71:6–12.
10. Yunis EJ, Awdeh Z, Raum D et al. The MHC in human bone marrow allotransplantation. Clin Haematol 1983;12:641–680.
11. Bidwell JL, Bidwell EA, Bradley BA. HLA class II genes: Typing by DNA analysis. Clin Haematol 1990;3:355–384.
12. Hurley CK, Schreuder GM, Marsh SG et al. The search for HLA-matched donors: A summary of HLA-A*, -B*, -DRB1/3/4/5* alleles and their association with serologically defined HLA-A, -B, -DR antigens. Tissue Antigens 1997;50:401–418.
13. Little AM, Marsh SG, Madrigal JA. Current methodologies of human leukocyte antigen typing utilized for bone marrow donor selection. Curr Opin Hematol 1998;5:419–428.
14. Baxter-Lowe LA. Molecular techniques for typing unrelated marrow donors: Potential impact of molecular typing disparity on donor selection. Bone Marrow Transplant 1994;14(Suppl 4):S42–S50.
15. Dyer PA, Jawaheer D, Ollier B et al. HLA allele detection using molecular techniques. Dis Markers 1993;11:145–160.
16. Hurley CK. Acquisition and use of DNA-based HLA typing data in bone marrow registries. Tissue Antigens 1997;49:323–328.
17. Akimoto S, Abe M, Ishikawa O et al. HLA-DRB1 and DQB1 genes in anticentromere antibody positive patients with SSc and primary biliary cirrhosis. Ann Rheum Dis 2001;60:639–640.
18. Schreuder GM, Hurley CK, Marsh SG, et al. The HLA Dictionary 2001: A summary of HLA-A, -B, -C, -DRB1/3/4/5 and -DQB1 alleles and their association with serologically defined HLA-A, -B, -C, -DR and -DQ antigens. Eur J Immunogenet 2001;28:565–596.
19. Marsh SG, Bodmer JG, Albert ED et al. Nomenclature for factors of the HLA system, 2000. Eur J Immunogenet 2001;28:377–424.
20. Mori M, Graves M, Milford EL et al. Computer program to predict likelihood of finding an HLA-matched donor: Methodology, validation, and application. Biol Blood Marrow Transplant 1996;2:134–144.
21. Beatty PG, Mori M, Milford E. Impact of racial genetic polymorphism on the probability of finding an HLA-matched donor. Transplantation 1995;60:778–783.
22. Confer DL. Unrelated marrow donor registries. Curr Opin Hematol 1997;4:408–412.
23. Sierra J, Anasetti C. Marrow transplantation from unrelated donors. Curr Opin Hematol 1995;2:444–451.
24. Beatty PG, Boucher KM, Mori M et al. Probability of finding HLA-mismatched related or unrelated marrow or cord blood donors. Hum Immunol 2000;61:834–840.

# PART *II*

# SPECIAL CONSIDERATIONS

# CHAPTER IV

# Counseling Before Stem Cell Transplantation

VICKI L. FISHER AND PAULETTE MEHTA

Patients referred to a blood and marrow transplant program for consideration of transplantation require a comprehensive clinical evaluation and in-depth counseling by an experienced multidisciplinary team. This evaluation and counseling period occurs even before the first visit to the transplant center.

It is vital that the transplant team is able to communicate the potential curative nature of the transplant procedure as well as the significant risk to life with transplant-related morbidity and mortality.

## REFERRAL

Most blood and marrow transplant candidates are referred by hematologists, oncologists, or immunologists to the center where the transplant procedure will be performed.[1] Chauvenet et al. showed that much of the pretransplant counseling is done by the referral non-transplant oncologist. In their survey of 24 pediatric oncologists from 21 institutions not performing bone marrow transplants, they found that families made the decision for transplantation almost always before arriving at the transplant center. Thus, referring physicians begin the process and should do so with complete information at hand.[1]

One of the most critical factors for a smooth transition from the referring institution to the transplant center is communication of information between the health care providers and the family.[2] The nursing committee of the Children's Cancer Study Group showed that good communication between local and referral centers was critical to the long-term success of patients. Not only will this help maintain consistency, but also it fosters the family's trust in the transplant program. The necessary information required from the referring center is listed in ▼ Table 4.1. Information about the blood and marrow transplant process as well as specific daily routines used by the transplant center must be accurate and detailed. Differences in techniques or routines between the referring center and the transplant program must be presented in a way that does not prejudice the family or jeopardize the development of trust in the transplant center or referring center.

## CONSULTATIVE PROCESS

The consultative aspect of the referral often begins before the initial appointment, when the transplant coordinator or nurse practitioner contacts the patient and family to discuss

| TABLE 4.1 | Referral Process: Medical/Psychosocial Information Required from Referring Center |
| --- | --- |

Demographic data
Insurance data
Diagnostic information:
   Presentation of initial disease/relapsed disease
   Pathology reports/slides
   Radiographic reports/films
   Cytogenetic abnormalities
Chemotherapy road maps:
   Response to chemotherapy
   Acute and chronic toxicities
Radiation treatment:
   Radiation fields
   Total radiation dose
Infectious disease history:
   Transfusion history
   Compliance history
   School performance
   Lansky/Karnofsky score

the scheduled appointment. The family has the opportunity to ask general questions regarding the scheduled meeting. It is helpful if the transplant center sends a transplant information packet to the potential candidate prior to the initial consult. The initial meeting with the transplant team is important, as it may clarify the process of transplantation, resolve misconceptions, and establish trust. Often the first meeting occurs close to the initial diagnosis, for example, in patients with high-risk leukemia or patients with Stage IV neuroblastoma, or in some cases a few days after relapse. This initial discussion with the patient and family reviews the rationale for transplant options, type and source of stem cell transplant, potential risks, toxicities and complications, proposed preparatory regimen, timing of transplant, and expected outcomes. Then the transplant team will discuss the patient's eligibility, appropriateness for transplantation, potential stem cell sources, and best curative intent. This initial session is for "information only" so that the family can take the time to decide whether they wish to proceed. Once the patient and family agree with transplantation as their best option, the child is placed on the "new patient list."

In circumstances where the child is being considered for an allogeneic transplant process, HLA typing may have been performed and a family donor identified.

In the event that HLA typing did not yield a family donor, a preliminary search for an unrelated donor can be initiated prior to the family's consultation. Once all search results are available, the type of stem cell source, cell dose, and HLA parity are discussed, and all results are compared to determine the best source for the recipient's circumstances. In the case of autologous peripheral blood or marrow stem cell transplantation, dates for marrow and peripheral blood harvest are scheduled in conjunction with a planned date of transplantation.

## PRE-TRANSPLANT EVALUATION

Before the conditioning regimen or transplant admission, all prospective patients, donors, and their families participate in a comprehensive evaluation process (▼ Table 4.2). The pre-transplant evaluation includes a thorough clinical assessment of the child and donor (if relevant) and provides an introduction to the transplant center, transplant team, and the blood and marrow transplant process. This evaluation is performed a maximum of four weeks before the actual day of the transplant to ascertain the most representative clinical, organ, and performance status. Appropriate baseline tests confirm the recipients overall clinical condition and disease status.

The child undergoes medical tests to determine that he is in good medical condition in order to tolerate the transplant toxicity and also to ascertain that his disease is in the best possible remission prior to the transplant. The child also undergoes a full psychosocial evaluation to determine if special interventions will be necessary to help him tolerate the rigors of the procedure. Pfefferbaum et al. have shown that there are predictable stages of stress during the transplant and that these can be anticipated.[3,4] In their studies of approximately 30 children at the UCLA Medical Center, they identified 11 stages including awareness of the procedure, preadmission evaluation, psychosocial assessment, introduction into isolation, donor's hospitalization, the transplant per se, and the various reactions to treatment. Each of these stages carries with it special stresses that can be anticipated, and sometimes prophylactically treated. Even discharge from the unit, when one "graduates" from his transplant, is fraught with fear and stress.[5,6] Surprisingly some children and their families do well during and after transplant and some experience improved spirituality and gratitude and empathy after transplant.[7] Much of the child's reaction is dependent on family resilience, although reasons for family resilience are not well understood.[8]

In allogeneic transplants, the family donor also undergoes a rigorous evaluation including a physical exam, laboratory testing, and psychological/educational preparation to insure that this is an appropriate candidate who is willing and able to undergo the harvest process. This same evaluation process is performed on the unrelated adult donor through numerous agencies.

The donor may also need counseling as well as psychosocial preparation and sometimes even long-term follow-up.[9,10] ▼ Table 4.3 delineates the steps in a psychological assessment of the pediatric transplant candidate. Each of these issues should be explored with the child and his or her family. Surprisingly when a sibling is chosen as the donor, non-donor siblings may be singularly left out as neither patient nor donor and this can create its own set of psychosocial problems.[11] Much research is still needed in this area.[8]

A thorough psychosocial assessment of the patient and family is undertaken to evaluate financial resources, social support, religious, cultural and ethnic variables, and family dynamics. Additionally, issues surrounding compliance, follow-up, and aftercare demands are explored with the family. Decision-making styles are accessed so that physicians can help patients agree, and not just acquiesce, to treatment.[12] A psychological assessment of the family will identify areas of needed support or allocation of resources.

**TABLE 4.2**    Comprehensive Pre-Blood and Marrow
Stem Cell Transplant Evaluation

Staging disease-related tests as appropriate:
   Bone marrow aspirate/biopsies
   Cerebral spinal fluid analysis via spinal tap
   Radiographic tests (CT, MRI, bone scan, x-ray, Gallium scan)
   Tissue biopsy
Tumor markers
Comprehensive assessment of organ performance status
   Cardiac evaluation:
      ECHO
      EKG
      MUGA scan
   Pulmonary evaluation:
      Chest x-ray
      Pulmonary function tests with DLCO
      Sinus films
   Renal evaluation:
      Creatinine clearance
      Glomerular filtration rate (GFR)
Central venous catheter access
Psychosocial assessment
Nutritional evaluation
Occupational/physical therapy evaluation
Transfusion history:
   Transfusion support planning
   Blood product donor, screening, and preparation
Significant drug intolerance/allergies
Genetic disease status evaluation, if applicable
Dental evaluation
Hearing evaluation
Laboratory testing:
   CBC
   Renal
   Hepatic
   Endocrine serum tests
   Hepatitis A,B,C
   HIV
   CMV
   Herpes simplex virus
   Human T cell lymphotrophic virus (HTLV)
   Rapid plasma reagin (RPR)
   Syphilis screening
   Coagulation tests

| TABLE 4.3 | Psychological Assessment of the Pediatric Transplant Candidate |
|---|---|

Assent/consent to undergo transplant
Understanding of diagnosis, treatment plan, and prognosis
History of sexual/physical abuse or neglect
Past psychiatric histories/substance abuse
Developmental assessment
Interests/hobbies and coping strategies
Behavioral/school problems
Problems with peers/family relationships
Compliance issues
Problems with prior hospitalization experiences
Previous methods of coping with treatment and hospitalizations
Pain tolerance/experiences
Understanding of advance directives
Awareness of aftercare/follow-up demands posttransplant

Phipps and his colleagues at St Jude's Research Hospital have shown that family environment prior to the transplant was highly predictive of adjustment after stem cell transplantation.[13,14] Children in families where there is cohesiveness and expressiveness are more resilient than children who have less family support or from families in which there is conflict.[14] Children from this latter type of environment should be watched more closely and offered intervention therapy early if necessary. Regardless of family cohesiveness, most families will suffer stress during transplantation. Rodrigue et al., for example, showed that mothers of children undergoing stem cell or solid organ transplantation suffered from increased parenting stress, financial strain, caregiver burden, and family stress and this often persisted for months after the transplant was completed.[15]

It is very rare for patients needing bone marrow transplantation to be denied a transplant because of non-medical need. Unlike solid organ transplantation, stem cells are available, renewable, and for most individuals, at this time, usually not scarce. Thus, the rationing of resources in stem cell transplantation is minimal compared to what occurs necessarily in solid organ transplantation. Accordingly, few patients are denied transplants for psychosocial problems. Moreover, whereas gender discrimination sometimes has been incriminated in solid organ transplantation; this does not occur in bone marrow transplantation.[16]

The pre-blood and marrow transplant evaluation period is a time of anxiety and uncertainty for the child and the family. Their fears are only heightened if the transplant is delayed or if the evaluation test indicates that the transplant is contraindicated, for example, due to significant organ damage or relapse.

Obtaining insurance coverage or raising necessary funds can delay the transplant process, compounding the already existing anxiety and leading to tremendous frustration for everyone involved. A letter of medical necessity is formulated and information is communicated to the payer, family, and referring physician. Insurance benefits are reviewed and authorization for transplantation is obtained before scheduling the transplant surgery.

| TABLE 4.4 | Transplant Education Plan |
|-----------|---------------------------|

Extensive discussions with patients and families and provision of supportive educational materials, which can be written, computer based, and/or audiovisual
    Orientation to transplant team unit in process
    Role and rationale of stem cell transplant
    Type of transplant
    Preparatory/conditioning regimen
    Role of the pre-transplant testing
    PBSCs vs marrow stem cells
    If peripheral: stem cell transplantation cannulas vs apheresis catheter
    Donor evaluation
    Peripheral stem cell harvest information:
        Transplant related restrictions and routines
        Discussion of stem cell infusion and its effects
        Peri-transplant complications/toxicities
        DNR and intensive care unit issues
        Advance directives
        Graft-versus-host disease
        Immunosuppressive therapy
        Discharge guidelines/planning process
        Homecare management
        Potential posttransplant complications
        Posttransplant aftercare demands
        Follow-up expectations
        Family/sibling issues
        Financial counseling
        Lodging/transportation resources
        Community- and hospital-based resources
        Potential long-term effects of therapy

## EDUCATION AND COUNSELING

Educating and preparing the patient before transplantation are critical factors for his or her subsequent adjustment and adaptation during and after transplantation (▲ Table 4.4). Many patients already have had initial discussions with their primary referring physicians, received written materials, and/or obtained information or misinformation from the Internet before meeting the transplant team. Visual pictures and videotapes are extremely helpful to orient families to the transplant process for the first time. The first meeting focuses on information sharing and establishing the patient as a potential transplant candidate, and is not a decision-making session. It should be a general, well-organized session individualized to the needs of the particular patient and family. Families may elect to tape record the conversation or have an additional family member present to listen and take notes. Families are then given time to absorb and validate the information, discuss it with other family members and friends, and consider seeking a second or third opinion if desired. Subsequent meetings usually are held with the transplant nurse practitioner or coordinator, who share protocol and informed consent information, make necessary decisions, and schedule the transplant-related tests. During this preparatory time, patient and family coping strategies are identified, a psychological assessment is completed, and resource and support systems are activated. Multiple visits and counseling sessions are scheduled in the weeks following the referral to consolidate the preparation/evaluation of the patient and the family. Extensive verbal and written information and education are provided to the family and referring physician institution.

## SUMMARY

Through the educational and counseling efforts of the transplant team as well as the informed consent process, the patient and family should acquire a solid level of understanding of the transplant process. Unfortunately, many patients and their families tend to focus on the immediate effects of having a transplant and not dwell on the many late effects that are seen particularly in children. As health care providers, we must remind our patients and their families that there is much more to transplantation than the preparative regimen and infusion of the hematopoietic stem cells. Numerous medical and social circumstances arise as our patients go through life, which cannot be described in detail or even anticipated. However, a well-functioning communication system that involves the patient, the referring physician, and the transplant center is priceless.

Not all bone marrow transplant centers have complete facilities recognizing specific needs for potential psychosocial intervention before the transplant begins. As part of the Pediatric Blood and Bone Marrow Transplantation Consortium, Mehta et al.[16] recently studied the availability of routine screening for quality-of-life deficits in different pediatric bone marrow transplant units. To do this, a brief survey was distributed via e-mail to the 65 geographically diverse centers enrolled in this consortium. The consortium is part of the larger Clinical Trials Consortium recently established by the National Institutes of Health. A preliminary survey addressed provision of routine screening (quality-of-life domains evaluated, staff responsible, assessment modalities used), availability of supportive care services (e.g., support groups, arts-in-medicine), and use of long-term follow-up clinics (e.g., duration of follow-up, use of separate specialty clinics, estimated attrition), as well as characteristics of the center.

Preliminary results indicated that most centers provided routine screening for a number of quality-of-life domains, including psychological difficulties (90.9%), cognitive deficits (72.7%), pain and fatigue (both 81.8%). However, many fewer provided screening for sleep deficits (45.0%) or spiritual concerns (36.4%). The majority of screening was conducted via interview, with very few centers making use of standardized instruments, even when assessing cognitive deficits (18.2%). In terms of intervention services, roughly half of centers offered support groups for pediatric BMT patients (54.5%) or provided arts-in-medicine programs (45.5%). All centers provided extended follow-up care after completion of active treatment. Provision of quality-of-life screening, intervention services, or extended follow-up did not seem strongly influenced by the size of the transplant center or whether it was academically affiliated or community-based.

If substantiated by additional data, these findings suggest that preparation for bone marrow transplantation may need to include anticipatory problems, which may occur long after transplant has been completed. Moreoever, it may establish means of early intervention, attention to new problems that may not yet be recognized at this time, and could lead to more extensive use of validated screening measures to supplement interview information. Greater use of standardized measures would also facilitate comparisons across centers and help establish base rates for difficulties during and after bone marrow transplantation. The proportion of centers that provide long-term follow-up care is encouraging and needs to be extended to all centers.

In addition to excellent facilities for psychosocial support before, during, and after the transplant, there is also a need for creative new approaches and interventions and for research.[17] One group has used songwriting as a method for expressing stress and for guiding intervention techniques,[17] while other programs have integrated all of the creative arts in arts-in-medicine programs.[18-20] More research into this area should allow for better means of predicting outcome, intervening early, and promoting a good quality of life after stem cell transplantation.

# REFERENCES

1. Chauvenet AR, Smith NM. Referral of pediatric oncology patients for marrow transplantation and the process of informed consent. Med Pediatr Oncol 1988;16:40–44.
2. Wakerwitz MJ, Wiley FM, Perin GA. Nursing communication between local and referral cancer centers for pediatric bone marrow transplant patients. A report on the outcome of a project undertaken by the Children's Cancer Study Group Nursing Committee. J Assoc Pediatr Oncol Nurses 1984;1:26–29.
3. Pfefferbaum B, Lindamood MM, Wiley FM. Pediatric bone marrow transplantation: psychosocial aspects. Am J Psychiatry 1977;134:1299–1301.
4. Pfefferbaum B, Lindamood M, Wiley FM. Stages in pediatric bone marrow transplantation. Pediatrics 1978;61:625–628.
5. Atkins DM, Patenaude AF. Psychosocial preparation and follow-up for pediatric bone marrow transplant patients. Am J Orthopsychiatry 1987;57:246–252.
6. Freund BL, Siegel K. Problems in transition following bone marrow transplantation: psychosocial aspects. Am J Orthopsychiatry 1986;56:244–252.
7. McConville BJ, Steichen-Asch P, Harris R et al. Pediatric bone marrow transplants: psychological aspects. Can J Psychiatry 1990;35:769–775.
8. Weisz V, Robbennolt JK. Risks and benefits of pediatric bone marrow donation: a critical need for research. Behav Sci Law 1996;14:375–391.
9. Shama WI. The experience and preparation of pediatric sibling bone marrow donors. Soc Work Health Care 1998;27:89–99.
10. Spinetta JJ, Jankovic M, Eden T et al. Guidelines for assistance to siblings of children with cancer: report of the SIOP Working Committee on Psychosocial Issues in Pediatric Oncology. Med Pediatr Oncol 1999;33:395–398.
11. Packman WL, Crittenden MR, Schaeffer E et al. Psychosocial consequences of bone marrow transplantation in donor and nondonor siblings. J Dev Behav Pediatr 1997;18:244–253.
12. Mehta P, Rodrigue J, Nejame C et al. Acquiescence to adjunctive experimental therapies may relate to psychological distress: pilot data from a bone marrow transplant center. Bone Marrow Transplant 2000;25:673–676.
13. Phipps S, Brenner M, Heslop H et al. Psychological effects of bone marrow transplantation on children and adolescents: preliminary report of a longitudinal study. Bone Marrow Transplant 1995;15:829–835.
14. Phipps S, Mulhern RK. Family cohesion and expressiveness promote resilience to the stress of pediatric bone marrow transplant: a preliminary report. J Dev Behav Pediatr 1995;16:257–263.
15. Rodrigue JR, MacNaughton K, Hoffmann RG III et al. Transplantation in children. A longitudinal assessment of mothers' stress, coping, and perceptions of family functioning. Psychosomatics 1997;38:478–486.
16. Mehta P, Pollock BH, Nugent M et al. Access to stem cell transplantation: do women fare as well as men? Am J Hematol 2003;72:99–102.
17. Robb SL, Ebberts AG. Songwriting and digital video production interventions for pediatric patients undergoing bone marrow transplantation, part II: an analysis of patient-generated songs and patient perceptions regarding intervention efficacy. J Pediatr Oncol Nurs 2003;20:16–25.
18. Graham-Pole JR. The marriage of art and science in health care. Yale J Biol Med 2001;74:21–27.
19. Lane MT, Graham-Pole J. Development of an art program on a bone marrow transplant unit. Cancer Nurs 1994;17:185–192.
20. Lane MT, Graham-Pole J. The power of creativity in healing: a practice model demonstrating the links between the creative arts and the art of nursing. NLN Publ 1994;(14-2611):203–222.

# CHAPTER V

# Nutrition for the Child Undergoing Stem Cell Transplantation

INDIRA SAHDEV AND MIRIAM A. BOTWINICK

Hematopoietic stem cell transplantation (HSCT) has become a widely accepted treatment for several malignant and nonmalignant disorders such as leukemia, lymphoma, selected metastatic solid tumors, aplastic anemia, congenital disorders, bone marrow failure syndromes, and immunodeficiency disorders. In the last three decades, the prognosis of children with various malignancies has improved dramatically.[1]

HSCT can be classified into two main categories: allogeneic and autologous. In allogeneic transplantation, the patient receives hematopoietic stem cells from a donor other than himself. In autologus transplatation, the patient receives his own stem cells after he receives drugs, which would otherwise be toxic or lethal to his bone marrow. These hematopoietic stem cells can be obtained from bone marrow,[2] peripheral blood[3], or cord blood.[4] Most recipients of allogeneic transplant get cells collected from the bone marrow. When the patient receives an infusion of stem cells through peripheral blood, the hematopoietic progenitor cells in the peripheral blood are increased in number by administering hematopoietic growth factors. Then these mobilized stem cells are collected by leukophoresis. When derived from a donor and infused into the patient after receiving chemotherapy and/or radiation, the process is known as an allogeneic peripheral blood stem cell transplant (PBSCT). In autologous PBSCT, cells are collected from the patient and later reinfused after administration of chemotherapy. At present, the majority of patients with solid tumors receive autologous PBSCT instead of bone marrow infusion.[5] Since umbilical cord blood is rich in hematopoietic stem cells, it is also being utilized as a source of allogeneic stem cells for patients without a marrow donor.[4,6]

## PHASES OF THE HEMATOPOIETIC STEM CELL TRANSPLANT

The initial course of the HSCT can be divided into three phases: preparatory, pancytopenic, and engraftment. During the preparatory phase, the patient receives high dose or non-myeloablative chemotherapy with or without total body irradiation(TBI). The choice of the treatment regimen depends upon the disease. Most patients who undergo an autologous transplant receive chemotherapy without irradiation and usually have non-hematological malignancies. Complications commonly encountered during the pancytopenic phase include mucositis, infections, and organ related toxicities. During the engraftment phase, there is a slow resolution of pancytopenia. However, other complications still can be seen, such as graft-versus-host disease (GVHD), venoocclusive disease (VOD) of the liver, and other liver, renal, lung, and heart toxicities. Any organ toxicity can compromise the nutritional status of the patient. Malnutrition in these patients is multifactorial and can be seen in all three phases. Therefore, it is necessary to assess and maintain the nutritional status of the recipient before, during, and after the transplant.

## FACTORS AFFECTING NUTRITIONAL STATUS

The complications affecting the nutritional status of the patient can be divided into two stages: acute and long term. The acute complications that occur during the preparatory phase are nausea, vomiting, and anorexia. Patients typically eat very little during the conditioning period.[7] The etiology of anorexia is often difficult to define. Occasionally patients have had a history of poor oral intake and are characterized as picky eaters before admission for transplant. Some patients are afraid to eat because of fear of vomiting. This may stem from the severe nausea and vomiting that occur due to the side effects of chemotherapy and results in suboptimal p.o. intake. Chemotherapy and total body irradiation also cause dysgeusia, hypogeusia (alterations in taste), and alterations in smell. For example, cyclophosphamide is associated with a metallic taste.[8]

Patients may be profoundly pancytopenic for one to three weeks following the preparatory regimen. Anorexia and dysgeusia persist during this phase. In addition, mucositis, esophagitis, diarrhea, infections, and VOD are observed. The change in microbial flora and composition of the saliva can cause painful mucositis in the oro-pharynx and esophagus.[9] Chemotherapy-induced acid reflux also can cause esophagitis. As a result, the patient's p.o. intake is drastically limited. These changes affecting the oro-pharynx and esophagus may persist for three to four weeks post-transplant. High dose chemotherapy and/or radiation have a profound effect on the gastrointestinal mucosa,[10,11] delaying repair and resulting in malabsorption.[10,12] Watery diarrhea occurs and may last for weeks post-transplant because of the reversal of salt and water absorption.[13] This causes a transient increase in exudative protein loss into the feces and a loss of vitamins and minerals.[14]

During this phase, patients are also at high risk for bacterial and fungal infections. Due to mucositis, the damaged intestine may serve as a portal of entry for organisms or can be affected with bacterial or fungal overgrowth.[15] Narcotics used to alleviate mucositis-related pain also predispose to bacterial overgrowth because of intestinal stasis. Infection exacerbates the tissue damage and nitrogen mobilization from protein breakdown. The cytokines that are released during systemic infection also can cause altered nutrient utilization.[16]

During the engraftment phase, resolution of pancytopenia occurs and healing of the mucosa begins. Recipients of PBSCT engraft faster (10 to 15 days) than patients receiving bone marrow transplant (14 to 21 days).[17,18] This reduces the period of neutropenia and therefore lessens the risk for infection.[19] Oral intake continues to be limited because of the association of eating with painful mucositis and the fear of vomiting. Eating also can become a battleground between parent and child when the child attempts to gain control over his or her environment.[20] The isolation and dietary restrictions enforced can also play a role in inadequate intake. As in the pancytopenic phase, acute complications that occur include anorexia, nausea, vomiting, dysgeusia, esophagitis, diarrhea, infections, and VOD. In addition, GVHD may occur.

## Acute Graft-Versus-Host Disease

Acute GVHD is a major complication following allogeneic HSCT and affects as many as 30% to 60% of patients.[21,22] Although it generally occurs within three months, it can be seen as early as seven to ten days posttransplant.[11,21] This complication is mediated by donor T cells. Immune competent T-lymphocytes contained in the donor marrow proliferate and differentiate in response to disparate HLA antigens on the host tissues and attack recipient cells.[21,22] Targeted organs in GVHD most commonly affect the skin, gastrointestinal (GI) tract, and liver.[22]

## Graft-Versus-Host Disease of the Gut

The symptoms of acute GVHD of the gut include anorexia, nausea, vomiting, altered intestinal motility, abdominal cramping, and secretory diarrhea. The amount of fluid in the stool is an excellent predictor of the degree and extent of mucosal damage.[23] Edema of the bowel wall and alteration of the mucosal integrity occurs as the gut GVHD becomes severe. This facilitates the migration of bacteria into the blood stream and may cause generalized sepsis.[24,25]

Total parenteral nutrition (TPN) plays a very important role in the management of acute intestinal GVHD. The intestinal tract first needs to be adequately healed in order for the patient to tolerate oral feeds. This requires total gut rest, which is defined as restriction of all foods and fluids. When abdominal pain subsides and stool volume is reduced, oral supplements can be introduced to stimulate intestinal regeneration. As long as the patient remains symptom free, different foods are gradually introduced and TPN is decreased. The Fred Hutchinson Cancer Research Center empirically developed a five-phase regimen in treating GVHD.[26] The initial phase is complete bowel rest with TPN, followed by a gradual advancement of a low residue, low lactose, low fiber, and low fat diet. In our experience, approximately 15% of pediatric patients with acute gastrointestinal GVHD require TPN for longer than two months.

## Diarrhea

Diarrhea occurs in approximately 70% of the children undergoing HSCT.[27] Patients who have diarrhea have greater weight loss, hypoalbuminemia, and zinc deficiency.[28] The etiology of this complication is multifactorial. For example, the cytoreductive regimen, such as chemotherapy and radiation, may cause diarrhea. In addition, it has been reported that radiation therapy causes varying degrees of villous atrophy[29] associated with functional changes such as disaccharide and fat malabsorption.[30] Infections such as rotavirus, c. difficile, enterovirus, and cytomegalovirus (CMV) gastroenteritis also may give rise to this condition. In addition, multiple antibiotics used to prevent or treat infection can contribute to this problem. Acute GVHD of the gut is also a major cause of diarrhea. The medications used to prevent or treat GVHD (e.g., cyclosporine, methotrexate, tacrolimus, corticosteroids) can be toxic to the GI tract, cause diarrhea, and may result in additional increases in protein metabolism and nitrogen loss.[31]

## Protein-losing Enteropathy

Protein-losing enteropathy (PLE) may contribute to low serum albumin levels.[32] The etiology of this hypoalbuminemia is multifactorial. The loss can be due to abnormal or inflamed mucosal surface.[33] Some of the causes are high dose chemotherapy, radiation, GVHD,[34] CMV, rotavirus,[35] and c. difficile. Papadopoulou et al.[31] noted that 91% of the diarrheal episodes were associated with PLE; however, PLE was more severe in children who had GVHD when compared with other causes such as CMV or rotavirus enteritis.

## Pancreatic Insufficiency

In a study of 47 pediatric stem cell transplant recipients, impaired pancreatic exocrine function was found in 40% of the children.[36] The majority of children (74%) had pancreatic insufficiency during diarrheal episodes.[36] Pancreatic insufficiency is thought to be caused by gallbladder sludge,[37] TBI, chemotherapy, and drugs (e.g. cyclosporine, opiates, steroids).[38] GVHD[39] and certain viral infections such as CMV[40] and adenovirus[39] also have been implicated. Careful management, including gut rest and special attention to fluid, electrolyte balance, and nutrition is mandatory.

## Acute Graft-Versus-Host Disease of the Liver

Acute GVHD of the liver is associated with abnormal liver function tests, jaundice, mild hepatomegaly, ascites, and, in severe cases, encephalopathy. Nutritional management in liver GVHD depends on the degree of hepatic involvement. Cycling the TPN solution may help to reduce the stress placed on the liver.[41] The distribution of macronutrients is similar to that used in VOD of the liver. In some centers a plasma acid profile is used to determine whether elevated aromatic amino acid and methionine levels are contributing to the observed encephalopathy.[42] If the levels of these amino acids are elevated to two to three times their normal values, a trial of a hepatic failure amino acid formulation may be useful.[42]

## Venoocclusive Disease of the Liver

The preparatory therapy used for HSCT may result in VOD of the liver. This is a clinical and histologic process characterized by occlusion of small hepatic veins that results in hepatomegaly, fluid retention, jaundice, and elevated liver function enzymes. The clinical symptoms of VOD develop one to three weeks after transplant and cause right upper quadrant pain, significant weight gain, and ascites.[43,44] If VOD continues to progress, more symptoms of liver failure are seen, including encephalopathy and coagulopathy, which may lead to multiorgan failure.[43,44] Nutritional status is profoundly compromised by the necessary restrictions of fluid, protein, and glucose. In order to minimize the risk of encephalopathy, the patient may require specific substrates, such as branched-chain amino acids.[45] The limitation of intravenous fluids, including the TPN formula, in an attempt to minimize edema and ascites, is frequently complicated by intravascular volume depletion and deterioration of renal function. Conversely, repleting the intravascular space with intravenous solutions often results in pulmonary edema and massive ascites. Daily monitoring of weight, abdominal girth, and liver function tests such as serum alanine aminotransferase (ALT), serum aspartate aminotransferase (AST), serum bilirubin, serum albumin, and blood chemistries are important to alert the clinician to the early development of VOD.[42] Restriction of sodium and the use of spironolactone helps promote negative sodium balance and the reduction of total fluid accumulation. Therefore, TPN solutions should be concentrated to reduce total volume while providing adequate calories. It is essential to strictly monitor lipid utilization in patients who have VOD, especially if patients have elevated serum bilirubin levels.

## Acute Renal Failure

Acute renal disease in recipients of HSCT may be caused by hypotension secondary to severe GI losses, septic shock, severe hemorrhage, and capillary leak syndrome. The use of nephrotoxic drugs such as cyclosporine, tacrolimus, aminoglycosides, antivirals, and antifungals also may contribute to renal complications.[46] This results in extracellular fluid, intravascular volume depletion, hypoperfusion of the organs, fluid and electrolyte disorders, pulmonary edema, acidosis, and uremia. Dialysis often is required as renal function deteriorates. The primary goal of nutrition therapy in acute renal failure is to minimize uremic toxicity, while providing nutrition.[47,48] However, nutritional management is dependent upon the general clinical state of these patients, including metabolic and volume status and type and degree of the organ function.

## Pulmonary Edema

Pulmonary edema may be associated with rapid and significant weight gain. The pathogenesis is attributed to capillary permeability changes caused by various clinical occurrences, and medications, including chemotherapy and radiation damage.[49] This also is compounded by iatrogenic fluid overload. Management of pulmonary edema includes reducing primary sources of sodium, which include oral intake, intravenous fluids, and medications. Similar to treatment of VOD of the liver, TPN formula should be concentrated to decrease the total fluid volume, while providing optimum calories. Serum electrolytes and renal function must be monitored closely, particularly if the patient is on diuretics. During ventilator support, nutrition should be provided at energy substrate levels adequate to reduce the muscle break down.[42] The initial goal should be to provide estimated baseline energy requirement (1.3 to 1.5 × basal energy expenditure). If additional support is clinically indicated because of infection or trauma, additional calories should be provided to account for stress.[42]

## Infection

Severe neutropenia and immunosuppressive drugs predispose the allogeneic HSCT recipient to severe life-threatening complications, including bacterial, fungal, and viral infections.[50] Bacterial pathogens account for more than 90% of the first infection that occurs during neutropenia. Gram-negative bacteria are the most virulent pathogens during this period.[50] In recent years, gram-positive bacteria also have emerged as major pathogens.[51] Infections can be caused by fungal species as well. The presence of GVHD and the use of immunosuppressive agents to prevent or treat this complication may make these patients susceptible to viral infections such as herpes, CMV pneumonia, and gastroenteritis. The use of multiple antibiotics to prevent or treat these infections may cause anorexia, nausea, vomiting, diarrhea, and electrolyte imbalance.[11,52,53] Esophagitis is common and may be due to chemotherapy, acid reflux, chemotherapy-induced ulcers, or GVHD.[11,52,53] High rates of morbidity and mortality are associated with these infections despite the aggressive treatment with antibiotics, anti-fungal, and/or anti-viral agents.[54,55] Nutritional support of these debilitated and immunocompromised patients is very important during this period and is a standard posttransplant treatment modality.

## Chronic Graft-Versus-Host Disease

Chronic GVHD is a condition that may present de novo or follow acute GVHD. It behaves like an autoimmune disorder, and alloreactivity is considered to be the cause of its pathogenesis. The incidence of chronic GVHD in patients who receive HLA-identical HSCT is 13% in children less than 10 years of age and 28% in 10- to 19-year-old children, which is lower than that found in adult patients.[56] However, the incidence is much higher among both pediatric and adult recipients of unrelated transplant or HLA non-identical donors.

Chronic GVHD can affect any organ of the body, such as the skin, liver, mouth, esophagus, lungs, intestine, eyes, and vagina.[57,58] Since the majority of patients are on immunosuppressive therapy, they have persistent cell-mediated and humoral immune deficiencies resulting in sinu-pulmonary, bacterial, fungal, and viral infections, such as candida, herpes, and CMV.[59] Although the data are not clear, there may be a relationship between chronic GVHD and the development of viral infections such as herpes or CMV.[60] The most common clinical manifestations affecting the nutritional status of the patients are loss of appetite, taste alterations, mucositis, dysphagia, xerostomia, esophagitis, strictures of the esophagus, liver disease, diarrhea, and steatorrhea.[61] Weight loss is also a common problem that can present between three and twelve months posttransplant. Oral mucosa seems to be a major target organ affected by chronic GVHD. Lenssen et al. conducted a retrospective chart review of 121 long-term survivors of allogeneic HSCT with chronic GVHD and found that 70% of the patients had oral cavity involvement.[61] Many patients complained of oral sensitivity, which manifested itself in pain, burning, increased soreness, and loss of taste sensation. Other complaints involving the oral cavity include erythema, ulceration, and lesions on the buccal mucosa, gingiva, hard palate, and lips.[62] This may be caused by herpetic lesions or candidiasis secondary to immunosuppression. Reflux symptoms and esophageal involvement are found in 12% to 13% of patients with extensive chronic GVHD,[63] resulting in difficulty swallowing and retro-sternal pain. This is thought to be caused by the thinning of the esophageal wall and generalized desquamation of the epithelium of the upper- and mid-esophagus.[64,65] All these symptoms lead to decreased food intake and subsequent weight loss.[66] Some patients also are found to have diarrhea, which is thought to be due to the prolongation of acute GVHD of the gut, drugs, and/or bacterial overgrowth.[61] In addition, steatorrhea caused by hepatic involvement is seen in approximately 21% of patients with extensive chronic GVHD, which may lead to anorexia and eventually weight loss.[61]

Extensive chronic GVHD also may cause hypoalbuminemia and may be due to inadequate nutrition, protein-losing enteropathy, ongoing malabsorption, or ineffective protein synthesis secondary to liver dysfunction.[61] Abnormal values of AST, gamma-glutamyl transferase, alkaline phosphatase, and bilirubin are commonly seen in extensive chronic GVHD.

Patients with low weight and eating problems should be referred to the nutrition specialist. Evaluation of nutritional status such as history, food intake, GI complaints, activity level, and psychosocial evaluation are very important, as all of these factors influence dietary intake. Patients should have their weight monitored weekly. Special intervention may be necessary for patients who have prednisone-related obesity or diabetes.

## DELAYED GROWTH AND DEVELOPMENT

Delayed growth and development in children are late effects of the HSCT. This impairment of growth and development in children is multifactorial. It may be due to the disease and its treatment (e.g., steroids), the cytoreductive regimen (chemotherapy and/or total body irradiation), or chronic GVHD.[67,68] Anorexia, depression, and persistent alterations of taste result in inadequate nutrition and may contribute to the slow growth. The long-term use of large doses of steroids also can alter the growth pattern.

## GOALS OF NUTRITION THERAPY

The main goals of nutrition therapy in HSCT are to maintain or improve nutritional status, prevent or reverse protein-energy malnutrition, and maximize quality of life.[69] Children are at greater risk for developing malnutrition than adults since they have a higher metabolic rate and require more energy for growth and development. Younger children who are smaller have even fewer reserves and are therefore at higher risk of developing malnutrition.[70] It has been demonstrated that poor nutritional status has an adverse effect on outcome in children with cancer. For example, increased rates of infection were found in malnourished children with leukemia and metastatic bone disease.[71,72] Shorter remission rates and treatment delays were observed in malnourished children with neuroblastoma.[73] In pediatric HSCT patients, it was observed that poor nutritional status correlated with delayed marrow recovery[74] and length of hospital stay.[69]

## NUTRITION ASSESSMENT

Nutrition assessment is an ongoing process in the HSCT patient. It is necessary to detect any pre-existing signs of nutritional deficiency, correct them if possible before the transplant, and monitor the patient in the hospital and in the outpatient setting. A thorough assessment includes obtaining information regarding the patient's clinical status, anthropometric and laboratory values, and diet. Anthropometric assessment includes obtaining weight, length or height, and head circumference (if appropriate), and plotting these values on the appropriate growth charts. Some centers also obtain additional measures of triceps skinfolds (TSF) and arm-muscle circumferences to determine degree of fatness and skeletal muscle mass, respectively. Laboratory values of albumin and prealbumin are evaluated to determine visceral protein stores. Other routine questions include the child's medical history, diet, and feeding ability. This includes questions about specific food allergies or intolerances, feeding history, psychosocial factors, and the use of complementary and alternative medicine.

However, it is important to realize that weight, TSF, and mid-arm circumferences may not be the most reliable measures of body composition in the HSCT patient because of fluid shifts resulting from aggressive hydration, diarrhea, or vomiting. For example, in a study of nine children and adults following transplant, it was observed that weight correlated poorly with body cell mass and fluid volume changes, but change in arm muscle area correlated well with changes in body cell mass and lean body mass.[75] Serum albumin is also not a good indicator of nutritional status because it has a long half-life of 20 days and is influenced easily by hydration. Prealbumin has a very short half-life of two days and therefore is a good indicator of nutritional status and repletion. It was determined that, although albumin has been found to be an established vector of the severity of illness, it is relatively unresponsive to changes in nutritional status. Instead, prealbumin was found to be the easiest to measure and the most free of interference of all the rapid turnover proteins,[76] although its value decreases in the presence of severe liver dysfunction and vitamin A or zinc deficiency and rises in the presence of renal disease and steroids. It has been recommended that the trend of prealbumin values be followed since prealbumin responds to both over- and underfeeding.[77] Several studies in children undergoing HSCT have demonstrated the benefit of using prealbumin to mark clinical changes.[75,78,79]

## NUTRITION THERAPY

Nutrition counseling initially begins with encouraging nutrient dense foods and beverages while the patient is able to eat with minimal difficulty. Guidelines are given to manage nutrition complications from treatment and to increase calories and protein intake. However, children at high risk for malnutrition usually require enteral or parenteral nutrition support.

Different criteria have been used to initiate nutritional intervention. In general, if p.o. intake is less than 70% of the caloric needs required for normal growth, intervention should be initiated.[80] Other criteria being recommended by a Task Force Report formed by the American Academy of Pediatrics to the Food and Drug Administration regarding the special nutritional needs of children with malignancies are:[80]

- Weight loss of > 5% of admission weight.
- Weight/height percentile < 10th percentile as determined from the National Center for Health Statistics.
- The current percentile has fallen two percentile channels for weight and/or height.
- Serum albumin is < 3.2 mg/dL.

### Indications for Parenteral Nutrition

Total parenteral nutrition (TPN) is indicated when there is an inability to consume adequate calories orally or enterally, or there is a nonfunctioning GI tract.[81] Children undergoing HSCT may benefit from TPN if they have intractable vomiting or GI problems secondary to chemotherapy and/or radiation.

## Initiating Total Parenteral Nutrition

Although TPN is not an absolute contraindication during the preparative regimen, most patients will not begin TPN until after they complete the cytoreductive regimen. This is due to the large fluid administration required during some of the chemotherapy regimens, such as cyclophosphamide. Fluid requirements per kilogram of body weight are greater in infants and children compared with adults because of the relatively higher body surface area and increased metabolic rate found in this population. However, additional fluid is required during fever, diarrhea, or GI losses. Fluid may need to be restricted during episodes of hepatic, renal, pulmonary, and/or cardiac dysfunction.

## Energy Needs

Energy needs vary widely among individuals and depend mainly on the patient's age, activity, and health status. Several methods are available to calculate caloric requirements. The most common method used is that of the Recommended Dietary Allowances (RDA; ▼ Table 5.1).[82] However, the RDA is based on the healthy active individual and is not geared for the ill patient; it takes into account the basal metabolic rate (BMR), activity, growth, diet-induced thermogenesis, fecal losses, and the maintenance of body temperature.[82] Therefore, the RDA may overestimate the caloric needs of the HSCT patient due to reduced activity while in the hospital. In addition, caloric needs for the patient on TPN are about 10 to 15% lower than enteral needs, due to decreased energy necessary for digestion and absorption and reduced fecal losses.[83]

| TABLE 5.1 | Recommended Dietary Allowances for Energy and Protein | | |
|---|---|---|---|
| *Category* | *Age (years)* | *Energy (kcal/kg/d)* | *Protein (g/kg/d)* |
| Infants | 0.0–0.5 | 108 | 2.2 |
|  | 0.5–1.0 | 98 | 1.6 |
| Children | 1–3 | 102 | 1.2 |
|  | 4–6 | 90 | 1.1 |
|  | 7–10 | 70 | 1.0 |
| Females | 11–14 | 47 | 1.0 |
|  | 15–18 | 40 | 0.8 |
| Males | 11–14 | 55 | 1.0 |
|  | 15–18 | 45 | 0.9 |

Reprinted from Recommended Dietary Allowances (10th ed.) 1989, with permission of National Academy Press, Washington, D.C.

Another method used to determine caloric requirements is to calculate the BMR (▼ Table 5.2)[84] and add a stress factor. In general, stress factors of 1.25 for mild stress, 1.50 for nutritional depletion, and 2.0 for high stress are used to determine energy needs. Most stable patients who are post-stem cell transplant and with hematologic evidence of engraftment, without infection, or GVHD require 1.3 to 1.5 times the estimated BMR.[45,85]

## Macronutrients

### Dextrose

Dextrose is used to provide the majority of non-protein calories in the TPN solution. Dextrose concentrations are to be increased gradually to allow an appropriate endogenous insulin response and to avoid glycosuria.[11] Symptomatic hyperglycemia is usually treated with reduction of the infusion rate, adding regular insulin to the TPN bag, and/or by decreasing the dextrose and increasing the lipid content so as not to jeopardize the nutritional status of the patient by providing inadequate calories.

**TABLE 5.2    Basal Metabolic Rates: Infants and Children**

| Age 1 week to 10 months | | Age 11–36 months | | | Age 3–16 years | | |
|---|---|---|---|---|---|---|---|
| Weight (kg) | Kcal/hr (M/F) | Weight (kg) | Kcal/hr Male | Kcal/hr Female | Weight (kg) | Kcal/hr Male | Kcal/hr Female |
| 3.5 | 8.4 | 9.0 | 22.0 | 21.2 | 15 | 35.8 | 33.3 |
| 4.0 | 9.5 | 9.5 | 22.8 | 22.0 | 20 | 39.7 | 37.4 |
| 4.5 | 10.5 | 10.0 | 23.6 | 22.8 | 25 | 43.6 | 41.5 |
| 5.0 | 11.6 | 10.5 | 24.4 | 23.6 | 30 | 47.5 | 45.5 |
| 5.5 | 12.7 | 11.0 | 25.2 | 24.4 | 35 | 51.3 | 49.6 |
| 6.0 | 13.8 | 11.5 | 26.0 | 25.2 | 40 | 55.2 | 53.7 |
| 6.5 | 14.9 | 12.0 | 26.8 | 26.0 | 45 | 59.1 | 57.8 |
| 7.0 | 16.0 | 12.5 | 27.6 | 26.9 | 50 | 63.0 | 61.9 |
| 7.5 | 17.1 | 13.0 | 28.4 | 27.7 | 55 | 66.9 | 66.0 |
| 8.0 | 18.2 | 13.5 | 29.2 | 28.5 | 60 | 70.8 | 70.0 |
| 8.5 | 19.3 | 14.0 | 30.0 | 29.3 | 65 | 74.7 | 74.0 |
| 9.0 | 20.4 | 14.5 | 30.8 | 30.1 | 70 | 78.6 | 78.1 |
| 9.5 | 21.4 | 15.0 | 31.6 | 30.9 | 75 | 82.5 | 82.2 |
| 10.0 | 22.5 | 15.5 | 32.4 | 31.7 | | | |
| 10.5 | 23.6 | 16.0 | 33.3 | 32.6 | | | |
| 11.0 | 24.7 | 16.5 | 34.0 | 33.4 | | | |

Reprinted from Metabolism 1968. By PL Altman and DS Dittmer, with permission of the Federation of American Societies for Experimental Biology.

## Protein

Protein requirements are related to age, body size, organ function, and state of catabolism. Although proteins are also a source of calories, they are given primarily to support protein synthesis and maintain lean body mass. Children undergoing HSCT may require more than the RDA of protein because of the severe stress they are undergoing during the time of the transplant. Lenssen et al.[86] conducted a study investigating the use of branched-chain amino acids in patients with leukemia who had undergone allogeneic HSCT. They did not find any improvement in nitrogen balance during the first month following transplant. However, these solutions may benefit patients with hepatic insufficiency or VOD.[45]

## Lipids

Lipids are used as an energy source of non-protein calories and to provide essential fatty acids. The American Society for Parenteral and Enteral Nutrition recommends providing 25 to 30% of total calories as lipids in TPN[41] and most transplant centers follow this recommendation. It is recommended also that triglyceride (TG) levels should be obtained prior to initiating TPN and thereafter weekly. Serum TG levels should be $< 250$ mg/dL four hours after lipid infusion for piggybacked lipids and $< 400$ mg/dL for continuous lipid infusion.[87] TG values also should be monitored carefully in patients who have hepatic dysfunction (e.g., bilirubin $> 10$ mg).[88]

There has been some thought that intravenous (IV) lipids may be immunosuppressive,[89,90] and therefore harmful to the patient undergoing HSCT. Potential difficulties with lipid emulsions in TPN are the slow clearance and oxidation of long-chain triglycerides (LCT) from the blood stream.[91] The accumulation of oil droplets may inhibit the clearance capacity of the reticuloendothelial system (RES), which in turn is thought to promote bacteremia, and result in sepsis and infection. LCT may decrease the T helper/T suppressor ratio, inhibiting neutrophil migration, chemotaxis, endotoxin clearance, and complement synthesis.[90] Some experimental studies have suggested that IV lipid emulsions from LCT depress phagocytosis and diminish bacterial defenses in animal models.[92,93] Although there has been little evidence in humans, some reservations remain due to a report of increased risk of coagulase-negative staphylococcal bacteremia with the use of lipids in neonates.[94] However, an increased risk of bacterial or fungal infection was not found in 482 HSCT patients, ranging in age from infancy through adulthood, randomized to either a low dose (6 to 8% of kcal) or standard dose (25 to 30% of kcal) of lipids intravenously infused over 12 hours.[95]

However, essential fatty acid deficiency can ensue if lipids are eliminated from the TPN solution.[96] Essential fatty acid deficiency is not only associated with immunosuppression, but is also associated with bacterial translocation.[97] Insufficient lipids may increase production of interleukin-2 and possibly stimulate GVHD. Muscaritoli et al. found a lower incidence of lethal acute GVHD in 60 allogeneic HSCT patients placed on an 80% lipid solution compared with patients on a glucose-only TPN solution.[98] However, they did not find a difference in the incidence of acute GVHD nor in the rate of disease relapse.

In addition to providing a minimal fat dose to prevent essential fatty acid deficiency, lipids are also useful in that they provide a rich source of energy, spare protein, and limit the hyperglycemic and hepatic effects of excessive dextrose administration.[90,95] Providing adequate calories from fat may be especially beneficial in patients who are fluid restricted since lipids are a high-density caloric source. They also can benefit the immune system with its role in eicosanoid regulation and cytokine production.[99]

There has been some recent thought that a combination of medium chain triglycerides (MCT) and LCT are more beneficial than LCT or MCT alone.[100] Demirer et al. conducted a randomized study comparing the efficacy of MCT and LCT with LCT alone in TPN solutions in 36 patients who underwent allogeneic PBSCT.[90] However, they found that the LCT group had fewer days of febrile neutropenia and antibiotic administration.

### Cyclosporine and Lipids

Cyclosporine, well known to reduce the incidence of GVHD after HSCT, has been associated with hypertriglyceridemia.[101] In a retrospective study of 38 HSCT patients, more than half developed hypertriglyceridemia, which was significantly correlated with administration of cyclosporine.[101] However, different results were observed in a prospective randomized crossover trial of ten patients undergoing allogeneic transplant and receiving TPN secondary to severe mucositis: one group received TPN for four days with a 50:50 mixture of medium and long chain triglycerides, and the other group received TPN without lipids.[102] It was observed that the lipid group did not affect cyclosporine parameters, but there was a higher systemic clearance rate of cyclosporine in the TPN group without lipids. The authors hypothesized that this might be due to a possible binding of cyclosporine to triglycerides with a delay in clearance. In fact, they suggest that providing lipid emulsions may minimize complications associated with TPN and have a stabilizing effect on the hepatic cytochrome p-450 system, known to influence the metabolism of cyclosporine.

## Enteral versus Parenteral Nutrition

TPN provided to children undergoing HSCT has been found to maintain body weight,[74] and improve visceral protein status as determined from prealbumin and retinol-binding protein levels.[79] Until recently it has been considered the preferred method of nutrition support for transplant patients because of concerns of vomiting, mucositis, and bleeding (due to low platelet counts) when using a nasogastric tube. However, recent studies have been successful in using tube feeding in the transplant setting.[69,103–107] Several studies have found that both enteral nutrition and TPN were no different in time to engraftment or length of hospital stay.[69,103] Although Weisdorf et al.[108] found a benefit of TPN on long-term survival, Szeluga et al.[103] did not find any benefit when comparing TPN to enteral feeds. However, while previous studies have shown that both parenteral[109,110] and enteral[107] nutrition can maintain body mass in children, oral supplements and intense nutrition counseling combined with peripheral parenteral nutrition or nasogastric feeds without TPN may be inadequate during intense chemotherapy or HSCT.[105,106,111]

It has been suggested that enteral feeds are safer, more physiologic, and more economical. While it is indubitable that enteral feeds are less costly[103,105] the literature is not as clear regarding safety in children following HSCT. For example, while one study found that TPN caused a 31% infectious rate from central venous catheters,[112] another study found no difference in positive blood cultures when comparing TPN to tube feeding.[69] Also, a study by Roberts and Miller[104] found that 11 of 16 patients who had undergone placement for percutaneous endoscopic gastrostomy around the time of transplant had positive blood cultures. In addition, while TPN is associated with mechanical, infectious, and metabolic complications, enteral nutrition also has its risks. For example, if nasogastric tubes are not placed properly, it may result in pneumonia or pneumothorax, and gastrostomy runs the risk of bowel perforation. Furthermore, while it is proposed that enteral nutrition is more physiologic than TPN, both are provided in a non-volitional manner. Oral intake of food is completely bypassed with both methods, so there is no cephalic or oral phase of digestion.[113]

## Vitamins and Trace Elements

Special attention should be paid to vitamin K when the patient is on broad-spectrum antibiotics[114,115] and should be added to the TPN solution when the p.o. intake is < 50% of usual. Some centers also add more vitamin C to the TPN solution following chemotherapy to promote tissue repair.[116] Additional zinc may be required in patients with copious diarrhea.[117] Additional potassium may be necessary with amphotericin B[88] and supplementary magnesium may be needed with patients on cyclosporine.[118]

# CYCLING TPN

When a child is transitioned from TPN to enteral or oral feeds, it is first necessary to evaluate the clinical status, GI function, and patient motivation. Cyclic TPN may be used if the patient will require long-term TPN in the hospital, when transitioning the child to an oral diet, or if the patient is to be discharged home on TPN. In fact, it has been proposed that cyclic TPN is a more physiologic approach to continuous 24-hour TPN.[119] It is thought that cyclic TPN minimizes hyperinsulinism and allows for the mobilization and use of calories stored as fat, reduces glycogen and fat deposition in the liver and possibly lessens TPN-associated cholestasis.[120,121] The infusion-free period also provides a period of time when blood products and medications can be administered without interfering with the child's food intake.

# DISCONTINUING TPN

It is also essential to evaluate the child's appetite as well as the ability to take food by mouth before discontinuing TPN. TPN should be discontinued when p.o. intake is at least 50% of the usual intake.[122] At our transplant center, we try to wean patients off TPN when their food intake provides 50 to 60% of their caloric needs. It has been observed that recipients of autologous PBSCT require fewer calories from TPN compared with patients undergoing allogeneic transplant.[123] This is thought to occur because autologous patients are found to have a shorter hospital stay, a quicker engraftment period, and fewer days on antimicrobial and antiviral therapy compared with allogeneic patients.[123] It is hard to motivate children to restart their oral intake in the hospital setting and a challenge for the nutrition support team, because of taste alterations, food aversions, and fear of eating due to the remembrance of pain when the patient had mucositis. In addition, the dislike of hospital food compared with the meals patients are accustomed to eating at home, and discomfort with remaining in the hospital setting compared to the home environment may limit the child's p.o. intake. It also has been observed that TPN may delay the resumption of oral intake. For example, Clamon et al. found that oral intake was transiently depressed in lung cancer patients who had been on TPN for 30 days.[124] Sriram et al. found that voluntary food intake proportionately increased within three days when TPN was decreased by 50% in ten patients who were transitioned to an oral diet.[125] More recently, a double-blind randomized study compared outpatient TPN with IV hydration in children and adults following HSCT and found that resumption of at least 85% of oral intake was seen six days sooner in the hydration group.[126]

## DIETARY RESTRICTIONS

Infection is one of the greatest threats a patient undergoing HSCT encounters. Most of these infections are due to organisms that are either present at the time of therapy or are acquired from the hospital environment. Because the preparative regimen causes mucosal damage throughout the gastrointestinal tract and allows access of otherwise nonpathogenic organisms, the introduction of new and potentially resistant organisms into the GI tract from food is of great concern.[127] There is limited research in this area and no clear guidelines regarding this issue. Some argue that due to the high costs and inadequate research there is no need to implement these diets, but others state that despite the paucity of clinical research, it is still more prudent to err on the side of caution.[128]

Currently, the three levels of food restriction that are commonly used for the HSCT patient are the sterile diet, low microbial diet, and a modified diet.[129] The sterile diet was initially used for HSCT patients. Foods were sterilized by autoclaving, prolonged baking, irradiation, or canning in order to be sure that food did not have bacterial or fungal growth. With this method very few foods can remain palatable and only a limited number of foods can be fully sterilized. This method was also very expensive and cost prohibitive for many centers.

The low-microbial diet is most commonly used, and entails the use of well-cooked foods. Although foods permitted vary widely, individually packaged foods may be used, but raw fruit and salad are not allowed. The rationale for this kind of diet is that it decreases the total bacterial count and eliminates pathogens while providing greater palatability and flexibility than the sterile diet. This type of diet also may meet the needs of more people than the sterile diet.

The modified diet permits food to be prepared in the hospital kitchen. Restrictions continue to be variable but usually exclude salad, unpeeled fruits, and uncooked vegetables. The rationale for this type of diet is that patients are not being cared for in strict protective isolation and do not require specific restrictions other than hygienic food practices.

Some controversial areas surrounding food are tap water, fruits and vegetables, dairy products, eggs, and cooking with microwave ovens. Some centers recommend sterile, boiled, and cooled water.[129] Others only allow specific brands of mineral water since they are not subject to the same level of microbial stringency as tap water and are therefore subject to greater levels of contamination.[129] Although cooked fruit and vegetables are usually permitted, most centers prohibit fresh fruit and vegetables, since it has been demonstrated that enteric viruses and bacteria cannot be removed from the surface of vegetables from washing alone,[130] for example, hepatitis A from watercress; *Escherichia coli, Staphylococcus aureus,* and *Klebsiella* from salad, and *pseudomonas* from bananas.[129] Only well-cooked eggs are permitted because of salmonella.[129] Many units do not allow ripened soft cheeses such as Brie, Camembert, blue-veined cheeses, and goat's cheese since they may be associated with bacterial contamination (e.g., *Listeria monocytogenes, salmonella paratyphoid, Brucella melitensis*).[131] In general, cream cheese and hard and processed cheese are considered to be less risky.[129] Although many people mistakenly believe that microwave cooking sterilizes food, research has found that foods cooked in a microwave oven have more gram-positive bacteria [e.g., *salmonella*[132] Listeria[133]] than food cooked in a conventional oven. Also, it is recommended that microwave ovens be limited to reheating canned foods since they cook unevenly.[129]

Most centers today follow some version of the low microbial diet.[128,134,135] This practice is based on the lack of evidence supporting the efficacy of stringent dietary restrictions.

## APPETITE STIMULANTS

Two appetite stimulants commonly used to promote weight gain in the pediatric oncology patient are cyproheptadine hydrochloride (Periactin) and megestrol acetate (Megace). Cyproheptadine hydrochloride (CPH) is an antihistamine with antiserotonergic properties, and has been used traditionally for treatment of allergies, but also has been associated with increased appetite and weight gain.[136] Its main side effect is drowsiness. Megestrol acetate (MA) is a synthetic progesterone agent, and traditionally has been used as a hormonal treatment for breast and endometrial cancer. It was observed that one of the side effects was weight gain,[137,138] which led to its use as an appetite stimulant. Other side effects include adrenal suppression, hyperglycemia, edema, impotence, and thrombophlebitis.

Although most pediatric studies using CPH found increased appetite, weight gain, and linear growth.[136,139,140] one study found increased appetite and weight gain, but no change in linear growth.[141] Weight gain was found also in studies of pediatric patients on MA who had cancer or were HIV+.[142-144] In one randomized study conducted over a three-month period comparing MA and CPH in 14 HIV+ patients, it was found that more of the subjects gained weight in the MA group than in the CPH group.[145] However, it is reported in the literature that incidences of glucocorticoid-like activity occur secondary to the use of MA.[146] Several studies investigated the possibility of adrenal suppression with the use of MA.[142,147,148] Therefore, it has been recommended that patients be screened by testing basal cortisol levels, that the dose be tapered before discontinuing, and that cortisol replacement should be considered when tapering.[147,148]

## GLUTAMINE

Glutamine has recently generated much interest in the field of nutrition. It is the most abundant amino acid in plasma and muscle.[149] It is important for cell growth, is an essential nutrient for rapidly dividing cells, and is the major energy source for intestinal epithelium.[150] The mechanisms of the beneficial effects of glutamine in patients undergoing chemotherapy and HSCT are not entirely clear.[151] Glutamine may result in improved nitrogen retention,[152] which may contribute to improved function of the immune system and resistance to infection. Glutamine also is thought to help maintain the gut mucosal barrier,[153] and improve tissue antioxidant glutathione status.[151,154,155] Decreased mucositis in some studies may be related to the antioxidant effects of glutamine[155] and/or the use of this particular amino acid as an energy source for epithelial cells.

## Glutamine and TPN

Glutamine-enriched parenteral nutrition has been found to be safe and efficacious in HSCT patients. A double-blind randomized study of patients undergoing allogeneic transplant and receiving glutamine-supplemented TPN found improved nitrogen balance, decreased rates of infection, and shortened hospital stay, although no relationship was observed between glutamine-supplemented TPN and engraftment or mucositis.[152] In another double-blind randomized trial of allogeneic and autologous HSCT patients, Schloerb and Amare observed a shorter hospital stay for those supplemented with glutamine, but there was no difference between the two groups in infection or mucositis.[156]

## Oral Glutamine

To evaluate the beneficial effects of glutamine, Schloerb and Skikne evaluated oral (added to liquids) and parenteral glutamine in a randomized double-blind study of 66 patients undergoing allogeneic or autologous HSCT.[157] All patients were initially started on oral glutamine and if they required TPN, they were then switched from oral glutamine to IV glutamine. In this study, a decreased need for TPN was found in the glutamine-supplemented group, but no significant differences were observed for length of hospital stay, infection, engraftment, mucositis, or diarrhea. In another double-blind randomized study, Coghlin Dickson et al. did not find any benefit of oral glutamine when provided as a powder in liquid or soft foods in 58 HSCT patients.[158]

## Glutamine and Mucositis

Although it has been observed that IV or oral glutamine did not influence the incidence or severity of mucositis after HSCT,[152,156–158] some recent studies suggest that oral glutamine when given in a swish and swallow preparation is beneficial.[159,160] For example, glutamine as a swish and swallow preparation was associated with decreased severity and duration of mucositis in autologous HSCT patients,[159,160] but not in allogeneic patients.[160] Anderson et al. speculated that perhaps the difference in results between autologous and allogeneic patients was the use of methotrexate to prevent graft-versus-host disease in allogeneic patients.[160] Glutamine has been found to inhibit renal clearance of methotrexate, resulting in increased methotrexate concentrations and therefore increased mucositis.[161]

## CONCLUSIONS

Nutrition plays a major role in the management of patients undergoing HSCT. Since the overall goal is to prevent malnutrition and optimize quality of life, it is vital that nutrition evaluation be done continuously; before, during, and posttransplant. Treatment needs to be individualized, and special attention to psychosocial factors is mandatory. Although novel therapies such as glutamine, MCT/LCT products, and immunomodulatory formulas[162–164] have been suggested for critically ill and/or oncology patients, further research is necessary. Nutritional support in the HSCT patient often can be labor intensive and exasperating, but its role in improving the quality of life and healing process ultimately is gratifying.

# REFERENCES

1. Horowitz MM. Uses and growth of hematopoietic cell transplantation. In: Thomas ED, Blume KG, Forman SJ, eds. Hematopoietic Cell Transplantation (2nd ed). Boston: Blackwell Science, 1999:12–18.
2. Thomas ED, Strob R, Clift RA et al. Bone marrow transplantation. N Engl J Med 1975;292:832–843, 895–902.
3. Antman KH, Rowlings PA, Vaughan WP et al. High dose chemotherapy with autologous HSC support for breast cancer in North America. J Clin Oncol 1997;15:1870–1879.
4. Kurtzberg J, Laughlin M, Graham ML et al. Placental blood as a source of hematopoietic stem cells for transplantation into unrelated recipients. N Engl J Med 1996;335:157–166.
5. Kessinger A, Armitage JO, Landmark JD et al. Reconstitution of human hematopoietic function with autologus cryopreserved circulating cells. Exp Hematol 1986;14:192–196.
6. Gluckman E. The therapeutic potential of fetal and neonatal hematopoietic stem cells. N Engl J Med 1996;335:1839–1840.
7. Aker SN. Oral feedings in the cancer patient. Cancer 1979;43:2103–2107.
8. Nunnally C. Taste alterations. In:Yasko JM, ed. Guidelines for Cancer Care, Symptom Management. Reston: Reston Publishing Company, 1983:224–229.
9. Bondi E, Baroni C, Prete A et al. Local antimicrobial therapy of oral mucositis in pediatric patients undergoing bone marrow transplantation. Oral Oncol 1997;33:322–326.
10. Wolford JL, McDonald GB. A problem-oriented approach to intestinal and liver disease after marrow transplantation. J Clin Gastroenterol 1988;10:419–433.
11. Keenan AM. Nutritional support of the bone marrow transplant patient. Nurse Clin North Am 1989;24:383–393.
12. Liddell S, Applebaum JR, Buckner CD et al. High-dose cytarabine and total body irradiation with or without cyclophosphamide as a preparative regimen for marrow transplantation for acute leukemia. J Clin Oncol 1988;6:576–582.
13. Bearman SI, Appelbaum FR, Buckner CD et al. Regimen-related toxicity in patients undergoing bone marrow transplantation. J Clin Oncol 1988;6:1562–1568.
14. Weisdorf SA, Salati LM, Longsdorf JA et al. Graft-versus-host disease of the intestine: a protein losing enteropathy characterized by fecal alpha-1 antitrypsin. Gastroenterology 1983;85:1076–1081.
15. King CE, Toskes PP. Breath tests in the diagnosis of small intestine bacterial overgrowth. Crit Rev Clin Lab Sci 1984;21:269–281.
16. Weisdorf SA, Schwarzenberg SJ. Nutritional support of hematopoietic skin cell recipients. In: Thomas ED, Blume KG, Forman SJ (eds). Hematopoietic Cell Transplantation. Boston: Blackwell Science, 1999:723–732.
17. Walker F, Roethke SK, Martin A. An overview of the rationale, process and nursing implications of peripheral blood stem cell transplantation. Cancer Nurs 1994;17:141–148.
18. Champlin RE. Peripheral blood progenitor cells: a replacement for marrow tranplantation? Semin Oncol 1996;23:15–21.
19. Wright D. Peripheral stem cell transplantation. Med Surg Nurs 1994;3:36–41.
20. Costlow N. Pediatric oncology nutrition support. In: Bloch A (ed). Nutrition Management of the Cancer Patient. Gaithersburg: Aspen Publishers, 1990:135–139.
21. Storb R. Critical issues in bone marrow transplantation. Transplant Proc 1987;19:2774–2781.
22. Deeg HJ, Storb R. Graft versus host disease: patho-physiological and clinical aspects. Annu Rev Med 1984;35:11–24.
23. Sale GE, Shulman HM, McDonald GB et al. Gastrointestinal graft versus host disease in man: a clinico-pathologic study of the rectal biopsy. Am J Surg Pathol 1979;3:291–299.
24. Fegan C, Poynton CH, Whittaker JA. The gut mucosal barrier in bone marrow transplantation. Bone Marrow Transplant 1990;5:373–377.
25. Spencer GD, Shulman HM, Myerson D et al. Diffuse intestinal ulceration after marrow transplantation. A clinical-pathological study of 13 patients. Hum Pathol 1986;17:621–633.
26. Gavreau JM, Lenssen P, Cheney CL et al. Nutritional management of patients with intestinal graft-versus-host disease. J Am Diet Assoc 1981;79:673–677.
27. Papadapoulou A, Nalhavitharana KA, Williams MD et al. Diarrhea and weight loss after bone marrow transplantation in children. Pediatr Hematol Oncol 1994;11:601–611.
28. Antila HM, Salo MS, Kirvela O et al. Serum trace element concentration and iron metabolism in allogeneic marrow transplant recipients. Ann Med 1992;24:55–59.
29. Donaldson SS, Jundt S, Ricour C et al. Radiation enteritis in children. Cancer 1975;35:1167–1178.
30. Beer WH, Fan A, Halsted CH. Clinical and nutritional implications of radiation enteritis. Am J Clin Nutr 1985;41:85–91.
31. Papadopoulou A, Lloyd DR, Williams MD et al. Gastrointestinal and nutritional sequelae of bone marrow transplantation. Arch Dis Child 1996;75:208–213.
32. Comelius EA. Protein-losing enteropathy in the graft-versus-host reaction. Transplantation 1970;9:247–252.

33. Buell MG, Harding RK. Proinflammatory effects of local abdominal irradiation on rat gastrointestinal tract. Dig Dis Sci 1989;34:390–399.
34. Appleton AL. The need for endoscopic biopsy in the diagnosis of upper gastrointestinal graft-versus-host disease. J Pediatr Gastroenterol Nutr 1993;16:183–185.
35. Willoughby RE, Wee SB, Volken RH. Non-group A rotavirus infection associated with severe gastroenteritis in a bone marrow transplant patient. Pediatr Infect Dis J 1988;7:133–135.
36. Thomas A, Seemayer JG, Bartner EC et al. Acute graft versus host reaction in the pancreas. Transplantation 1983;35:72–77.
37. Teefy SA, Hallister MS, Lee SP et al. Gallbladder sludge formation after bone marrow transplant: sonographic observations. Abdom Imaging 1994;19:57–60.
38. Underwood TW, Frye CB. Drug induced pancreatitis. Clin Pharm 1993;12:440–448.
39. Washington K, Gossage DL, Gottfried R. Pathology of the pancreas in severe combined immunodeficiency and DiGeorge syndrome: acute graft versus host disease and unusual viral infections. Hum Pathol 1994;25:908–914.
40. Margreiter R, Schmid T, Dunser M et al. Cytomegalovirus (CMV) pancreatitis: a rare complication after pancreas transplantation. Transplant Proc 1991;23:1619–1622.
41. Roberts S. Bone marrow transplantation. In: Nutrition Support Dietetics Core Curriculum (2nd ed). Rockville: ASPEN Publishers Inc, 1993:423–432.
42. Aker SN. Bone marrow transplantation: nutrition support and monitoring. In: Bloch A (ed). Nutrition Management of the Cancer Patient. Gaithersburg: ASPEN Publishers, 1990:199–225.
43. Jones RJ, Lee KSK, Beschorner WE et al. Venoocclusive disease of the liver following bone marrow transplantation. Transplantation 1987;44:778–783.
44. McDonald GB, Sharma P, Mathews et al. The clinical course of 53 patients with venoocclusive disease of the liver after marrow transplantation. Transplantation 1985;39:603–608.
45. Herrmann VM, Petruska PJ. Nutritional support in bone marrow transplant recipients. Nutr Clin Pract 1993;8:19–27.
46. Zager RA. Acute renal failure in the setting of bone marrow transplantation. Kidney Int 1994;46:1443–1458.
47. Feinstein EI, Kopple JD, Silberman H et al. Total parenteral nutrition with high or low nitrogen intakes in patients with acute renal failure. Kidney Int 1983;(Suppl 16):S319–S323.
48. Kopple JD. The nutrition management of the patient with acute renal failure. JPEN J Parenter Enteral Nutr 1996;20:3–12.
49. Trigg ME, Finlay JL, Bozdech M et al. Fatal cardiotoxicity in bone marrow transplant patients receiving cytosine arabinoside, cyclophosphamide and total body irradiation. Cancer 1987;59:38–42.
50. Wingard JR. Prevention and treatment of bacterial and fungal infections. In: Forman SJ, Blume KG, Thomas DE (eds). Bone Marrow Transplantation. Boston: Blackwell Scientific Publications, 1994:363–375.
51. Rubin M, Hathorn JW, Marshall D et al. Gram positive infections and the use of vancomycin in 550 episodes of fever and neutropenia. Ann Intern Med 1988;108:30–35.
52. McDonald GB, Sharma P, Hackman RC et al. Esophageal infections in immunosuppressed patients after marrow transplantation. Gastroenterology 1985;88:1111–1117.
53. Schubert MM, Sullivan KM, Truelove EL. Head and neck complications of bone marrow transplantation. In: Peterson ED, Sonis SB, Elias EG (eds). Head and Neck Management of Cancer Patients. Boston: Martenus Nijhoff, 1986;401–427.
54. Tutschka PJ. Complications of bone marrow transplantation. Am J Med Sci 1987;294:86–90.
55. Santos GW, Kaizer H. Bone marrow transplantation in acute leukemia. Semin Hematol 1982;19:227–237.
56. Sullivan KM, Agura E, Anssetti C et al. Chronic graft versus host disease and other late complications of bone marrow transplantation. Semin Hematol 1991;28:250–259.
57. Sullivan KM, Deeg HJ, Sanders JE et al. Late complications after marrow transplantation. Semin Hematol 1984;21:53–63.
58. Corcoran B. Long term complications of allogeneic bone marrow transplantation; nursing implications. Oncol Nurs Forum 1986;13:61–70.
59. Sullivan KM. Acute and chronic graft versus host disease in man. Int J Cell Cloning 1986;4(Suppl 1):42–93.
60. Lonnquist B, Ringden O, Wahrren B et al. Cytomegalovirus infection associated with and preceding chronic graft versus host disease. Transplantation 1984;38:465–468.
61. Lenssen P, Sherry ME, Cheney CL et al. Prevalence of nutrition-related problems among long term survivors of allogeneic marrow transplantation. J Am Diet Assoc 1990;90:835–842.
62. Schubert MM, Sullivan KM, Morton TH et al. Oral manifestations of chronic graft-versus-host disease. Arch Intern Med 1984;144:1591–1595.
63. McDonald GB, Shulman HM, Sullivan KM et al. Intestinal and hepatic complications of human bone marrow transplantation. Gastroenterology 1986;90:770–784.
64. McDonald GB, Sullivan KM, Schuffler MD et al. Esophageal abnormalities in chronic graft versus host disease in humans. Gastroenterology 1981;80:914–921.
65. McDonald GB, Sullivan KM, Pulmley TF et al. Radiographic features of esophageal involvement in chronic graft versus host disease. Am J Roentgenol 1984;142:501–506.

66. Nims JW, Strom S. Late complications of bone marrow transplant recipients. Nursing care issues. Semin Oncol Nurs 1988;4:47–54.
67. Cohen A, Duell T, Socie G et al. Nutritional status and growth after bone marrow transplantation (BMT) during childhood: EBMT Late-Effects Working Party retrospective data. European Group for Blood and Marrow Transplantation. Bone Marrow Transplant 1999;23:1043–1047.
68. Sanders JE, Pritchard S, Mahoney P et al. Growth and development following marrow transplantation for leukemia. Blood 1986;68:1129–1135.
69. Papadopoulou A, Williams MD, Darbyshire PJ et al. Nutritional support in children undergoing bone marrow transplantation. Clin Nutr 1998;17:57–63.
70. Pencharz PB. Aggressive oral enteral or parenteral nutrition: Prescriptive decisions in children with cancer. Int J Cancer 1998;(Suppl 11):73–75.
71. Taj MM, Pearson AD, Mumford DB et al. Effect of nutritional status on the incidence of infection in childhood cancer. Pediatr Hematol Oncol 1993;10:283–287.
72. van Eys J, Copeland EM, Cangir A et al. A clinical trial of hyperalimentation in children with metastatic malignancies. Med Pediatr Oncol 1980;8:63–73.
73. Rickard KA, Detamore CM, Coates TD et al. Effect of nutrition staging on treatment delays and outcome in Stage IV neuroblastoma. Cancer 1983;52:587–598.
74. Yokoyama S, Fujimoto T, Mitomi T et al. Use of total parenteral nutrition in pediatric bone marrow transplantation. Nutrition 1989;5:27–30.
75. Cheney CL, Abson KG, Aker SN et al. Body composition changes in marrow transplant recipients receiving total parenteral nutrition. Cancer 1987;59:1515–1519.
76. Bernstein L, Bachman TE, Meguid M et al. Measurement of visceral protein status in assessing protein and energy malnutrition: Standard of care. Prealbumin in Nutritional Care Consensus Group. Nutrition 1995;11:169–171.
77. Spiekerman AM. Proteins used in nutritional assessment. Clin Lab Med 1993;13:353–369.
78. Reed MD, Lazarus HM, Herzig RH et al. Cyclic parenteral nutrition during bone marrow transplantation in children. Cancer 1983;51:1563–1570.
79. Uderzo C, Rovelli A, Bonomi M et al. Total parenteral nutrition and nutritional assessment in leukaemic children undergoing bone marrow transplantation. Eur J Cancer 1991;27:758–762.
80. Mauer AM, Burgess JB, Donaldson SS et al. Special nutritional needs of children with malignancies: A review. JPEN J Parenter Enter Nutr 1990;14:315–324.
81. American Society for Parenteral and Enteral Nutrition. Guidelines for the use of parenteral and enteral nutrition in adult and pediatric patients. Nutrition support for infants and children with specific diseases and conditions: Cancer. JPEN J Parenter Enter Nutr 1993;17(Suppl 4): 39SA–41SA.
82. Recommended Dietary Allowances (10th ed). Washington, DC: National Academy Press, 1989.
83. Hovasi Cox J, Cooning SW. Parenteral nutrition. In: Queen PM, Lang CE (eds). Handbook of Pediatric Nutrition. Gaithersburg: Aspen Publishers, Inc., 1993;279–314.
84. Altman PL, Dittmer DS. Metabolism. Bethesda: Federation of American Societies for Experimental Biology, 1968.
85. Dickson B, Barale KV. Nutritional assessment. In: Lenssen P, Aker SN (eds). Nutritional Assessment and Management during Marrow Transplantation: A Resource Manual. Seattle: Fred Hutchinson Cancer Research Center, 1985:5–14.
86. Lenssen P, Cheney CL, Aker SN et al. Intravenous branch chain amino acid trial in marrow transplant recipients. JPEN J Parenter Enter Nutr 1987;11:112–118.
87. Matarese LE. Metabolic complications of parenteral nutrition therapy. In: Gottschlich MM, Editor-in-Chief. The Science and Practice of Nutrition Support; a Case-Based Core Curriculum. American Society for Parenteral and Enteral Nutrition. Dubuque: Kendall/Hunt Publishing Co, 2001;269–279.
88. Charuhas PM, Gautier ST. Parenteral nutrition in pediatric oncology. In: Baker R, Baker S, Davis A, eds. Pediatric Parenteral Nutrition. New York: Chapman & Hall, 1997:331–352.
89. Monson JR, Sedman PC, Ramsden CW et al. Total parenteral nutrition adversely influences tumour-directed cellular cytotoxic responses in patients with gastrointestinal cancer. Eur J Surg Oncol 1988;14:935–943.
90. Demirer S, Aydintug S, Ustun C et al. Comparison of the efficacy of medium chain triglycerides with long chain triglycerides in total parenteral nutrition in patients with hematologic malignancies undergoing peripheral blood stem cell transplantation. Clin Nutr 2000;19:253–258.
91. Wan JM, Tiew TC, Babayan VK et al. Invited comment: lipids and the development of immune dysfunction and infection. JPEN J Parenter Enter Nutr 1988;12(Suppl 6):43S–52S.
92. Wiernik A, Jarstand C, Julander I. The effect of intralipid on mononuclear and polymorphonuclear phagocytes. Am J Clin Nutr 1983;37:256–261.
93. Fischer GW, Hunter KW, Wilson SR et al. Diminished bacterial defenses with intralipid. Lancet 1980;2:819–820.
94. Freeman J, Goldmann DA, Smith NE et al. Association of intravenous lipid emulsion and coagulase-negative staphylococcal bacteremia in neonatal intensive care units. N Engl J Med 1990;323:301–308.

95. Lenssen P, Bruemmer BA, Bowden RA et al. Intravenous lipid dose and incidence of bacteremia and fungemia in patients undergoing bone marrow transplantation. Am J Clin Nutr 1998;67:927–933.
96. Clemans GW, Yamanaka W, Flournoy N et al. Plasma fatty acid patterns of bone marrow transplant patients primarily supported by fat-free parenteral nutrition. JPEN J Parenter Enter Nutr 1981;5:221–225.
97. Barton RG, Cerra FB, Wells CL. Effect of a diet deficient in essential fatty acids on the translocation of intestinal bacteria. JPEN J Parenter Enter Nutr 1992;16:122–128.
98. Muscaritoli M, Conversano L, Torelli GF et al. Clinical and metabolic effects of different parenteral nutrition regimens in patients undergoing allogeneic bone marrow transplantation. Transplantation 1998;66:610–616.
99. Yamanaka WK, Tilmont G, Aker S. Plasma fatty acids of marrow transplant recipients on fat-supplemented parenteral nutrition. Am J Clin Nutr 1984;39:607–611.
100. Dennison AR, Ball MJ, Growe PJ. The metabolic consequences of infusing emulsions containing medium chain triglycerides for parenteral nutrition: a comparative study. Ann R Coll Surg Eng 1986;68:111–121.
101. Carreras E, Villamor N, Reverter JC et al. Hypertriglyceridemia in bone marrow transplant recipients: another side effect of cyclosporine A. Bone Marrow Transplant 1989;4:385–388.
102. Santos P, Lourenco R, Camilo ME et al. Parenteral nutrition and cyclosporine: do lipids make a difference? A prospective randomized crossover trial. Clin Nutr 2001;20:31–36.
103. Szeluga DJ, Stuart RK, Brookmeyer R et al. Nutritional support of bone marrow transplant recipients: a prospective, randomized clinical trial comparing total parenteral nutrition to an enteral feeding program. Cancer Res 1987;47:3309–3316.
104. Roberts SR, Miller JE. Success using PEG tubes in marrow transplant recipients. Nutr Clin Pract 1998;13:74–78.
105. Pietsch JB, Ford C, Whitlock JA. Nasogastric tube feedings in children with high-risk cancer: a pilot study. J Pediatr Hematol Oncol 1999;21:111–114.
106. Langdana A, Tully N, Bourke B et al. Intensive enteral nutrition support in paediatric bone marrow transplantation. Bone Marrow Transplant 2001;27:741–746.
107. Barron MA, Duncan DS, Green GJ et al. Efficacy and safety of radiologically placed gastrostomy tubes in paediatric haematology/oncology patients. Med Pediatr Oncol 2000;34:177–182.
108. Weisdorf SA, Lysne J, Wind D et al. Positive effect of prophylactic total parenteral nutrition on long-term outcome of bone marrow transplantation. Transplantation 1987;43:833–838.
109. Rickard KA, Kirksey A, Baehner RL et al. Effectiveness of enteral and parenteral nutrition in the nutritional management of children with Wilms' tumors. Am J Clin Nutr 1980;33:2622–2629.
110. Rickard KA, Becker MC, Loghmani E et al. Effectiveness of two methods of parenteral nutrition support in improving muscle mass of children with neuroblastoma or Wilms' tumor. A randomized study. Cancer 1989;64:116–125.
111. Rickard KA, Godshall BJ, Loghmani ES et al. Integration of nutrition support into oncologic treatment protocols for high and low nutritional risk children with Wilm's tumor. A prospective randomized study. Cancer 1989;64:491–509.
112. Uderzo C, D'Angelo P, Rizzari C et al. Central venous catheter-related complications after bone marrow transplantation in children with hematological malignancies. Bone Marrow Transplant 1992;9:113–117.
113. Lipman TO. Grains or veins: Is enteral nutrition really better than parenteral nutrition? A look at the evidence. JPEN J Parenter Enteral Nutr 1998;22:167–182.
114. Conly J, Suttie J, Reid E et al. Dietary deficiency of phylloquinone and reduced serum levels in febrile neutropenic cancer patients. Am J Clin Nutr 1989;50:109–113.
115. Carlin A, Walker WA. Rapid development of vitamin K deficiency in an adolescent boy receiving total parenteral nutrition following bone marrow transplantation. Nutr Rev 1991;49:179–183.
116. Cunningham BA. Parenteral management. In: Lenssen P, Aker SN (eds). Nutritional Assessment and Management during Marrow Transplantation: A Resource Manual. Seattle: Fred Hutchinson Cancer Research Center, 1985;45–61.
117. Papadopoulou A, Nathavitharana K, Williams MD et al. Diagnosis and clinical associations of zinc depletion following bone marrow transplantation. Arch Dis Child 1996;74:328–331.
118. June CH, Thompson CB, Kennedy MS et al. Profound hypomagnesemia and renal magnesium wasting associated with the use of cyclosporine for marrow transplantation. Transplantation 1985;39:620–624.
119. Just B, Messing B, Darmaun D et al. Comparison of substrate utilization by indirect calorimetry during cyclic and continuous total parenteral nutrition. Am J Clin Nutr 1990;51:107–111.
120. Maini B, Blackburn GL, Bistrian BR et al. Cyclic hyperalimentation: an optimal technique for preservation of visceral protein. J Surg Res 1976;20:515–525.
121. Benotti PN, Bothe A Jr, Miller JD et al. Cyclic hyperalimentation. Comp Ther 1976;2:27–36.
122. Lenssen P, Moe GL, Cheney CL et al. Parenteral nutrition in marrow transplant recipients after discharge from the hospital. Exp Hematol 1983;11:974–981.
123. Chamouard Cogoluenhes V, Chambrier C, Michallet M et al. Energy expenditure during allogeneic and autologous bone marrow transplantation. Clin Nutr 1998;17:253–257.

124. Clamon G, Gardner L, Pee D et al. The effect of intravenous hyperalimentation on the dietary intake of patients with small cell lung cancer. A randomized trial. Cancer 1985;55:1572–1578.
125. Sriram K, Pinchcofsky G, Kaminski MV Jr. Suppression of appetite by parenteral nutrition in humans. J Am Coll Nutr 1984;3:317–323.
126. Charuhas PM, Fosberg KL, Bruemmer B et al. A double-blind randomized trial comparing outpatient parenteral nutrition with intravenous hydration: effect on resumption of oral intake after marrow transplantation. JPEN J Parenter Enter Nutr 1997;21:157–161.
127. Aker SN, Cheney CL. The use of sterile and low microbial diets in ultraisolation environments. JPEN J Parenter Enter Nutr 1983;7:390–397.
128. French MR, Levy-Milne R, Zibrik D. A survey of the use of low microbial diets in pediatric bone marrow transplant programs. J Am Diet Assoc 2001;101:1194–1198.
129. Henry L. Immunocompromised patients and nutrition. Prof Nurse 1997;12:655–659.
130. Kominos SD, Copeland CE, Konowalchuk J et al. Survival of enteric viruses on fresh vegetables. J Milk Food Technol 1975;38:469–472.
131. Rampling A. Raw milk, cheese and salmonella. BMJ 1996;312:67–68.
132. Gessner BD, Beller M. Protective effect of conventional cooking versus use of microwave ovens in an outbreak of salmonellosis. Am J Epidemiol 1994;139:903–909.
133. Farber JM, D'Aoust JY, Diotte M et al. Survival of Listeria spp. on raw whole chickens cooked in microwave ovens. J Food Prot 1998;61:1465–1469.
134. Todd J, Schmidt M, Christain J et al. The low-bacteria diet for immunocompromised patients. Reasonable prudence or clinical superstition? Cancer Pract 1999;7:205–207.
135. Fierini D. Is the low microbial diet effective? Can this question be answered? Marrow Transplant Nutrition Network Newsletter 1995;3:1–5.
136. Lavenstein AF, Dacaney EP, Lasagna L et al. Effect of cyproheptadine on asthmatic children. JAMA 1962;180:912–916.
137. Ansfield FJ, Kallas GJ, Singson JP. Clinical results with megestrol acetate in patients with advanced carcinoma of the breast. Surg Gynecol Obstet 1982;155:888–890.
138. Alexieva-Figusch J, van Gilse HA, Hop WC et al. Progestin therapy in advanced breast cancer: megestrol acetate-an evaluation of 160 treated cases. Cancer 1980;46:2369–2372.
139. Penfold JL. Effect of cyproheptadine and a multivitamin preparation on appetite stimulation, weight gain, and linear growth: a clinical trial of 40 children. Med J Aust 1971;1:307–310.
140. Kaplowitz PB, Jennings S. Enhancement of linear growth and weight gain by cyproheptadine in children with hypopituitarism receiving growth hormone therapy. J Pediatr 1987;110:140–143.
141. Bergen SS. Appetite stimulating properties of cyproheptadine. Am J Dis Child 1964;108:270–273.
142. Azcona C, Castro L, Crespo E et al. Megestrol acetate therapy for anorexia and weight loss in children with malignant solid tumors. Aliment Pharmacol Ther 1996;10:577–586.
143. Brady MT, Koranyi KI, Hunkler JA. Megestrol acetate for treatment of anorexia associated with human immunodeficiency virus infection in children. Pediatr Infect J 1994;13:754–755.
144. Clarick RH, Hanekom WA, Yogev R et al. Megestrol acetate treatment of growth failure in children infected with human immunodeficiency virus. Pediatrics 1997;99:354–357.
145. Summerbell CD, Youle M, McDonald V et al. Megestrol acetate vs cyproheptadine in the treatment of weight loss associated with HIV infection. Int J STD AIDS 1992;3:278–280.
146. Mann M, Koller E, Murgo A et al. Glucocorticoidlike activity of megestrol. A summary of Food and Drug Administration experience and a review of the literature. Arch Intern Med 1997;157:1651–1656.
147. Naing KK, Dewar JA, Leese GP. Megestrol acetate therapy and secondary adrenal suppression. Cancer 1999;86:1044–1049.
148. Stockheim JA, Daaboul JJ, Yogev R et al. Adrenal suppression in children with the human immunodeficiency virus treated with megestrol acetate. J Pediatr 1999;134:368–370.
149. Bergstrom J, Furst P, Noree LO et al. Intracellular free amino acid concentration in human muscle tissue. J Appl Physiol 1974;36:693–697.
150. Windmueller HG. Glutamine utilization by the small intestine. Adv Enzymol Relat Areas Mol Biol 1982;53:201–237.
151. Ziegler TR. Glutamine supplementation in cancer patients receiving bone marrow transplantation and high dose chemotherapy. J Nutr 2001;131:2568S–2584S.
152. Ziegler TR, Young LS, Benfell K et al. Clinical and metabolic efficacy of glutamine-supplemented parenteral nutrition after bone marrow transplantation: a randomized, double-blind, controlled study. Ann Int Med 1992;116:821–828.
153. Yoshida S, Matsui M, Shirouzu Y et al. Effects of glutamine supplements and radiochemotherapy on systemic immune and gut barrier function in patients with advanced esophageal cancer. Ann Surg 1998;227:485–491.
154. Klimberg VS, McClellan JL. Glutamine, cancer, and its therapy. Am J Surg 1996;172:418–424.

155. Ziegler TR, Bazargan N, Leader LM et al. Glutamine and the intestinal tract. Curr Opin Clin Nutr Metab Care 2000;3:355–362.
156. Schloerb PR, Amare M. Total parenteral nutrition with glutamine in bone marrow transplantation and other clinical applications (a randomized, double-blind study). J Parenter Enteral Nutr 1993;17:407–413.
157. Schloerb PR, Skikne BS. Oral and parenteral glutamine in bone marrow transplantation: a randomized, double-blind study. J Parenter Enter Nutr 1999;23:117–122.
158. Coghlin Dickson TM, Wong RM, Negrin RS et al. Effect of oral glutamine supplementation during bone marrow transplantation. J Parenter Enter Nutr 2000;24:61–66.
159. Cockerham MB, Weinberger BB, Lerchie SB. Oral glutamine for prevention of oral mucositis associated with high dose paclitaxel and melphalan for autologous bone marrow transplantation. Ann Pharmacother 2000; 34:300–303.
160. Anderson PM, Ramsay NKC, Shu XO et al. Effect of low-dose oral glutamine on painful stomatitis during bone marrow transplantation. Bone Marrow Transplant 1998;22:339–344.
161. Charland SL, Bartlett DL, Torosian MH. A significant methotrexate-glutamine pharmokinetic interaction. Nutrition 1995;11:154–158.
162. Braga M, Gianotti L, Radaelli G et al. Perioperative immunonutrition in patients undergoing cancer surgery: results of a randomized double-blind phase 3 trial. Arch Surg 1999;134:428–433.
163. Gianotti L, Braga M, Fortis C et al. A prospective, randomized double-blind clinical trial on perioperative feeding with an arginine-, omega-3 fatty acid-, and RNA-enriched enteral diet: effect on host response and nutritional status. J Parenter Enteral Nutr 1999;23:314–320.
164. Riso S, Aluffi P, Brugnani M et al. Postoperative enteral immunonutrition in head and neck cancer patients. Clin Nutr 2000;19:407–412.

# CHAPTER VI

# Pediatric Stem Cell Transplantation: Ethical Concerns

PUNEET CHEEMA AND PAULETTE MEHTA

Pediatric stem cell transplantation presents unique challenges because children unable to make independent decisions are usually transplanted with cells from other children also unable to make independent decisions, by parents who may have deep conflicts of interests in trying to save their sick child's life. Moreover, the field is changing quickly and is becoming so highly technical that patients may be bewildered by the variety of options available and may only partially understand what they hear. Furthermore, the emotional turmoil surrounding a child's illness also clouds the ability to think clearly.

The dilemma of ethical issues in pediatric stem cell transplant will surely increase as more children undergo, and survive, stem cell transplantation. Indications are increasing from aplastic anemia and leukemia alone from several years ago, to a wide variety of malignant and benign conditions at the present time.[1-3] These include diseases of metabolism, bone formation, immune deficiency, and of auto-immunity.[4-7] The advent of umbilical cord blood transplantation banking has greatly increased the chances of finding a donor, thereby making transplantation realizable for patients of common and uncommon human lymphocyte antigen (HLA) types. Globalization has added to the number of available donors also, making a match more likely for patients of minority groups in this country. Along with the increasing number of children being transplanted and those expected to be transplanted is the anticipated greater survival for these children. Survival from stem cell transplantation as well as from underlying diseases and their complications all are improving secondary to better supportive care, far improved antiviral and antifungal therapies, and growth factors to hasten engraftment.[1,4,8,9] Moreover, the use of non-myeloablative regimens, allowing for mixed chimersim for hematologic disease, and of gradual full chimerism through donor lymphocyte infusions for patients with malignant disease have reduced morbidity and mortality.[5,10]

Many chapters in this book address the scientific developments in each of these areas of pediatric stem cell transplantation. However, even as these questions become answered scientifically, they raise concerns in the private and public arena about ethical issues. These issues are described in the remainder of this chapter.

## ISSUES RELATED TO INFORMED CONSENT

Informed consent has been considered by some as an oxymoron. In the throes of a catastrophic disease affecting a child, few patients can truly remain sufficiently detached to render a fully conscious, considered decision, and few patients or families can remain uninfluenced by their physician's opinion.[11-14] Thus, the entire process of informed consent as a knowing, conscious reflection of the field and as a conscious, detached process for making a reasoned decision must be questioned. Rather, informed consent may allow for eventual acceptance of a needed treatment, may spark the interest of the patient, and may solidify the patient–physician relationship. It is improbable that any decision making in this setting will be impartial. Also, informed consent is not an event as it is currently ritualized, but rather a process of learning, understanding, releasing control, and accepting. In some ways it resembles and complements the cycle of grief.

A primary principle of bioethics is patient autonomy. Yet in the setting of pediatric stem cell transplantation, parents do not have complete autonomy in making decisions in their child's behalf, despite any appearance.[15-18] No child with a life-threatening illness is entitled to be untreated, and decisions not to treat ordinarily would invoke child welfare services. All parents know this at some level. The appearance that the family can choose therapy for their child is a façade; they cannot. The law insists that children be treated if there are sufficient grounds for benefit of treatment, and for certain harm without treatment. In the case of cancer in children, at least for those who present with low risk disease, parents are in effect forced to consent to treatment. Thus, the presence of autonomy is replaced by the principle of beneficence and is decided in effect by society as spoken through the courts.

The real reasons for decision making relate to factors other than factual information presented during the informed consent signing. Rather, it usually relates to trust in a physician, faith in the treatment, and a need to "do something."[16,19,20] Our earlier study found that informed consent to the greatest number of supportive care trials within a bone marrow transplant setting was related to the amount of emotional distress, thus often resulting in "acquiescence to treatment" rather than "acceptance of treatment."[20]

Regardless of the reasons for making decisions, most families already have accepted bone marrow transplantation as the treatment of choice by the time they arrive at a bone marrow transplant center.[21] Chauvenet and Smith[21] surveyed 24 pediatric oncologists from 21 institutions not performing bone marrow transplants and found that the opinion of the pediatric oncologist was the deciding factor in whether or not a family would consent to bone marrow transplantation. Thus, the decisions appear to lie with the primary treating physician rather than the subspecialist. Subspecialists need to be aware of this information and make sure that their referring pediatricians and pediatric oncologists are fully informed about their patients' progress in bone marrow transplant regimens.

## ROLE OF THE CHILD IN THE INFORMED CONSENT PROCESS

Children are becoming increasingly precocious with the use of the Internet and other electronic equipment connecting them to the world at young ages. Although young children will normally comply with their parent's wishes, not knowing differently and not understanding differently, older children and adolescents may not agree with their parents, although they have no legal grounds for independent decision-making in most cases.[17,22] In rare cases when children have fought their way for their decision-making power in treatment decisions, they have occasionally swayed judges that they deserve to have that power. However, it is rare.

Assent has been proposed and is used as a way to overcome the awkward situation whereby children are not given the right of consent for their own treatment to their own bodies.[22] Thus, assent is always requested from patients who are over 6 and under 21 years of age. Such assent then gives the child the opportunity to participate in the process and to have his or her voice heard. However, assent or lack of assent in detriment to the child's welfare is not legally allowable. Thus, the whole concept of consent and assent in childrens' decisions remain relative to what the state insists is in the child's best interest. Our society has supported this stand and this has major impact on the dynamics of signing informed consent.

## TRANSPLANTATION FOR IMPROVING, RATHER THAN SAVING, LIFE

An interesting variation of this theme arises when the need for the transplant is not necessary to save life, but rather to improve life.[23,24] Patients with sickle cell disease fit into this category, as the benefit to these patients is the possibility of fewer complications of sickle cell disease after bone marrow transplantation. Often it is difficult to know how serious the complications will be for each case and, therefore, in whom bone marrow transplantation would have the most benefit. This is especially true since children optimally should be selected before a serious complication occurs and yet there no accurate ways of predicting severity of disease. In the face of these abstract benefits, the risks of 10% to 20% mortality and 60% to 100% morbidity is more difficult to reconcile. When the physician is clear about the benefit/risk ratio, counseling is not difficult. Where there is insufficient evidence-based information, counseling is much more difficult.

## SIBLING DONOR ISSUES

The relative autonomy of informed consent is further complicated in the case of the sibling child asking to donate for an ailing sibling.[25,26] Here, there is no benefit to the donor child, yet there may be significant potential harm in terms of venipuncture, invasion of privacy even of most intimate details of his being, and subjection to a burdensome procedure of either bone marrow harvesting or of peripheral blood stem cell pheresis. Bone marrow harvesting can be done quickly but requires general anesthesia with its incumbent side effects. Peripheral blood stem cell pheresis is generally preferred since anesthesia is not required, overnight stay in the hospital is not usually recommended, and because it provides the greatest number of stem cells for the recipient. Nevertheless, this procedure entails placement of a large catheter, treatment with growth stimulating factors for at least five days to mobilize stem cells from bone marrow to peripheral blood, and may take many days of sitting quietly while pheresis is performed.

The question of who is in the proper position to decide what is in the donor child's best interest has been raised in many centers.[27,28] The child who is most involved usually has no legal right to decide as he or she is usually under a legal age. Here, assent is an important way of hearing the child's voice and of inviting full participation in the decision making process. However, non-consent on the part of the child is not binding. Rather, the parents are almost always left to decide whether they will or will not consent to the pheresis. Yet they have a deep sense of conflict since their ill child, for whom this child is donating, is in dire need of matched cells. Some hospitals have transcended this paradox by appointing hospital guardians for the donor sibling, in order to make decisions and to set limits to the extent to which the child can be used to offer the cells for his or her siblings, and other procedures that may be needed after the transplant such as matched blood transfusions, matched platelet transfusions, subsequent donor lymphocyte infusions, etc.[27,28] Nevertheless, the child is usually under duress at least from conscience, fear of repercussions, and for wanting to please parents by donating cells.

The emotional suffering of the donor child has been well explored.[29] These children often feel burdened by life-threatening processes early in life and may suffer from the complications of the sick child, especially if his or her own bone marrow cells were not sufficient to save the sibling. This is likely to be much more burdensome in the child who is born for the purpose of donating cord blood stem cells for the sick child, although this issue has not been studied yet.

The other siblings who are in the family also may be affected adversely by the transplant and the donation. Some investigators have suggested that the siblings not asked to donate may suffer more than the ones who are asked to donate, because they do not receive any share of the pride or publicity of having saved a sibling, and also receive less family attention than either the sick child or the healthy donor.[29] In most cases, decision making, at least for the physician, is based on a benefit/risk ratio. For children who are in first remission of acute myelogenous leukemia or second or higher remission of acute lymphoblastic leukemia, or with aplastic anemia, the benefits of a matched sibling donor transplant ordinarily far outweighs the risks.

## CONCEIVING A CHILD FOR SPARE PARTS: DOES BENEFICENCE TO ONE CHILD OUTWEIGH JUSTICE TO THE OTHER?

Another concern is when a child is specifically conceived in order to provide stem cells for a sibling in need.[30] It is intuitive that a child born to provide stem cells for a sibling may be deprived of his inalienable right to define and defend his own reason for living, rather than be born for a cause which he has not chosen and over which he has no control. The child so conceived who does not have a close HLA match with his sibling may have failed for life even as he is born. Worse, the child who does match with the sibling, but whose sibling nevertheless succumbs to disease, may feel he has disappointed his family in ways outside of his control. Ethicists are wary of this situation, yet it is impossible to judge another person's actions without fully understanding the motives. Moreover, there are many worse reasons for conceiving children. Clearly, however, this is a case in which beneficence towards one child may occur at the expense of justice to the other. The physician's role may be used best in this situation by advising the family to help the child find his own happiness in the world, regardless of the fate of the ailing sibling.

## ISSUES RELATED TO UMBILICAL CORD BANKING

An interesting development in the field of bone marrow transplantation has arisen with the advent of umbilical cord banking.[31,32] Public banks have been developed through NIH grants and have been successful in finding donors for patients for whom other sources may not be available. Donation to a public bank asserts the principle of beneficence to society as well as generosity. In giving stem cells, parents must sign away any subsequent claims that they could use these cells even if such need arose later in their child's life. In return, the family may earn the satisfaction of altruism and joy of contributing to science. The rise of private umbilical cord centers is fed in part by fears that a person may need cells for their own child due to some catastrophic event, at a future point in time.[31,33,34] Companies ready to save, store, and distribute umbilical cells for a fee now abound throughout the country.

This industry of "blood money" probably appeals to parents who fear that they may need the cells someday for their own child. In practice, the risk of needing one's own umbilical cells is exceedingly rare. Moreover, if a baby does develop leukemia in childhood (the most common cause for which bone marrow transplantation would be needed), allogeneic bone marrow transplantation would be preferred to profit from the graft-versus-leukemia effect. Moreover, the recognition that children with leukemia may have malignant cells in their newborn blood renders use of such autologous cells undesirable for themselves, or for others. The duty to inform would appear to be a moral imperative for parents whose child develops leukemia and who had previously donated cord blood stem cells from their same child's umbilical cord. Yet this issue has not been addressed formally or legally.

This interesting juxtaposition of public and private banks remains at tension with each other and may require legislation to establish one system or the other. In the meantime, a compromise solution used by many companies is the reservation of cells for the child if needed, with a provision to release such blood cells to the public banks when and if the family relinquishes rights on the cells.

## WHO PROFITS FROM DISCOVERIES FROM CHILDRENS' STEM CELLS?

Donation of umbilical cells for research also raises the ethical concern of ownership of cells in the event of discovery of a new gene.[35,36] Who owns such cells and their genetic products, which may be used for further research or for commercialization in the form of diagnostic tests? If such cells generate profits, to whom do these profits rightfully belong? These are as yet unanswered, and perhaps unanswerable, questions.

## IS THERE A DUTY TO WARN?

Umbilical cord blood banking has led to other interesting ethical considerations. One is the duty to warn biological parents if a genetic mutation or other abnormality is found in the cord stem cells donated to the other child.[35,37] At the present time, no such duty has been declared and information related to the fetus after his birth is strictly confidential even to biological parents. A condition of cord blood donation at the present time is that parties will not be disturbed by findings from the blood cells later. However, as genetic tests improve and as therapies become available for genetic abnormalities, this policy may change.

## ETHICAL PRINCIPLE OF PRIVACY

Another interesting dilemma arises in the case of a child who receives cord blood from an umbilical cord blood donor and who subsequently needs cells from the same donor. This need could arise either if the patient relapses after initial response, or if the patient requires donor lymphocyte infusions to complete full donor chimerism. At the present time, the patient and family are not allowed to contact the family of origin, or even to obtain information about the family. The anguish of families in such desperate need of one particular person's cells needs to be balanced against the rights of the privacy of the family who already made a contribution by donating the cord. Yet some such families needing follow-up cells from the original cord blood donor have argued that not contacting the family deprives them of the right to life, and of the family to again offer and benefit from an act of courage and altruism.

## CHOOSING THE EMBRYO TO SAVE FOR SPARE PARTS

Another interesting twist of cord blood transplantation was recently highlighted by the media. Parents sought cord blood stem cells by in vitro fertilization to obtain choices of embryos from which to choose the closest HLA match for their child with Fanconi's anemia.[30,35] The choice in this case was made on the basis of HLA similarities to the HLA of the sick child. Ethicists have decried this situation that deprives the newborn of his right to autonomy and raises a potential situation in which he can be blamed for, and suffer from, not succeeding in his mission in life, i.e., to save the sibling. Despite the unaesthetic nature of such a choice, it is made frequently by couples who are desperate to save the lives of their children. Although one can decry the concept of birth of a child to save a sibling's life, it is nonetheless more noble than many other causes for which babies are born and as such should be respected.

Of course, another consideration is that in vitro fertilization always requires the choice of a single embryo among many to save and nurture. Since a decision is needed, one based on closeness of HLA type to save another child is more defendable than other reasons for which embryos may be discarded, including gender preference.

## CONCLUSIONS

Modern medicine has created innumerable benefits along with new ethical concerns. Many of these ethical dilemmas are present in the everyday life of a busy pediatric hematology oncology bone marrow transplant center. Some of the ethical concerns relate simply to the nature of informed consents, while others concern benefit/risk ratios, donors who suffer consequences without any personal benefit and who do so without their consent, and to the emerging world of umbilical cord blood transplantation. Each generation of patients and families will need to discover their own path and their truth, while society searches to find a common moral ground. Although the principles of autonomy have been relative in the sphere of pediatric decisions, the principle of beneficence remains a primary principle by which to steer ourselves in a highly evolving world of highly specialized and technically advanced medicine.

# REFERENCES

1. Gluckman E, Rocha V, Chastang C. Cord blood banking and transplant in Europe. Eurocord. Vox Sang 1998;74(Suppl 2):95–101.
2. Kline RM, Bertolone SJ. Umbilical cord blood transplantation: providing a donor for everyone needing a bone marrow transplant? South Med J 1998;91:821–828.
3. Mills A. Experimental treatments in end-stage leukaemia. Lancet 1978;2:1310.
4. Locatelli F, Burgio GR. Transplant of hematopoietic stem cells in childhood: where we are and where we are going. Haematologica 1998;83:550–563.
5. Slavin S, Nagler A, Aker M et al. Non-myeloablative stem cell transplantation and donor lymphocyte infusion for the treatment of cancer and life-threatening non-malignant disorders. Rev Clin Exp Hematol 2001;5:135–146.
6. Slavin S, Or R, Aker M et al. Nonmyeloablative stem cell transplantation for the treatment of cancer and life-threatening nonmalignant disorders: past accomplishments and future goals. Cancer Chemother Pharmacol 2001;48(Suppl 1):S79–S84.
7. Uderzo C. Indications and role of allogeneic bone marrow transplantation in childhood very high risk acute lymphoblastic leukemia in first complete remission. Haematologica 2000;85(Suppl 11):9–11.
8. Barker JN, Wagner JE. Umbilical cord blood transplantation: current state of the art. Curr Opin Oncol 2002;14:160–164.
9. Matthay KK. Intensification of therapy using hematopoietic stem-cell support for high-risk neuroblastoma. Pediatr Transplant 1999;3(Suppl 1):72–77.
10. Slavin S, Morecki S, Weiss L et al. Donor lymphocyte infusion: the use of alloreactive and tumor-reactive lymphocytes for immunotherapy of malignant and nonmalignant diseases in conjunction with allogeneic stem cell transplantation. J Hematother Stem Cell Res 2002;11:265–276.
11. Jacoby LH, Maloy B, Cirenza E et al. The basis of informed consent for BMT patients. Bone Marrow Transplant 1999;23:711–717.
12. Rosenberg HL. Informed consent. Mother Jones 1981;6:31–37, 44.
13. Smith DL, Levine MD. Informed consent and medical ethics. J Pediatr Surg 1975;87:327–328.
14. Williams TE. Legal issues and ethical dilemmas surrounding bone marrow transplantation in children. Am J Pediatr Hematol Oncol 1984;6:83–88.
15. Davies S. Bone marrow transplant raises issues of privacy. BMJ 1997;314:1356.
16. Dermatis H, Lesko LM. Psychosocial correlates of physician-patient communication at time of informed consent for bone marrow transplantation. Cancer Invest 1991;9:621–628.
17. Grochowski EC, Bach S. The ethics of decision making with adolescents: what a physician ought to know. Adolesc Med 1994;5:485–495.
18. Taylor B. Parental autonomy and consent to treatment. J Adv Nurs 1999;29:570–576.
19. Crawford SW. Decision making in critically ill patients with hematologic malignancy. West J Med 1991;155:488–493.
20. Mehta P, Rodrigue J, Nejame C et al. Acquiescence to adjunctive experimental therapies may relate to psychological distress: pilot data from a bone marrow transplant center. Bone Marrow Transplant 2000;25:673–676.
21. Chauvenet AR, Smith NM. Referral of pediatric oncology patients for marrow transplantation and the process of informed consent. Med Pediatr Oncol 1988;16:40–44.
22. Ross LF. Justice for children: the child as organ donor. Bioethics 1994;8:105–126.
23. Davies SC. Bone marrow transplant for sickle cell disease—the dilemma. Blood Rev 1993;7:4–9.
24. Kodish E, Lantos J, Siegler M et al. Bone marrow transplantation in sickle cell disease: the trade-off between early mortality and quality of life. Clin Res 1990;38:694–700.
25. Korins JB. Curran v. Bosze: toward a clear standard for authorizing kidney and bone marrow transplants between minor siblings. Vt Law Rev 1992;16:499–539.
26. Massimo L. Ethical problems in bone marrow transplantation in children. Bone Marrow Transplant 1996;18(Suppl 2):8–12.
27. Kent G. Volunteering children for bone marrow donation. Studies show large discrepancies between views of surrogate decision makers and patients. BMJ 1996;313:49–50.
28. Serota FT, August CS, O'Shea AT et al. Role of a child advocate in the selection of donors for pediatric bone marrow transplantation. J Pediatr 1981;98:847–850.
29. Packman W. Psychosocial impact of pediatric BMT on siblings. Bone Marrow Transplant 1999;24:701–706.
30. Alby N. The child conceived to give life. Bone Marrow Transplant 1992;9(Suppl 1):95–96.
31. Fasouliotis SJ, Schenker JG. Human umbilical cord blood banking and transplantation: a state of the art. Eur J Obstet Gynecol Reprod Biol 2000;90:13–25.

32. Sugarman J, Kaalund V, Kodish E et al. Ethical issues in umbilical cord blood banking. Working Group on Ethical Issues in Umbilical Cord Blood Banking. JAMA 1997;278:938–943.
33. Butler D. US company comes under fire over patent on umbilical cord cells. Nature 1996;382:99.
34. Varadi G, Elchalal U, Shushan A et al. Umbilical cord blood for use in transplantation. Obstet Gynecol Surv 1995;50:611–617.
35. Auerbach AD. Umbilical cord blood transplants for genetic disease: diagnostic and ethical issues in fetal studies. Blood Cells 1994;20:303–309.
36. Hehlmann R, Odenbach E, Hofschneider PH et al. Round table discussion 'gene therapy and society'—summary and conclusions. Leukemia 1995;9(Suppl 1):S7–S8.
37. Sugarman J, Reisner EG, Kurtzberg J. Ethical aspects of banking placental blood for transplantation. JAMA 1995;274:1783–1785.

# Psychosocial Adjustment After Stem Cell Transplantation

ALLEN C. SHERMAN, STEPHANIE SIMONTON, AND UMAIRA LATIF

Within the past two decades bone marrow and peripheral stem cell transplantation (SCT) have been used to treat a growing range of childhood diseases. As survival rates are extended, a larger number of patients are confronted by the complexities of adjusting to life after transplant. Increasing attention has focused on quality of life for these children and their families. What kinds of challenges and burdens do they face, and how do these change over the course of illness? This chapter briefly reviews the research literature concerning psychosocial adjustment for pediatric transplant patients. We discuss quality of life changes during the acute posttransplant period and over the longer term, examining outcomes for patients and family members. We also consider which children may be most vulnerable to psychosocial difficulties and which most resilient. Psychosocial interventions are briefly noted. Each section reviews some of the gaps in the literature and offers recommendations for further research.

## ASSESSING QUALITY OF LIFE AND ADJUSTMENT

Health-related quality of life is generally viewed as encompassing a number of different spheres of functioning, including physical symptoms, functional status, emotional well-being, and social functioning.[1] There is a growing consensus that investigators should assess each of these domains. Moreover, a developmental frame of reference is particularly important in understanding adjustment among children. For example, how do the demands of illness and treatment affect the transition to elementary school for a preschool child, or the establishment of peer relationships for a third grader, or pursuit of a drivers license and growing independence for a teenager, or comfort with intimacy and identity for a young adult? In addition, health investigators have expressed increasing interest in the possibility of positive consequences of illness or treatment. Although traditionally psychosocial oncology research has focused on areas of deficit and vulnerability, there is growing recognition that serious illness brings opportunities for growth as well as morbidity.[2,3] A comprehensive understanding of quality of life outcomes thus would include evaluation of positive changes, such as heightened maturity or enhanced competence, as well as negative sequelae. An additional challenge in assessing children's adjustment is the fact that different respondents provide different perspectives.[4] The picture provided by the mother, for example, who is the major informant in most studies, may not conform closely with that of the child or his or her teachers. From a systems perspective, these differences reflect more than simply imprecise measurement or error variance—they capture the multiplicity of perceptions inherent in dynamic social systems. Ideally, therefore, studies should encompass multiple voices, including that of the child, though logistic constraints often make this difficult to achieve.

## PSYCHOSOCIAL DIMENSIONS OF STEM CELL TRANSPLANTATION

Notwithstanding significant advances in supportive care (such as improved use of growth factors, graft-versus-host disease prophylaxis, and anti-emetics), SCT remains an aggressive, debilitating treatment. The particular burdens that confront transplant recipients and their families shift over the trajectory of illness, from the initial crisis of diagnosis through the ambiguities of long-term survivorship. These challenges include adapting to a life-threatening illness and an uncertain future, accommodating disruptions in family and school routines, and enduring protracted periods of hospitalization and isolation, often at specialized facilities located far from home. During conditioning treatment, patients are exposed to an array of demanding toxicities (e.g., mucositis, nausea, and immunosuppression) and heightened risk of fatal complications. For some children this debilitating treatment follows many years of prior therapies, which carried their own toxicities and unfulfilled hopes. Stress may be compounded further by periodic painful procedures (e.g., bone marrow biopsies) and demanding regimens of mouth and skin care that are required after transplantation.[5] Clearly then, the transplant process is an extremely taxing one for the entire family. Children's emotional reactions are colored by their level of development, but anxiety, regressive behavior, and compliance problems are fairly common.[5,6] Worry, strain, and exhaustion are characteristic for parents.[7]

After transplantation and early engraftment, school attendance and contact with peers remain sharply curtailed during prolonged periods of convalescence. Common problems include fatigue, appetite disturbance, and continued risk of infectious complications. Children or their families may be quite anxious about leaving the safety of the hospital,[7,8] or exhausted by the ongoing need for frequent medical appointments and multiple medications. Over the long-term, children may experience a number of medical late effects including chronic graft-versus-host disease (GVHD), endocrine abnormalities, cataracts, bone necrosis, and second malignancies.[9] Some of these complications may retard growth or alter the child's physical appearance, and most would be expected to disrupt school attendance, athletic activity, and peer relationships. Financial pressures associated with the daunting costs of treatment and frequent absences from work may have enduring effects on the family's lifestyle long after active treatment has ended. For most families, long-term recovery is also marked by an unsettling fear of recurrence.[10] Some families become paralyzed by a vigilant watch for the next medical crisis. Family life may remain organized around acute illness long after this arrangement is no longer adaptive;[11,12] normal routines and plans for the future remain deferred, and members may have difficulty moving toward greater autonomy and independence.

## RESEARCH ON PSYCHOSOCIAL ADJUSTMENT AND QUALITY OF LIFE AMONG TRANSPLANT PATIENTS

Unfortunately, despite growing interest in psychosocial adjustment for children treated with SCT, research has been quite limited. In contrast to the growing database concerning behavioral and psychosocial outcomes for adult transplant recipients, few studies have focused on children. Among the studies that have been completed, several examined adjustment in the acute-to-intermediate posttransplant period (i.e., up to 6-12 months following transplant; ▼ Table 7.1). In the largest prospective study to date, Phipps and colleagues[6] followed 153 children with varying diagnoses from pretransplant admission to six months after transplant. These children displayed high levels of physical symptoms, activity limitations, and emotional distress upon entering the hospital, and each of these difficulties increased sharply in the immediate aftermath of conditioning treatment and transplantation. By four or five weeks after transplant, however, these problems had receded to their levels at admission, and they continued to decline through the sixth month follow-up assessment. The patterns of change over time were similar whether based on reports from the parents or the patients. Other prospective studies have been based on much smaller samples. In these investigations, as in the study by Phipps et al., physical and functional status improved 6–12 months after transplant, relative to pretransplant levels.[13,15] At the same time, however, participants demonstrated declines in psychological adjustment, such as self-concept and emotional well-being.[17,20] They also displayed declines in social competence, assessed by parent ratings[17] in conjunction with mild-to-moderate symptoms of posttraumatic stress (e.g., avoidance of reminders, intrusive thoughts, irritability), based on clinical interviews.[15] Behavioral problems were noted in some studies[20] but not others.[13,17]

Not surprisingly then, the two to three week interval immediately following conditioning and transplant seems to be the time of greatest distress for children;[6] despite subsequent marked improvement, there are indications that adjustment problems may not be uncommon over the next 6–12 months.[15,17,20] Are psychosocial difficulties enduring or are they limited to the transitional period after transplant? Some investigations have focused on long-term outcomes, assessed several years after transplant (▼ Table 7.2). Findings are not uniform, but they suggest several areas of difficulty. In a study of social functioning among school-aged children (age 8–16), transplant recipients had significantly fewer reciprocated friendships and fewer best friends than age- and gender-matched peers.[25] They also were viewed by their classmates as more socially isolated and withdrawn, less attractive, and less athletic, as well as more ill and more likely to miss school. These social limitations were evident despite that fact that all patients were in remission and were assessed, on average, 3½ years posttransplant. Moreover, social difficulties were not associated with time since transplant, implying that these challenges may be enduring rather than transient.[25]

A small study of older transplant survivors also suggested heightened risk for social and emotional difficulties.[23] Participants in this investigation were teenagers and young adults (mean age 19.5), who were assessed on average seven years after transplant. Compared to a historical control group of bone cancer survivors, transplant patients reported higher levels of anxiety and sensitivity/vulnerability, and greater difficulty achieving their goals with respect to intimate relationships and school or work. In most of these areas, these concerns reached clinical levels of severity more often among the transplant patients than among the bone cancer patients or the general population. Difficulties were not evident in the other domains assessed (i.e., depression, self-esteem, relationships with family and peers). The control group was older than the transplant patients in this study, but age was not significantly associated with the outcomes evaluated. A similar picture emerged from a study of pediatric survivors of allogeneic transplant, who had undergone treatment an average of seven years earlier.[21] Relative to population norms, these survivors demonstrated difficulties with social competence, as rated by their parents, and internalizing behavior problems

**TABLE 7.1    Selected Studies Examining Acute and Intermediate Psychosocial Outcomes Among Pediatric BMT Patients**

| Study | Sample | Measures | Design | Time of Assessment |
|---|---|---|---|---|
| Barerra et al.[13] | 26 patients with diverse diseases | *Child:* Vineland Adaptive Behavior Scales; Child Behavioral Checklist; Pediatric Oncology QOL Scale | Prospective | Pre-BMT and 6-mos post-BMT |
| | Mean age = 8.5 yrs (range: 10 mons–17.5 yrs) | | | |
| | 46.1% female | *Parent/Family:* Beck Depression Inventory; State-Trait Anxiety Inventory (State); FACES III | | |
| Lee et al.[14] | 6 patients with neuroblastoma or acute myelogenous leukemia, and 7 healthy controls | *Child/Parent:* 20-minute videotapes of parent-child interactions, coded using Family Interaction Q-Sort | Prospective, with healthy control group | Patients: Pre-BMT, 3, 6, 12, and 24 mos post-BMT |
| | Age range: 3.9–6.9 yrs | *Child:* PTSD Reaction Index | | Controls: assessed once |
| | 50% female | | | |
| | 16.67% allo | *Parent:* Ways of Coping– Cancer Interview | | |
| | 83.33% auto | | | |
| Stuber et al.[15] | Same as Lee et al.[14] (No controls) | *Child:* PTSD Reaction Index; Play Performance Scale | Prospective | Pre-BMT, 3, 6, 12 mos post-BMT |
| McConville et al.[16] | 15 patients who survived BMT to 1 yr and 17 who did not. | *Child:* Brief Psychiatric Rating Scale; Global Assessment Scale; DSM-III diagnoses | Retrospective ratings by staff of hospital period, as recalled at 1-yr follow-up | Retrospective recall of hospitalization period |
| | No data provided re: sample characteristics | *Parents:* Brief Psychiatric Rating Scale; Global Assessment Scale | | |
| | | *Family:* Author-derived measure of family interactions (no psychometric data provided); Family functioning | | |

**TABLE 7.1    Selected Studies Examining Acute and Intermediate Psychosocial Outcomes Among Pediatric BMT Patients—cont'd**

| Study | Sample | Measures | Design | Time of Assessment |
|---|---|---|---|---|
| Phipps & DeCuir-Whalley[5] | 54 patients with diverse diseases<br><br>Mean age = 9.1 yrs (range: 1 mon–20 yrs)<br><br>46% female<br><br>66.7% allo<br>33.3% auto | Chart review of compliance problems during hospitalization | Retrospective chart review | During hospitalization |
| Phipps et al.[17] | 25 patients with diverse diseases<br><br>Age <3.0 to >18.0 yrs<br><br>44% female<br><br>76.0% allo<br>24.0% auto | Child Behavior Checklist<br>Piers-Harris Self-Concept<br>Play Performance Scale<br>Bayley Scales of Infant Development,<br>WPPSI-R, WISC-R, WISC-III, or WAIS-R<br>WRAT-R, Beery VMI, Test of Visual-<br>Perceptual Skills, Rey AVLT<br>Symbol Digits Modality Test | Prospective | Pre-BMT, 6–12 mos post-BMT<br>(mean = 8.2 mos) |
| Phipps & Mulhern[18] | 25 patients, overlaps with sample from Phipps et al. 1995.[17] Ages 4–16, no descriptive data provided for this subsample. | Child:<br>Child Behavior Checklist<br>Piers-Harris Self-Concept | Prospective | Pre-BMT, 6–12 mos post-BMT<br>(mean = 8.2 mos) |
| Phipps et al.[6]<br>Phipps et al.[19] | 153 patients with diverse diseases<br><br>Mean age = 8.9 yrs (range: <1–20 yrs)<br><br>45% female<br><br>66.7% allo<br>33.3% auto | Family:<br>Family Environment Scale<br>Behavioral, Affective, and Somatic Experiences Scales, completed by child, parent, and nurse | Prospective | Pre-BMT (admission), weekly to 6 weeks post-BMT, and monthly to 6 mos post-BMT |

Note: Table does not include studies that focused exclusively on neurocognitive functioning.

Abbreviations: allo = allogeneic; auto = autologous; AVLT = Auditory-Verbal Learning Task; BMT = bone marrow transplant; mo = month; VMI = Visual-Motor Integration; WAIS-R = Wechsler Adult Intelligence Scale-Revised; WISC-R = Wechsler Intelligence Scale for Children-Revised; WPPSI-R = Wechsler Preschool and Primary Scales of Intelligence-Revised; yr = year.

**TABLE 7.2    Selected Studies Examining Long-Term Psychosocial Outcomes Among Pediatric BMT Patients**

| Study | Sample | Measures | Design | Time of Assessment |
|---|---|---|---|---|
| Arvidson et al.[21] | 26 patients with acute lymphoblastic leukemia, acute myelocytic leukemia, or lymphoma, in complete remission, at least 2 yrs post BMT<br><br>Median age = 16.1 (range: 6.9–22.7 yrs)<br><br>31% female<br><br>100% auto | I Think I Am (self-concept)<br>Somatic complaints<br>Disease- or Treatment-related Somatic Symptoms (author-derived measure)<br>Child Behavior Checklist<br>Rutter Teacher Questionnaire | Cross sectional | Median = 7.0 yrs post-BMT |
| Badell et al.[22] | 98 patients with diverse diseases, currently disease-free, at least 3 yrs post-BMT, >age 17, and 58 healthy controls<br><br>Mean age for patients = 21.8 yrs (range: 16.8–33.0 yrs)<br><br>39% female among patients, 64% female among controls<br><br>73.5% allo<br>26.5% auto | QOL questionnaire | Cross sectional, with healthy comparison group (no info on how recruited) | Mean = 8.9 yrs post-BMT |
| Felder-Puig et al.[23] | 26 patients with diverse diseases at least 2 yrs post-allo stem cell transplant, ages 14-30, and historical control group of 60 bone cancer survivors<br><br>Mean age for BMT patients = 19.5 yrs (range: 15-27 yrs).<br><br>54% female for BMT patients<br><br>100% allo | Depressive Mood from Questionnaire on Subjective Well-Being<br>State-Trait Anxiety Inventory (Trait)<br>Frankfurt Self-Concept<br>Items from Questionnaire on Life Goals and Satisfaction with Life<br>Author-derived measure of living arrangements, disease-related problems | Cross sectional, with control group of bone cancer survivors | Mean = 7 years post-BMT |

**TABLE 7.2    Selected Studies Examining Long-Term Psychosocial Outcomes Among Pediatric BMT Patients—cont'd**

| Study | Sample | Measures | Design | Time of Assessment |
|---|---|---|---|---|
| Parsons et al.[4] | 54 patients with diverse diseases, ages 5–12, receiving care at a post-transplant clinic<br><br>Mean age = 9 yrs (range: 5.0–12.9 yrs)<br><br>40% female<br><br>57.3% allo<br>42.7% auto | Child Health Rating Inventory; Disease Impairment Inventory-BMT (rated by child, parent, and physician) | Cross sectional | Range = 24 days - 8.4 yrs post-BMT |
| Schmidt et al.[24] | 50 patients with diverse diseases at least 1 yr post-allo BMT<br><br>Mean age = 18 yrs (range: 7–27 yrs)<br><br>44% female<br><br>100% allo | Structured interview (author-derived, no psychometric data) | Cross sectional | Mean = 6 yrs post-BMT |
| Vannatta et al.[25] | 48 patients with diverse diseases, post-BMT, enrolled in school full-time, and 48 demographically-matched healthy controls in same classroom<br><br>Mean age = 11.7 yrs (range: 8–16 yrs)<br><br>44% female<br><br>72.9% allo<br>27.1% auto | Revised Class Play (ratings by self, peers, and teacher)<br>2 Best Friends<br>Liking Rating Scale | Cross sectional, with age- and gender-matched healthy controls | Mean = 3.6 yrs post-BMT |

Note:  Table does not include studies that focused exclusively on neurocognitive functioning.
Abbreviations: allo = allogeneic; auto = autologous; BMT = bone marrow transplant; mo = month; yr = year.

(e.g., withdrawal, neuroticism), as rated by parents and teachers. They did not express problems with self-esteem or somatic symptoms on self-report measures.

In contrast, other investigations have suggested more favorable long-term adaptation. Schmidt and colleagues[24] assessed survivors who were at least one-year posttransplant; their sample included a subgroup of 50 pediatric patients (median age 18). Pediatric survivors reported good global quality of life and functional status, and an absence of major difficulties with appearance, current school enrollment, or employment. Conclusions are somewhat limited, however, because this study did not employ validated measures, assessed school and vocational involvement in only a rudimentary fashion, and did not examine emotional or social functioning at all. A Spanish study evaluated adolescents and young adults (median age 22) an average of 8.5 years after transplant.[22] Interestingly, transplant survivors reported better adjustment than a healthy control group on measures of global quality of life, depression, interpersonal difficulties, and leisure activities. On the other hand, survivors reported significantly greater difficulties with appearance and with work or school, findings that are consistent with problems noted among adult transplant patients. The significant gender difference between patients and controls in this study, and the limited psychometric support for the assessment instrument, limit conclusions.

In addition to its impact on emotional and social adjustment, there has been great interest in the effects of transplant on cognitive performance. In particular, there have been concerns that cognitive or academic functioning may be disrupted as a result of exposure to total body irradiation (TBI) or high dose chemotherapy.[26] Findings have been mixed, but a recent large prospective study[26] using individually administered test batteries found generally stable neurocognitive functioning through a three-year follow-up. There was no evidence of serious declines in cognitive or academic performance for the sample as a whole, although there were trends for more circumscribed declines in attention, concentration, and fine-motor functioning. There were no indications that TBI, prior central nervous system (CNS) therapy, or acute or chronic GVHD were associated with adverse changes in IQ. However, younger children, particularly those under age 3 at transplant, did demonstrate declines in global IQ. The greater vulnerability of younger children is consistent with findings from an earlier prospective study.[27]

In sum, although findings are variable, on balance the few studies that have been completed raise concerns about psychosocial adjustment for children, both in the acute aftermath of transplant and over the course of long-term recovery. Social functioning appears to be among the pockets of continued vulnerability. As highlighted by Noll and colleagues,[28] the quality of social interactions during childhood may be a fundamental aspect of psychosocial development, and in turn may predict future adjustment during adolescence and adulthood. Other areas of concern among at least some pediatric transplant patients include emotional distress,[17,20,23] posttraumatic stress disorder (PTSD) symptoms,[15] goal achievement in academic and vocational spheres,[23] and, for very young children, neurocognitive functioning.[26,27] Further research is needed to clarify the prevalence, intensity, and chronicity of these difficulties.

The pioneering investigations that have been conducted with pediatric transplant patients have made important contributions, but much of the research is characterized by methodological limitations. First, the range of outcomes that has been assessed is rather narrow. Little is known about children's adjustment in several important domains of functioning, such as fatigue, body image, treatment adherence, or school re-entry. Our understanding of adjustment difficulties is especially limited as children grow older. To what extent do survivors experience disruption in basic developmental tasks, such as identity formation, independence from parents, establishment of intimate relationships, or pursuit of career goals? How do they cope with treatment-related infertility, and for those who eventually become parents, how do their experiences with illness shape their own parenting? Does surviving a SCT affect their subsequent health practices, such as smoking, alcohol use, unprotected sex, or risk-taking? In general, research with adolescent survivors of cancer has not demonstrated an increased prevalence of risk behaviors,[29–31] but even rates of substance use comparable to that of the general adolescent population might pose special risks for transplant survivors.[30] Finally, we are aware of no studies that have explored the possibility of positive changes or personal growth in the aftermath of pediatric transplant. Over the long term, does their experience with illness and transplant early in life leave some children with enhanced maturity, deeper relationships, greater zest for life, or stronger spiritual ties as they grow older? Such changes have begun to emerge in research with adult SCT recipients[2] and survivors of childhood cancer who have not undergone transplantation.[38]

Another problem that characterizes most of the literature involves reliance on very small samples, which limits the prospects for detecting significant results; there is an obvious need to move toward multi-center collaborative group investigations. Moreover, samples tend to be quite heterogeneous, mixing patients who differ widely across age, disease type and severity, pretransplant treatment history, conditioning regimen, type of transplant, and phase of recovery. The reliance on diverse samples is understandable given the small numbers of patients that have been available to study in any one institution, but it obscures potentially important distinctions among patients from varying developmental levels receiving different treatments for different illnesses. Several prospective studies have examined short-term outcomes,[6,13,17,20] but as yet we are aware of no longitudinal research concerning longer-term adjustment. The reliance on cross-sectional designs (i.e., patients assessed on one occasion) limits information about how outcomes change over time or how they may be influenced by other factors. Moreover, some of the research is undermined by measurement problems. Some investigations have used unvalidated or minimally validated measures, which limit confidence in the findings and inhibit comparison across studies. There has been minimal use of health-related quality of life instruments to supplement information from measures of behavioral or emotional adjustment. Recently, several of these instruments have been developed for use with children (e.g., Behavioral, Affective and Somatic Experiences Scale,[33] Pediatric Quality of Life Inventory[34]) which should facilitate future investigations.

How do findings from research on pediatric transplant recipients compare to the broader literature on adjustment to childhood cancer? Results from childhood cancer survivors (who have not undergone SCT) are conflicting. On balance, many studies suggest favorable global adjustment; overall psychosocial functioning for cancer survivors is not worse than that of healthy peers or population test norms.[35–37] However, some children experience more marked or enduring distress. Moreover, specific areas of difficulty may be more common than broad indicators of psychopathology.[35] For example, problems with identity formation have been noted among adolescent cancer survivors.[38,39] Relative to healthy peers, cancer survivors were more likely to display a "foreclosed" identity status, expressing commitment to goals and values without having questioned them or explored alternative beliefs.[39] These adolescents appeared to prematurely adapt the values and beliefs of adults in their lives, avoiding the uncertainty of exploring other possibilities. Other studies have suggested a tendency toward excessive compliance, caution, or conformity.[40] Some have highlighted a proclivity to minimize or blunt emotional distress (i.e., repressive coping[41,42]), which is a coping style that may be characteristic of children with a number of chronic illnesses.[42] Though findings are not invariant, other areas of concern for some survivors include social functioning,[32,43,44] body image, sexuality, fertility,[32,40] and PTSD symptoms.[45,46] Additional studies are needed to examine these outcomes specifically among SCT patients, with due attention to differences in children's treatment history, phase of recovery, and level of development.

## FACTORS ASSOCIATED WITH PSYCHOSOCIAL RISK AND RESILIENCE

Notwithstanding the difficulties noted above, it appears that many transplant patients and their families adapt remarkably well to a daunting treatment. Which children may be most vulnerable to adjustment problems and which are most resilient? Clues are limited, given that few studies have focused on pediatric transplant recipients, and even fewer have explored predictors of outcomes. Several theoretical models have been offered to help explain the wide disparities in adjustment noted among children with chronic illnesses. Varni and Wallender,[47] for example, delineated a number of risk and resistance factors drawn from stress and coping theory. Most conceptual frameworks incorporate medical and demographic characteristics (e.g., disease severity), personal resources (e.g., premorbid adjustment, coping), and family/social context (e.g., family adaptability, concomitant stressors).

Research with adult transplant patients has yielded inconsistent findings concerning the effects of basic medical variables such as diagnosis, allogeneic versus autologous transplant, quality of graft, and chronic GVHD. Among pediatric recipients, children who received autologous transplants experienced significantly fewer somatic difficulties, better activity level, and marginally less mood disturbance during the posttransplant period compared with those who received allogeneic transplants.[19] Younger children displayed significantly fewer somatic problems, better activity level, and marginally fewer mood problems than older children. And those from families with greater socioeconomic resources had better outcomes in each of these areas than those from poorer families. Other studies have not found strong effects for these variables among pediatric recipients,[13,18,22] perhaps due in part to small sample sizes.

Although young children may display less emotional distress in response to SCT than their older counterparts, very young children (i.e., age 3 and younger) are more vulnerable to cognitive deficits.[26,27] Those receiving cranial irradiation also have been thought to be at greater risk for cognitive impairment, but a number of studies have not confirmed this expectation.[26] The effects of CNS-directed treatment on psychosocial as opposed to neurocognitive functioning have rarely been investigated. Interestingly, however, several studies hint that CNS treatment may contribute to vulnerability to social difficulties.[21,25] For example, children who had received TBI or whole brain radiation therapy an average of 3.6 years earlier were perceived by their classroom peers as more socially withdrawn and isolated (though not less well liked[25]). Adjustment has not been strongly associated with other basic medical and demographic variables, such as gender,[18,19] pretransplant symptom severity,[13] or, among long-term survivors, time since transplant.[25] Clearly, however, additional research is needed to examine the potential impact of demographic and medical variables at various phases of treatment.

Adjustment would be expected to be influenced not only by characteristics of the illness and treatment, but by the resources of the child and family as well. For example, in a recent prospective study, children who displayed better adaptive functioning shortly after diagnosis (i.e., better communication, socialization, and daily living skills) subsequently developed fewer emotional and behavioral problems six months after transplant.[13] In other words, personal strengths seemed to have protective value. Adjustment is also powerfully shaped by family context. Children who came from families characterized by greater cohesion or closeness subsequently demonstrated better quality of life (i.e., better role functioning, emotional functioning, and physical functioning) at the six-month follow-up assessment.[13] They also demonstrated higher behavior problem scores, though still within normal limits, which the investigators interpreted as healthy "acting out." Similarly, in another recent study,[18] greater cohesion and expressiveness within the family prior to transplant were associated with better emotional well-being, self-concept, and social competence for the child 6–12 months following transplant. Conversely, higher levels of family conflict prior to transplant were associated with greater anxiety, less social competence, and greater behavior problems following transplant. Outside the SCT setting, the considerable impact of the family system on children's adjustment to cancer (and in turn, the impact of the child's illness on the family) has been a consistent theme in the literature.[11,48]

Taken together, these preliminary findings begin to sketch an initial picture of children who may be most at risk for adjustment difficulties, and for whom intervention efforts may be most pressing. These patients include older children or adolescents, those receiving allogeneic transplants or perhaps intensive CNS treatment, and those from families characterized by fewer economic resources or greater conflict or disengagement. The contours of this portrait are tentative, however, and considerable work is needed to broaden its outlines and define its features. Among children with cancer, for example, negative perceptions of physical appearance have been associated with greater anxiety and depression;[49] one would anticipate similar findings among SCT patients, for whom alterations in appearance are not uncommon. Similarly, limited social support, particularly from classmates, has been linked to greater adjustment problems among children with recently diagnosed cancer.[50] Other contextual factors that may influence children's response to transplant but have yet to be explored include the family's parenting practices (e.g., overprotectiveness[51]), health beliefs[52] (e.g., fatalism, self-efficacy), and cultural and religious commitments (e.g., God health locus of control[53]). It may be especially instructive to examine connections between these variables and specific transplant-related outcomes (e.g., adherence to mouth care, anxious avoidance of bone marrow biopsies, difficulty returning to school) rather than global measures of adjustment.

## FAMILY ADJUSTMENT

The patient's illness and transplant have a profound impact on the entire family. Having a gravely ill child is one of the most jarring experiences a parent can face. In addition to confronting the possibility of losing their child, parents of transplant patients must mobilize the family for clinic visits and hospitalizations, arrange time away from work or other responsibilities, and negotiate new roles and priorities within the family, while continuing to provide for the needs of other children or elderly members.[54] Nodal events such as the search for a donor (if autologous transplant is not an option), hospitalization,[55] and the wait for engraftment after transplantation are periods of heightened stress and anxiety.[56,57] Access to family and friends—critical sources of support—may be disrupted by lengthy treatments at facilities far from home. The demands of treatment may be especially burdensome for single-parent families. Even after the active phase of treatment has been successfully completed, chronic stressors may include ongoing follow-up appointments, anxiety about recurrence, and delayed complications and late medical effects.[58] In our experience, distress or delayed grief are not uncommon after a successful transplant; these reactions may be particularly hard to cope with because they are generally unexpected (at this point the family expects an emotional "uplift" rather than a "letdown"), and because by now social support may begin to recede.[10,59]

Few studies have focused specifically on the experience of parents of SCT patients,[55,60] but there is a large amount of literature concerning adjustment among parents of children with cancer. Not surprisingly, following the acute crisis of diagnosis, parents demonstrate heightened emotional distress, such as anxiety, depression, and marital distress.[61,62] In most studies[63,64] distress is less pronounced one year or more after diagnosis, though some investigations[65] continue to find elevated symptoms. In particular, parents experience higher levels of posttraumatic stress symptoms (though not necessarily posttraumatic stress disorder) than do parents of healthy children, even when assessed several years after treatment has been completed.[58,66] Interestingly, posttraumatic stress reactions are more pronounced among parents than among the child survivors,[58] which underscores the dramatic impact of illness on the family.

Predictors of parents' adjustment include some of the same risk and resource variables identified as important among children with cancer. Objective characteristics of the illness (e.g., relapse vs. remission;[64] functional impairment[62]) have been associated with parental adjustment, but more robust correlates include subjective beliefs about the illness (e.g., perceived life threat[48,58] and positive expectations for recovery[64]), family resources (e.g., family cohesion, satisfaction,[58] parenting stress[67]), and social support (e.g., network size,[48,58] perceived support,[68] and social constraints[68]). Some correlates of adjustment (e.g., coping[65]) differ for mothers and fathers.

Siblings are also powerfully affected by the transplant experience. They may feel neglected by busy parents, dismayed by the toxic side effects they witness, anxious about the patient's recovery, and disgruntled by frequent separations from the patient and parents during extended treatment intervals. Normal family routines are disrupted, new roles and responsibilities may be required, and opportunities outside the home may be constrained. Efforts to adapt to these changes may be undermined by fears that they too may get sick, and by the limited medical information that children often receive from their well-meaning parents.[7] At the same time, illness in the family may pave the way toward positive changes as well, such as enhanced empathy, self-reliance, or family closeness.[69]

Siblings who donate marrow or stem cells for allogeneic transplants may have a different experience than those who do not. There have been concerns that some young donors may perceive the process as an invasion of their body integrity or identity;[70] others may be burdened by an unrealistic sense of responsibility for the outcome (e.g., GVHD or death).[71,72] As highlighted by Weisz and Robbennolt,[73] outcomes are more important than good intentions in shaping moral judgments and feelings of guilt among younger children. Non-donors, on the other hand, may feel alternately envious of the heroic role their donor sibling gets to play, relieved that they are not needed, or neglected and ignored.[7,70]

Thus far, there has been very little research concerning siblings of pediatric SCT patients. Preliminary findings hint at greater adjustment difficulties for donors compared to non-donors.[56,72] For example, among children and adolescents assessed several years after transplant, donor siblings displayed greater anxiety, lower self-esteem, and more developmental difficulties than non-donor siblings, although teachers rated the donors more favorably.[72] Moderate PTSD symptoms were evident in approximately one-third of children from both groups. During interviews, participants reported that they had received very little information about transplantation, and the donors expressed a desire to be included more actively in the decision-making process.[7] Research among adult marrow donors similarly has suggested that siblings may have more troubled reactions to the experience (i.e., more pain and depressive symptoms) than unrelated donors.[74]

On the other hand, highly positive experiences have been noted among both children[73] and adult[75] donors, including a sense of altruism, greater closeness in the family, and enhanced meaning in life. Participating in the care of a loved one can be enormously gratifying. Most child sibling donors interviewed several years after transplant noted that they felt like a better person after the experience and that they would make the same choice again.[7] Obviously, the risk of adjustment difficulties would be expected to be much more pronounced if the patient dies than if the transplant is successful.[73] Interestingly, however, when evaluated one year after harvest, adult sibling donors whose recipient had died demonstrated better psychological adjustment compared to sibling donors whose recipient remained alive.[75] It is not clear whether children would react to these circumstances in the same way. Clearly, there is a need for further research concerning adjustment among donor and non-donor childhood siblings, in cases where treatment is successful as well as those where it is not.

## PSYCHOSOCIAL INTERVENTIONS

Most transplant centers include pediatric psychologists and social workers as members of the interdisciplinary treatment team. Ideally, all patients and families should be seen for preliminary screening and support during their initial medical work-up, as a routine part of comprehensive care. These interviews help educate families about psychosocial aspects of illness, and facilitate identification and preemptive treatment of problems before they develop into more serious complications that might compromise care. A range of services should be available to families as they transition through active treatment and long-term follow-up. Access to individual and family counseling, psychopharmacological services, and pastoral care are basic aspects of supportive care. For some children, neuropsychological testing is important in order to identify and track specific cognitive deficits. In addition, support groups can be helpful in diminishing feelings of isolation and enhancing adjustment to a rigorous treatment. Different types of group interventions have been designed for patients, parents, and siblings. Many transplant programs are not large enough to sustain group services solely for SCT patients, so where they are available, these groups are often open to patients with mixed oncologic or hematologic disorders.

Thus far, interventions to improve adjustment and coping have received very little empirical study either in the transplant setting or among pediatric cancer patients more generally. Documenting outcomes and delineating which children are most responsive to which interventions remains a pressing agenda for future research. Among some of the more innovative interventions that have begun to be tested are use of massage and humor during active treatment,[76] social skills training to facilitate the transition back to school,[77] and multi-family group therapy to enhance long-term recovery.[11,59]

Psychological interventions also may play a useful role in symptom management. These strategies have been used as adjunctive treatments to help ameliorate pain or chemotherapy-related nausea.[78] They also have been employed to diminish distress and adherence problems associated with invasive procedures (e.g., bone marrow aspiration, lumbar puncture, venipuncture[79]). Regrettably, in our experience these services are often either unavailable or greatly underutilized. Typically interventions include relaxation training, imagery, hypnosis, modeling, or distraction using video games or cartoons. More comprehensive programs to address procedure-related distress have included use of distracting, relaxing activities (e.g., computer games), reinforcement through praise and stickers, and behavioral rehearsal beginning with noninvasive routines (e.g., blood pressure measurement) and simulated procedures (e.g., fake needles), followed by exposure to the actual feared procedure.[80] Parents and medical staff are trained to serve as coaches. The efficacy of these types of approaches for procedure-related pain is well established in the pediatric literature,[81] although few studies have focused specifically on SCT patients. In contrast to the growing number of studies targeting symptom management and adherence among pediatric patients during active treatment, little attention has been directed toward improving long-term psychosocial outcomes. One of several areas that merit further exploration involves health practices and self-care. It remains unclear whether the prevalence of poor health behaviors (e.g., smoking, alcohol use, unprotected sex) is elevated among SCT survivors, but the risks of these practices may be greater, warranting concerted efforts toward prevention.[30,31]

## CONCLUSIONS

Stem cell transplantation presents considerable challenges to children and their families. From the acute treatment phase through long-term recovery, it affects multiple dimensions of quality of life. Research is in its early stages, but investigators have began to trace the outlines of this terrain, enhancing our understanding of which spheres of functioning are most affected at which points in the trajectory of treatment. We anticipate that the growing emphasis on quality of life will intensify research efforts in this area, extending our appreciation of the myriad obstacles that families face over time, the factors that contribute to risk, and the important resources that facilitate adaptation and growth. These efforts may be bolstered by the availability of improved assessment instruments for children, and by greater opportunities for multi-center collaboration.

# REFERENCES

1. Ganz PA. Quality of life and the patient with cancer: individual and policy implications. Cancer 1994;74:1445–1452.
2. Andrykowski MA, Cordova MJ, Hann DM et al. Patients' psychosocial concerns following stem cell transplantation. Bone Marrow Transplant 1999;24:1121–1129.
3. Tedeschi RG, Park CL, Calhoun LG (eds). Posttraumatic Growth: Positive Changes in the Aftermath of Crisis. Mahwah: Lawrence Erlbaum, 1998.
4. Parsons SK, Barlow SE, Levy SL et al. Health-related quality of life in pediatric bone marrow transplant survivors: according to whom? Int J Cancer Suppl 1999;12:46–51.
5. Phipps S, DeCuir-Whalley S. Adherence issues in pediatric bone marrow transplantation. J Pediatr Psychol 1990;15:459–475.
6. Phipps S, Dunavant M, Garvie PA et al. Acute health-related quality of life in children undergoing stem cell transplant: I. descriptive outcomes. Bone Marrow Transplant 2002;29:425–434.
7. Packman WL, Crittenden MR, Fischer J et al. Siblings' perceptions of the bone marrow transplantation process. J Psychosoc Oncol 1997;15:81–105.
8. Sourkes BM. Psychological aspects of leukemia and other hematological disorders. In: Nathan D, Oski F, eds. Hematology of Infancy and Childhood. Philadelphia: WB Saunders, 1992:1754–1768.
9. Buchsel PC, Leum EW, Randolph SR. Delayed complications of bone marrow transplantation: an update. Oncol Nurs Forum 1996;23:1267–1291.
10. Sherman AC, Simonton S. Family therapy for cancer patients: clinical issues and interventions. Family J 1999;7:39–50.
11. Ostroff J, Ross S, Steinglass P. Psychosocial adaptation following treatment: a family systems perspective on childhood cancer survivorship. In: Baider L, Kaplan De-Nour A (eds). Cancer and the Family (2nd ed). New York: John Wiley, 2000:155–173.
12. Sherman AC, Simonton S. Coping with cancer in the family. Family J 2001;9:193–200.
13. Barrera M, Pringle L-AB, Sumbler K et al. Quality of life and behavioral adjustment after pediatric bone marrow transplantation. Bone Marrow Transplant 2000;26:427–435.
14. Lee ML, Cohen SE, Stuber ML et al. Parent-child interactions with pediatric bone marrow transplant patients. J Psychosoc Oncol 1994;12:43–60.
15. Stuber ML, Nader K, Yasuda P et al. Stress responses after pediatric bone marrow transplantation: preliminary results of a prospective longitudinal study. J Am Acad Child Adolesc Psychiatry 1991;30:952–957.
16. McConville BJ, Steichen-Asch P, Harris R et al. Pediatric bone marrow transplants: psychological aspects. Can J Psychiatry 1990;35:769–775.
17. Phipps S, Brenner M, Heslop H et al. Psychological effects of bone marrow transplantation on children and adolescents: preliminary report of a longitudinal study. Bone Marrow Transplant 1995;15:829–835.
18. Phipps S, Mulhern RK. Family cohesion and expressiveness promote resilience to the stress of pediatric bone marrow transplant: a preliminary report. J Dev Behav Pediatr 1995;16:257–263.
19. Phipps S, Dunavant M, Lensing S et al. Acute health-related quality of life in children undergoing stem cell transplant: II. medical and demographic determinants. Bone Marrow Transplant 2002;29:435–442.
20. Pot-Mees CC. The Psychosocial Effects of Bone Marrow Transplantation in Children. Delft: Eburon Publishers, 1989.
21. Arvidson J, Larsson B, Lonnerholm G. A long-term follow-up study of psychosocial functioning after autologous bone marrow transplantation in childhood. Psychooncology 1999;8:123–134.
22. Badell I, Igual L, Gomez P et al. Quality of life in young adults having received a BMT during childhood: a GETMON study. Bone Marrow Transplant 1998;21(Suppl 2):S68–S71.
23. Felder-Puig R, Peters C, Matthes-Martin S et al. Psychosocial adjustment of pediatric patients after allogeneic stem cell transplantation. Bone Marrow Transplant 1999;24:75–80.
24. Schmidt GM, Niland JC, Forman SJ et al. Extended follow-up in 212 long-term allogeneic bone marrow transplant survivors: issues of quality of life. Transplantation 1993;55:551–557.
25. Vannatta K, Zeller M, Noll RB et al. Social functioning of children surviving bone marrow transplantation. J Pediatr Psychol 1998;23:169–178.
26. Phipps S, Dunavant M, Srivastava DK et al. Cognitive and academic functioning in survivors of pediatric bone marrow transplantation. J Clin Oncol 2000;18:1004–1011.
27. Kramer JH, Crittenden MR, DeSantes K et al. Cognitive and adaptive behavior 1 and 3 years following bone marrow transplantation. Bone Marrow Transplant 1997;19:607–613.
28. Noll RB, Bukowski WM, Rogosch FA et al. Peer relationships and adjustment in children with cancer. J Pediatr Psychol 1991;16:307–326.
29. Haupt R, Byrne J, Connelly RR. Smoking habits in survivors of childhood and adolescent cancer. Med Pediatr Oncol 1992;20:301–306.

30. Hollen PJ, Hobbie WL. Decision-making and risk behaviors of cancer-surviving adolescents and their peers. J Pediatr Oncol Nurs 1996;13:121–134.
31. Mulhern RK, Tyc VL, Phipps S et al. Health-related behaviors of survivors of childhood cancer. Med Pediatr Oncol 1995;25:159–165.
32. Gray RE, Doan BD, Shermer P et al. Surviving childhood cancer: a descriptive approach to understanding the impact of life-threatening illness. Psychooncology 1992;1:235–246.
33. Phipps S, Dunavant M, Jayawardene D et al. Assessment of health-related quality of life in acute in-patient settings: use of the BASES instrument in children undergoing bone marrow transplantation. Intl J Cancer Suppl 1999;12:18–24.
34. Varni JW, Seid M, Kurtin PS. PedsQL 4.0: reliability and validity of the Pediatric Quality of Life Inventory Version 4.0. Generic core scales in healthy and patient populations. Med Care 2001;39:800–812.
35. Eiser C. Practitioner review: long-term consequences of childhood cancer. J Child Psychol Psychiatry 1998;39:621–633.
36. Eiser C, Hill JJ, Vance YH. Examining the psychological consequences of surviving childhood cancer: systematic review as a research method in pediatric psychology. J Pediatr Psychol 2000;25:449–460.
37. Elkin TD, Phipps S, Mulhern RK et al. Psychological functioning of adolescent and young adult survivors of pediatric malignancy. Med Pediatr Oncol 1997;29:582–588.
38. Gavaghan MP, Roach JE. Ego identity development of adolescents with cancer. J Pediatr Psychol 1987;12:203–213.
39. Madan-Swain A, Brown RT, Foster MA et al. Identity in adolescent survivors of childhood cancer. J Pediatr Psychol 2000;25:105–115.
40. Madan-Swain A, Brown RT, Sexson SB et al. Adolescent cancer survivors: psychosocial and family adaptation. Psychosom 1994;35:453–459.
41. Canning EH, Canning RD, Boyce WT. Depressive symptoms and adaptive style in children with cancer. J Am Acad Child Adolesc Psychiatry 1992;31:1120–1124.
42. Phipps S, Steele R. Repressive adaptive style in children with chronic illness. Psychosom Med 2002;64:34–42.
43. Mulhern RK, Wasserman AL, Friedman AG et al. Social competence and behavioral adjustment of children who are long-term survivors of cancer. Pediatrics 1989;83:18–25.
44. Stern M, Norman SL, Zevon MA. Adolescents with cancer: self-image and perceived social support as indices of adaptation. J Adolesc Res 1993;8:124–142.
45. Hobbie WL, Stuber M, Meeske K et al. Symptoms of posttraumatic stress in young adult survivors of childhood cancer. J Clin Oncol 2000;18:4060–4066.
46. Pelcovitz D, Libov BG, Mandel F et al. Posttraumatic stress disorder and family functioning in adolescent cancer. J Trauma Stress 1998;11:205–221.
47. Varni JW, Wallander JL. Pediatric chronic disabilities. In: Routh DK, ed. Handbook of Pediatric Psychology. New York: Guilford; 1988:190–221.
48. Kazak AE, Stuber ML, Barakat LP et al. Predicting posttraumatic stress symptoms in mothers and fathers of survivors of childhood cancers. J Am Acad Child Adolesc Psychiatry 1998;37:823–831.
49. Varni JW, Katz ER, Colegrove R Jr et al. Perceived physical appearance and adjustment of children with newly diagnosed cancer: a path analytic model. J Behav Med 1995;18:261–278.
50. Varni JW, Katz ER, Colegrove R Jr et al. Perceived social support and adjustment of children with newly diagnosed cancer. J Dev Behav Pediatr 1994;15:20–26.
51. Thomasgard M, Shonkoff JP, Metz WP et al. Parent-child relationship disorders: part II. The vulnerable child syndrome and its relation to parental overprotection. J Dev Behav Pediatr 1995;16:251–256.
52. Rosenstock IM, Strecher VJ, Becker MH. Social learning theory and the health belief model. Health Educ Q 1988;15:175–183.
53. Wallston KA, Malcarne VL, Flores L et al. Does God determine your health? The God Locus of Health Control Scale. Cogni Ther Res 1999;23:131–142.
54. Varni JW, Katz ER, Colegrove R Jr et al. Family functioning predictors of adjustment in children with newly diagnosed cancer: a prospective analysis. J Clin Psychol Psychiatry 1996;3:321–328.
55. Sormanti M, Dungan S, Rieker PP. Pediatric bone marrow transplantation: psychosocial issues for parents after a child's hospitalization. J Psychosoc Oncol 1994;12:23–42.
56. Pott-Mees CC, Zeitlin H. Psychosocial consequences of bone marrow transplantation in children: a preliminary communication. J Psychosoc Oncol 1989;5:73–81.
57. Phipps S, Barclay D. Psychosocial consequences of pediatric bone marrow transplantation. Int J Pediatr Hematol/Oncol 1996;3:171–182.
58. Barakat LP, Kazak AE, Meadows AT et al. Families surviving childhood cancer: a comparison of posttraumatic stress symptoms with families of healthy children. J Pediatr Psychol 1997;22:843–859.
59. Kazak AE, Simms S, Barakat L et al. Surviving Cancer Competently Intervention Program (SCCIP): a cognitive-behavioral and family therapy intervention for adolescent survivors of childhood cancer and their families. Fam Process 1999;38:175–191.

60. Dermatis H, Lesko LM. Psychological distress in parents consenting to child's bone marrow transplantation. Bone Marrow Transplant 1990;6:411–417.
61. Dahlquist L, Czyzewski D, Copeland K et al. Parents of children newly diagnosed with cancer: anxiety, coping, and marital distress. J Pediatr Psychol 1993;18:365–376.
62. Manne SL, Lesanics D, Meyers P et al. Predictors of depressive symptomatology among parents of newly diagnosed children with cancer. J Pediatr Psychol 1995;20:491–510.
63. Dahlquist LM, Czyzewski DI, Jones CL. Parents of children with cancer: a longitudinal study of emotional distress, coping style, and marital adjustment two and twenty months after diagnosis. J Pediatr Psychol 1996;21:541–554.
64. Grootenhuis MA, Last BF. Predictors of parental emotional adjustment to childhood cancer. Psychooncology 1997;6:115–128.
65. Hoekstra-Weebers JEHM, Jaspers JPC, Kamps WA et al. Gender differences in psychological adaptation and coping in parents of pediatric cancer patients. Psychooncology 1998;7:26–36.
66. Kazak AE, Barakat LP, Meese K et al. Posttraumatic stress, family functioning, and social support in survivors of childhood leukemia and their mothers and fathers. J Consult Clin Psychol 1997;65:120–129.
67. Kazak AE, Barakat LP. Brief report: parenting, stress and quality of life during treatment for childhood leukemia predicts child and parent adjustment after treatment ends. J Pediatr Psychol 1997;22:749–758.
68. Manne SL, Duhamel K, Redd WH. Association of psychological vulnerability factors to post-traumatic stress symptomatology in mothers of pediatric cancer survivors. Psychooncology 2000;9:372–384.
69. Houtzager BA, Grootenhuis MA, Last BF. Adjustment of siblings to childhood cancer: a literature review. Support Care Cancer 1999;7:302–320.
70. Wiley FM, Lindamood M, Pfefferbaum-Levine B. Donor-patient relationship in pediatric bone marrow transplantation. J Assoc Pediatr Oncol Nurses 1984;1:8–14.
71. Rappaport BS. Evolution of consultation-liaison services in BMT. Gen Hosp Psychiatry 1988;10:346–351.
72. Packman WL, Crittenden MR, Schaeffer E et al. Psychosocial consequences of bone marrow transplantation in donor and nondonor siblings. J Dev Behav Pediatr 1997;18:244–253.
73. Weisz V, Robbennolt JK. Risks and benefits of pediatric bone marrow donation: a critical need for research. Behav Sci Law 1996;14:375–391.
74. Chang G, McGarigle C, Spitzer TR et al. A comparison of related and unrelated marrow donors. Psychosom Med 1998;60:163–167.
75. Switzer GE, Dew MA, Magistro CA et al. The effects of bereavement on adult sibling bone marrow donors' psychological well-being and reactions to donation. Bone Marrow Transplant 1998;21:181–188.
76. Phipps S. Behavioral research in pediatric stem cell transplantation. Paper presented at Oncology Ground Rounds, Arkansas Cancer Research Center, Little Rock, AR, Jan. 30, 2002.
77. Varni JW, Katz ER, Colegrove R Jr et al. The impact of social skills training on the adjustment of children with newly diagnosed cancer. J Pediatr Psychol 1993;18:751–767.
78. McQuaid EL, Nassau JH. Empirically supported treatments of disease-related symptoms in pediatric psychology: asthma, diabetes, and cancer. J Pediatr Psychol 1999;24:305–328.
79. Blount RL, Powers SW, Cotter MW et al. Making the system work: training pediatric oncology patients to cope and their parents to coach them during BMA/LP procedures. Behav Modif 1994;18:6–31.
80. Slifer KJ, Babbitt RL, Cataldo MD. Simulation and counterconditioning as adjuncts to pharmacotherapy for invasive pediatric procedures. Dev Behav Pediatr 1995;16:133–141.
81. Powers SW. Empirically supported treatments in pediatric psychology: procedure-related pain. J Pediatr Psychol 1999;24:131–145.

# CHAPTER VIII

# Medically Indicated Banking of Sibling Donor Cord Blood

WILLIAM REED AND BERTRAM H. LUBIN

Umbilical cord blood has become an important alternative source of hematopoietic stem cells for transplantation for children who have either malignant or non-malignant diseases.[1-6] A very low risk to the donor coupled with decreased risk of graft-versus-host disease (GVHD), especially in the matched sibling setting,[7] support wider exploration of cord blood (CB) as an alternative stem cell source. However, most activity in the CB banking field has focused on CB banking for the support of unrelated recipients. These efforts have resulted in widespread banking of high quality CB stem cell products[8-12] and these products have been useful as a stem cell source for transplantation.[2,3,13-15] Despite these activities with unrelated CB donors, many families caring for a child with a transplant-treatable illness experience an additional pregnancy. Because there is approximately a 25% probability that a new sibling will be human leukocyte antigen (HLA)-identical to the existing full sibling, parents and physicians often wish to preserve the CB from that birth, but the options available to accomplish this have been limited. Because women of these relatively few families give birth at a variety of smaller hospitals across the United States, it is a considerable logistical challenge to provide access to specialized high quality sibling donor cord blood banking (SDCB) services for them. Many of the operational procedures and medical policies appropriate for national comprehensive SDCB banking contrast sharply with those that have been established recently for unrelated donor CB banking. This chapter summarizes some of these differences based upon our experience in developing a sibling CB program.[1]

## MEDICAL ELIGIBILITY AND SCOPE OF NEED

Cord blood banking follows three separate banking models: autologous, unrelated, and sibling. SDCB banking differs markedly from autologous or commercial family CB banking where there is no existing transplant recipient. We agree with other experts who have questioned the medical value of CB banking services whose primary orientation is commercial rather than medical.[16,17] A comparison of some essential features among these three models for CB banking is presented in ▼ Table 8.1.

Because, in sibling CB banking, one important goal is to obtain an acceptably HLA-matched CB unit for a child with a disease that can be treated by hematopoietic stem cell transplantation, medical eligibility for SDCB banking must address both the genetic

| TABLE 8.1 | Comparative Features Among Three Models for Cord Blood Banking | | |
|---|---|---|---|
| | **Autologous** | **Unrelated** | **Sibling** |
| **Operating Model** | | | |
| Financial status | for-profit | non-profit | non-profit |
| Donation | business transaction | voluntary act | motivated act |
| Donor's status | payer | neutral | non-fiduciary benefit |
| Product ownership | contingent upon payment? | public | family |
| Operating location | remote sites | few specified sites | remote sites |
| Potential size/market | very large | large | small |
| **Safety and QA** | | | |
| Eligibility | all who can pay | medical and lab deferrals | defined medical eligibility with few absolute deferrals |
| ID testing | unpublished | full blood donor ± NAT | donor re-tested ± NAT |
| Genetic disease testing | unpublished | variable | established, often specific to family's mutation |
| Deliberate maneuvers to facilitate CB collection volume | no | no | not excluded |
| Donor-recipient linkage | defining property | usually no or limited | intrinsic |
| Trained collectors | no | yes | limited training at the time of collection |
| Quality Assurance | unpublished | established | under development using blood center model |
| **Disposition of Units** | | | |
| Likelihood of complete histocompatibility | 100% | low | ~25% |
| Likelihood of use for transplant | low to nil | moderate | relatively high |
| Research potential | low to nil | high | high |
| Crossed-over for public use | no | n/a | under discussion |

Abbreviation: NAT = nucleic acid testing for HIV and HCV.

relationship between donor and recipient and the recipient's disease entity. In our program eligibility criteria are constantly being re-examined because stem cell transplantation is a rapidly evolving field. In order to achieve a reasonable probability for collection of an HLA-identical SDCB unit for medically eligible families, we have asked that the parents stipulate a full-sibling relationship between the donor and the potential recipient. Exceptions may be considered on an individual basis for selected half-sibling collections if the medical condition of the recipient is grave and other donor options are limited. The eligible disease entities in the sibling recipient are also the subject of continuing debate. In our program, severe hemoglobinopathies and hematopoietic malignancies are clearly eligible conditions. We have also considered a large assortment of rare non-malignant disorders to be eligible if it is plausible that the condition may be effectively treated by CB transplantation.

Children with solid tumors (other than lymphomas) generally have not been considered eligible by our group.

Far fewer families participate in SDCB banking services compared with either the autologous or unrelated CB banking. Approximately 80,000 patients with sickle cell disease (SCD) live in the Unites States (US). We estimate that each year approximately several hundred full siblings are born and thus may be eligible for SDCB banking (details of this calculation are available from the authors upon request). Transfusion dependent thalassemia is a much less common disorder in the US than SCD and it is more difficult to estimate the number of potentially eligible births. In part, this results from a relative paucity of accurate newborn screening data for thalassemia syndromes; only approximately 5–10% of enrollments in our program have been for thalassemia. In contrast to these numbers, approximately 5000 children in the US age 0–14 are newly diagnosed each year with a malignant process and approximately 40% of these represent hematopoietic malignancies.[18] Actuarial calculations indicate that approximately 1 in 900 individuals in the US population may now be a survivor of childhood cancer.[18] Enrollment in our SDCB program has been consistent with these statistics; more than half of the enrollments are by families caring for a child with a hematopoietic malignancy who are expecting the birth of a new full sibling. A partial list of other conditions that have been treated by SDCB transplantation or for which we have banked sibling CB is shown in ▼ Table 8.2.

## TRACKING THE DONOR'S PREGNANCY: A CASE MANAGEMENT MODEL

Families enrolling in the Children's Hospital Oakland Research Institute (CHORI) SDCB Program are enrolled in a research protocol and sign an informed consent that has been reviewed and approved by an Institutional Review Board.

---

**TABLE 8.2**    **Partial List of Diseases Treated by Transplantation of Umbilical Cord Blood or for Which Directed SDCB Banking Has Been Undertaken**

| | | |
|---|---|---|
| *Malignant diseases:* | Refractory anemia | Hurler syndrome |
| | Thalassemia major | Hunter syndrome |
| Acute lymphocytic leukemia | Sickle cell anemia | Gunther disease |
| Acute myeloid leukemia | Amegakaryocytic thrombocytopenia | Osteopetrosis |
| Juvenile chronic myeloid leukemia | Kostman's syndrome | Globoid cell leukodystrophy |
| Chronic myeloid leukemia | Diamond-Blackfan anemia | Adrenoleukodystrophy |
| Neuroblastoma | Severe combined immunodeficiency | Metachromatic leukodystrophy |
| Myelodysplastic syndrome | X-linked lymphoproliferative | Lesch-Nyhan syndrome |
| Lymphoma | disorder | IPEX syndrome |
| Refractory anemia with excess | X-linked agammaglobulinemia | LDL receptor deficiency |
| blasts | Wiscott-Aldrich syndrome | |
| | Chronic granulomatous disease | |
| *Non-malignant diseases:* | Juvenile dermatomyositis (severe) | |
| | Schwachman-Diamond syndrome | |
| Fanconi anemia | DiGeorge syndrome | |
| Severe aplastic anemia | | |

In the SDCB model, families enroll during pregnancy and their progress is tracked prospectively through gestation. At various stages after enrollment specific tasks must be accomplished including: detailed family education; establishment of a working relationship with the mother's obstetrician; informed consent; donor and family medical history; blood draws for HLA typing and infectious disease testing; assembly, shipping, and receipt of the CB collection kit; and many others. In our case management model, these responsibilities are carefully coordinated among the family, the obstetrician, and the referring physician, usually a pediatric hematologist.

The enrolled family and their child's referring physician must participate actively and bear certain defined responsibilities if a SDCB collection is to be successful. The family must be available to receive a collection kit that contains everything needed to collect, label, and return ship the CB in a validated temperature-stabilized manner back to our laboratories for processing. The family also must accept responsibility to bring this kit with them to the hospital when the mother is admitted in labor and avail themselves for needed blood sampling. The referring physician is asked to provide demographic data and to complete a form summarizing the clinical status of the potential transplant recipient.

## DONOR EVALUATION IN THE SIBLING SETTING

Community donations of whole blood or CB are voluntary and unremunerated; a detailed medical history, focused on risk factors for transmissible diseases (genetic as well as infectious), coupled with an abbreviated physical examination, results in the deferral of donors who present even minimal or (sometimes) theoretical risk. Finally, sophisticated immunological and nucleic acid-based testing procedures detect nearly all established infections for which testing is available. With SDCB banking, however, many of these risk-diminishing strategies cannot operate in exactly the same manner. A mother whose child has an eligible condition participates out of a desire to assist the child, making the donation motivated rather than voluntary. Second, although an identical medical history instrument may be used in unrelated and sibling CB banking, discovered risk factors lead only to documentation rather than automatic donor deferral; the SDCB is collected but held in medical quarantine until its use is contemplated for the designated sibling. In summary, while elimination of risk is usually the goal in unrelated donor CB banking, medical policies for SDCB banking must be designed to discover, document, and manage risk rather than to eliminate it.

## ISSUES IN COLLECTION METHODOLOGY UNIQUE TO THE SIBLING SETTING

Two general methods, with many variations in equipment and style, are in common use for cord blood collection. Most unrelated donor CB programs have a technician trained and specifically assigned to collect CB and perform the donor evaluation. The collection may take place from the delivered placenta in an area separate from the delivery room (ex utero method) or, in some programs, the obstetrician or midwife who is delivering the infant performs the collection during the third stage of labor (in utero method). These methods have proven appropriate and satisfactory, but the ex utero method cannot be applied easily to most sibling collections because many of these collections occur at community hospitals where neither the dedicated personnel nor the equipment and other infrastructure needed for ex utero CB collection is available.

To accomplish a SDCB collection away from the few centers that have an existing CB infrastructure, the obstetrician or midwife who delivers the baby must be willing to participate by collecting and labeling the CB using appropriate equipment and in accordance with specific standard operating procedures. In our program, the vast majority of SDCB births have been at hospitals that identify themselves as "community" rather than "academic." The collection is accomplished during the third stage of labor (after the baby is born but before the placenta is delivered) by the medical professional delivering the infant. While many devices are available for CB collection, simplicity and reliability are at a substantial premium for a sibling CB collection because there is only one chance to correctly accomplish training and collection, and the individual performing the collection may or may not have experience with CB collection. For these reasons, we prefer a single standard 250 mL blood bag with 35 mL citrate-phosphate-dextrose (CPD) anticoagulant and a single needle attached; this set up is among the simplest for CB collection in a closed system.

For autologous and unrelated donor CB collections, it is a well established norm that CB collection should be a painless procedure that does not interfere with or alter the birthing process.[8] In the sibling setting, however, there is a brother or sister with a life-threatening disease and the family is often highly motivated to assure collection of an amount of CB adequate to transplant the sibling. In this setting, insistence on a collection that incurs nearly no risk may not provide the appropriate balance between risk and benefit. Some families, with support from their obstetrician or midwife, may choose to employ a maneuver, such as delivery of the infant to the mother's abdomen prior to cord clamping, in order to safely maximize the CB collection volume. Limited preliminary experience with this technique suggests that is safe and may significantly increases the volume of CB recovered.[19] However, in our experience during a pilot investigation, collections volumes were not significantly different when this maneuver was employed.[1] While this disappointing result may be due to the variability among CB collectors in our experience (different from the Grisaru study), carefully controlled investigation of other maneuvers that may safely augment CB collection volume may be pursued in the future.

With unrelated donor CB collections, women whose pregnancy presents risk of fetal anemia (e.g. maternal-fetal isoimmunization, α-thalassemia, Diamond-Blackfan anemia, and others) are usually deferred from donation whereas in the sibling setting, these women are not deferred because the family history of such a condition may constitute the primary reason the collection is undertaken. We have specifically recommended against any maneuver intended to facilitate the CB collection volume where there is a discernable possibility of fetal anemia.

▼ Figure 8.1 presents one possible analysis of the choices in CB collection methodology depending upon several variables including timing of consent, whether there is a trained collector available, whether the collection represents a public donation or is for an ill sibling, and whether there is a defined risk of fetal anemia.

## DONOR TESTING FOR INFECTIOUS AND GENETIC DISEASES

All participating mothers in the CHORI SDCB Program are tested for transmissible infectious diseases using a panel of serologic donor screening assays as is standard with community blood donors. Infectious disease testing is performed on blood samples from the mother. These assays include: hepatitis B surface antigen (HBsAg), antibody to hepatitis C virus (anti-HCV 3.0), antibody to human immunodeficiency virus (anti-HIV 1/2),

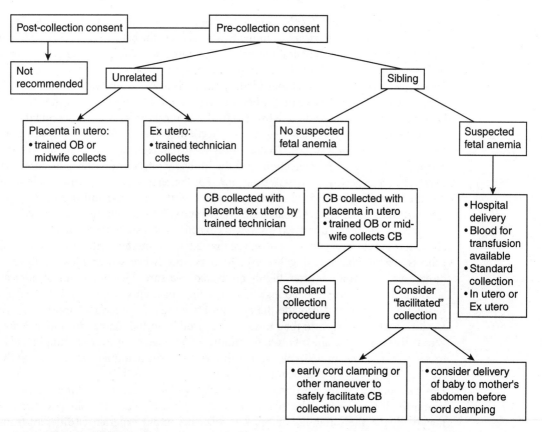

**FIGURE 8.1** Methodological options for the collection of cord blood (CB) from related and unrelated donors. Informed consent and methodological options in the collection of CB from sibling and unrelated donors are illustrated in one possible decision algorithm. It considers the timing of informed consent, whether the collection is medically indicated for a sibling, whether trained collection technicians are available, whether there is suspicion of fetal anemia, and whether the family wishes to utilize maneuvers designed to attempt to augment CB collection volume.

human immunodeficiency virus antigen (HIV p24), antibody to hepatitis B core protein (anti-HBc), antibody to cytomegalovirus (anti-CMV), and antibody to human T cell lymphotropic virus (anti-HTLV I/II). Neither blood grouping nor direct antiglobulin testing is performed on the maternal sample. Nucleic acid testing (NAT) is being added to this battery.

The population of mothers participating in a SDCB Program is not culled by donor deferrals based on medical history and they thus represent, as a group, a higher risk population than do community CB donors. It is likely that rates of seroconversion for transfusion-transmitted viral infections, while low, are higher than the blood donor population, and this may have consequences both for assay performance and medical policy. To reduce the residual risk for infectious disease transmission due to window-period infections in the mother, a second maternal sample is requested for repeat testing >4 months from parturition as has been done with fresh frozen plasma (donor retested strategy). This strategy is employed when a CB unit is being released for transplant and is feasible because of the intrinsic linkage between donor and recipient siblings. Risk for transmission of other infectious diseases must be weighed individually, sometimes with additional testing, at the time a SDCB unit is requested for release. Examples of such potential infectious risks may include families with a travel history to malaria-endemic areas,[20,21] extended European travel, or origin in countries associated with serogroup O HIV.[22,23]

Because many families participating in SDCB collections already have had a child with a hemoglobinopathy, we screen all collections for hemoglobin phenotype with isoelectric focusing. Supplemental techniques such as citrate agar electrophoresis, high performance liquid chromatography, and tandem mass spectroscopy may be utilized when needed to confirm zygosity or the identity of a variant hemoglobin. Thalassemia syndromes may require molecular testing specific for the individual family's globin mutations in order to exclude a clinically significant condition in the CB donor. Testing to exclude other genetic diseases from the CB donor (e.g. chronic granulomatous disease, Diamond Blackfan anemia, severe combined immunodeficiency, etc.) must be individualized and, in our program, is considered only if the CB unit is requested for transplant. Because most transplants for genetic disease are non-emergent, they do not occur until the CB donor reaches more than six months of age. This may allow marrow or mobilized peripheral blood to be obtained as a back-up stem cell source if needed, and also allows some longitudinal assessment of the donor's clinical and hematological characteristics that may be pivotal to the ascertainment or exclusion of a clinically significant genetic disease.

# CELL PROCESSING AND CRYOPRESERVATION OF SIBLING CORD BLOOD

Cell processing and cryopreservation are not fundamentally different for sibling CB units as compared with the unrelated donor CB units. Most CB programs have used a variation on the method of Rubinstein et al.[10] However, certain issues present unique challenges for sibling CB units: completion of cell processing within 48 hours, defining when a sibling CB unit is "too small" to process, and how best to balance cell loss and volume reduction. We shall consider each of these issues individually.

Regulatory guidance in the US from professional organizations such as the Foundation for the Accreditation of Hematopoietic Cell Therapy (FAHCT) and the American Association of Blood Banks (AABB) calls for processing and cryopreservation of CB units to be completed within 48 hours from collection.[24,25] Because, as noted above, many sibling CB units are collected at unpredictable times and at sites often quite remote to the cell processing lab, reliable express shipping must be utilized (at significant cost) to assure that the CB unit reaches the lab and that lab personnel are available to complete processing as soon as practical within the 48 hours.

Because nucleated cell dose has been related to engraftment,[2] it is critically important for an unrelated donor CB bank to store the highest cell count CB units possible. In practice, CB units containing less than $6-8 \times 10^8$ total nucleated cells (TNC) may be discarded rather than being allowed to reach final storage where they have been HLA typed and are accessible to donor searches. While high TNC counts are certainly desirable in the sibling setting, we have chosen to set the storage standard considerably lower than has been customary for unrelated donor CB units. This policy reflects the fact that the sibling CB unit may be of unique value to the family because of HLA identity. Only sibling CB units containing $< 3 \times 10^8$ TNC are discarded. In practice, for our program, this has represented well under 10% of collected CB units. A CB unit containing $3.0 \times 10^8$ TNC will supply a cell dose of $2.5 \times 10^7$ TNC/kg to a 12 kg child; a weight of 12 kg is reached at ages of 21 and 24 months by the average male and female, respectively. Thus, even a "small" sibling CB unit containing only $3.0 \times 10^8$ TNC (which would fall far short of the storage standard for an unrelated CB unit) is capable of delivering an acceptable cell dose for some sibling recipients.

Most cell processing methods for CB have been developed specifically to achieve significant volume reduction for maximally efficient cryostorage of very large numbers of CB units. The average cell loss ($\sim 15\%$) associated with these volume reduction methods may not be optimal for sibling CB banking because they are balanced toward volume reduction. Since, even in a substantial sibling CB program, only a few hundred CB units per year must be stored, alternative cryopreservation methods that place heightened emphasis on cell preservation and less emphasis on volume reduction should be investigated.

## RELEASE OF SDCB UNITS FROM MEDICAL QUARANTINE

All SDCB units are held in medical quarantine pending release for transplantation. Appropriate physical quarantine is also maintained for CB units with a positive infectious marker. Because each recipient's specific illness and clinical situation is different, the release and utilization of a SDCB unit for transplantation is an individual medical decision. This decision can be very complex and requires close collaboration between the SDCB Bank, which provides all relevant information concerning the CB unit, and the child's transplant physician who provides all relevant information concerning the child's particular clinical situation and various treatment options.

In our SDCB model, donors are not routinely deferred according to the usual criteria for public CB banking.[26,27] Instead, any departure from standard community donor suitability criteria is documented, and any issues relevant to safety and effectiveness are addressed individually and in the context of the recipient's specific medical situation at the time a SDCB unit is considered for release. Medical release thus requires a specific written request to the bank's medical director from the transplant physician, and this request must acknowledge a review of all characteristics unique to the particular CB unit. These issues include: the clinical status of the recipient; potential alternate treatment options; characteristics of the mother's pregnancy, labor, and delivery that may bear on risk for transmission of genetic or infectious disease; review of the family medical and donor history; the circumstances of collection; packaging and shipment documentation; graft characteristics; histocompatibility with the intended recipient; and any other circumstances unique to the case. Documents and conditions for release of a SDCB unit from our bank to a transplant center are shown in ▶ Table 8.3.

## QUALITY ASSURANCE AND COMPLIANCE

When CB is collected from unrelated donors, as with the collection of whole blood from community donors, strategies to diminish risk for transmissible disease operate at several levels and within the context of a detailed quality assurance plan.[28,29] Although a regulatory structure for human cellular and tissue-based products has not yet been finalized by the Food and Drug Administration (FDA),[30–32] we chose to adopt the blood center model for operations and quality assurance for the SDCB project at CHORI and to comply with standards promulgated by professional organizations[24,25] wherever possible, given the unique challenges encountered with remote site SDCB collections in the sibling setting. Specifically, our project's quality plan includes process control and error management, standards for supplier qualifications, and training of staff. Process control is achieved with standard operating procedures and policies (SOPPs), which address document control, label control, validation, inventory control, data integrity, and safety as well as other important areas of policy and operations. A system of internal audits and error management is also utilized to assess compliance with SOPPs.

## CONCLUSIONS

Banking of CB for siblings comprises a unique directed donation banking activity for a very limited number of medically eligible families. Many aspects of this unique banking activity are different from either the unrelated donor or the autologous models of CB banking. While many important issues have yet to be fully resolved with respect to medical and regulatory policy, the scope of and need for SDCB banking services is becoming more apparent as clinical progress is reported with transplantation of sibling CB. Perhaps most exciting is the prospect that a national comprehensive SDCB bank will be able to serve as the first research resource able to support prospective clinical trials in SDCB transplantation. Our group is currently initiating such a phase 1-2 trial for matched sibling CB transplantation of children with clinically severe hemoglobinopathies. Preliminary results upon which this trial is based have been very exciting.[2]

| TABLE 8.3 | Requirements for the Release of a SDCB Unit at Children's Hospital Oakland to a Transplant Center |
|---|---|

Copy of the transplant protocol to be used
Copy of the transplant center's Institutional Review Board (IRB) approval for the transplant protocol to be used
Copy of the family's signed informed consent for transplantation on this protocol
Copy of the CBU thawing SOP to be used if it is other than that recommended by SDCB Program
Post-thaw graft characterization data
Clinical outcome data in a timely manner

## ACKNOWLEDGMENTS

Support of the authors is from a Research Resource Grant (1-U24-HL61877-01) from the National Heart, Lung, and Blood Institute and in part by a Pediatric Clinical Research Center Grant (M-O1-RRO1271-16) from the National Institutes of Health; Support is also provided in part by gifts from the Children's Hospital Branches, the Y&H Soda Foundation, the McGowan Foundation, and through a contract with the state of California Genetic Disease Branch.

# REFERENCES

1. Reed W, Smith R, Dekovic F et al. Comprhensive banking of sibling donor cord blood for children with malignant and nonmalignant disease. Blood 2003;101:351–357.
2. Locatelli F, Rocha V, Reed W et al. Related umbilical cord blood transplantation in patients with thalassemia and sickle cell disease. Blood 2003;101:2137–2143.
3. Kurtzberg J, Laughlin M, Graham ML et al. Placental blood as a source of hematopoietic stem cells for transplantation into unrelated recipients. N Engl J Med 1996;335:157–166.
4. Gluckman E, Rocha V, Boyer-Chammard A et al. Outcome of cord-blood transplantation from related and unrelated donors. Eurocord Transplant Group and the European Blood and Marrow Transplantation Group. N Engl J Med 1997;337:373–381.
5. Rubinstein P, Carrier C, Scaradavou A et al. Outcomes among 562 recipients of placental-blood transplants from unrelated donors. N Engl J Med 1998;339:1565–1577.
6. Rubinstein P, Adamson JW, Stevens C. The placental/umbilical cord blood program of the New York Blood Center. A progress report [In Process Citation]. Ann N Y Acad Sci 1999;872:328–334; discussion 334–335.
7. Rocha V, Cornish J, Sievers EL et al. Comparison of outcomes of unrelated bone marrow and umbilical cord blood transplants in children with acute leukemia. Blood 2001;97:2962–2971.
8. Gluckman E, Rocha V, Chevret S. Results of unrelated umbilical cord blood hematopoietic stem cell transplant. Transfus Clin Biol 2001;8:146–154.
9. Rocha V, Wagner JE Jr., Sobocinski KA et al. Graft-versus-host disease in children who have received a cord-blood or bone marrow transplant from an HLA-identical sibling. Eurocord and International Bone Marrow Transplant Registry Working Committee on Alternative Donor and Stem Cell Sources. N Engl J Med 2000; 342:1846–1854.
10. Fraser JK, Cairo MS, Wagner EL et al. Cord Blood Transplantation Study (COBLT): cord blood bank standard operating procedures (see comments). J Hematother 1998;7:521–561.
11. Gluckman E, Wagner J, Hows J et al. Cord blood banking for hematopoietic stem cell transplantation: an international cord blood transplant registry. Bone Marrow Transplant 1993;11:199–200.
12. Rubinstein P, Dobrila L, Rosenfield RE et al. Processing and cryopreservation of placental/umbilical cord blood for unrelated bone marrow reconstitution. Proc Natl Acad Sci USA 1995;92:10119–10122.
13. Rubinstein P, Rosenfield RE, Adamson JW et al. Stored placental blood for unrelated bone marrow reconstitution. Blood 1993;81:1679–1690.
14. Harris D, Schumacher M, Rychlik S et al. Collection, separation and cryopreservation of umbilical cord blood for use in transplantation. Bone Marrow Transplant 1994;13:135–143.
15. Wagner J, Rosenthal J, Sweetman R et al. Successful transplantation of HLA-matched and HLA-mismatched umbilical cord blood from unrelated donors: analysis of engraftment and acute graft-versus-host disease. Blood 1996;88:795–802.
16. Rocha V, Chastang C, Souillet G et al. Related cord blood transplants: the Eurocord experience from 78 transplants. Eurocord Transplant group. Bone Marrow Transplant 1998;21(Suppl 3):S59–S62.
17. Wagner JE, Kernan NA, Steinbuch M et al. Allogeneic sibling umbilical-cord-blood transplantation in children with malignant and non-malignant disease (see comments). Lancet 1995;346:214–219.
18. Annas GJ. Legal issues in medicine: waste and longing — the legal status of placental-blood banking. N Engl J Med 1999;340:1521–1524.
19. Johnson FL. Placental blood transplantation and autologous banking—caveat emptor. J Pediatr Hematol Oncol 1997;19:183–186.
20. Nathan DG, Orkin SH (eds). Hematology of Infancy and Childhood (vol. 2, 5th ed). Philidelphia: W.B. Saunders, 1998.
21. Grisaru D, Deutsch V, Pick M et al. Placing the newborn on the maternal abdomen after delivery increases the volume and CD34 cell content in the umbilical cord blood collected: an old maneuver with new applications. Am J Obstet Gynecol 1999;180:1240–1243.
22. Brochstein J, Reed W, Smith RS et al. Sibling-donor cord blood transplantation in a 23 month old with severe sickle cell disease (Abstr). Philidelphia: National Sickle Cell Disease Program, 2000.
23. Kleinman S, Lugo J, Litty C et al. Transfusion-transmitted malaria. MMWR 1999;48:254–256.
24. First HIV-1 group O patient identified in the US. MMWR 1996;
25. Zoon K. Interim recommendations for deferral of donors at increased risk for HIV group O infection. FDA Memorandum to Registered Blood and Plasma Establishments. 1996:1–3.
26. Menitove J, Chambers LA, Gjertson DW et al. AABB Standards for Cord Blood Services (1st ed). Bethesda: American Association of Blood Banks, 2001.
27. FACT. Draft: Standards for Hematopoietic Progenitor Cell Collection, Processing, and Transplantation (2nd ed). Foundation for the Accreditation of Cellular Therapy; 2001.
28. Jefferies LC, Albertus M, Morgan MA et al. High deferral rate for maternal-neonatal donor pairs for an allogeneic umbilical cord blood bank. Transfusion 1999;39:415–419.

29. Lecchi L, Ratti I, Lazzari L et al. Reasons for discard of umbilical cord blood units before cryopreservation. Transfusion 2000;40:122–124; discussion 124–125.

30. Sirchia G, Rebulla P, Lecchi L et al. Implementation of a quality system (ISO 9000 series) for placental blood banking. J Hematother 1998;7:19–35.

29. Sirchia G, Rebulla P, Mozzi F et al. A quality system for placental blood banking. Bone Marrow Transplant 1998;21(Suppl 3):S43–S47.

31. Harvath L. Food and Drug Administration's proposed approach to regulation of hematopoietic stem/progenitor cell products for therapeutic use. Transfus Med Rev 2000;14:104–111.

32. Proposed rule: Suitability determination for donors of human cellular and tissue-based products (21 CFR Parts 210, 211, 820, and 1271). Fed Regist 1999;64:52,696–723.

33. Proposed rule: Current good tissue practices for manufacturers of human cellular and tissue based products: inspection and enforcement (21 CFR Part 1271). Fed Regist 2001;66:1508–1559.

# PART *III*

## DISEASE SPECIFIC PEDIATRIC CELL TRANPLANTS

CHAPTER *IX*

# Neuroblastoma

JOAN MORRIS

Neuroblastoma, a neoplasm of the sympathetic nervous system, is the most common extracranial solid tumor of childhood, with an annual incidence of 8 per million children in the United States.[1] Children of any age with localized neuroblastoma and infants younger than one year of age with advanced disease have been shown to have a good prognosis with surgical resection with or without conventional chemotherapy.[2-4] Unfortunately, 60% of children with neuroblastoma present with advanced stage disease that has disseminated to distant sites such as the bone, bone marrow, lymph nodes, and liver or have other unfavorable features such as undifferentiated histology or amplified expression of the *N-myc* gene.[5-7] The treatment of advanced stage neuroblastoma presents a challenge even with intensive chemotherapy regimens combined with aggressive surgical resection and irradiation. These aggressive approaches to advanced stage neuroblastoma have improved short-term but not long-term survival.[8-11]

In this chapter, I will give an overview of the known biologic and prognostic characteristics, the current staging system, the various therapeutic approaches for the advanced stage disease, and the future strategies to improve treatment.

## BIOLOGIC AND CLINICAL CHARACTERISTICS OF NEUROBLASTOMA

A number of biologic variables have been studied in neuroblastoma. The most relevant biologic variables are Shimada histology, amplification of N-myc oncogene, and tumor DNA ploidy, since they are used to stratify patients to a particular therapeutic regimen. Unfavorable Shimada histopathology, diploid tumors, and amplification of the N-myc oncogene have associated with high-risk tumors.[12-16] Other high-risk features include age >1 year, age <1 year with amplification of N-myc oncogene, deletion of chromosome 1p, gain of chromosome 17q, lack of expression of gp140proto-trk (the gene encoding one of the high-affinity neurotropin receptors), increased telomerase RNA expression, expression of P-glycoprotein, overexpression of nm23/nucleoside diphosphate kinase, elevated serum lactate dehydrogenase, elevated serum ferritin, and advanced clinical stage of the tumor at presentation.[17-30]

The clinical staging of the tumor is defined by the International Neuroblastoma Staging System (INSS), which is a worldwide staging system that provides common criteria to identify distinct prognostic groups (▼ Table 9.1).[31]

Based on the biologic characteristics and the clinical staging of the tumor at presentation, risk groups have been established by the Children's Cancer Study Group–Pediatric Oncology Group for stratification of therapeutic approaches (▶ Table 9.2).[32] Low risk patients will be treated with surgery alone unless symptomatic, intermediate risk with surgery and chemotherapy, and high risk with intensive treatment, including myeloablative therapy.

## TREATMENT FOR HIGH RISK NEUROBLASTOMA

High risk neuroblastoma has a poor outcome (<15% survival at 3 years) using conventional therapy.[33] The introduction of high-dose therapy strategies is showing promise in improving the disease-free survival in this group of patients. Cheung and Heller have reported the importance of dose intensity on response rate and survival. They demonstrated that the response rate and survival duration correlated with the "intensity of dose" they obtained, not only with higher drug doses but also shorter intervals between courses.[34]

This concept of dose intensity is the approach used in treating high risk neuroblastoma. Initially, therapy for this group of patients included using a combination of non-cross resistant agents at very high doses and at short intervals.[35–37] Another approach that is more widely used at this time is megatherapy, which destroys residual disease by using high doses

| TABLE 9.1 | International Neuroblastoma Staging System |
|---|---|
| Stage I | Localized tumor confined to the area of origin; complete gross excision, with or without microscopic residual disease; identifiable ipsilateral and contralateral lymph nodes negative microscopically. |
| Stage 2A | Unilateral tumor with incomplete gross excision; identifiable ipsilateral and contralateral lymph nodes negative microscopically. |
| Stage 2B | Unilateral tumor with complete or incomplete gross excision; with positive ipsilateral regional lymph nodes; identifiable contralateral lymph nodes negative microscopically. |
| Stage 3 | Tumor infiltrating across the midline with or without regional lymph node involvement; or unilateral tumor with contralateral regional lymph node involvement; or midline tumor with bilateral regional lymph node involvement. |
| Stage 4 | Dissemination of tumor to distant lymph nodes, bone, bone marrow, liver, and/or other organs (except as defined by stage 4S). |
| Stage 4S | Localized primary tumor as defined for stage 1 or 2 with dissemination limited to liver, skin, and/or bone marrow. |

| TABLE 9.2 | Risk Groups Based on Biologic and Clinical Staging |
|---|---|

Low Risk (survival >80–100% with surgery alone)
  INSS 1
  INSS 2
    Without amplification of N-myc oncogene
  INSS 2
    Amplification of N-myc oncogene, FH
  INSS 4-S
    Without amplification of N-myc oncogene, DI >1, FH

Intermediate Risk (survival >80% with surgery, conventional chemotherapy, ± local irradiation)
  INSS 3
    ≥1 year, without amplification of N-myc oncogene, FH
  INSS 3
    <1 year, without amplification of N-myc oncogene
  INSS 4
    <1 year, without amplification of N-myc oncogene
  INSS 4-S
    without amplification of N-myc oncogene, UH or DI = 1

High risk (survival <10–15% with conventional chemotherapy, surgery, ± local irradiation)
  INSS 2
    ≥1 year, amplification of N-myc oncogene, UH
  INSS 3
    >1 year or amplification of N-myc oncogene
  INSS 4
    <1 year, amplification of N-myc oncogene
  INSS 4
    ≥1 year
  INSS 4-S
    Amplification of N-myc oncogene

Abbreviations: DI = DNA index; INSS = International Neuroblastoma Staging System; UH = unfavorable histopathology; FH = favorable histopathology.

of chemotherapy with and without irradiation, and requires stem cells to rescue patients from fatal injury to bone marrow.[38–40] This therapeutic approach usually includes three phases: the induction phase, the consolidation phase, and the postconsolidation phase. The induction phase consists of a multidrug approach using agents that have non–cross-resistant mechanisms to decrease the risk of treatment failure due to tumor cell drug resistance. The purpose of this phase is to attempt to decrease the tumor burden; insure the bone marrow graft is free of tumor cells; and shrink the tumor to attempt to render it surgically resectable. Patients who achieve a complete response or very good partial response at the end of induction have been shown to have the best long-term survival.[41,42] The consolidation phase uses very intensive megatherapy requiring stem cell support. This phase is meant to achieve a minimal residual disease (MRD) state. Postconsolidation is the phase where minimal residual disease is treated using biologic or immunotherapy agents.

## Induction Chemotherapy

There are a variety of chemotherapeutic agents that have been shown to be useful in the treatment of neuroblastoma. The induction regimen is composed of a multidrug approach that has non-cross-resistant agents to prevent the emergence of drug-resistant disease using agents that work by different mechanisms.

Dose intensification by utilizing intensive doses of non-myeloablative chemotherapy in close intervals, may result in a high complete remission (CR) or very good partial remission (VGPR) state prior to consolidation therapy. Achieving a CR or VGPR state prior to consolidation therapy is associated with better overall survival. ▼ Table 9.3 shows the

| **TABLE 9.3** | **International Neuroblastoma Response Criteria** |
|---|---|

| Response | Primary Tumor* | Metastatic Sites |
|---|---|---|
| CR | No tumor | No tumor; catecholamines normal. |
| VGPR | Decreased by 90–99% | No tumor; catecholamines normal; residual 99Tc bone changes allowed. |
| PR | Decreased by >50% | All measurable sites decreased by >50%. Bones and bone marrow: number of positive bone sites decreased by >50%; no more than 1 positive bone marrow site allowed. |
| MR | No new lesions; >50% reduction of any measurable lesion (primary or any metastases) with <50% reduction in any other; <25% increase in existing lesion. | |
| NR | No new lesions; <50% reduction but <25% increase in any existing lesion. | |
| PD | Any new lesion; increase of any measurable lesion by >25%; previous negative marrow positive for tumor. | |

*3-dimensional measurements by computed tomography or magnetic resonance imaging.
Abbreviations: CR = complete remission; VGPR = very good partial remission; PR = partial remission; MR = mixed response; NR = no response; PD = progressive disease.

International Neuroblastoma Response Criteria that have been developed to allow comparisons of treatment results.[31]

The most common chemotherapeutic agents used during induction are cyclophosphamide, doxorubicin, cisplatin, teniposide (VM26), etoposide (VP16), carboplatin, vincristine, dacarbazine, and thiotepa. The combination of chemotherapy agents utilized in the various induction regimens is based on cell kinetic data, dose responsiveness of neuroblastoma, and toxicity considerations.[43–48] Some of the most common combinations of agents used for induction therapy are shown in ▼ Table 9.4.

## Surgery and Local Irradiation

Intensive induction chemotherapy is usually supplemented with surgical resection and local irradiation to achieve a complete or very good partial remission prior to undergoing myeloablative regimens and stem cell transplantation.

Surgical resection has been shown by investigators to be safer to undertake after induction chemotherapy has been given.[53–57] Chemotherapy changes the character of the tumor, usually making the tumor more fibrous, less vascular, and smaller in size resulting in easier surgery with fewer complications. Aggressive surgical resection has been shown to be effective in the control of relapse at the primary site, and in overall survival.[57–60] Haase et al. evaluated 104 patients with metastatic high risk or stage II neuroblastoma with amplification of the N-myc oncogene treated with the same induction chemotherapy. In addition, 42 patients went on to receive a bone marrow transplant after surgical resection. Patients who had complete primary tumor resection had a better overall survival (▼ Figure 9.1).[60]

Local irradiation to the primary and metastatic tumor sites has been utilized in a variety of studies if residual tumor was still present at the completion of induction therapy and surgical resection. The purpose of the irradiation is to render the patient disease-free prior to starting myeloablative therapy.[61–63] Local irradiation to residual tumor may decrease local recurrence. High-dose chemotherapy requires stem cell resuce to bypass lethal damage to bone marrow stem cells.[40,63]

## Stem Cell Source

Stem cells are usually collected after the third to fifth cycle of induction therapy. Initial trials using autologous stem cell transplantation, utilized bone marrow cells as the source of stem cells. More recently, peripheral blood stem cells (PBSC) are being used as the stem cell source. There are several advantages of utilizing autologous PBSC over autologous bone marrow cells. They can be collected as an outpatient without the trauma of a bone marrow harvest or general anesthesia.[64,65,66] PBSC result in a more rapid hematologic recovery, thus reducing the cytopenic period after myeloablative therapy.[64,67,68] Finally, there are data suggesting that the incidence of tumor cell contamination is lower in PBSC than in bone marrow grafts, although tumor cells can still be detected in PBSC.[64,68,69]

Brenner and Rill demonstrated that contaminating tumorigenic cells in a bone marrow stem cell graft can contribute to relapse. In their study, a neomycin resistance gene in a retroviral vector was used to mark the bone marrow graft containing neuroblasts. Marked tumor cells were seen at the site of relapse.[70] This demonstration that tumor cell contami-

| TABLE 9.4 | Selected Induction Chemotherapy Regimens for Advanced Stage Neuroblastoma |  |  |

| Investigators | Therapy Regimen | CR/VGPR | Patients |
|---|---|---|---|
| Kushner et al.[47] (MSKCC) | cyclophosphamide 140 mg/m$^2$<br>vincristine 0.1 mg/kg<br>doxorubicin 45 mg/m$^2$ | 64% | 14 |
| Lanino et al.[35] (Italian Cooperative Group) | (alternating)<br>PTC 360 mg/m$^2$<br>cisplatin 90 mg/m$^2$<br>VM 26 100 mg/m$^2$<br><br>cyclophosphamide 1050 mg/m$^2$<br>doxorubicin 35 mg/m$^2$<br>PTC 180 mg/m$^2$<br>cisplatin 90 mg/m$^2$<br>VM 26 100 mg/m$^2$ | 31% | 89 |
| Lanino et al.[35] (Italian Cooperative Group) | (alternating)<br>PTC 450 mg/m$^2$<br>cisplatin 200 mg/m$^2$<br>vincristine 1.5 mg/m$^2$<br>cyclophosphamide 600 mg/m$^2$<br><br>doxorubicin 45 mg/m$^2$<br>VM 26 375 mg/m$^2$ | 55% | 103 |
| Philip et al.[8] (LMEC 1) | (alternating)<br>cisplatin<br>VM 26 or VP 16<br><br>cyclophosphamide or ifosfamide<br>doxorubicin<br>vincristine | 32% | 72 |
| Donfrancesco et al.[49] | deferoxamine<br>cyclophosphamide 600 mg/m$^2$<br>carboplatin 1000 mg/m$^2$<br>thiotepa 30 mg/m$^2$ | 88% | 8 |
| Cambell et al.[37] (CCSG) | cisplatin 160 mg/m$^2$<br>VP 16 500 mg/m$^2$<br>doxorubicin 40 mg/m$^2$<br>ifosfamide 10 grams/m$^2$ | 43% | 35 |

| TABLE 9.4 | Selected Induction Chemotherapy Regimens for Advanced Stage Neuroblastom—cont'd | | |

| Investigators | Therapy Regimen | CR/VGPR | Patients |
|---|---|---|---|
| Kushner et al.[50] (MSKCC-N6) | (alternating) cyclophosphamide 140 mg/kg doxorubicin 75 mg/kg vincristine 1.6 mg/m$^3$ cisplatin 200 mg/m$^2$ VP 16 600 mg/m$^2$ | 88% | 24 |
| Hero et al.[51] (German Cooperative Neuroblastoma Study Group) | (alternating) vincristine 1.5 mg/m$^2$ adriamycin 35 mg/m$^2$ cyclophosphamide 1050 mg/m$^2$ dacarbazine 1000 mg/m$^2$ cisplatin 100 mg/m$^2$ cyclophosphamide 1000 mg/m$^2$ VM 26 100 mg/m$^2$ ifosfamide 10 grams/m$^2$ VP 16 300 mg/m$^2$ | 32% | 88 |
| Keneko et al.[52] (Study Group of Japan) | cyclophosphamide 1200 mg/m$^2$ vincristine 1.5 mg/m$^2$ tetrahydro-pyranyl adriamycin 40 mg/m$^2$ cisplatin 90 mg/m$^2$ | 69% | 168 |

Abbreviations: VM 26 = teniposide; VP 16 = etoposide; PTC = peptichemio; CCSG = Childen's Cancer Study Group; POG = Pediatric Oncology Group; MSKCC = Memorial Sloan Kettering; CR = complete remission; VGPR = very good partial remission.

nation of the stem cell graft can result in relapse has led to investigations of methods to purge stem cells from tumor cells. Two types of purging techniques have been studied. The cells can be purged either by a positive selection[71–74] where progenitor cells needed for engraftment (CD + 34 cells) are purified from the stem cell product, or by a negative selection in which tumor cells are selectively removed from the harvest. Negative selection purging has been accomplished using a variety of techniques such as 6-hydroxydopamine,[75] monoclonal antibodies,[76] immunomagnetic microspheres,[76] density sedimentation,[77] and mafosfamide (Asta-Z-7557).[78] The efficacy of purging PBSC is presently the focus of the most recent Children's Oncology Study Group protocol for high risk neuroblastoma.

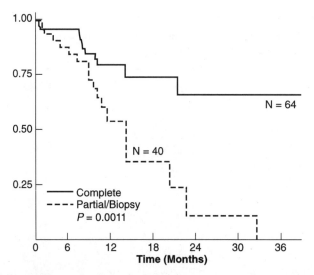

**FIGURE 9.1** Progression-free survival curve comparing patients who received complete tumor resection with those who received lesser procedures.[10]

## CONSOLIDATION THERAPY

### Myeloablative Regimens Used for Stem Cell Transplantation

Myeloablative regimens are used in consolidation therapy. Initially melphalan, an alkylating agent, was used alone or in combination with total body irradiation (TBI). Hartmann et al. reported on 15 patients who received high dose melphalan followed by autologous bone marrow transplant.[79] In this early study, five patients were free of disease at +29 to +54 months after transplantation. This study showed that this therapeutic modality was both tolerable and effective in the treatment of advanced stage neuroblastoma.

Other agents that have been included in consolidation regimens include cisplatin, teniposide, etoposide, vincristine, doxorubicin, carmustine, thiotepa, cyclophosphamide, and busulfan. Cisplatin was used in early trials but was replaced by carboplatin to decrease both renal and ototoxicity. However, Parsons has reported that severe ototoxicity can occur with carboplatin in patients who received platinum therapy if it was also exposed to other ototoxins such as aminoglycosides and diuretics.[80] TBI was used in early studies and has shown to have many toxicities including poor growth and development, second malignancies, and damage to other organs.[81] Thus, fractionated TBI and non-TBI containing regimens have been instituted. ▶ Table 9.5 outlines some of these studies.

### Is Consolidation Megatherapy with Stem Cell Rescue Better Than Continued Intensive Chemotherapy?

Initial studies comparing Myeloablative chemotherapy to conventional chemotherapy resulted in conflicting data.[35,39,90] The German Cooperative Neuroblastoma Group described

| TABLE 9.5 | Current Results of Myeloablative Regimens Followed by Stem Cell Transplantation (SCT) for Advanced Stage Neuroblastoma | | | |
|---|---|---|---|---|
| **Investigator** | **Number of Patients** | **Preparative Regimen** | **Outcome** | **Purging** |
| Hartmann et al.[39] | 33 | BCNU 300 mg/m$^2$ VM 26 1000 mg/m$^2$ melphalan 180 mg/m$^2$ | 16/33 CR at 28 months | |
| Franzone et al.[83] | 39 | vincristine 4 mg/m$^2$ melphalan 140 mg/m$^2$ TBIf 10 Gy | For 32 patients in CR at BMT DFS 28% at 30 months For 7 patients in CR at BMT DFS 14% at 25 months | unpurged |
| Philip et al.[84] | 62 | vincristine 4 mg/m$^2$ melphalan 180 mg/m$^2$ TBIf 12 Gy | PFS 40% at 2 years, 20% at 4 years, and 13% at 7 years | 54-immunomagnetic 1–6 hydroxydopamine 2–Asta Z 7557 |
| Kushner et al.[40] | 25 | cisplatin 1200 mg/m$^2$ XRT 21 Gy to primary and adjacent lymph nodes BCNU 200 mg/m$^2$ melphalan 180 mg/m$^2$ or thiotepa 900 mg/m$^2$ VP 16 900 mg/m$^2$ | 16-CR, PR: EFS 44% at 24 months 9-PD: 2 alive at 24 and 41 months | 4–6 hydroxydopamine |
| Lanino et al.[35] | 22 | vincristine 4 mg/m$^2$ melphalan 140 mg/m$^2$ TBIf | PFS 23% at 5 years | unpurged |
| Graham-Pole et al.[85] | 81 | melphalan 180 mg/m$^2$ TBIf 12 Gy | EFS 32% at 2 years in 1st CR EFS 43% at 2 years in 1st PR EFS 33% at 2 years in 2nd CR EFS 5% at 2 years in 2nd PR | 64-immunomagnetic |
| Garaventa et al.[30] | 39 | vincristine 4 mg/m$^2$ TBIf 10 Gy melphalan 140 mg/m$^2$ | PFS 12% at 6 years | 18-immunomagnetic 21-unpurged |

*Continued*

| TABLE 9.5 | Current Results of Myeloablative Regimens Followed by Stem Cell Transplantation (SCT) for Advanced Stage Neuroblastoma—cont'd | | | |

| Investigator | Number of Patients | Preparative Regimen | Outcome | Purging |
|---|---|---|---|---|
| Matthay et al.[86] | 147 | cisplatin 90 mg/m$^2$<br>VM 26 300 mg/m$^2$<br>doxorubicin 45 mg/m$^2$<br>melphalan 210 mg/m$^2$<br>TBI$f$ 10 Gy<br><br>cisplatin 120 mg/m$^2$<br>VP 16 400 mg/m$^2$<br>melphalan 210 mg/m$^2$<br>TBI$f$ 10 Gy<br><br>carboplatin 640–1200 mg/m$^2$<br>melphalan 210 mg/m$^2$<br>VP 16 500–800 mg/m$^2$ | PFS 38% at 4 years | immunomagnetic |
| Kamani et al.[62] | 27 | VM 26 360 mg/m$^2$<br>    or VP 16 500 mg/m$^2$<br>thiotepa 600–900 mg/m$^2$<br>±TBI$f$ 12 Gy | DFS 48% at 3 years | immunomagnetic |
| Hero et al.[51] | 39 | melphalan 180 mg/m$^2$<br>    or<br>melphalan 180 mg/m$^2$<br>vincristine 4.5 mg/m$^2$<br>    or<br>melphalan 180 mg/m$^2$<br>cisplatin 120 mg/m$^2$<br>BCNU 200 mg/m$^2$<br>VP 16 900 mg/m$^2$<br>$f$ irradiation to primary 21 Gy | EFS 18% | 22-immunomagnetic<br>17-unpurged |
| Villablanca et al.[63] | 58 | carboplatin 1700 mg/m$^2$<br>VP 16 800–1350 mg/m$^2$<br>melphalan 210 mg/m$^2$<br>$f$ irradiation to primary 21 Gy | survival 68% at 2 years | immunomagnetic |
| Kletzel et al.[61] | 51 | thiotepa 900 mg/m$^2$<br>cytoxan 6000 mg/m$^2$ | PFS 20% at 2 years for purged<br>PFS 60% at 2 years for unpurged | 15-immunomagnetic<br>1–4-hydroxycytoxan<br>35-unpurged |

*Continued*

| | | TABLE 9.5 | Current Results of Myeloablative Regimens Followed by Stem Cell Transplantation (SCT) for Advanced Stage Neuroblastoma—cont'd |
| --- | --- | --- | --- |

| Investigator | Number of Patients | Preparative Regimen | Outcome | Purging |
| --- | --- | --- | --- | --- |
| Matthay et al.[10] | 129 | carboplatin 1000 mg/m$^2$<br>VP 16 640 mg/m$^2$<br>TBI$f$ 10 Gy | EFS 43% at 3 years | immunomagnetic |
| Park et al.[87] | 14 | topotecan 5–10 mg/m$^2$<br>carboplatin 15 mg/m$^2$<br>thiotepa 900 mg/m$^2$ | EFS 41% at 220 days | unpurged |
| Kushner et al.[88] | 11 | topotecan 10 mg/m$^2$<br>carboplatin 15 mg/m$^2$<br>thiotepa 900 mg/m$^2$ | 10/11 in CR at<br>6 to 16 months post-BMT | unpurged |

Abbreviations: CR = complete remission; PR = partial remission; DFS = disease-free survival; PD = progressive disease; BCNU = carmustine; VM 26 = teniposide; VP 16 = etoposide; TBI$f$ = total body irradiation fractionated; XRT = irradiation; BMT = bone marrow transplant; PFS = progression-free survival; EFS = event-free survival.

a nonrandomized retrospective analysis where overall survival in the megatherapy group was 23% compared to 14% in the chemotherapy group.[51] However, these studies were retrospective and were not randomized. A Children's Cancer Study Group trial, CCG-321-P2, used intensive induction chemotherapy for five to seven courses. The chemotherapy was continued for 13 courses for some patients, while other patients received megatherapy with stem cell rescue per CCG-321-P3 for consolidation therapy. This was a nonrandomized study, and the choice of continuing chemotherapy versus consolidation with megatherapy was made by the parents and the treating physician. Intensive induction chemotherapy followed by megatherapy with stem cell rescue was more effective (estimated EFS at 4 years 40%) than continuing conventional chemotherapy (estimated EFS at 4 years 19%). This study also suggested that there was a significant benefit of megatherapy with stem cell support for a subgroup of very high risk patients: those patients with only a partial tumor response to induction chemotherapy (EFS at 4 years of 29% vs. 6% for continuation of chemotherapy) and to the group of patients whose tumors that had amplification of the N-myc oncogene (EFS 67% vs. 0% for continuation of chemotherapy).[41]

To remove selection bias in the previous study, the Children's Cancer Study Group then did a prospective randomized trial, CCG 3891, in which a combination of megatherapy with stem cell rescue was compared to nonmyeloablative chemotherapy. The three-year EFS was 43% for the megatherapy with stem cell rescue arm compared to 27% for the intensive nonmyeloablative chemotherapy arm ($P = .027$). This study also demonstrated that the subgroup of patients who were older than two years at diagnosis ($P = .01$) and the subgroup with amplification of the N-myc oncogene ($P = .03$) were significantly improved with the megatherapy with stem cell rescue when compared to the intensive nonmyeloablative chemotherapy arm (▼ Figure 9.2).[10]

## Allogeneic Versus Autologous Stem Cell Transplantation (SCT): Does One Offer a Better Chance for a Cure?

The advantage of allogeneic versus autologous SCT for treatment of advanced stage neuroblastoma has been evaluated by a variety of investigators.[91–93] The theoretical advantage of allogeneic SCT are graft-versus-tumor effect, and lack of tumor cell contamination. To date, these studies have shown no statistical advantage in overall disease-free survival or difference in the incidence of toxicity between these two modalities.

The Children's Cancer Study Group's (CCSG) trial was a retrospective, nonrandomized study of intensive chemotherapy followed by either a purged autologous or allogeneic SCT from September 1988 to July 1991.[91] The choice of proceeding to myeloablative therapy (allogeneic or autologous SCT) or continuation of chemotherapy was given to the physician and the parents prior to entering the study. Patients with identified human leukocyte antigen (HLA)-compatible sibling donors were given the option of allogeneic SCT or continuation of chemotherapy. The patients without a donor were given the option of autolo-

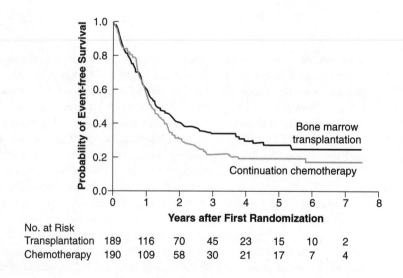

**FIGURE 9.2** Probability of Event-Free Survival among Patients Assigned to Bone Marrow Transplantation of Continuation Chemotherapy.[10]

Follow-up began at the the time the first randomization (eight weeks after diagnosis). The difference in survival between the two groups was significant at three years ($P = 0.034$).

gous stem cell transplant or continuation with chemotherapy. All patients received the same induction chemotherapy and ablative chemoradiotherapy. Allogeneic patients also received methotrexate for graft-versus-host disease (GVHD) prophylaxis. The progression-free survival (PFS) at four years was 49% in autologous SCT patients and 25% in the allogeneic group ($P = .051$). This study concluded that the toxicity and overall rate of relapse did not differ in the allogeneic or autologous SCTs.

The European Group for Bone Marrow Transplantation (EBMT) reported a case-controlled, retrospective analysis of 51 patients, reported to the registry, who received SCT for advanced stage neuroblastoma between March 1981 and January 1991.[92] Nineteen patients received allogeneic grafts and 34 patients received autologous grafts. A variety of myeloablative regimens were used. In addition, not all of the autologous grafts were purged of tumor cells (20 purged and 8 unpurged). The overall survival at five years was 29% in autologous SCT patients and 21% in the allogeneic group. The PFS at two years was 41% in autologous SCT patients and 35% in the allogeneic group. This analysis did not show any advantage of allogeneic over autologous SCT.

Both reports demonstrate no difference in PFS and toxicity of allogeneic SCT from autologous SCT. These studies, however, had small patient sizes and were not randomized, making it difficult to come to confirm the optimal donor source. In addition, the incidence of GVHD was low and mild. Therefore, an adequate antitumor effect may not have been achieved in the patients who received allogeneic SCTs. Future studies using immune modulation in conjunction with allogeneic SCT may result in the improvement of PFS.

## Tandem Transplantation: A Method to Further Dose Intensify Therapy

Dose intensification with autologous stem cell transplantation using high dose chemotherapy and chemoradiotherapy has been shown to improve overall survival in pediatric patients with solid tumors.[7,10,32,34] Tandem autologous stem cell transplantation allows further dose intensification of therapy with the goal being further improvement in disease-free survival. Theoretical advantages of tandem stem cell transplantation include: (1) exposure to multiple effective agents at maximal-tolerated doses; (2) exposure to non-cross-resistant therapies in rapid sequence; and (3) changes in the tumor microenvironment during the initial stem cell transplantation may allow for better tumor cell kill with the second stem cell transplantation.

Tandem transplants for advanced stage neuroblastoma were described initially by Philip et al. in the LMCE2 protocol.[94] Patients entered in the study had refractory disease in partial response after second line treatment or had relapsed. All patients had double bone marrow harvests and two different preparative therapy regimens. The first preparative therapy regimen consisted of tenoposide (VM 26), bichloronitrosurea (BCNU), cisplatin (CDDP), or carboplatin (CBDCA). The second therapy regimen contained vincristine, melphalan, and 1200 cGy total body irradiation (TBI). The first bone marrow harvest was performed four weeks after the last chemotherapy course. The second bone marrow harvest was 60 to 90 days after the first stem cell transplantation. All bone marrows were purged in vitro by an immunomagnetic technique. This study included 33 patients treated between 1985 and 1988. The overall survival at five years was 32%. Despite the encouraging survival rate, this treatment approach had a high toxic death rate (7 of 33 patents) and delayed engraftment (median time to reach an absolute neutrophil count [ANC] of greater than 500 was 43 days for the second stem cell transplantation).

Tandem bone marrow transplantation also was studied by Kawa-Ha et al. in Japan.[95] In their study, the bone marrow stem cells were harvested for both transplants on recovery from the last chemotherapy course (prior to any high dose chemotherapy for transplantation). The first preparative therapy regimen consisted of ifosfamide and melphalan. The second therapy consisted of busulfan and thiotepa. The bone marrow cells were purged if the bone marrow was positive for tumor cells by cytology (this occurred in half the patients). Neutrophil recovery was not delayed in these patients, however, prolonged thrombocytopenia occured. While the number of patients in this study was too small to make conclusions on progressive-free survival, this approach was shown to be feasible.

Vassal et al. demonstrated that tandem stem cell transplantation utilizing PBSC instead of bone marrow stem cells was tolerated well with little toxicity.[96] This study included patients with primitive neuroectodermal tumors of the brain and advanced stage neuroblastoma. Melphalan 100 mg/m$^2$ was given at 21-day intervals. This therapy was well tolerated with the median time to achieve an ANC of greater than 500 in six days. The major toxicity was prolonged thrombocytopenia. Influence on survival was not examined in this small study, but it was shown that repeated high dose chemotherapy with PBSC transplantation was tolerated with low toxicity.

The use of tandem transplants to treat patients with advanced stage neuroblastoma was also described by Grupp et al.[97] This study was designed to utilize PBSC instead of bone marrow as the stem cell source to help expedite engraftment. The PBSC were collected early in induction therapy (after documentation of no tumor contamination) to insure that the stem cells were viable. CD 34+ selected cells were obtained and saved. Patients received carboplatin, etoposide (VP16), and cyclophosphamide for the first high dose chemotherapy regimen. If the patients did not show signs of life-threatening organ toxicity, then six weeks later they proceeded to the second high dose chemotherapy that consisted of melphalan and TBI. Of 55 patients who entered this study 46 patients completed both SCTs. Engraftment was found to be rapid, with median ANC greater than 500/$\mu$L in 11 days. This demonstrated that PBSC engraft quickly and that CD 34 selection did not delay engraftment. Four toxic deaths occurred in this study, with all the deaths occurring after the second high dose chemotherapy transplant. The deaths were caused by bacterial sepsis, cytomegalovirus infection, adenovirus infection, and Epstein-Barr virus lymphoproliferative disease. The event-free survival was 50% at three years. This study demonstrated that tandem rapid-sequence PBCS transplantation is feasible and presents a method that will allow further dose intensification of therapy for advanced stage neuroblastoma.

Kletzel et al.[98] further intensified consolidation therapy by having patients undergo triple-tandem transplants. Twenty-five consecutive, newly diagnosed neuroblastoma patients and one patient with recurrent disease underwent this therapy. The therapy was well tolerated with a three-year event-free survival of 57%.

The impact of tandem PBSC transplantation on advanced stage neuroblastoma will be the focus of the next high risk neuroblastoma randomized trial conducted by the Children's Oncology Group. This study will compare single and tandem PBSC transplants for this disease.

# Radioimmunotherapy in Combination with Stem Cell Transplantation: Will It Improve Disease-Free Survival?

## $^{131}I$ Metaiodobenzylguanidine Therapy

$^{131}$I metaiodobenzylguanidine ($^{131}$I MIBG) is a catecholamine analogue that is selectively taken up by cells of neural crest origin. In low doses, it is useful as an imaging modality for both neuroblastoma and pheochromocytoma. At high doses, it has been used therapeutically as a targeted radionuclide for tumors of neural crest origin. The advantage of therapeutic $^{131}$I MIBG over standard radiation therapy is that it allows high concentration of radiation to the tumor site while sparing the surrounding normal tissue. Initial therapeutic trials utilizing $^{131}$I MIBG therapy were complicated by dose-limiting bone marrow suppression.[99–104] In addition, the tumor must be greater than 2 mm for this therapy to be useful. Micrometastases smaller than 1 mm diameter are not easily treated by $^{131}$I MIBG because the radionuclide disintegration energy is absorbed inefficiently in small tumors whose diameter is less than the mean range of the $^{131}$I beta particles.[105] These obstacles have been overcome by combining $^{131}$I MIBG therapy with high dose chemotherapy followed by stem cell rescue.[106–110]

Gaze et al. showed in a small series of advanced stage neuroblastoma patients that it was feasible to combine $^{131}$I MIBG therapy with high dose chemoradiotherapy and stem cell rescue.[106] They reported the results of two autologous and three allogeneic stem cell transplant patients treated with this multimodality megatherapy after having received chemotherapy and surgical resection of the primary tumor. Patients were treated with an $^{131}$I MIBG dose to give a whole body absorbed radiation dose of about 2 cGy on day 0, melphalan 140 mg/m$^2$ on day 10, and 12.6 cGy total body irradiation (TBI) in eight fractions on days 12 to 15. All the patients were found to tolerate this multimodality megatherapy well, with all patients engrafting. One patient remained alive without relapse at 32 months after treatment.

Ability to achieve engraftment after myeloablative doses of $^{131}$I MIBG followed by autologous bone marrow transplantation was also demonstrated in phase 1 studies by Goldberg and Matthay.[107,108] Goldberg et al. focused on whether hematopoietic reconstitution would be affected by myeloablative doses of $^{131}$I MIBG.[107] All patients had advanced stage $^{131}$I MIBG positive neuroblastoma tumors refractory to conventional therapy. Patients received conventional chemotherapy prior to bone marrow harvest. Bone marrow cells were purged by sedimentation, filtration, and immunomagnetic purging at the Children's Cancer Group purging laboratory. Twelve patients were administered $^{131}$I MIBG in one to four doses, ranging from 3 to 18 mCi/kg. The median cumulative dose of $^{131}$I MIBG administered was 18.0 mCi/kg and the median cumulative dose of TBI from the $^{131}$I MIBG dose was 426 cGy. The median time to an absolute neutrophil count (ANC) of greater than 500 was 19 days. Five patients achieved red cell transfusion independence at a median of 44 days and four patients achieved a platelet count of >20,000 without transfusions in a median of 27 days. Initially, seven patients achieved a partial response (PR), three patients had stable disease, and two patients had progression of their disease. By a median of nine months all patients had died of progressive disease (9), toxicity (2), or secondary leukemia (1). Matthay et al. studied dose limiting toxicity of $^{131}$I MIBG with and without autologous bone marrow support.[108] Thirty relapsed neuroblastoma patients were treated with escalating doses of $^{131}$I MIBG (3 to 18 mCi/kg). Patients receiving 12 mCi/kg or greater were supported with bone marrow cells that had been purged by sedimentation, filtration, and immunomagnetic purging at the Children's Cancer Group purging laboratory. Grade 4 thrombocytopenia and/or neutropenia occurred in 80% of patients receiving 12 mCi/kg of [131]I MIBG. At 15 mCi/kg dose-limiting hematologic toxicity was achieved. A therapeutic response occurred in 37% of the patients, with a majority of these patients receiving a minimum of 12 mCi/kg of [131]I MIBG. These two studies demonstrated that the main toxicity of [131]I MIBG was hematologic toxicity that could be overcome with bone marrow rescue. In addition, the high response rate in refractory neuroblastoma patients suggested that this therapy could be efficacious for improving the outcome of advanced stage neuroblastoma if used in combination with myeloablative chemotherapy and autologous bone marrow rescue.

Klingebiel et al. also showed that it was feasible to combine [131]I MIBG therapy with high dose chemoradiotherapy, stem cell rescue, and immunotherapy with antiGD2 antibody in a small series of advanced stage neuroblastoma patients.[109] Of the 11 patients studied, the progression-free survival was demonstrated to be $0.70 \pm 0.15$ with a median survival time of 19 months.

[131]I metaiodobenzylguanidine therapy followed by autologous bone marrow transplant also was shown to be a feasible therapeutic strategy by Miano et al.[110] This study included seventeen patients with advanced stage neuroblastoma who had [131]I MIBG-positive residual disease. The patients received 4.1 to 11.1 mCi/kg [131]I MIBG seven to ten days before starting chemotherapy for stem cell transplant. Stem cell transplant regimen consisted of busulphan 16 mg/kg and melphalan 140 mg/kg. The patients then received PBSC with a median of $4.7 \times 10^6$/kg CD34+ cells. Gastrointestinal toxicity was greater in this group of patients when compared to patients receiving the same chemotherapy without the [131]I MIBG therapy. Two patients on the study developed lung complications (interstitial pneumonitis and pneumonia).

Recently, Yanik et al.[111] reported on a pilot study of 12 patients treated with [131]I MIBG therapy after relapse (5 patients) or after induction therapy (seven patients). The patients received 12 mCi/kg bone marrow transplant (BMT) on day –21, followed by melphalan, carboplatin, and etoposide BMT on days –7 to –4. The patients received autologous stem cells on BMT day 0. This study concluded that it was feasible to perform this procedure and it warranted a larger scale study to determine the efficacy of this therapeutic approach.

### 3F8-Targeted Radioimmuno therapy

3F8 is a murine IgG monoclonal antibody selective for ganglioside GD2 that is expressed intensely on neuroblastoma tumors. Cheung et al.[38] described a novel use of this antibody in the treatment of neuroblastoma. In their study, the 3F8 monoclonal antibody was labeled with [131]I and delivered targeted radiation to the tumor bed. The cumulative blood radiation dose was 20 Gy, with the marrow dose estimated to be 500 to 700 cGy, much less than the exposure with total body irradiation. This therapy was well tolerated and was used in conjunction with high dose chemotherapy.

These studies all suggest that combining [131]I MIBG or [131]I 3F8 with high dose chemotherapy followed by stem cell rescue is a feasible approach to the treatment of advanced stage neuroblastoma. Further studies to determine the efficacy of this therapeutic approach needs to be evaluated in a large prospective trial.

## Postconsolidation Therapies

Treatment of neuroblastoma utilizing high dose chemotherapy regimens with stem cell transplantation combined with local irradiation and aggressive surgery has resulted in better control of bulky disease. Despite improvements in remission rates, relapse remains a common problem suggesting that minimal residual disease state may be responsible for tumor recurrences.[112–114] The focus of therapy for this aggressive disease is now therefore being redirected to treatment of minimal residual disease (MRD). These postconsolidation therapies, directed at eradicating MRD, include differentiation inducers,[10,115–117] immune therapies, genetically engineered monoclonal antibodies,[118] and vaccinations[119,120] with cytokine-expressing tumor cells or tumor-lysate pulsed dendritic cells.

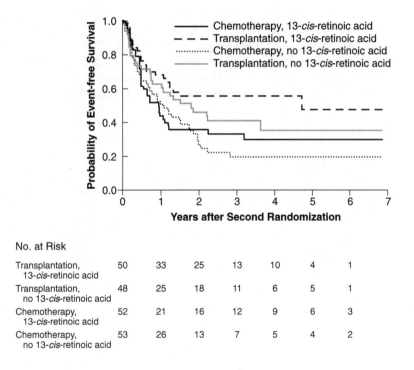

**FIGURE 9.3** Probability of Event-Free Survival among Patients Who entered Both Phases of the Study and Who Were Randomly Assigned to Receive a Bone Marrow Transplant plus 13-cis-Retinoic Acid, Transplant without 13-cis-Retinoic Acid, Continuation Chemotherapy plus 13-cis-Retinoic Acid, or Continuation Chemotherapy without 13-cis-Retinoic Acid.[10]

Follow-up began at the time of the second randomization (34 weeks after diagnosis). Overall event-free survival was significantly better in the group treated with transplantation plus 13-cis-retinoic acid than in the group assigned to continuation chemotherapy without the 13-cis-retinoic acid ($P = 0.02$).

## Retinoids

13-*cis*-retinoic acid (RA) is a synthetic retinoid derived from naturally occurring all-*trans*-retinoic acid. In vitro studies have shown that neuroblastoma cell lines exposed to *cis*-RA or *trans*-RA in cell culture demonstrate decreased proliferation, decreased expression of the N-myc oncogene, and morphologic differentiation.[115,121] Since the main effect of RA is on differentiation, it optimally can be used as a therapeutic agent in a minimal disease state. A phase I trial by Villablanca and Khan has demonstrated that 13-*cis* RA can be safely used in the postconsolidation stage of stem cell transplant on an intermittent schedule with little toxicity.[116] A recently published phase III trial by the Children's Cancer Study Group has demonstrated that 13-*cis*-RA, used in the posttransplant and postchemotherapy setting in advanced stage neuroblastoma, improves event-free survival in patients without progressive disease at the time of therapy (▼ Figure 9.3).[10] 13-*cis*-RA is used at 160 mg/m$^2$/day divided into two doses a day for 14 consecutive days in a 28-day cycle for six cycles.

Fenretinide [N-(4-hydroxyphenyl)retinamide] is a retinoid that induces apoptosis in neuroblastoma cell lines instead of differentiation.[117] In vitro studies have shown that even if a neuroblastoma cell line is resistant to 13-*cis*-RA or all-*trans*-RA, it will undergo apoptosis with fenretinide.[122] A phase I trial to determine the maximal tolerated dose of fenretinide is presently being performed by the Children's Oncology Group.

## Immunotherapy

Monoclonal antibodies to antigens on neuroblastoma tumor cells, is presently under investigation as a method to eradicate minimal residual disease.[38,118,123–125] GD$_2$, an antigen expressed with high density on neuroblastoma tumors and restricted to neuroectodermal tissue, is the most commonly used antibody.[126] Therapeutic responses have been shown to occur in phase I/II clinical studies utilizing a murine IgG$_3$ monoclonal antibody, 3F8[38,125] murine IgG$_2$ monocolonl antibody, 14G2a,[127] and a human-mouse chimeric monoclonal antibody, ch14.18.[123,124] Toxicities in these studies include pain (due to expression of GD$_2$ on peripheral pain fibers), hyper- and hypotension, tachycardia, fever, and urticaria.[38,123–126] The mechanism by which monoclonal antibodies destroy neuroblastoma tumor cells is through complement-mediated cytotoxicity and antibody-dependent cell-mediated cytotoxicity (ADCC).[128]

Cytokines, such as granulocyte-macrophage colony-stimulating factor (GM-CSF) and interleukin (IL)-2, have been shown to augment the immune system in vitro and in vivo.[129–132] GM-CSF can enhance antitumor immunity through direct activation of dendritic cells, macrophages, monocytes, and augmentation of ADCC. GM-CSF indirectly activates T cells via tumor necrosis factor (TNF), interferon (IFN), and interleukin (IL)-1.[131,133] IL-2 has been shown to activate natural killer (NK) cells, lymphokine-activated killer (LAK) cells, and augments ADCC.[129,132,134,135] Phase I/II clinical trials have been conducted combining anti-GD$_2$ monoclonal antibody with GM-CSF or IL-2 alone, or GM-CSF alternating with IL-2.[118,124] These studies demonstrated an antitumor response. More recently, a fusion protein, ch14.18-IL-2, was developed so the 14.18 anti-GD$_2$ antibody-mediated tumor cells recognize and bind to tumor cells while the IL-2 component activates cells expressing IL-2 receptors on lytic cells.[136] Studies on the ch14.18-IL-2 fusion protein have demonstrated that it has a longer half-life than IL-2 alone, resulting in higher and more sustained concentrations of IL-2 in the tumor microenvironment.[137] The downside of this fusion protein is that it is immunogenic, and so patients may develop high human antimouse antibody (HAMA) titers and allergic symptoms.[138] To overcome the problems with development of HAMAs, a humanized fusion protein was developed, called hu14.18-IL-2.[139] This fusion protein is presently the focus of a phase I trial in the Children's Oncology Group.

Tumor vaccination is another immunotherapy being developed to help eradicate minimal residual disease. Haight et al. performed a vaccination trial using IL-2 gene modified allogeneic neuroblastoma cells.[140] Five of the six patients studied demonstrated antitumor antibodies. Rousseau et al. created a vaccine combining lymphotactin and IL-2–secreting allogeneic neuroblastoma cells.[119] This vaccination was studied in 21 patients and revealed tumor responses that included two patients with complete remission and one with a partial remission. Six patients had an increase in NK cytolytic activity and 15 patients had immunoglobulin G antibodies that bound to the immunizing cell line. Geiger et al. created a dendritic cell vaccine from the patient's own peripheral blood monocytes.[120] The dendritic cells were pulsed with the neuroblastoma tumor cells in combination with the immunogenic protein keyhole limpet hemocyanin. Fifteen patients with a variety of solid tumors including neuroblastoma were treated. One patient had regression of tumor and five patients had stabilization of disease. These studies show that allogeneic tumor vaccines and dendritic-derived vaccines can induce an antitumor effect and may be a promising approach for the treatment of minimal residual disease in the future.

## Antiangiogenesis Agents

Aggressive neuroblastoma tumors are characteristically very vascular. Antiangiogenesis agents may play a therapeutic role in these very aggressive tumors by decreasing the blood supply to the tumor. TNP-470, a potent inhibitor of angiogenesis, has been studied in neuroblastoma pre-clinical trials in a mouse model. Katzenstein et al. demonstrated that the effectiveness of TNP-470 inversely correlates with tumor burden suggesting that it may be therapeutically useful in the MDR state.[141] Stern et al. studied the safety of TNP-470 in a poststem cell transplant state in a mouse model. This study showed no significant hematologic toxicity from the TNP-470, demonstrating that inhibitors of angiogenesis do not adversely impact engraftment after stem cell transplantation in a mouse model.[142] Future clinical trials to determine the role that antiangiogenesis agents can play in the postconsolidation phase, for the treatment of the MRD, needs to be investigated.

# REFERENCES

1. US incidence rates for selected childhood cancers. J Natl Cancer Inst 2001;93:1201.
2. Schmidt ML, Lukens JN, Seeger RC et al. Biologic factors determine prognosis in infants with stage IV neuroblastoma. A prospective Children's Cancer Group Study. J Clin Oncol 2000;18:1260–1268.
3. Matthay KK, Perez C, Seeger RC et al. Successful treatment of stage III neuroblastoma based on prospective biologic staging: a Children's Cancer Group Study. J Clin Oncol 1998;16:1256–1264.
4. Matthay KK, Sather HN, Seeger RC et al. Excellent outcome for stage II neuroblastoma is independent of residual disease and radiation therapy. J Clin Oncol 1989;7:236–244.
5. Bowman LC, Hancock ML, Santana VM et al. Impact of intensified therapy on clinical outcome in infants and children with neuroblastoma: the St Jude Children's Research Hospital experience, 1962 to 1988. J Clin Oncol 1991;9:1599–1608.
6. McWilliams NB, Hayes FA, Green AA et al. Cyclophosphamide/doxorubicin vs cisplatin/teniposide in the treatment of children older than 12 months of age with disseminated neuroblastoma: a Pediatric Oncology Group Randomized Phase II study. Med Pediatr Oncol 1995;24:176–180.
7. Matthay KK. Impact of myeloablative therapy with bone marrow transplantation in advanced neuroblastoma. Bone Marrow Transplant 1996;18(Suppl):S21–S24.
8. Philip T, Zucker JM, Bernard JL et al. Improved survival at 2 and 5 years in the LMCE1 unselected group of 72 children with stage IV neuroblastoma older than 1 year of age at diagnosis: is cure possible in a small subgroup? J Clin Oncol 1991;9:1037–1044.
9. Frappaz D, Michon J, Coze C et al. LMCE3 treatment strategy: results in 99 consecutively diagnosed stage 4 neuroblastomas in children older than 1 year at diagnosis. J Clin Oncol 2000;18:468–476.
10. Matthay KK, Villablanca JG, Seeger RC et al. Treatment of high-risk neuroblastoma with intensive chemotherapy, radiotherapy, autologous bone marrow transplantation, and 13-cis-retinoic acid. N Engl J Med 1999;341:1165–1173.
11. Castel V, Canete A, Navarro S et al. Outcome of high-risk neuroblastoma using dose intensity approach: Improvement in initial but not long-term results. Med Pediatr Oncol 2001;37:537–542.
12. Shimada H, Chatten J, Newton WA Jr et al. Histopathologic prognostic factors in neuroblastic tumors. Definition of subtypes of ganglioneuroblastoma and an age-linked classification of neuroblastomas. J Natl Cancer Inst 1984;73:405–416.
13. Chatten J, Shimada H, Sather HN et al. Prognostic value of histopathology in advanced stage neuroblastoma: A report from the Children's Cancer Study Group. Hum Pathol 1988;19:1187–1198.
14. Seefer RC, Brodeur GM, Sather H et al. Association of multiple copies of the N-myc oncogene and rapid progression of neuroblastomas. N Engl J Med 1985;313:1111–1116.
15. Look AT, Hayes FA, Shuster JJ et al. Clinical relevance of tumor cell ploidy and n-myc gene amplification in childhood neuroblastoma: A Pediatric Oncology Group Study. J Clin Oncol 1991;9:581–591.
16. Tonini GP, Boni L, Pession A et al. MYCN oncogene amplification in neuroblastoma is associated with worse prognosis, except in stage 4s: the Italian experience with 295 children. J Clin Oncol 1997;15:85–93.
17. Cotterill SJ, Pearson AD, Prichard J et al. Clinical prognostic factors in 1277 patients with neuroblastoma: results of The European Neuroblastoma Study Group "Survey" 1982–1992. Eur J Cancer 2000;36:901–908.
18. Brodeur GM, Azar C, Brother M et al. Neuroblastoma, effect of genetic factors on prognosis and treatment. Cancer 1992;70(6 Suppl):1685–1694.
19. Fong CT, White PS, Peterson K et al. Loss for heterozygosity for chromosome 1 or 14 defines subsets of advanced neuroblastomas. Cancer Res 1992;52:1780–1785.
20. Maris JM, Weiss MJ, Guo C et al. Loss of heterozygosity at 1p36 independently predicts for disease progression but not decreased overall survival probability in neuroblastoma patients: a Children's Cancer Group Study. J Clin Oncol 2000;18:1888–1899.
21. Brown N, Lastowska M, Cotterill S et al. UK Cancer Cytogenetics Group and the UK Children's Cancer Study Group: 17q gain in neuroblastoma predicts adverse clinical outcome. Med Pediatr Oncol 2001;36:14–19.
22. Brown N, Cotterill S, Lastowska M et al. Gain of chromosome arm 17q and adverse outcome in patients with neuroblastoma. N Engl J Med 1999;340:1954–1961.
23. Nakagawara A, Arima-Nakagawara M, Scavarda NJ et al. Association between high levels of expression of the TRK gene and favorable outcome in human neuroblastoma. N Engl J Med 1993;328:847–854.
24. Reynolds CP, Zuo JJ, Kim NW et al. Telomerase expression in primary neuroblastomas. Eur J Cancer 1997;33:1929–1931.
25. Chan HSL, Haddad G, Thorner PS et al. P-glycoprotein expression as a predictor of the outcome of therapy for neuroblastoma. N Engl J Med 1991;325:1608–1614.
26. Leone A, Seeger RC, Hong CM et al. Evidence for nm23 RNA overexpression, DNA amplification and mutation in aggressive childhood neuroblastomas. Oncogene 1993;8:855–865.
27. Shuster JJ, McWilliams NB, Castleberry R et al. Serum lactate dehydrogenase in childhood neuroblastoma. A Pediatrics Oncology Group recursive partitioning study. Am J Clin Oncol 1992;15:295–303.

28. Hann HW, Evans AE, Siegel SE et al. Prognostic importance of serum ferritin in patients with Stage III and IV neuroblastoma: the Children's Cancer Study Group experience. Cancer Res 1985;45:2843–2848.
29. Ladenstein R, Philip T, Lasset C et al. Multivariate analysis of risk factors in stage 4 neuroblastoma patients over the age of one year treated with megatherapy and stem-cell transplantation: A report from the European Bone Marrow Transplantation Solid Tumor Registry. J Clin Oncol 1998;16:953–965.
30. Garaventa O, Ladenstein R, Chauvin F et al. High dose chemotherapy with autologous bone marrow rescue in advanced stage IV neuroblastoma. Eur J Cancer 1993;29A:487–491.
31. Brodeur G, Pritchard J, Berthold F et al. Revisions of the international criteria for neuroblastoma diagnosis, staging, and response to treatment. J Clin Oncol 1993;11:1466–1477.
32. Matthay K. Intensification of therapy using hematopoietic stem-cell support for high-risk neuroblastoma. Pediatr Transplant 1999;3(Suppl 1):72–77.
33. Matthay KK. Neuroblastoma: biology and therapy. Oncology 1997;11:1857–1866.
34. Cheung NV, Heller G. Chemotherapy dose intensity correlates strongly with response, median survival, and median progression-free survival in metastatic neuroblastoma. J Clin Oncol 1991;9:1050–1058.
35. Lanino E, Boni L, Corciulo P, De Bernardi B. Did BMT change the clinical course of neuroblastoma? Bone Marrow Transplant 1991;7(Suppl 3):109–111.
36. Suita S, Zaizen Y, Kaneko M et al. What is the benefit of aggressive chemotherapy for advanced stage neuroblastoma with N-myc amplification? A report from the Japanese Study Group for the Treatment of Advanced Neuroblastoma. J Pediatr Surg 1994;29:746–750.
37. Campbell LA, Seeger RC, Harris RC et al. Escalating dose of continuous infusion combination chemotherapy for refractory neuroblastoma. J Clin Oncol 1993;11:623–629.
38. Cheung NK, Kushner BH, LaQuaglia M et al. N7: A novel multi-modality therapy of high risk neuroblastoma (NB) in children diagnosed over 1 year of age. Med Pediatr Oncol 2001;36:227–230.
39. Hartmann O, Benhamou E, Beaujean F et al. Repeated high dose chemotherapy followed by purged autologous bone marrow transplantation as consolidation therapy in metastatic neuroblastoma. J Clin Oncol 1987; 5:1205–1211.
40. Kushner BH, O'Rielly RJ, Mandell LR et al. Myeloablative combination chemotherapy without total body irradiation for neuroblastoma. J Clin Oncol 1991;9:274–279.
41. Stram DO, Matthay KK, O'Leary M et al. Consolidation chemoradiotherapy and autologous bone marrow transplantation versus continued chemotherapy for metastatic neuroblastoma: A report of two concurrent Children's Cancer Group studies. J Clin Oncol 1996;14:2417–2426.
42. Seeger RC, Reynolds CP, Gallego R et al. Quantitative tumor cell content of bone marrow and blood as a predictor of outcome in stage IV neuroblastoma: a Children's Cancer Group Study. J Clin Oncol 2000;18:4067–4076.
43. Hayes FA, Green AA, Caper J et al. Clinical evaluation of sequentially scheduled cisplatin and VM 26 in neuroblastoma. Cancer 1981;48:1751–1758.
44. Green A, Hayes FA, Husto HO. Sequential cyclophosphamide and doxorubicin for induction of complete remission in children with disseminated neuroblastoma. Cancer 1981;48:2310–2317.
45. Kushner BH, Helson L. Coordinated use of sequentially escalated cyclophosphamide and cell cycle-specific chemotherapy (N4SE protocol) for advanced neuroblastoma: experience with 100 patients. J Clin Oncol 1987;5:1746–1751.
46. Philip T, Ghalie R, Pinkerton R et al. A phase II study of high-dose cisplatin and VP-16 in neuroblastoma: a report from the Societe Francaise d'Oncologie Pediatrique. J Clin Oncol 1987;5:941–950.
47. Kushner BH, O'Rielly RJ, LaQuaglia M, Cheung NK. Dose intensive use of cyclophosphamide in ablation of neuroblastoma. Cancer 1990;66:1095–1100.
48. Bernard JL, Philip T, Zucker JM et al. Sequential cisplatin/VM26 and vincristine/cyclophosphamide/doxorubicin in metastatic neuroblastoma: An effective alternating non-cross-resistant regimen? J Clin Oncol 1987; 5:1952–1959.
49. Donfrancesco A, Deb G, Dominici C et al. Deferoxamine, cyclophosphamide, etoposide, carboplatin, and thiotepa (D-CECaT): a new cytoreductive chelation-chemotherapy regimen in patients with advanced neuroblastoma. Am J Clin Oncol 1992;15:319–322.
50. Kushner BH, LaQualghia MP, Bonillar MA et al. Highly effective induction treatment for stage IV neuroblastoma in children >1 year of age. J Clin Oncol 1994;12:2607–2613.
51. Hero B, Kremens B, Klingebiel T et al. Does megatherapy contribute to survival in metastatic neuroblastoma? Klin Padiatr 1997;209:196–200.
52. Kaneko M, Tsuchida Y, Uchino J et al. Treatment results of advanced stage neuroblastoma with the first Japanese Study Group protocol. J Pediatr Hematol Oncol 1999;21:190–197.
53. La Quaglia MP, Kushner BH, Heller G et al. Stage 4 neuroblastoma diagnosed at more than 1 year of age: Gross total resection and clinical outcome. J Pediatr Surg 1994;29:1162–1166.
54. Kameko M, Ohakawa H, Iwakawa M. Is extensive surgery required for treatment of advanced neuroblastoma? J Pediatr Surg 1997;32:1616–1619.
55. Kiely EM. The surgical challenge of neuroblastoma. J Pediatr Surg 1994;29:128–133.

56. Black CT, Haase GM, Azizkham RG et al. Optimal timing of primary resection in high risk neuroblastoma. Med Pediatr Oncol 1996;27:220.
57. Castel V, Tovar JA, Costa E et al. The role of surgery in stage IV neuroblastoma. J Pediatr Surg 2002;37:1574–1578.
58. Matthay KK, Atkinson JB, Stram DO et al. Patterns of relapse after autologous purged bone marrow transplantation for neuroblastoma: A Children's Cancer Group Pilot Study. J Clin Oncol 1993;11:2226–2233.
59. Yokoyama J, Ikawa H, Endow M et al. The role of surgery in advanced neuroblastoma. Eur J Pediatr Surg 1995;5:23–26.
60. Haase GM, O'Leary MC, Ramsey NK et al. Aggressive surgery combined with intensive chemotherapy improves survival in poor-risk neuroblastoma. J Pediatr Surg 1991;26:1119–1124.
61. Kletzel M, Abella EM, Sandler ES et al. Thiotepa and cyclophosphamide therapy for children with high-risk neuroblastoma: A phase I/II study of the Pediatric Blood and Marrow Transplant Consortium. J Pediatr Hematol Oncol 1998;20:49–54.
62. Kamani N, August CS, Bunin N et al. A study of thiotepa, etoposide and fractionated total body irradiation as a preparative regimen prior to bone marrow transplantation for poor prognosis patients with neuroblastoma. Bone Marrow Transplant 1996;17:911–916.
63. Villablanca JG, Reynolds CP, Swift PS et al. Phase I trial of carboplatin, etoposide, melphalan, local irradiation (CEM-LI) with purged autologous marrow transplantation for children with high risk neuroblastoma. Proc Am Soc Clin Oncol 1998;17:533a.
64. To L, Roberts M, Haylock D et al. Comparison of hematological recovery times and supportive care requirements of autologous recovery phase pheripheral blood stem cell transplants, autologous bone marrow transplants, and allogeneic bone marrow transplants. Bone Marrow Transplant 1992;9:277–284.
65. Huan S, Hester J, Splitzer G et al. Influence of mobilized peripheral stem cells on the hematopoietic recovery by autologous marrow and recombinant human granulocyte-macrophage colony-stimulating factor after high-dose cyclophosphamide, etoposide, and cisplatin. Blood 1992;79:3388–3393.
66. Lee JH, Klein HG. Collection and use of circulating hematopoietic progenitor cells. Hematol Oncol Clin North Am 1995;9:1–22.
67. Kletzel M, Longino R, Danner K et al. Peripheral blood stem cell rescue in children with advanced stage neuroblastoma. Prog Clin Biol Res 1994;389:513–519.
68. Miyajima Y, Horibe K, Fukuda M et al. Sequential detection of tumor cells in the peripheral blood and bone marrow of patients with stage IV neuroblastoma by the reverse-transcriptase polymerase chain reaction for tyrosine hydroxylase mRNA. Cancer 1996;77:1879–1883.
69. Cohn SL, Moss TJ, Hoover M et al. Treatment of poor-risk neuroblastoma patients with high-dose chemotherapy and autologous peripheral stem cell rescue. Bone Marrow Transplant 1997;20:543–551.
70. Brenner MK, Rill DA. Gene marking to improve the outcome of autologous bone marrow transplantation. J Hematother 1994;3:33–36.
71. Handgretinger R, Greil J, Shurmann U et al. Positive selection and transplantation of peripheral CD34+ progenitor cells: Feasibility and purging efficacy in pediatric patients with neuroblastoma. J Hematother 1997;6:235–242.
72. Lopez M, Beaujean F. Positive selection of autologous peripheral blood stem cells. Baillieres Best Pract Res Clin Haematol 1999;12:71–86.
73. Donovan J, Temel J, Zuckerman A et al. CD34 selection as a stem cell purging strategy for neuroblastoma: Preclinical and clinical studies. Med Pediatr Oncol 2000;35:677–682.
74. Kanold J, Yakouben K, Tchirkov A et al. Long term results of CD34+ cell transplantation in children with neuroblastoma. Med Pediatr Oncol 2000;35:1–7.
75. Kushner BH, Gulati SC, Kwon J-H et al. High-dose melphalan with 6-hydroxydopamine-purged autologous bone marrow transplantation for poor-risk neuroblastoma. Cancer 1991;68:242–247.
76. Kemshead JT, Heath L, Gibson FM et al. Magnetic microspheres and monoclonal antibodies for the depletion of neuroblastoma cells from bone marrow: experience, improvements, and observations. Br J Cancer 1986;54:771–778.
77. Reynolds CP, Billups CB, Moss TJ et al. Depletion of tumor cell clumps with sedimentation and filtration of bone marrow prior to other purging modalities. Proc Am Soc Clin Oncol 1989;8:309.
78. Beaujean F, Hartmann O, Benhamou E et al. Hematopoietic reconstitution after repeated autologous transplantation with mafosfamide-purged marrow. Bone Marrow Transplant 1989;4:537–541.
79. Hartmann O, Kaifa C, Benhamou E et al. Treatment of advanced stage neuroblastoma with high-dose melphalan and autologous bone marrow transplant. Cancer Chemother Pharmacol 1986;16:165–169.
80. Parsons SK, Neault MW, Lehmann LE et al. Severe ototoxicity following carboplatin containing conditioning regimen for autologous marrow transplantation for neuroblastoma. Bone Marrow Transplant 1998;22:669–674.
81. Hovi L, Saarinen-Pihkala UM, Vettenranta K et al. Growth in children with poor-risk neuroblastoma after regimens with or without total body irradiation in preparation for autologous bone marrow transplantation. Bone Marrow Transplant 1999;24:1131–1136.

82. Sander J, Sullivan K, Witherspoon K et al. Long-term effects and quality of life in children and adults after marrow transplantation. Bone Marrow Transplant 1989;4:27–29.

83. Franzone P, Scarpati D, Vitale V et al. Chemo-radiotherapy and autologous bone marrow transplantation in poor prognosis neuroblastoma. Radiother Oncol 1990;18(Suppl 1):102–104.

84. Philip T, Zucker J, Bernard J et al. Improved survival at 2 and 5 years in the LMCE1 unselected group of 72 children with stage IV neuroblastoma older than 1 year of age at diagnosis: is cure possible in a small subgroup? J Clin Oncol 1991;9:1037–1044.

85. Graham-Pole J, Casper J, Elfenbein G et al. High-dose chemoradiotherapy supported by marrow infusions for advanced neuroblastoma: a Pediatric Oncology Group Study. J Clin Oncol 1991;9:152–158.

86. Matthay KK, O'Leary MC, Ramsey NK et al. Role of myeloablative therapy in improved outcome for high risk neuroblastoma: review of recent Children's Cancer Group results. Eur J Cancer 1995;31A:572–575.

87. Park JR, Slattery J, Gooley T et al. Phase I topotecan preparative regimen for high-risk neuroblastoma, high-grade glioma, and refractory/recurrent pediatric solid tumors. Med Pediatr Oncol 2000;35:719–723.

88. Kushner BH, Cheung NK, Kramer K et al. Topotecan combined with myeloablative doses of thiotepa and carboplatin for neuroblastoma, brain tumors, and other poor-risk solid tumors in children and young adults. Bone Marrow Transplant 2001;28:551–556.

89. Shuster JJ, Cantor AB, McWilliams N et al. The prognostic significance of autologous bone marrow transplant in advanced neuroblastoma. J Clin Oncol 1991;9:1045–1049.

90. Ohnuma N, Taahashi H, Kaneko M et al. Treatment combined with bone marrow transplantation for advanced neuroblastoma: an analysis of patients who were pretreated intensively with the protocol of the Study Group of Japan. Med Pediatr Oncol 1995;24:181–187.

91. Matthay KK, Seeger RC, Reynolds CP et al. Allogeneic versus autologous purged bone marrow transplantation for neuroblastoma: a report from the Children's Cancer Group. J Clin Oncol 1994;12:2382–2389.

92. Ladenstein R, Lasset C, Hartmann O et al. Comparison of auto versus allografting as consolidation of primary treatments in advanced neuroblastoma over one year of age at diagnosis: Report from the European Group for Bone Marrow Transplantation. Bone Marrow Transplant 1994;14:37–46.

93. Graham-Pole J. Is there an advantage to allogeneic over autologous marrow transplantation in patients with metastatic neuroblastoma. Exp Hematol 1989;17:586.

94. Philip T, Ladenstein R, Zucker JM et al. Double megatherapy and autologous bone marrow transplantation for advanced neuroblastoma: the LMCE2 study. Br J Cancer 1993;67:119–127.

95. Kawa-Ha K, Yumura-Yagi K, Inoue M et al. Results of single and double autografts for high-risk neuroblastoma patients. Bone Marrow Transplant 1996;17:957–962.

96. Vassal G, Trabchand B, Valteau-Couanet D et al. Pharmacodynamics of tandem high-dose melphalan with peripheral blood stem cell transplantation in children with neuroblastoma and medulloblastoma. Bone Marrow Transplant 2001;27:471–477.

97. Grupp SA, Stern JW, Bunin N et al. Rapid-sequence tandem transplant for children with high-risk neuroblastoma. Med Pediatr Oncol 2000;35:696–700.

98. Kletzel M, Katzebstein HM, Haut PR et al. Treatment of high-risk neuroblastoma triple-tandem therapy and stem-cell rescue: Results of the Chicago Pilot II Study. J Clin Oncol 2002;20:2284–2292.

99. Sisson JC, Shapiro B, Beirealtes WH. Radiopharmaceutical treatment of malignant pheochromocytoma. J Nucl Med 1984;24:198–206.

100. Treuner J, Klingebiel T, Bruchelt G et al. Treatment of neuroblastoma with metaiodobenzylguanidine: results and side effects. Med Pediatr Oncol 1987;15:199–202.

101. Hartman O, Lumbroso J, Lemerle J et al. Therapeutic use of [131]I-metaiodobenzylguanidine (MIBG) in neuroblastoma: A phase II study in nine patients. Med Pediatr Oncol 1987;15:205–211.

102. Sisson JC, Hutchinson RJ, Carey JC et al. Toxicity from treatment of neuroblastoma with [131]I-metaiodobenzylguanidin. Eur J Nucl Med 1988;14:337–340.

103. Beierwaltes WH. Treatment of neuroblastoma with [131]I-MIBG: dosimetric problems and perspectives. Med Pediatr Oncol 1987;15:188–191.

104. Lashford LS, Lewis IJ, Fielding SL et al. Phase I/II study of iodine [131]metaiodobenzylguanidine in chemoresistant neuroblastoma: A United Kingdom Children's Cancer Study Group investigation. J Clin Oncol 1992;10:1889–1896.

105. Wheldon TE, O'Donoghue JA, Barrett A, Michalowski AS. The curability of tumours of differing size by targeted radiotherapy using [131]I or [90]Y. Radiother Oncol 1991;21:91–99.

106. Gaze MN, Wheldon TE, O'Donoghue JA et al. Multi-modality megatherapy with [[131]I]metaiodobenzylguanidine, high dose melphalan and total body irradiation with bone marrow rescue: feasibility study of a new strategy for advanced neuroblastoma. Eur J Cancer 1995;31:252–256.

107. Goldberg SS, DeSantes K, Huberty JP et al. Engraftment after myeloablative doses of [131]I-metaiodobenzylguanidine followed by autologous bone marrow transplantation for treatment of refractory neuroblastoma. Med Pediatr Oncol 1998;30:339–346.

108. Matthay KK, DeSantes K, Hasegawa J et al. Phase I dose escalation of [131]I-metaiodobenzylguanidine with autologous bone marrow support in refractory neuroblastoma. J Clin Oncol 1998;16:229–236.

109. Klingebiel T, Bader P, Bares R et al. Treatment of neuroblastoma stage 4 with [131]I-meta-iodo-benzylguanidine, high-dose chemotherapy and immunotherapy. A pilot study. Eur J Cancer 1998;34:1398–1402.

110. Miano MM, Garaventa A, Pizzitola MR et al. Megatherapy combining [131]I-metaiodobenzylguanidine and high-dose chemotherapy with haematopoietic progenitor cell rescue for neuroblastoma. Bone Marrow Transplant 2001;27:571–574.

111. Yanik GA, Levine JE, Matthay KK et al. Pilot study of iodine-[131]-metaiodobenzylguanidine in combination with myeloablative chemotherapy and autologous stem-cell support for the treatment of neuroblastoma. J Clin Oncol 2002;20:2142–2149.

112. Horibe K, Fukuda M, Miyajima Y et al. Outcome prediction by molecular detection of minimal residual disease in bone marrow for advanced stage neuroblastoma. Med Pediatr Oncol 2001;36:203–204.

113. Seeger RC, Reynolds CP, Gallego R et al. Qualitative tumor cell content of bone marrow and blood as predictor of outcome in stage IV neuroblastoma: A Children's Cancer Study Group Study. J Clin Oncol 2000; 18:4067–4076.

114. Burchill SA, Kinsey SE, Picton S et al. Minimal residual disease at the time of peripheral blood harvest in patients with advanced stage neuroblastoma. Med Pediatr Oncol 2001;36:213–219.

115. Reynolds CP, Kane DJ, Einhorn PA et al. Response of neuroblastoma to retinoic acid in vitro and in vivo. Prog Clin Biol Res 1991;366:203–211.

116. Villablanca JG, Khan AA, Avramis VI et al. Phase I trial of 13-cis-retinoic acid in children with neuroblastoma following bone marrow transplantation. J Clin Oncol 1995;13:894–901.

117. Mariotti A, Marcora E, Bunone G et al. N-(4-hydroxyphenylretinamide): a potent inducer of apoptosis in human neuroblastoma cells. J Natl Cancer Inst 1994;86:1245–1247.

118. Cheung NK. Monoclonal antibody-based therapy for neuroblastoma. Curr Oncol Rep 2000;2:547–553.

119. Rosseau RF, Haight AE, Hirschmann-Jax C et al. Local and systemic effects of an allogeneic tumor cell vaccine combining transgenic human lymphotactin with interleukin-2 patients with advanced or refractory neuroblastoma. Blood 2003;101:1718–1726.

120. Geiger JD, Hutchinson RJ, Hohenkirk LF et al. Vaccination of pediatric solid tumor patients with tumor lysate-pulsed dendritic cells can expand specific T cells and mediate tumor regression. Cancer Res 2001;61: 8513–8519.

121. Thiele CJ, Reynolds CP, Israel MA. Decreased expression of N-myc precedes retinoic acid-induced morphological of human neuroblastoma. Nature 1985;313:404–406.

122. Delia D, Aiello A, Lombardi L et al. N-(4-hydroxyphenyl) retinamide induces apoptosis of malignant hemopoietic cell lines including those unresponsive to retinoic acid. Cancer Res 1993;53:6036–6041.

123. Yu AL, Uttenreuther-Fischer MM, Huang C-S et al. A phase I trial of a human-mouse chimeric anti-disalo-ganglioside (GD2) monoclonal antibody ch14.18 in patients with refractory neuroblastoma and osteosarcoma. J Clin Oncol 1998;16:2169–2180.

124. Ozkaynak MF, Seeger R, Bauer M et al. A phase I study of ch14.18 with GM-CSF in children with neuroblastoma following autologous BMT. Children's Cancer Study Group. J Clin Oncol 2000;18:4077–4085.

125. Kushner BH, Kramer K, Cheung NK. Phase II trial of the anti-G(D2) monoclonal antibody 3F8 and granulocyte-macrophage colony-stimulating factor for neuroblastoma. J Clin Oncol 2001;1:4189–4194.

126. Schultz G, Cheresh DA, Varki NM et al. Detection of ganglioside GD2 in tumor tissues and sera of neuroblastoma. Cancer Res 1984;44:5914–5920.

127. Murray JL, Cunningham JE, Brewer H et al. Phase I trial of murine monoclonal antibody 14G2a administered by prolonged intravenous infusion inpatients with neuroectodermal tumors. J Clin Oncol 1994;12:184–193.

128. Bruchelt G, Hangretinger R, Fierlbeck G et al. Lysis of neuroblastoma cells by the ADCC-reaction: Granulocytes of patients with chronic granulomatous disease are more effective than those of healthy donors. Immunol Lett 1989;22:217–220.

129. Bonig H, Laws H-J, Wundes A et al. In vivo cytokine responses to interleukin-2 immunotherapy after autologous stem cell transplantation in children with solid tumors. Bone Marrow Transplant 2000;26:91–96.

130. Baker E, Reisfeld RA. A mechanism for neutrophil-mediated lysis of human neuroblastoma cells. Cancer Res 1993;53:362–367.

131. Baxevanis CN, Tsavaris NB, Papadhimitriou SI et al. Granulocyte-macrophage colony-stimulating factor improves immunological parameters in patients with refractory solid tumors receiving second-line chemotherapy: correlation with clinical responses. Eur J Cancer 1997;33:1202–1208.

132. Toren A, Nagler A, Rozenfeld-Granot G et al. Amplification of immunological functions by subcutaneous injection of intermediate-high dose interleukin-2 for 2 years after autologous stem cell transplantation in children with stage IV neuroblastoma. Transplant 2000;70:1100–1104.

133. Masucci G, Ragnhammer P, Werall P, Mellstedt H. Granulocyte-monocyte-colony-stimulating factor augments the cytotoxic capacity of lymphocytes and monocytes in antibody dependent cellular cytotoxicity. Cancer Immunol Immunother 1990;31:231–235.

134. Hank JA, Robinson RR, Surfus J et al. Augmentation of antibody dependent cell mediated cytotoxicty following in vivo therapy with recombinant interleukin-2. Cancer Res 1990;50:5234–5239.

135. Lotze MT, Grimm EA, Mazumder A et al. Lysis of fresh and cultured autologous tumor by human lymphocytes cultured in T cell growth factor. Cancer Res 1981;41:4420–4425.

136. Hank JA, Surfus JE, Gan J et al. Activation of human effector cells by a tumor reactive recombinant anti-ganglioside-GD2/interleukin-2 fusion protein (ch14.18-IL2). Clin Cancer Res 1996;2:1951–1959.

137. Gillies SD, Young D, Lo KM, Robert S. Biological activity and in vivo clearance of antitumor antibody/cytokine fusion proteins. Bioconjug Chem 1993;4:230–235.

138. Saleh MN, Khazaeli MB, Wheeler RH et al. Phase I trial of the chimeric anti-GD2 monoclonal antibody ch14.18 in patients with malignant melanoma. Hum Antibodies Hybridomas 1992;3:19–24.

139. Albertini MA, Hank JA, Surtus J et al. Antibody-cytokine fusion protein (HU14.18-IL2) retains biological activity in human serum following in vivo administration for treatment of melanoma (Abstr). Proc Am Soc Clin Oncol 1999.

140. Haight AE, Bowman LC, Ng CY et al. Humoral response to vaccination with interleukin-2 expressing allogeneic neuroblastoma cells after primary therapy. Med Pediatr Oncol 2000;35:712–715.

141. Katzenstein HM, Rademaker AW, Senger C et al. Effectiveness of the angiogenesis inhibitor TNP-470 in reducing the growth of human neuroblastoma in nude mice inversely correlates with tumor burden. Clin Can Res 1999;5:4272–4278.

142. Stern JW, Fang J, Shusterman S et al. Angiogenesis inhibitor TNP-470 during bone marrow transplant: safety in a preclinical model. Clin Cancer Res 2001;7:1026–1032.

# CHAPTER X

# Stem Cell Transplantation for Ewing's Sarcoma

ROBERT B. MARCUS, JR.

Ewing's sarcoma is the second-most common primary tumor of bone in childhood, and also occurs in soft tissues. The median age is 14 years, with 57% of the patients male and 43% female.[1] The malignancy is rare in African Americans and presents most commonly in the pelvis, femur, tibia, fibula, and ribs.[1,2]

The cell of origin of Ewing's sarcoma of bone was long in doubt, but the development of cytogenetics has shown that it is one of a family of tumors, with Ewing's sarcoma of bone and soft tissue the most undifferentiated members of the family.[3-5] These neoplasms share a common neuroectodermal precursor cell, but are arrested at different stages of differentiation.[6] Cytogenetically, 90%–95% of the Ewing's family of tumors have a translocation between the EWS gene on chromosome 22 and the FLI1 gene on chromosome 11 [t(11:22)(q24:q12)] or the ERG gene on chromosome 21 [t(21;22)(q22;q12)].[7] The translocations are present only in tumor cells and not in normal cells taken from the same patients.[7-9] They are present in both osseous and extraosseous variants as well as primitive neuroectodermal tumors (PNETs) of bone and soft tissue, peripheral primitive neuroectodermal tumors (pPNET), Askin tumors, some esthesioneuroblastomas in children, and some central nervous system (CNS) tumors.[8]

## LOCALIZED DISEASE

Ewing's sarcoma is a disease that responds well to chemotherapy and radiation therapy. The addition of chemotherapy to only local therapy in the late 1960s and early 1970s increased the survival rate from <10% to >40% at five years for patients without metastases at diagnosis. However, Ewing's sarcoma is a disease for which the ultimate cure rate may not be established for at least 10 years because of late recurrences and deaths from complications. ▼ Table 10.1 lists survival rates from major studies over the last 30 years where long-term follow-up was reported and patients with metastatic disease were excluded. For patients treated in the 1970s, two-year survival rates ranged from 66%–76%, five-year survival rates from 42%–60%, and ten-year survival rates from 38%–47%. Studies of patients treated in the 1980s did not show any definite improvement. Though studies from the 1990s have encouraging early survival rates, more follow-up is needed to determine if these will be confirmed.

| TABLE 10.1 | Overall Survival by Decade of Treatment for Patients with Localized Disease at Diagnosis | | |
|---|---|---|---|

| Institution (Reference) | Survival | | |
|---|---|---|---|
| | 2 Years | 5 Years | 10 Years |
| **Treated in the 1970s** | | | |
| National Cancer Institute[10] | 68 | 51 | 39 |
| Mayo Clinic[11] | 70 | 42 | 38 |
| Mass. General[12] | 76 | 60 | 47 |
| Univ. of FL[13] | 66 | 45 | 44 |
| **Treated in the 1980s** | | | |
| Gustave-Roussy[14] | 75 | 47 | 35 |
| POG 8346[15] | 70 | 62 | 48 |
| Univ. of FL[13 a] | 75 | 59 | 55 |
| CESS-86[16] | 70 | 65 | 47 |
| POG-CCG Intergroup[17] | — | 62 | — |
| **Treated in the 1990s** | | | |
| SE-91 CNR[18] | 87 | 65 | — |
| St. Jude[19] | 88 | — | — |

[a]Patients with large primary lesions received end-intensification

## STANDARD THERAPY

Both effective local and systemic therapy are necessary for the cure of Ewing's sarcoma. Over 90% of Ewing's sarcoma patients have either detectable or subclinical metastases at diagnosis; local therapy (either surgery, irradiation, or a combination), if delivered correctly, is probably not the critical event in determining survival. The majority of patients who relapse fail systemically and it is systemic therapy that primarily determines survival.

Most chemotherapy regimens are a combination of cyclophosphamide, doxorubicin HCl (Adriamycin), vincristine, dactinomycin, ifosphamide, and etoposide.[8–12,17,19–30] Other drugs have not been shown to be very active. Most regimens have an induction phase for two to four months, followed by local therapy and additional chemotherapy for up to 12 months.

The first Intergroup Ewing's Sarcoma Study (IESS-I) established VACA (vincristine, doxorubicin, cyclophosphamide, dactinomycin) as the best regimen.[28] A randomized POG/CCG Intergroup study starting in 1988 showed that the addition of the ifosphamide/etoposide combination to VACA improved the survival rates, particularly for patients with primary tumors of the pelvis.[17]

Unfortunately, no significant new drugs or drug combinations have been developed since ifosphamide/etoposide. Whereas the majority of older studies use a duration exposure concept, present strategies are based primarily on intensifying systemic therapy. IESS-II compared two regimens of VACA; the best arm delivered the chemotherapy using intensive pulses.[24] In 1991 Smith et al.[31] reported a direct relationship between survival and the doxorubicin dose intensity. More recently, Kushner et al.[32] reported short-term results of a quick, intensive protocol of HD-CAV (vincristine, doxorubicin, cyclophosphamide with mesna alternating with ifosfamide and etoposide) for peripheral neuroectodermal tumors (pPNET) of the soft tissues from Memorial Sloan-Kettering Cancer Center. Patients treated on the P6 protocol had a two-year event-free survival of 77%, perhaps producing better results than previously for this rare member of the Ewing's family.[32] Early results of dose-intensification from a St. Jude Research Hospital trial running from 1992 through 1996 are encouraging, with a two-year survival rate of > 88% and a two-year event-free survival rate of 80%.[19] Delepine et al.[33] reported that survival after treatment for Ewing's sarcoma depends upon the dose intensity of vincristine and dactinomycin.

A POG/CCG Intergroup study (CCG-7942, POG 9354) studied dose intensification by escalating the doses of the alkylating agents cyclophosphamide and ifosfamide. This study opened in 1995 and closed in 1998 but the results have not been released yet. The successor study, AEWS0031, which opened in 2001, is studying dose intensification by decreasing the interval between doses, comparing an interval of 21 days with an interval of 14 days. AEWS0031 is based upon a pilot study by Womer et al.,[34] where 30 patients with localized Ewing's sarcoma were treated with interval compression to 14 days between cycles. The overall survival at three years was 85%.[34] It remains to be seen whether any of these approaches will provide a significant increase in survival rates, but these early results do support the premise that intensifying systemic therapy warrants further investigation.

## END-INTENSIFICATION FOLLOWED BY STEM CELL RESCUE

One method of dose intensification that has been studied by a few institutions is ending systemic treatment with a course of myeloablative chemotherapy with or without total body irradiation (TBI), followed by hematopoietic stem cell transplant (HSCT), or originally an autologous bone marrow transplant (ABMT). One of the problems with this approach is that a group of high risk patients must be defined because patients with a more favorable prognosis should not be placed at risk until enough data are obtained to prove that the approach is feasible and beneficial. It is clear that patients with metastatic disease at diagnosis have a poor prognosis, but what about those with localized disease? There is no commonly utilized staging system for Ewing's sarcoma, but a number of prognostic factors have been reported for patients with localized disease at diagnosis. Primary tumors of the pelvis or trunk, a large primary tumor, the presence of a large soft-tissue mass, an older age at diagnosis, a high lactic dehydrogenase (LDH) level at diagnosis, poor response to induction chemotherapy, the lack of surgery as part of the treatment of the primary lesion, and a filigree histologic pattern all have been proposed as poor-prognostic factors.[1,9,12,29,30,35–40] Some of these have been utilized to select out a group of high risk patients for end-intensification trials. ▼ Table 10.2 shows five-year survival results contrasting patients with "small" and "large" primary tumors. Though the definition varies from institution to institution, the results for these studies reporting patients treated in the 1970s and 1980s show five-year survival rates of about 70% for "small" lesions and 30% for "large" lesions.

Institutions that have designed trials to test end-intensification with myeloablative regimens for patients with localized disease have used different criteria to define the high risk group. The following trials have enough follow-up to provide some useful data (▼ Table 10.3).

| Institution | Size Criteria for Large | Small | Large |
|---|---|---|---|
| **TABLE 10.2** | **Five-Year Survival by Tumor Size, Localized Patients Only** | | |
| University of Florida[13] | >8 cm max diameter | 78% | 30% |
| CESS-81[38] | > 100 mL volume | 78%[a] | 17%[a] |
| CESS 86 update[35] | > 200 mL volume | ~67% | 32% |
| Massachusetts General Hospital, MA[12] | > 500 mL volume | 70% | 34% |
| Memorial Sloan-Kettering Hospital, NY[30] | > 8 cm max diameter | 79% | 38% |

[a]Three-year event-free survival

## National Cancer Institute Trial

Between 1981 and 1986, 97 patients with primary small round cell tumors were treated on three successive protocols utilizing high dose consolidative therapy. Of these, 18 had localized Ewing's sarcoma with high risk primary lesions of the trunk, humerus, or femur, not further stratified. The majority of the patients were treated with five cycles of vincristine, doxorubicin, and cylcophosphamide (VAdrC), followed by a conditioning regimen consisting of an additional cycle of VAdrC in conjunction with 8 Gy TBI in two fractions. The marrow was harvested after two cycles of VAdrC. The local treatment was radiation therapy in most patients. Although the event-free survival (EFS) and the overall survival for the entire cohort of 97 patients was only 25% and 30%, respectively, at six years, the EFS and overall survival for the patients with localized Ewing's sarcoma of bone was 48%.[26] Complications were only reported for the entire 97 patients, but there were six therapy-related deaths, five directly related to the transplant: one viral pneumonia, one interstitial pneumonitis, and three with complications related to invasive aspergillosis. No patient developed leukemia after treatment.[26]

## University of Florida Trials

An attempt to improve survival utilizing end-intensification was begun in 1982 at the University of Florida. Because an analysis of patients treated from 1969 through 1981 showed a dramatic decrement in survival for patients with primary lesions greater than 8 cm in diameter, patients with localized disease were divided into standard-risk ($\leq$ 8 cm in maximum diameter) and high risk (>8 cm in maximum diameter) by tumor size.[39] Patients with metastases also were considered high risk. Patients on standard-risk protocols received what was considered to be standard chemotherapy at the time.[13,27,45] High risk patients received more intensive chemotherapy followed by end-intensification consisting of a conditioning regimen and an ABMT or HSCT.[13,27,46]

Sixty-seven patients with localized disease were treated from 1982 through 1998, 28 on standard-risk protocols and 39 on high risk protocols. Three separate regimens were used for high risk patients with localized disease at diagnosis during the time period of this analysis (▶ Table 10.3).

All three protocols started with two cycles of VAdrC, followed by a bone marrow or stem cell harvest, which was then stored. Treatment of the primary lesion was delayed until after

| TABLE 10.3 | Five-Year Survival of High Risk Patients With Localized Disease |

| Institution | Conditioning Regimen | Selection Criteria | N Pts | Survival |
|---|---|---|---|---|
| NCI (3 protocols)[26] (1981–1986) | VAdrC 8 Gy/2 Fx TBI | Humerus, femur, trunk | 18 | 48% |
| Univ. Florida[13] HR-2 (1982–1984) | Melphalan 60 mg/m² × 3 d | > 8 cm | 6 | 17% |
| Univ. Florida[13] HR-3 & HR-4 (1985–1998) | VAdrC (HR-3) 8 Gy/2 Fx TBI  VP-16/C (HR-4) 12 Gy/6 Fx TBI | > 8 cm | 33 | 63% |
| EBMT Registry[41] | Various | Large lesions or poor response to ChTx | 28 | 60% |
| Tom Baker Centre[42] (1985–1994) | Melphan ± 500 cGy/1 FX TBI | >8 cm or Femur | 6 | 33%[a] |
| Royal Marsden[43] (Not stated) | Busulphan Melphan | >100 mL | 7 | 100% |
| Madrid Collaboration[44] (1986–1995) | Busulphan Melphan | >100 mL | 15 | 50-71% |

Abbreviations: HR = high risk; Adr = Adriamycin (doxorubicin); C = Cytoxan (cyclophosphamide); V = vincristine; VP-16 = Vepesid (etoposide); Ifos = ifosfomide; TBI = total body irradiation.
[a]Two-year survival

the harvest; on the high risk protocols all patients received radiotherapy after the harvest, though expendable bones were surgically removed at the end of all systemic therapy. Melphalan alone was used as the conditioning regimen for protocol HR-2, whereas the other two high risk protocols used a combination of total body irradiation and chemotherapy.

Six patients were entered on the High Risk-2 (HR-2) protocol from 1982 to 1984. Patients placed on this protocol received four cycles of induction chemotherapy (Regimen A) consisting of oral cyclophosphamide (150 mg/m²) for seven days, followed by intravenous doxorubicin (35 mg/m²) on day 8. Starting with cycle five, two additional regimens (B and C) were added. Regimen B consisted of oral cyclophosphamide (150 mg/m²) for seven days, followed by intravenous dactinomycin (1.5 mg/m²) on day 8. Regimen C consisted of intravenous vincristine (1.5 mg/m²) on days 1, 8, and 15, with intravenous cyclophosphamide (1000 mg/m²) and intravenous doxorubicin (75 mg/m²) on day 2. These three regimens (A, B, and C) were alternated from cycle 5 to cycle 11 at a 28-day interval. Each cycle was started every 21 days. Following a one-month period for marrow recovery and scheduling, another reevaluation was performed. If no disease was detected, 60 mg/m$^2$ of intravenous melphalan was given on three consecutive days, followed by an ABMT. The treatment plan on this protocol extended over 10 months.[27]

The High Risk-3 (HR-3) protocol was used from 1985 through 1988. Twelve patients were placed on this protocol. The induction chemotherapy was composed of two cycles of VAdrC, which consisted of vincristine (2.0 mg/m$^2$), cyclophosphamide (900 mg/m$^2$), and doxorubicin (45 mg/m$^2$), all on day 1, followed by the same doses of cyclophosphamide and doxorubicin on day 2 (all given intravenously). During the radiological reevaluation (week 6), just prior to the initiation of local therapy, a bone marrow harvest was performed, followed by radiation therapy to the primary site, while VAdrC was continued for three more cycles every 28 days with each doxorubicin dose reduced to 30 mg/m$^2$. One month after the last cycle, the treatment was concluded with an ABMT after a preparatory regimen consisting of 400 cGy TBI on days -4 and -3, followed by an additional cycle of VAdrC on days -2 and -1.[27] This protocol was similar to the previously described NCI protocols.

Twenty-one patients were treated on the High Risk-4 (HR-4) protocol from 1989 through 1998. This protocol consisted of three cycles of VAdrC (weeks 1, 4, and 12) and two cycles of cyclophosphamide and etoposide (weeks 8 and 16). A stem cell harvest was taken after the second cycle of VAdrC (week 6), followed by local therapy as soon as possible. After the last cycle of cyclophosphamide and etoposide (week 16), a HSCT was done in four weeks if there was no evidence of persistent disease. The preparatory regimen was intravenous etoposide (300 mg/m$^2$) and cyclophosphamide (300 mg/m$^2$) on days -9, -8, -7, -6, -5, and -4 and TBI (2 Gy twice a day) on days -3, -2, and -1. To minimize bladder damage, 5 mg/kg of mesna was given before and after the cyclphosphamide (Marcus, unpublished data).

For high risk patients the results were protocol dependent. The survival rate for patients treated on the HR-2 was poor; only one of six patients with localized disease at diagnosis survived five years.[13] The results of subsequent protocols were better. For patients without metastases at diagnosis treated on protocols HR-3 and HR-4 from 1985 through 1998, the five-year survival was 63%.[13]

Tumor response to the first two cycles of induction chemotherapy was the most significant predictor of outcome on all protocols, with 80% of patients alive at five years after a complete response, 46% after a partial response, and 0% after no response. Patients who were not evaluable for response had a 58% five-year survival. These same results were true if patients were stratified into standard-risk and high risk protocols; that is, patients with complete response fared the best, and all patients with no response died.[13]

In addition to the expected side effects of the treatment, four patients died of complications secondary to end-intensification, all ABMT, none with PSCT. One patient died on HR-3, while three patients died after ABMT on HR-4. All occurred prior to 1992. No patients developed leukemia after treatment.[13]

## EBMT

In 1999, Ladenstein et al.[41] published the European Bone Marrow Transplantation Registry (EBMT) experience with high dose therapy in localized high risk Ewing's sarcoma. Twenty-eight patients were grafted because of a large tumor volume and/or a poor response to chemotherapy. The five-year survival was 60% for these patients with localized disease at diagnosis. The problem with this study is that it includes a number of high dose regimens and is not the experience of a single prospective protocol that follows and accounts for every patient entered.[41]

## Hospital Infantil Niño Jesus, Hospital Ramon y Cajal, and Hospital Valle Hebron

From 1986 to 1995, 30 patients with localized disease (out of 72 total patients) treated at three hospitals in Madrid and Barcelona were considered high risk and entered on a protocol that consolidated with myeloablative radiochemotherapy. The most common high dose therapy consisted of busulfan 4 mg/kg on days -5, -4, -3, and -2, with melphalan 140 mg/m$^2$ on days -7, -6, -5, and -4, carboplatin 500 mg/m$^2$ on days -4, -3, and -2, and etoposide 40 mg/m$^2$ on day -3. Five patients received TBI of 12 Gy at 2 Gy b.i.d. on days -5, -4, and -3 followed by melphalan 160 mg/m$^2$ on day -1. Although 30 patients were considered high risk, only 20 patients are described. Of the other ten patients, six were excluded because they did go into remission, and four refused the high dose therapy. Fifteen of the 20 high dose patients had localized disease at diagnosis, 12 with primary lesions > 100 mL, and three with pelvic primary lesions. For the localized patients who completed therapy, the five-year survival was 70.6%, with 11 of the 15 patients alive. Two patients died of toxicity after transplant. However, the five-year survival is probably much lower if all patients treated were considered in the final statistics. If all ten patients excluded prior to transplant had localized disease, then the five-year survival could be as low as 50%, assuming that all six patients who did not achieve remissions died, as well as 50% of the four responders that declined ABMT.[44]

## Other Trials

Other prospective trials have included patients with high risk localized disease as part of a larger trial. Unfortunately, the number of patients in each trial is small and the follow-up short (median ~ 2 years). Royal Marsden reported seven out of seven survivors with localized, high risk disease (primary lesions >100 mL).[42] Tom Baker Centre in Calgary reported two of six survivors with large (>8 cm) or femur lesions and no metastases at diagnosis. All were adults.[43] Royal Marsden used a conditioning regimen of busulphan 600 mg/m$^2$ on days -5, -4, -3, and -2, followed by melphalan 140-160 mg/m$^2$ on day -1; Tom Baker Centre utilized melphalan 140-200 mg/m$^2$, followed by TBI in some patients, 5 Gy/1 fraction.[42,43]

## METASTATIC DISEASE

Approximately 20% of patients present with metastatic disease.[1] In the EICESS (European Intergroup Cooperative Ewing's Sarcoma Studies) trials from 1977 to 1993, 44% of these patients presented with lung metastases only; 51% with bone or bone marrow involvement (with or without lung metastases); 5% presented with metastases in other organs.[1] Since about 50% of patients relapse after treatment for localized disease, approximately 60% of all Ewing's sarcoma patients eventually are treated for metastatic disease.

The prognosis of the patients with metastatic disease is poor, whether it is present at diagnosis or develops after treatment for apparent localized disease. Excluding patients with a pleural effusion as the only site of metastatic disease, only five patients with metastases at diagnosis became long-term survivors after treatment on IESS-I and IESS-II.[21] It may be better in more recent trials; in a report from the EICESS, the five-year relapse-free survival for patients with lung metastases only was 29%, for patients with bone and bone marrow metastases 19%, and for patients with both lung and bone metastases at diagnosis 8%.[1]

For patients who relapse after primary therapy the prognosis is even worse, though the results of salvage treatment are better with less aggressive initial therapy. Patients whose only site of failure is local warrant aggressive attempts at salvage.[47] Patients who relapse with only lung metastases can be occasionally salvaged with additional chemotherapy, lung irradiation, and resection.[48] Late relapses fare better than early relapses.[49] Patients who develop bone metastases, however, are essentially incurable with standard therapy.

Because of the poor results for these patients, a number of trials have used high dose therapy, followed by a HSCT, in an attempt to improve survival. For the group of patients with metastases at diagnosis, most regimens add this approach to the end of treatment after obtaining as much a remission as possible with more conventional chemotherapy. For patients who relapse, megatherapy is given more quickly, sometimes without any additional chemotherapy, but preferably after reinducing a remission with one or more cycles of additional chemotherapy.

## HIGH DOSE THERAPY FOR SALVAGE AFTER RELAPSE

Reports using megatherapy for salvage are anecdotal at best and usually only report results of patients who completed the high dose therapy, not giving results for all patients entered in the trial. In addition, the plethora of conditioning regimens used make it difficult to determine which one might be the best.

The largest study for relapsed patients was Ladenstein's review of patients from the EBMT. This study included both relapsed and de novo cases treated at a large number of major European institutions. Only patients referred for transplant were included; it is unknown how many patients were treated at the same institutions without a high dose therapy.

In this retrospective registry review, non-TBI regimens produced superior survival rates after relapse. Busulphan/melphalan conditioning regimens were best. The EFS were 19, 51 and 34% for TBI, busulphan-melphalan and miscellaneous regimens.[50]

## HIGH DOSE THERAPY FOR PATIENTS WITH METASTATIC DISEASE AT DIAGNOSIS

End-intensification with megatherapy and stem-cell rescue has been investigated by a large number of institutions for patients with metastatic disease at diagnosis. Unfortunately, none of the studies are randomized and few are prospective. The larger ones that report at least five-year follow-up are discussed in the next section (▶ Table 10.4).

### National Cancer Institute

The trial described previously for patients with localized disease also included small round-cell tumors with metastatic disease at diagnosis. Overall, 49 of 97 patients had metastases at diagnosis; the number with Ewing's sarcoma is not stated, but the six-year survival for

| TABLE 10.4 | Five-Year Survival of Patients With Bone/Bone Marrow Metastases at Diagnosis | | | | |
|---|---|---|---|---|---|
| **Institution** | **Conditioning Regimen** | **N Pts** | **Standard Therapy** | **High-Dose Therapy** | |
| Univ. of Florida[13,51]<br>HR-2 to 5 (1982–1998) | Melphalan (HR-2)<br>60 mg/m² × 3 d | 11 | — | 18% | |
| | VAdrC (HR-3)<br>8 Gy/2 Fx TBI | | | | |
| | VP-16/C (HR-4)<br>12 Gy/6 Fx TBI | | | | |
| | VP-16/C<br>13.5 Gy/9 Fx TBI | | | | |
| Vienna/Dusseldorf[52]<br>(1987–1993) | 12 Gy/8 Fx TBI<br>Melphalan/VP-16 | 7 | 2% (Matched Cohort) | 43% | |
| EICESS[53]<br>(1990–1995) | Melphalan/VP-16 | NS | 0% | 27% | |
| CCG-7951[54]<br>(1996–1998) | 12 Gy/6 Fx TBI<br>Melphalan/ VP-16 | 32 | 38%[a] | 38%[a] (Matched Cohort) | |

Abbreviations: HR = high risk; Adr = Adriamycin (doxorubicin); C = Cytoxan (cyclophosphamide); Act-D = dactinomycin; V = vincristine; VP = Vepesid (etoposide); Ifos = ifosfomide; ABMT = autologous bone marrow transplantation; ASCT = autologous stem cell transplantation; TBI = total body irradiation; NS = not stated.
[a]Two-year survival

patients with Ewing's sarcoma was only 14%. Survival results for different sites of metastatic disease are not stated.[26]

## University of Florida

The HR-2, HR-3 and HR-4 protocols at the University of Florida previously described also included patients with metastatic disease at diagnosis. In addition, in an effort to improve results for patients with metastatic disease, a specific protocol for these patients was opened in 1993 (HR-5).

HR-5 consisted of three courses each of two alternating chemotherapy regimens. The interval between each course was minimized using G-CSF (granulocyte-colony stimulating growth factor) 250 mg/m² per day until the AGC reached ≥ 500 and platelets ≥ 100 K/mL. Each course started as soon as these counts were reached. Courses #1, #3, and #5 consisted of vincristine (2 mg/m² IV), doxorubicin (120 mg/m², 48-hour continuous infusion), and cyclophosphamide (1200 mg/m² per day, 1-hour continuous infusion), all on day 1, and the same doses of doxorubicin and cyclophosphamide on day 2. Courses #2, #4, and #6 consisted of VP-16 (600 mg/m², 72-hour CI), ifosfamide (1.5 mg/m² per day) plus mesna (500 mg/m² twice a day) and carboplatin (100 mg/m² per day IVP, all given on days 1, 2, and 3. A stem cell harvest was performed following course #4. The preparatory regimen for transplant consisted of TBI (1.5 Gy TID) on days -8, -7, and -6 and cyclophosphamide, (500 mg/m² BID) and etoposide (500 mg/m²) on days -5, -4, -3, and -2. There was a rest period on day 1 and the stem cell reinfusion was administered on day 0. To minimize or prevent bladder damage, 5 mg/kg of mesna was given before and after cyclophosphamide. Interleukin-2 (IL-2) was started at the time of recovery from ABMT (about 4 weeks).[13,51]

Between 1982 and 1998, 26 patients with metastases at diagnosis were treated on the four protocols: four on HR-2, six on HR-3, seven on HR-4, and nine on HR-5. The mean age of patients was 14.4 years (range, 3-23 years). Twenty were male and six female. There were 15 patients with metastases to the lungs only, and 11 with bone or bone marrow involvement, with or without lung involvement.[13,51]

Eight patients did not go on to receive a transplant. Five patients developed progressive disease on chemotherapy, two patients developed cardiomyopathy during chemotherapy, and one patient refused transplant. Only one of these patients survived, a 16-year old male who developed severe cardiomyopathy on HR-3, eventually requiring a cardiac transplant.

The overall absolute survival rate was 42% at two years and 25% at five years. The five-year survival rate for the nine patients on HR-5 was 44% compared to 16% for the other three protocols (P = .0549).[13]

The survival rate for patients with only lung metastases was significantly higher than for patients with bone metastases and/or other metastases: 45% versus 9% at five years. Patients 16 years or younger had a better survival than older patients, 43% versus 11% at five years. Of the nine patients older than 16 who were entered on the four protocols, only one survived and only four completed the high dose therapy.

## EICESS

In an update on the multicenter European Intergroup Cooperative Ewing's Sarcoma Studies, Paulussen et al.[53] reported on 171 patients with metastatic disease at diagnosis registered between 1990 and 1995. The four-year EFS was slightly better than the previous report: 34% for patients with lung metastases only, 28% for bone/bone marrow metastases, and 14% for patients with both lung and bone/bone marrow metastases.[1,53] Thirty-six of the patients in the more recent report received myeloablative therapy with stem cell rescue following conventional chemotherapy. In patients with combined lung and bone/bone marrow metastases, the group with the worst survival rates overall, consolidation with high dose therapy (various regimens, ± whole lung irradiation) improved EFS from 0% to 27%.[53]

## Hospital Infantil Niño Jesus, Hospital Ramon y Cajal, and Hospital Valle Hebron

In this report from three hospitals in Madrid, 11 patients with metastatic disease at diagnosis were treated on a protocol that consolidated with high dose busulfan and melphalan, as previously described. Ten patients had lung metastases only and one had bone marrow involvement. Six of 11 are surviving, five with lung disease and one with bone marrow involvement.[44]

## Vienna St. Anna Children's Hospital and Düsseldorf University Children's Hospital

Between 1987 and 1992, seven patients with multifocal bone disease were consolidated with a radiochemotherapy conditioning regimen of 12 Gy TBI at 1.5 Gy b.i.d. on days -7, -6, -5, and -4 and melphalan 30-45 mg/m$^2$ on the same days. Three patients survived. A matched-cohort analysis of historic controls from the CESS-81 study produced a group of patients with only a 2% five-year survival rate.

## CCG-7951

In an attempt to determine the usefulness of high dose therapy at the end of conventional chemotherapy, CCG-7951 was designed to compare patients treated on this regimen with a matched historical control group from the predecessor study, INT-0091, all of whom were treated with more conventional therapy. Only patients with bone or bone marrow metastases were eligible. After five cycles of vincristine, doxorubicin, and cylcophosphamide alternating with ifosfamide and etoposide, a conditioning regimen of TBI (12 Gy at 2 Gy b.i.d.) on days -8, -7, and -6, followed by melphalan 60 mg/m$^2$/d with etoposide 250 mg/m$^2$/d on days -5, -4, and -3.[54]

Thirty-six patients were entered on study; 32 were declared eligible. The median age was 13 years, 20 were male and 12 were female. Twenty-two patients finished therapy. The two-year EFS and overall survival was 20% and 38%. The EFS was identical to the matched historical control set taken from INT-0091 for the first two years of follow-up. Longer follow-up is not yet available.[54]

## CONCLUSIONS

Including patients with metastatic disease at diagnosis, < 50% of all Ewing's sarcoma patients survive, and only small gains in survival have occurred during the last 20 years. Even for patients with localized disease at diagnosis, no study with long-term follow-up shows survival rates significantly above 50%. It is possible that more recent studies will show better long-term results, but clearly there is room for improvement.

There are patients who have a relatively favorable prognosis within the group with no detectable metastases at diagnosis. Most authors agree small lesions of the extremities have a more favorable prognosis. More recently, it has been established that a good response to induction chemotherapy is accompanied by a high chance of cure.[13,29,30,33,35,37,40]

However, what about the larger group, those with an unfavorable prognosis? Is consolidation with high dose chemo/radiation followed by stem cell rescue a useful tool? Is there any evidence that such an approach improves survival rates?

Clearly, it is difficult to compare results of small series between institutions and cooperative groups, particularly when the selection criteria for inclusion into the studies are different or are not accurately stated. If comparisons are to be made, they should be made between patients treated during the same eras. As shown in Table 10.2, patients with large primary lesions treated in the late 1970s, 1980s, and early 1990s had five-year survival rates of 17%–38%. The results of using high dose therapy for consolidation of patients with high risk, localized disease (Table 10.3) show a much better prognosis, with five-year survival rates of 48% and higher. Most of the patients in Table 10.3 also were treated in the 1980s and early 1990s, and are comparable by era. The results are worth further evaluation with additional studies.

There are other advantages to a short intensive regimen with high dose consolidation. Treatment is completed in less than 24 weeks, shorter even than the new COG protocol that is attempting to shorten treatment to 28 weeks with growth factor support. More standard chemotherapy protocols are almost a year in length. In addition, if the stem cell harvest is performed early in treatment, after only two cycles of VadrC (for patients with localized disease only) as reported in the University of Florida approach, there appears to be a very low risk of developing secondary leukemia from treatment, since these stem cells have never been exposed to etoposide or radiation.[13] Subsequent to the harvest, the regimen can be changed to include the ifosphamide/etoposide drug combination that has been shown to be beneficial.[17]

If one were to further explore consolidation with HSCT, the question of the optimal conditioning regimen remains. Although most of the data in Table 10.3 were produced by high dose regimens containing TBI, there is evidence in relapsed patients that non-TBI conditioning regimens may produce better results than those dependent upon TBI.[50] For localized, de novo patients, the small trials from the Royal Marsden and the Madrid collaboration that used busulfan/cyclosphosphamide support the use of non-TBI regimens. Such an approach may lower long-term morbidity from treatment.

For patients with metastatic disease at diagnosis, the results of previous studies are even more difficult to decipher. There has been no randomized study to date, and certainly there are far too few patients in the studies performed thus far to support a mega-analysis. Is the approach useful for these patients? Modern studies appear to show some improvement in survival for patients with metastases, particularly for those with only pulmonary metastases.[55] With pulmonary irradiation, survival is improved without high dose consolidation and has been reported to be as high as 42% EFS at five years.[55] Other patients may have a much worse prognosis; the initial EICESS studies report only an 8% five-year survival for patients with combined pulmonary and bone/bone marrow metastases, and 19% for patients with bone/bone marrow metastases only.[1] Table 10.4 shows the results for patients with bone/bone marrow metastases treated with high dose therapy described previously. Whereas CCG-7951 shows no advantage, the survival of the matched cohort from the previous United States Intergroup Study, INT-0091, is surprisingly high. In addition, follow-up is short. The Vienna/Dusseldorf collaboration shows better results but the number of patients treated de novo is small. The EICESS is a larger study, though the number of these patients is not stated, but shows a large difference between the high dose therapy patients and a simultaneously (but not randomized) group of patients treated with more conventional therapy. The University of Florida protocols produced a 43% five-year survival for all patients with metastases at diagnosis who were 16 years of age or younger at diagnosis. For patients with bone/bone marrow metastases at diagnosis, the five-year survival was 29% in the University of Florida trials, but the numbers are small.

Clearly, the results of high dose therapy from these trials appear better than results from the 1970s and 1980s, particularly for patients with bone/bone marrow metastases at diagnosis or both bone/bone marrow and lung metastases. It is more difficult to compare the results of high dose therapy with the results of patients treated more recently with conventional therapy. Paulussen et al., describing the EICESS patients treated between 1990 and 1995, reported a 0% five-year survival for patients with bone/bone marrow and lung metastases who were treated without high dose therapy. The United States Intergroup trial INT-0091 had a better result: a 38% two-year EFS for bone/bone marrow metastases treated with conventional systemic therapy between 1988 and 1993. Because the latter trial does include some patients with only bone/bone marrow metastases, potentially it is a slightly more favorable group, but is not more favorable enough to explain the difference. What is the survival for these patients treated conventionally? Which study is right?

It is necessary to know the answers to these questions to improve therapy for this disease. However, it is obvious that survival rates are low for every therapy reported, and it is important to continue to study every approach to the treatment of these very high risk patients in an attempt to improve survival. High dose therapy remains one treatment option that probably benefits some patients, and must be explored further.

# REFERENCES

1. Cotterill SJ, Ahrens S, Paulussen M et al. Prognostic factors in Ewing's tumor of bone: analysis of 975 patients from the European Intergroup Cooperative Ewing's Sarcoma Study Group. J Clin Oncol 2000;18:3108–3114.
2. Kissane JM, Askin FB, Foulkes M et al. Ewing's sarcoma of bone: clinicopathologic aspects of 303 cases from the Intergroup Ewing's Sarcoma Study. Hum Pathol 1983;14:773–779.
3. Cavazzana AO, Magnani JL, Ross RA et al. Ewing's sarcoma is an undifferentiated neuroectodermal tumor. In: Advances in Neuroblastoma Research. New York: Alan R. Liss, 1988;487–498.
4. Sandberg AA. Chromosomes in human cancer and leukemia. Mutat Res 1991;247:231–240.
5. Whang-Peng J, Freter CE, Knutsen T et al. Translocation t(11:22) in esthesioneuroblastoma. Cancer Genet Cytogenet 1987;29:155–157.
6. Sandberg AA, Bridge JA. The Cytogenetics of Bone and Soft Tissue Tumors. Austin: R.G. Landes Company, 1994;303.
7. Womer RB. The cellular biology of bone tumors. Clin Orthop 1991;262:12–21.
8. Arai Y, Kun LE, Brooks MT et al. Ewing's sarcoma: Local tumor control and patterns of failure following limited-volume radiation therapy. Int J Radiat Oncol Biol Phys 1991;21:1501–1508.
9. Bacci G, Picci P, Gherlinzoni F et al. Localized Ewing's sarcoma of bone: ten years' experience at the Istituo Ortopedico Rizzoli in 124 cases treated with multimodal therapy. Eur J Cancer Clin Oncol 1998;21:163–173.
10. Kinsella TJ, Miser JA, Waller B et al. Long-term follow-up of Ewing's sarcoma of bone treated with combined modality therapy. Int J Radiat Oncol Biol Phys 1991;20:389–395.
11. Wilkins RM, Pritchard DJ, Burgert EO Jr et al. Ewing's sarcoma of bone: experience with 140 patients. Cancer 1986;58:2551–2555.
12. Sailer SL, Harmon DC, Mankin HJ et al. Ewing's sarcoma: surgical resection as a prognostic factor. Int J Radiat Oncol Biol Phys 1988;15:43–52.
13. Marcus RB Jr, Berrey BH, Graham-Pole J et al. The treatment of Ewing's sarcoma of bone at the University of Florida. Clin Ortho Relat Res 2002;397:290–297.
14. Fizazi K, Dohollou N, Blay JY et al. Ewing's family of tumors in adults: multivariate analysis of survival and long-term results of multimodality therapy in 182 patients. Journal of Clinical Oncology 1998;16:3736–3743.
15. Donaldson SS, Torrey M, Link MP et al. A multidisciplinary study investigating radiotherapy in Ewing's sarcoma: end results of POG #8346. Pediatric Oncology Group. Int J Radiat Oncol Biol Phys 1998;42:125–135.
16. Paulussen M, Ahrens S, Dunst W et al. Localized Ewing tumor of bone: final results of the Cooperative Ewing's Sarcoma Study CESS 86. J Clin Oncol 2001;19:1818–1829.
17. Grier HE, Krailo MD, Tarbell NJ et al. Addition of ifosfamide and etoposide to standard chemotherapy in Ewing's sarcoma and primitive neuroectodermal tumor of bone. N Engl J Med 2003;348(8):747–749.
18. Rosito P, Mancini AF, Rondelli R et al. Italian Cooperative Group Study for the treatment of children and young adults with localized Ewing's sarcoma of bone: a preliminary report of 6 years of experience. Cancer 1999;86:421–428.
19. Marina NM, Pappo AS, Parham DM et al. Chemotherapy dose-intensification for pediatric patients with Ewing's family of tumors and desmoplastic small round-cell tumors: a feasibility study at St. Jude Children's Research Hospital. J Clin Oncol 1999;17:180–190.
20. Burgert EO Jr, Nesbit ME, Garnsey LA et al. Multimodal therapy for the management of nonpelvic, localized Ewing's sarcoma of bone: Intergroup Study IESS-II. J Clin Oncol 1990;8:1514–1524.
21. Cangir A, Vietti TJ, Gehan EA et al. Ewing's sarcoma metastatic at diagnosis: Results and comparisons of two Intergroup Ewing's Sarcoma Studies. Cancer 1990;66:887–893.
22. Capanna R, Toni A, Sudanese A et al. Ewing's sarcoma of the pelvis. Int Orthop 1990;14:57–61.
23. Dunst J, Sauer R, Burgers JMV et al. Cooperative Ewing's Sarcoma Study Group Radiation therapy as local treatment in Ewing's sarcoma: Results of the Cooperative Ewing's Sarcoma Studies CESS 81 and CESS 86. Cancer 1991;67:2818–2825.
24. Evans RG, Nesbit ME, Gehan EA et al. Multimodal therapy for the management of localized Ewing's sarcoma of pelvic and sacral bones: A report from the Second Intergroup Study. J Clin Onco 1991;19:1173–1180.
25. Hayes FA, Thompson EI, Meyer WH et al. Therapy for localized Ewing's sarcoma of bone. J Clin Oncol 1989;7:208–213.
26. Horowitz ME, Kinsella TJ, Wexler LH et al. Total-body irradiation and autologous bone marrow transplant in the treatment of high risk Ewing's sarcoma and rhabdomyosarcoma. J Clin Oncol 1993;11:1911–1918.
27. Marcus RB Jr, Graham-Pole JR, Springfield DS et al. High risk Ewing's sarcoma: End-intensification using autologous bone marrow transplantation. Int J Radiat Oncol Biol Phys 1988;15:53–59.
28. Nesbit ME Jr, Gehan EA, Burgert EO Jr et al. Multimodal therapy for the management of primary, non-metastatic Ewing's sarcoma of bone: A long-term follow-up of the first intergroup study. J Clin Oncol 1990;8:1664–1674.
29. Oberlin O, Patte C, Demeocq F et al. The response to initial chemotherapy as a prognostic factor in localized Ewing's sarcoma. Eur J Cancer Clin Oncol 1985;21:463–467.

30. Wunder JS, Paulian G, Huvos A et al. The histologic response to chemotherapy as a predictor of the oncologic outcome of operative treatment of Ewing's sarcoma. J Bone Joint Surg 1998;7:1020–1033.
31. Smith MA, Ungerleider RS, Horowitz ME et al. Influence of doxorubicin dose intensity on response and outcome for patients with osteogenic sarcoma and Ewing's sarcoma. J Natl Cancer Inst 1991;83:160–170.
32. Kushner BH, Meyers PA, Gerald WL et al. Very-high dose short-term chemotherapy for poor-risk peripheral primitive neuroectodermal tumors, including Ewing's sarcoma, in children and young adults. J Clin Oncol 1995;13:2794–2804.
33. Delepine N, Delepine G, Cornille H et al. Prognostic factors in patients with localized Ewing's sarcoma: the effect of survival of actual received drug dose intensity and of histologic response to induction therapy. J Chemother 1997;9:352–363.
34. Womer RB, Daller RT, Fenton JG et al. Granulocyte colony stimulating factor permits dose intensification by interval compression in the treatment of Ewing's sarcoma and soft tissue sarcomas in children. Eur J Cancer 2000;36:87–94.
35. Ahrens S, Hoffmann C, Jabar S et al. Evaluation of prognostic factors in a tumor volume-adapted treatment strategy for localized Ewing's sarcoma of bone: the CESS 86 experience. Med Pediat Oncol 1999;32:186–195.
36. Aparicio J, Munarriz B, Pastor M et al. Long-term follow-up and prognostic factors in Ewing's sarcoma. A multivariate analysis of 116 patients from a single institution. Oncology 1998;55:20–26.
37. Bacci G, Picci P, Mercuri M et al. Predictive factors of histological response to primary chemotherapy in Ewing's sarcoma. Acta Oncol 1998;37:671–676.
38. Jürgens H, Exner U, Gadner H et al. Multidisciplinary treatment of primary Ewing's sarcoma of bone: A 6-year experience of a European cooperative trial. Cancer 1988;61:23–32.
39. Marcus RB Jr, Million RR. The effect of primary tumor size on the prognosis of Ewing's sarcoma (Abstr #24). Int J Radiat Oncol Biol Phys 1984;10(Suppl 2):88.
40. Picci P, Bohling T, Ferrari L et al. Chemotherapy-induced tumor necrosis as a prognostic factor in localized Ewing's sarcoma of the extremities. J Clin Oncol 1997;15:1553–1559.
41. Ladenstein R, Hartmann O, Pinkerton R et al. A multivariate and matched pair analysis on high risk Ewing tumor patients treated by megatherapy and stem cell reinfusion in Europe (Abstr. #555). Am Soc Clin Oncol 1999;18:555a.
42. Stewart DA, Gyonyor E, Paterson AH et al. High dose melphalan ± total body irradiation and autologous hematopoietic stem cell rescue for adult patients with Ewing's sarcoma or peripheral neuroectodermal tumor. Bone Marrow Transplant 1996;18:315–318.
43. Atra A, Whelan JS, Calvagna V et al. High dose busulphan/melphalan with autologous stem cell rescue in Ewing's sarcoma. Bone Marrow Transplant 1997;20:843–846.
44. Madero L, Munoz A, Sanchez de Toledo J et al. Megatherapy in children with high risk Ewing's sarcoma in first complete remission. Bone Marrow Transplant 1998;21:795–799.
45. Bolek TW, Marcus RB Jr, Mendenhall NP et al. Local control and functional results after twice-daily radiotherapy for Ewing's of the extremities. Int J Radiat Oncol Biol Phys 1995;35:687–692.
46. Marcus RB Jr, Cantor A, Heare TC et al. Local control and function after twice-a-day radiotherapy for Ewing's sarcoma of bone. Int J Radiat Oncol Biol Phys 1991;21:1509–1515.
47. Hayes FA, Thompson EI, Kumar M et al. Long-term survival in patients with Ewing's sarcoma relapsing after completing therapy. Med Pediatr Oncol 1987;15:254–256.
48. Lanza LA, Miser JS, Pass HI et al. The role of resection in the treatment of pulmonary metastases from Ewing's sarcoma. J Thor Cardiovas Surg 1987;94:181–187.
49. Craft A, Cotterill S, Malcolm A et al. Ifosfamide-containing chemotherapy in Ewing's sarcoma: the Second United Kingdom Children's Cancer Study Group and the Medical Research Council Ewing's Tumor Study. J Clin Oncol 1998;16:3628–3633.
50. Ladenstein R, Lasset C, Pinkerton R et al. Impact of megatherapy in children with high risk Ewing's tumours in complete remission: a report from the EBMT solid tumours registry. Bone Marrow Transplant 1995;15:697–705.
51. Taeb P, Sharda S, Marcus R et al. Results of an ablative-dose stem cell rescue protocol for patients with Ewing's sarcoma, metastatic at diagnosis: results of a 20-year experience at the University of Florida (Abstr. #423). Blood 2000;96:423a.
52. Burdach S, Jurgens H, Peters C et al. Myeloablative radiochemotherapy and hematopoietic stem-cell rescue in poor-prognosis Ewing's sarcoma. J Clin Oncol 1993;11:1482–1488.
53. Paulussen M, Ahrens S, Burdach S et al. Primary metastatic (stage IV) Ewing tumor: survival analysis of 171 patients from the EICESS studies. European Intergroup Cooperative Ewing's Sarcoma Studies. Ann Oncol 1998;9:275–281.
54. Meyers PA, Krailo MD, Ladanyi M et al. High dose melphalan, etoposide, total-body irradiation, and autologous stem-cell reconstitution as consolidation therapy for high risk Ewing's sarcoma does not improve prognosis. J Clin Oncol 2001;19:2812–2820.
55. Paulussen M, Ahrens S, Craft AW et al. Ewing's sarcoma with primary lung metastases: survival analysis of 114 (European Intergroup) Cooperative Ewing's Sarcoma Studies patients. J Clin Oncol 1998;16:3044–3052.

# CHAPTER XI

# High Dose Chemotherapy and Stem Cell Rescue for Treatment of Brain Tumors

Naomi Moskowitz, Jonathan Finlay, and Sharon Gardner

Brain tumors are the second most common type of malignant tumors in children and the most common solid tumor.[1] They are also the most common cause of cancer-related death in children.[2] Although the number of survivors of childhood brain tumors is improving, the children are often left with significant long-term sequelae. A great deal of research has been performed over the past several years to try to improve the survival and quality of life of children with these tumors.

Surgery has played a key role in the treatment of brain tumors in numerous ways. Samples obtained at the time of surgery have enabled precise histological diagnosis that has aided prognosis and management. When possible, removal of bulky tumor has been helpful in relieving symptoms resulting from increased intracranial pressure and in prolonging survival. Numerous improvements in neurosurgical techniques and instruments have helped to improve survival, but the efficacy of this treatment relies on the location and extent of the tumor. For most brainstem and widely infiltrative tumors, surgery is not an option.

Radiation therapy is often used to treat brain tumors because of their radiosensitivity. While radiation therapy has proven efficacy for many brain tumors, it also has proven adverse effects such as impaired cognitive ability, impaired growth (especially with craniospinal irradiation), and impaired endocrine function.[3] The toxic effects are more pronounced in young children since their brains are still developing.[4] Furthermore, once radiation therapy is given, there are few options left for treating relapses. Therefore, attempts to delay or give less radiation (by fractionating and/or giving more focused therapy) have been made, but with few improvements in long-term survival.[5,6]

Because of the limitations of surgery and radiation therapy, many investigators have explored the use of a variety of chemotherapy regimens in the treatment of children with brain tumors. Alkylating agents have been the focus of many chemotherapeutic trials for several reasons. These agents can penetrate the blood brain barrier and have a linear-log dose-response curve.[7] The main dose-limiting toxicity for many of these agents is myelosuppression. However, with the development of hematopoietic growth factors and stem cell transplantation techniques, myelosuppression is no longer an obstacle and doses can be optimized with fewer adverse effects. Another chemotherapeutic agent that has been used in the treatment of brain tumor is the topoisomerase II inhibitor, etoposide. It is thought that this drug might be synergistic with alkylating agents by preventing the repair of DNA that has been damaged by alkylating agents.[8]

Numerous studies have focused on the use of high dose chemotherapy and stem cell transplantation in the treatment of brain tumors. In the following sections of this chapter, a number of these studies conducted in pediatric patients will be summarized, followed by a discussion of the adverse effects of such therapy and the conclusions to be drawn from these studies.

## MEDULLOBLASTOMA

Medulloblastomas are neuroectodermal in origin and comprise 10% to 20% of all childhood brain tumors and 40% of tumors in the posterior fossa.[6] The median age at diagnosis is five to six years with the majority of patients diagnosed in the first decade of life. Over the past 70 years, the treatment of medulloblastoma has evolved significantly from surgical resection to a multidisciplinary approach with surgery, craniospinal irradiation, and multidrug chemotherapy. With these changes the five-year event-free survival has risen from 2% to almost 90% in children with localized disease.[9,10] Unfortunately, results using standard dose therapy for patients with metastatic or recurrent disease are less encouraging, with five-year survival rates of 65% and essentially 0%, respectively.[10–12] Several investigators have used high dose chemotherapy with autologous stem cell rescue in an attempt to improve survival in these patients.

Kalifa et al. published one of the earliest studies using high dose chemotherapy with autologous bone marrow rescue in 42 children previously treated for medulloblastoma/ primitive neuroectodermal tumors (PNET).[13] Prior therapy included surgery in all patients with irradiation in the 13 oldest patients and conventional chemotherapy in the 29 youngest children. High dose chemotherapy consisted of busulfan 150 mg/m$^2$/day for four days and thiotepa 350 mg/m$^2$/day for three days. Four patients who underwent high dose chemotherapy for isolated relapse following irradiation were alive without disease recurrence one to six years following stem cell reinfusion. There were four (10%) toxic deaths.

Mahoney et al. reported the Pediatric Oncology Group experience using high dose chemotherapy in children with recurrent or progressive malignant brain tumors.[14] The primary aim of the study was to determine the maximum tolerated dose of cyclophosphamide with a fixed dose of melphalan and autologous bone marrow rescue. Bone marrow was harvested just prior to the initiation of high dose chemotherapy. The dose of cyclophosphamide ranged from 750 to 1500 mg/m$^2$/day for four days followed by melphalan 60 mg/m$^2$/day for three days. There were eight children with medulloblastoma enrolled on this study. All eight children had received prior craniospinal irradiation and seven also had received multidrug chemotherapy. All of the children had measurable disease at the time of the consolidation therapy. The dose of cyclophosphamide for these eight patients ranged from 750 to 1200 mg/m$^2$/day. Four children had responses (1 complete and 3 partial responses). Two children were alive with disease 24 and 25 months following high dose chemotherapy. There were four (22%) toxic deaths in the entire cohort; three of whom had medulloblastoma. The cause of death included *Staphylococcus epidermidus* (1 patient), cardiomyopathy, capillary leak syndrome and *E. coli* sepsis (1 patient), and fungal infection with hemorrhage (2 patients).

Graham et al. used three different high dose chemotherapy regimens in patients with recurrent or high risk brain tumors.[15] Eighteen patients had recurrent medulloblastoma and had a median age of 12 years (range, 1 to 32 years). All patients had received prior irradiation and chemotherapy. Fifteen patients received a fixed dose of cyclophosphamide (1.5 $g/m^2$/day for 4 days) followed by melphalan ranging from 25 to 60 $mg/m^2$/day for three days. Two patients received carboplatin 700 $mg/m^2$/day alternating every other day with etoposide 500 $mg/m^2$/day for a total of three days for each drug. One patient received oral busulfan 37.5 $mg/m^2$ every six hours for 16 doses followed by melphalan 180 $mg/m^2$ for one dose. Four patients who had recurrences isolated to the posterior fossa and had no evidence of disease prior to the high dose chemotherapy remain event-free survivors 27 to 49 months following autologous stem cell rescue. There was one (2%) toxic death from pulmonary aspergillosis in the entire cohort.

In the study reported by Dunkel et al., 23 patients with recurrent medulloblastoma with a median age of 13 years (range, two to 44 years) were treated with a three drug regimen including carboplatin, thiotepa, and etoposide.[16] Carboplatin was administered at a dose of 500 $mg/m^2$/day or dosed using the Calvert formula with an area under the concentration curve of 7 mg/mL-min/day for three days followed by thiotepa 300 $mg/m^2$/day and etoposide 250 $mg/m^2$/day for three days. Four patients received irradiation (craniospinal in three patients and focal irradiation in one patient) following recovery from the high dose chemotherapy. Event-free survival was 30% at a median of 54 months following autologous stem cell rescue. The toxic mortality rate was 13%. The deaths were due to multiorgan system failure in two patients and *Aspergillus* infection and venooclusive disease in one patient.

Vassal et al. reported results using tandem courses of high dose chemotherapy with autologous stem cell rescue in children newly-diagnosed with metastatic medulloblastoma.[17] The tandem courses of high dose chemotherapy included two courses of melphalan 100 $mg/m^2$/day for two days with a planned interval of 21 days between each course. The sequential melphalan therapy was part of an intensive chemotherapy protocol that included two courses of carboplatin and etoposide given prior to the sequential melphalan treatment. Following recovery from the second high dose melphalan, patients received a third high dose course with busulfan and thiotepa. Eleven of 14 evaluable patients had partial responses.

Strother et al. also used sequential autologous stem cell reinfusions to enhance hematopoietic recovery following multiple cycles of intensive chemotherapy in 53 patients newly diagnosed with medulloblastoma or supratentorial primitive neuroectodermal tumors.[18] Thirty-four patients had average-risk disease and 19 patients had high-risk disease. Patients with average-risk disease underwent surgical resection followed by craniospinal irradiation. Six weeks following completion of irradiation, patients received four cycles of chemotherapy including cisplatin 75 $mg/m^2$ and vincristine 1.5 $mg/m^2$ on day -4 followed by cyclophosphamide 2 $g/m^2$ on days -3 and -2 with stem cell infusion on day 0. Patients with high-risk disease received the same therapy with the addition of a phase II topotecan window prior to irradiation.

Fifty patients proceeded to intensive chemotherapy following irradiation. Several patients had reductions in the chemotherapy due to toxicity, but there were no toxic deaths. The two-year progression-free survival from the start of therapy for average and high-risk patients was 93.6% ± 4.7% and 73.7% ± 10.5%, respectively.

## OTHER PRIMITIVE NEUROECTODERMAL TUMORS

Primitive neuroectodermal tumors (PNETs) outside the posterior fossa comprise 2% to 3% of all childhood tumors. These tumors are divided into two major categories: supratentorial PNETs and pineoblastomas. Most investigators have combined results of all patients with PNETs in the same report, since historically the treatment has been the same and because of the small number of noncerebellar tumors. Histologically noncerebellar tumors resemble medulloblastomas.[19] However, several investigators have suggested that they behave differently and recent data from microarray analyses support this observation.[20,21]

Results from a Children's Cancer Group study indicate that three-year progression-free survival rates of 45% can be achieved in children newly-diagnosed with supratentorial PNETs treated with surgery, irradiation, and standard dose chemotherapy.[22] Unfortunately, therapeutic options are more limited for patients with recurrent disease.

Several investigators have reported results of high dose chemotherapy in patients with recurrent supratentorial PNETs. Most of these studies include small numbers of patients and are reported along with patients with cerebellar PNETs. Broniscer et al. have compiled the results of seventeen patients with non-cerebellar tumors (pineal gland, 8 patients; other supratentorial areas, 8 patients; cauda equina, 1 patient) treated with high dose chemotherapy (A. Broniscer, in press, Medical Pediatric Oncology, 2003). The median age of the patients was 3.9 years (range 1.5 to 32.5 years). Conditioning therapy consisted of thiotepa 300 mg/m$^2$/day and etoposide 250 to 500 mg/m$^2$/day for three days with or without carboplatin 500 mg/m$^2$/day or dosed using the Calvert formula with an area under the concentration curve of 7 mg/mL-min/day for three days. Two patients received the two drug regimen and 15 received the three-drug regimen. The five-year event-free survival for patients with pineoblastoma and other PNETs was 0% and 62.5% $\pm$ 27%, respectively. There were two toxic deaths: one from septic shock and a second from multiorgan system failure and meningitis.

## GLIOMAS

Although gliomas comprise nearly 40% of the central nervous system tumors in adults, their frequency is less than 12% in children.[23,24] Unfortunately, the prognosis is as poor in children as it is in adults. Several investigators have used high dose chemotherapy with autologous stem cell rescue in an attempt to improve upon the dismal survival rates seen in patients treated with surgery, irradiation, and conventional dose chemotherapy.

The earliest studies involved carmustine given as a single agent at high doses with autologous bone marrow rescue to adults with malignant glioma.[25-27] The dose of carmustine ranged from 600 to 1400 mg/m$^2$. Although there were some responses seen, there also was significant pulmonary, hepatic, and neurologic toxicity, particularly at the highest doses of carmustine.

The majority of high dose chemotherapy approaches in children with glioma have involved multidrug regimens. Several different combinations have been used including thiotepa/cyclophosphamide, melphalan/cyclophosphamide, and thiotepa/etoposide alone and with the addition of carmustine or carboplatin.

Heideman et al. treated 13 children with malignant glioma (11 newly diagnosed; 2 recurrent) using thiotepa 300 mg/m$^2$/day and cyclophosphamide 2 g/m$^2$/day.[28] The drugs were given twelve hours apart on three consecutive days. Prior to chemotherapy, three patients had near total resections (>90% tumor removal); four patients had subtotal resections (>50% but <90% tumor removal); six patients had biopsy only. The eleven patients who had at least stable disease at day 60 received hyperfractionated ($N = 9$) or conventional external beam radiation ($N = 2$). One complete response and three partial responses were seen. After combined modality therapy, the median progression free survival was nine months (range, 0 to 30 + months).

Kedar et al. also used the combination of thiotepa 250 to 300 mg/m$^2$/day for three days and cyclophosphamide 750 to 975 mg/m$^2$/day for four days in three patients with newly diagnosed high grade astrocytoma.[29] Hyperfractionated radiation therapy was given following recovery from chemotherapy. One patient survived disease-free 22 months from diagnosis.

The Pediatric Oncology Group used melphalan 60 mg/m$^2$/day for three days and cyclophosphamide 750 to 1500 mg/m$^2$/day for four days in children with recurrent/progressive malignant brain tumors.[14] Four children had high grade gliomas: two had anaplastic astrocytoma; one had glioblastoma multiforme; one had a brainstem glioma. All four children died within seven months of high dose therapy, one from treatment related toxicity and three from disease.

Bouffet et al. treated 22 pediatric patients with high grade gliomas.[30] Thirteen were newly diagnosed; nine had recurrent disease. High dose chemotherapy consisted of etoposide 500 mg/m$^2$/day for three days and thiotepa 300 mg/m$^2$/day for three days followed by autologous bone marrow reinfusion. Two patients died of toxicity. Seventeen patients died of disease 1.5 to 23 months posttreatment. Three patients have survived 54 to 65 + months posttreatment, although two of these have seizure disorders and all three have schooling difficulties. All three of these patients were newly diagnosed, received prior radiation therapy, and had tumors that were not located in the brainstem.

Finlay et al. also used the combination of etoposide 500 mg/m$^2$/day for three days and thiotepa 300 mg/m$^2$/day on the same three days in children and young adults with recurrent central nervous system tumors.[31] At the time of the report, five of 18 patients (28%) with high grade gliomas were disease free at 39+, 44+, 49+, 52+, and 59+ months following bone marrow rescue.

Because of these encouraging results, Finlay's group added carmustine to the thiotepa/etoposide combination.[32] The dose of carmustine was 600 mg/m$^2$ given over three or four days followed by thiotepa 300 mg/m$^2$/day and etoposide 250 or 500 mg/m$^2$/day on the same three days. Papadakis et al. reported the results of 42 patients (29 newly diagnosed; 13 recurrent) treated with this regimen. Diagnoses included high grade glioma ($N = 37$), medulloblastoma ($N = 2$), and nonbiopsied tumors ($N = 3$). Twenty-one patients with newly diagnosed disease received irradiation post-high dose chemotherapy. Patients ranged in age from 0.7 to 46.8 years (median 12.2 years). Three newly diagnosed patients and one patient treated for recurrent disease were alive without disease progression 64, 67, 86, and 110 months, respectively, following autologous bone marrow rescue. Unfortunately, toxicity was significant with nine early deaths. The deaths were due to multiorgan system failure. The preceding event included respiratory failure (3 patients), pulmonary hemorrhage (1 patient), renal failure (1 patient), brainstem necrosis (1 patient), infection (2 patients), and tumor invasion (1 patient). Patients older than 18 years of age had a significantly higher toxic mortality rate (50%) compared with those less than 18 years of age (15%).

Grovas et al. reported similar results for the Children's Cancer Group using the same approach in children newly diagnosed with glioblastoma multiforme.[33] Eleven children received carmustine 100 mg/m$^2$ every twelve hours for six doses followed by thiotepa 300 mg/m$^2$/day and etoposide 250 mg/m$^2$/day with 5400 cGy radiotherapy beginning 42 days following autologous stem cell rescue. Two-year progression-free survival was 46% ± 14%. Three children (27%) had complete radiographic response 2.9, 3.9, and 5.1 years post-autologous bone marrow rescue. However, once again toxicity was significant with five patients (45%) developing grade III or IV pulmonary and/or neurologic toxicity and a toxic mortality rate of 18%.

## BRAINSTEM TUMORS

Brainstem tumors are located in the area between the aqueduct of Sylvius and the fourth ventricle and comprise approximately 10% to 20% of central nervous system tumors in childhood.[34] They occur most commonly in children between five and ten years of age. The histology of these tumors is most often anaplastic astrocytoma or glioblastoma multiforme.[35] Their location prohibits surgical resection including, in most cases, even a biopsy. Historically radiation therapy has been the primary treatment. However, even with irradiation, most patients die within two years of diagnosis.[36,37]

Dunkel et al. explored the efficacy of high dose chemotherapy with autologous bone marrow rescue in 16 patients with diffuse pontine tumors.[38] Ten patients with recurrent or refractory disease had previously received irradiation. Five of these patients also had received chemotherapy and one had received beta-interferon. Three different regimens were used to treat the ten patients with recurrent/refractory disease. Six patients received three days of thiotepa 300 mg/m$^2$/day and etoposide 250 to 500 mg/m$^2$/day; two patients received carmustine 100 mg/m$^2$/dose q12 hours for three days followed by thiotepa and etoposide; and two patients received carboplatin 500 mg/m$^2$/day for three days followed by thiotepa and etoposide. Six newly-diagnosed patients had received no prior therapy. These patients received the carmustine/thiotepa/etoposide regimen with hyperfractionated irradiation (7200 to 7800 cGy) beginning approximately six weeks following autologous bone marrow rescue. Two patients (13%) died of toxicity; one with multiorgan system failure and one with *Candida* septicemia. The remaining patients died of disease. Median survival for patients with recurrent or refractory disease was 4.7 months (range 0.1 to 18.7) and 11.4 months (range 7.6 to 17.1) for newly-diagnosed patients.

The French Society of Pediatric Oncology performed a pilot study using irradiation followed by high dose chemotherapy with autologous bone marrow rescue in children newly diagnosed with diffuse intrinsic pontine tumors.[39] The median age at diagnosis was seven years (range 3 to 17 years) and 35 children were enrolled and met eligibility criteria. Only 24 children proceeded to high dose chemotherapy following irradiation. The median time between irradiation and high dose chemotherapy was 54 days (range 25 to 95 days). One child died during irradiation, eight children experienced disease progression that prevented consolidation, and two children were removed from the study at their parents' request prior to the high dose chemotherapy. The high dose chemotherapy included oral busulfan 150 mg/m$^2$/day as four divided doses given over four days followed by thiotepa 300 mg/m$^2$/day for three days. Three patients died from toxicity during the consolidation phase. The deaths were due to *Aspergillus fumigatus* pneumonia (1 patient), toxic exfoliative dermatitis (1 patient), and venoocclusive disease and interstitial pneumonitis followed by multiorgan failure (1 patient). The remaining 21 children died of disease progression. Median survival was ten months.

## EPENDYMOMA

Ependymomas account for 8% to 10% of pediatric central nervous system tumors resulting in approximately 170 new cases each year.[1] These tumors usually originate from the ependymal lining of the ventricular system in the brain and central canal of the spinal cord. Nearly all of the tumors are intracranial, with only 10% occurring in the spinal cord. The primary therapy for patients newly diagnosed with ependymoma is maximal surgical resection without causing unacceptable neurologic complications followed by postoperative irradiation with or without chemotherapy. This approach has resulted in ten-year overall survival rates of 40% to 50%. Progression-free survival has been reported as approximately 35% to 40%.[40,41] Most recurrences are local and late relapses are not uncommon.

There have been two studies published using high dose chemotherapy with autologous stem cell rescue in children with recurrent ependymoma. Mason et al. reported the Children's Cancer Group experience in 15 children with recurrent intracranial ependymoma.[42] The initial patients were treated with thiotepa 300 mg/m$^2$/day and etoposide 500 mg/m$^2$/day for three days. The dose of etoposide was later decreased to 250 mg/m$^2$/day because of multiorgan toxicity. Ten of these children also received carboplatin initially at a dose of 500 mg/m$^2$/day and later were dosed using the Calvert formula to give an area under the concentration curve of 7 cc/min-mL/day for an additional three days prior to autologous stem cell rescue. All patients had maximal surgical resection prior to treatment. Fourteen children had received prior chemotherapy and 13 had received prior irradiation. Five children (33%) died of toxicity within 62 days of marrow reinfusion. Eight children died of progressive disease 4 to 34 months following high dose chemotherapy and one child died from unrelated causes. One child was alive 25 months following high dose chemotherapy, but had recurrent disease requiring additional surgery, irradiation, and maintenance chemotherapy.

Grill et al. treated sixteen children with refractory or recurrent ependymoma in a phase II study including busulfan 150 mg/m$^2$/day for four days and thiotepa 300 to 350 mg/m$^2$/day for three days.[43] All patients had received prior chemotherapy and eight had received prior irradiation. There was one toxic death. Ten children died of progressive disease seven to 45 months following treatment including five children who received irradiation after stem cell reinfusion. Five children were alive 15 to 66 months posttreatment. Three had no evidence of disease. There were no radiographic responses seen.

## GERM CELL TUMORS

Germ cell tumors (GCT) make up half of the tumors found in the pineal region, although overall, pineal region tumors account for less than 2% of childhood tumors. The majority of patients with GCT in the central nervous system are diagnosed between 10 and 14 years of age.[6] The diagnosis is often made based upon elevation of tumor markers including alpha-fetoprotein and beta human chorionic gonadotropin (HCG). However, if these markers are not elevated, biopsies or surgical resection should be performed to distinguish

GCT from other tumors that can occur in the pineal region including pineal parenchymal tumors and astrocytomas.

Central nervous system GCT can be divided into two primary categories: germinomas and nongerminomatous germ cell tumors. Irradiation has been the primary therapy for most patients with germinomas.[44] However, because of the absence of the blood brain barrier and the chemosensitivity of these tumors, chemotherapy has recently been added to many treatment regimens. Several pilot studies have suggested efficacy of combining postoperative chemotherapy with reduced dose and reduced volume irradiation.[45,46]

Investigators have begun to explore the use of high dose chemotherapy with autologous stem cell rescue in the treatment of GCT for a variety of reasons. These include the efficacy of high dose chemotherapy in non-central nervous system GCT, the limitation of radiation therapy as an option in patients with recurrent germinomas who were previously irradiated and the relative refractoriness of nongerminomatous GCT to irradiation and standard dose chemotherapy.

The results of the French Society of Pediatric Oncology using high dose chemotherapy with autologous stem cell rescue were initially published by Baranzelli et al.[47] and later updated by Bouffet et al.[48] Twenty children with recurrent ($N = 18$) or refractory ($N = 2$) intracranial GCT were treated. Thirteen patients had nongerminomatous GCT and seven had germinomas. All of the children had previously received carboplatin-based chemotherapy. Fifteen had previously received irradiation. High dose chemotherapy consisted of etoposide 1500 mg/m$^2$ and thiotepa 900 mg/m$^2$. Following the high dose chemotherapy, three patients underwent surgical resection, four patients received craniospinal irradiation, and three patients received focal irradiation. At the time of the report, 16 patients were alive at a median of 29 months following high dose chemotherapy. Thirteen patients were in continuous complete remission (CCR), one patient was in complete remission after salvage craniospinal irradiation, and two patients were alive with disease. Patients who were in complete remission prior to the high dose chemotherapy fared the best. Eight of nine patients in complete remission prior to the high dose chemotherapy remained in CCR. Five of nine patients with a partial response achieved a complete response to high dose chemotherapy. No patients with progressive disease prior to the high dose chemotherapy had a complete response. There were no toxic deaths.

Modak et al. also used thiotepa-based regimens in their treatment of eight patients with recurrent GCT.[49] Three patients had germinomas and five had nongerminomatous germ cell tumors. All patients had received irradiation and standard dose chemotherapy prior to the high dose chemotherapy. Four patients were supposed to receive carboplatin 500 mg/m$^2$/day or dosed using the Calvert formula with an area under the concentration curve of 7 mg/mL-min/m$^2$, followed by thiotepa 300 mg/m$^2$/day and etoposide 250 mg/m$^2$/day for three days. Two of the four patients did not receive the intended thiotepa and etoposide because of reduced renal function. Two patients received thiotepa 300 mg/m$^2$/day and etoposide 500 mg/m$^2$/day for three days. One patient received etoposide 500 mg/m$^2$/day for three days with autologous stem cell rescue followed by thiotepa 200 mg/m$^2$/day for three days with a second stem cell rescue. One patient received thiotepa alone at a dose of 200 mg/m$^2$/day for three days with autologous stem cell rescue. Three patients with germinoma were event-free survivors at two, four, and nine months following stem cell rescue. All patients with nongerminomatous GCT died of disease. There were no toxic deaths.

Tada et al. treated six children with nongerminomatous GCT (3 with choriocarcinoma, 2 with embryonal carcinoma, and 1 with a yolk sac tumor).[50] All patients were in first complete remission prior to the high dose chemotherapy. Complete remission was achieved with irradiation and four to seven courses of standard dose chemotherapy including cisplatin 20 mg/m$^2$/day for five days and etoposide 100 mg/m$^2$/day for five days. Five of six children also underwent surgical resection either at diagnosis or during induction therapy. One child achieved a complete remission without the need for surgical resection. High dose chemotherapy included cisplatin 40 mg/m$^2$/day and etoposide 250 mg/m$^2$/day for five days. ACNU was given at a dose of 150 mg/m$^2$ only on the first day. Two patients received carboplatin 160 mg/m$^2$/day for four days instead of cisplatin to avoid renal dysfunction. At the time of the report, all of the patients were alive without recurrence one to seven years from diagnosis.

# INFANTS

Review of Surveillance, Epidemiology, End Results (SEER) registries indicate that approximately 10% of childhood tumors occur in patients under two years of age.[51] The histology is most often medulloblastoma/PNET, ependymoma, or low grade glioma. Several studies have shown that infants with brain tumors do not do as well as older children.[51–53] The etiology of the poor outcome includes a reluctance to pursue aggressive therapy in such young children as well as the long-term sequelae associated with irradiation in these patients. As investigators have become more comfortable with the use of high dose chemotherapy with autologous stem cell rescue in older children and adults, this approach has been applied to the treatment of young children and infants with brain tumors in an attempt to decrease or avoid the use of irradiation.

Dupuis-Girod et al. were among the first groups to use high dose chemotherapy with autologous stem cell rescue in very young children.[54] The children ranged in age from five to 71 months (median, 23 months). All of the children had medulloblastoma whose disease had recurred or was refractory following standard dose chemotherapy. They were treated with oral busulfan 37.5 mg/m$^2$/dose every six hours for 16 doses followed by thiotepa 300 mg/m$^2$/day for three days. Following recovery from the high dose chemotherapy eleven patients with local recurrences received cranial irradiation (45 to 55 Gy). Six children with metastatic disease at the time of recurrence received craniospinal irradiation with 25 to 35 Gy to the spine and a boost of 45 to 55 Gy to the posterior fossa. Two children died of disease and one child died of interstitial pneumonitis prior to irradiation. Eleven of 20 patients (55%) were alive at a median of 31 months following stem cell reinfusion with no evidence of disease.

Gururangan et al. also used high dose chemotherapy in young children with malignant brain tumors who had recurrent disease following standard dose chemotherapy.[55] The diagnoses included medulloblastoma/PNET in five patients, pineal PNET in five patients, cerebral PNET in three patients, glioblastoma multiforme in four patients, and one patient each with anaplastic astrocytoma, choroid plexus carcinoma, and ependymoma. Patients ranged in age from 0.7 to 5.9 years (median, 2.9 years) at the time of autologous bone marrow rescue. No children received irradiation during the initial treatment and only two children received gamma knife surgery at the time of relapse prior to the high dose chemotherapy. Three different consolidation regimens were used. Sixteen children received carboplatin 500 mg/m$^2$/day or dosed using the Calvert formula with an area under the concentration curve of 7 mg/mL-min daily for three days followed by thiotepa 300 mg/m$^2$/day and etoposide 250 mg/m$^2$/day for three days. Three children received the same regimen but without the carboplatin. One patient received thiotepa 300 mg/m$^2$/day and etoposide 500 mg/m$^2$/day for three days followed by carmustine 150 mg/m$^2$/day for four days. Twelve children received irradiation approximately six weeks following autologous bone marrow reinfusion. Six received focal irradiation (54 to 59.4 Gy), five received focal (50.2 to 54 Gy) and reduced-dose (18 to 19.2 Gy) craniospinal irradiation, and one received focal (54 Gy) with craniospinal irradiation (36 Gy). Progression-free survival for the entire cohort was 50% at a median of 37.9 months following autologous bone marrow rescue.

In an effort to avoid irradiation, Mason et al. used high dose chemotherapy with autologous bone marrow rescue as consolidation therapy in young children newly diagnosed with malignant brain tumors.[56] All children initially underwent maximal possible surgical resection. This was followed by five cycles of induction chemotherapy that included cisplatin vincristine, cyclophosphamide, and etoposide. Patients proceeded to consolidation chemotherapy if they had minimal residual disease. Consolidation chemotherapy consisted of carboplatin 500 mg/m$^2$/day or dosed using the Calvert formula with an area under the concentration curve of 7 mg/mL-min for three days followed by thiotepa 300 mg/m$^2$/day and etoposide 250 mg/m$^2$/day daily for three days. Autologous bone marrow was reinfused on the third day following completion of the chemotherapy. All patients were less than 72 months of age. Sixty-two children were enrolled in the study. Diagnoses included medulloblastoma ($N = 13$); other PNET ($N = 14$); ependymoma ($N = 10$); malignant glioma ($N = 9$); brainstem glioma ($N = 6$); atypical teratoid tumor ($N = 5$); anaplastic astroblastoma ($N = 3$); choroid plexus carcinoma ($N = 1$); and primary central nervous system sarcoma ($N = 1$). Thirty-seven children proceeded to consolidation therapy. The five-year event-free survival was 41%, 39%, and 22% for patients with medulloblastoma, noncerebellar PNET and ependymoma, respectively. The five-year overall survival was 64%, 43%, and 42% for these same patients.

## TOXICITY

Myelosuppression is the most common toxicity and is similar to high dose chemotherapy for any disorder. As a result of the myelosuppression, patients usually require broad spectrum antibiotics and transfusions with red cells and platelets. In addition, mucositis often requires the use of pain medication and parenteral nutrition. Fortunately, the development of new antimicrobial and antifungal drugs has significantly decreased the infectious complications seen with this therapy. Furthermore, the use of growth factors and peripheral blood stem cells rather than bone marrow stem cells has decreased toxicity by enhancing hematopoietic recovery.[57] Because of these advances, the toxic mortality rate associated with the use of high dose chemotherapy with autologous stem cell rescue in patients with malignant brain tumors has decreased to less than 5% in most centers.

In addition to the side effects seen in nearly all patients treated with intensive therapy, there are some toxicities that are unique for patients with malignant brain tumors. Because of the location of their primary tumors, these patients are more susceptible to bleeding in the central nervous system. Many of these patients are on dexamethasone, which puts them at increased risk of developing fungal infections.

Studies performed by Faulkner et al. revealed that patients treated with spinal irradiation had decreased numbers of stem cells in their posterior iliac crests.[58] Therefore, if stem cells are collected following spinal irradiation, patients should undergo peripheral blood stem cell harvest or have bone marrow harvested from the anterior iliac crests.

Unfortunately, some of the drugs with the most activity against central nervous system tumors have significant nonhematopoietic toxicities at very high doses. Several studies using carmustine as a single agent as well as in combination have confirmed the pulmonary, hepatic and neurotoxicity associated with this drug.[25-27] Severe ototoxicity is another complication often seen in patients with malignant brain tumors following high dose chemotherapy. It is due to a number of factors including platinum drugs such as carboplatin and cisplatin as well as aminoglycosides and irradiation. The lipophilic property of thiotepa results in good central nervous system penetration but is associated with encephalopathy at very high doses, particularly in older patients and patients who have had prior cranial irradiation.[59]

## CONCLUSIONS AND FUTURE GOALS

Until recently the diagnosis of malignant brain tumor in childhood was associated with a dismal prognosis no matter what the histology. However, over the past several years advances in surgical techniques, radiation therapy, and chemotherapy have resulted in long-term survival for many of these children. The use of high dose chemotherapy with autologous stem cell rescue has increased the survival rate further, especially in children with medulloblastoma and central nervous system germ cell tumors. This therapy also has helped to improve the quality of life for many infants and young children with malignant brain tumors through the use of lower doses of irradiation or in some cases total avoidance of irradiation, thereby resulting in fewer long-term sequelae associated with this treatment.

Unfortunately, the use of high dose chemotherapy has had little impact to date on survival in children with brainstem gliomas and ependymomas. For these children, survival may be improved with the use of new chemotherapeutic agents such as temozolomide as well as the combination of high dose chemotherapy with other approaches such as antiangiogenesis, monoclonal antibody therapy, and/or differentiating agents.

# REFERENCES

1. Gurney JF, Severson RK, Davis S, Robison LL. Incidence of cancer in children in the United States. Cancer 1995;75:2186–2195.
2. Young J, Miller R. Incidence of malignant tumors in U.S. children. J Pediatr 1975;86:254–258.
3. Long-Term Clinical Effects. In: Cohen ME, Duffner PK (eds). Brain Tumors In Children (2nd ed). New York: Raven Press, 1994:455–481.
4. Chin H, Maruyama Y. Age at treatment and long term performance results in medulloblastoma. Cancer 1984;53:1952–1958.
5. Duffner PK, Horowitz ME, Krischer JP et al. Post-operative chemotherapy and delayed radiation in children less than 3 years of age with malignant brain tumors. N Engl J Med 1993;328:1725–1731.
6. Strother DR, Pollack IF, Fisher PG et al. Tumors of the central nervous system. In: Pizzo PA, Poplack DG (eds). Principles and Practice of Pediatric Oncology (4th ed). Philadelphia: Lippincott-Raven Publishers, 2002:751–824.
7. Frei E III, Teicher BA, Holden SA et al. Preclinical studies and clinical correlation of the effect of alkylating dose. Cancer Res 1988;48:6417–6423.
8. Hirota H, Gosky D, Berger NA, Chatterjee S. Interference with topoisomerase II alpha potentiates melphalan cytotoxicity. Int J Oncol 2002;20:311–318.
9. Cushing H. Experiences with cerebellar medulloblastoma: A critical review. Acta Pathol Microbiol Scand 1930;7:1–86.
10. Packer RJ, Sutton LN, Elterman R et al. Outcome for children with medulloblastoma treated with radiation and cisplatin, CCNU, and vincristine chemotherapy. J Neurosurg 1994;18:690–698.
11. Torres CF, Rebsamen S, Silber JH et al. Surveillance scanning of children with medulloblastoma. N Engl J Med 1994;330:892–895.
12. Belza MG, Donaldson SS, Steinberg GK et al. Medulloblastoma: Freedom from relapse longer than 8 years— a therapeutic cure? J Neurosurg 1991;75:575–582.
13. Kalifa C, Hartmann O, Demeocq F et al. High-dose busulfan and thiotepa with autologous bone marrow transplantation in childhood malignant brain tumors: A phase II study. Bone Marrow Transplant 1992;9:227–233.
14. Mahoney DH, Strother D, Camitta B et al. High dose melphalan and cyclophosphamide with autologous bone marrow rescue for recurrent/progressive malignant brain tumors in children: a pilot pediatric oncology group study. J Clin Oncol 1996;14:382–388.
15. Graham ML, Herndon JE, Casey JR et al. High-dose chemotherapy with autologous stem-cell rescue in patients with recurrent and high-risk pediatric brain tumors. J Clin Oncol 1997;15:1814–1823.
16. Dunkel IJ, Boyett JM, Yates A et al. High-dose carboplatin, thiotepa, and etoposide with autologous stem-cell rescue for patients with recurrent medulloblastoma. J Clin Oncol 1998;16:222–228.
17. Vassal G, Tranchand B, Valteau-Couanet D et al. Pharmacodynamics of tandem high-dose melphalan with peripheral blood stem cell transplantation in children with neuroblastoma and medulloblastoma. Bone Marrow Transplant 2001;27:471–477.
18. Strother D, Ashley D, Kellie SJ et al. Feasibility of four consecutive high-dose chemotherapy cycles with stem-cell rescue for patients with newly diagnosed medulloblastoma or supratentorial primitive neuroectodermal tumor after craniospinal radiotherapy: results of a collaborative study. J Clin Oncol 2001;19: 2696–2704.
19. Rorke LB. Primitive Neuroectodermal Tumor- A Concept Requiring an Apologia? In: Vincken PJ, Bruyn GW (eds). Tumors of the Brain and Skull, part III. New York: Elsevier, 1975:5–15.
20. Rubinstein LJ. Justification for a cytogenetic scheme of embryonal central neuroepithelial tumors. In: Fields WS (ed). Primary Brain Tumors: A Review of Histologic Classification. New York: Springer-Verlag, 1989:16-27.
21. Pomeroy SL, Tamayo P, Gaasenbeek M et al. Prediction of central nervous system embryonal tumour outcome based on gene expression. Nature 2002;415:436–442.
22. Cohen BH, Zeltzer PM, Boyett JM et al. Prognostic factors and treatment results for supratentorial primitive neuroectodermal tumors in children using radiation and chemotherapy: a Children's Cancer Group randomized trial. J Clin Oncol 1995;13:1687–1696.
23. Duncan, GG, Goodman, GB, Ludgate, CM, Rheaume DE. The treatment of adult supratentorial high grade astrocytoma. J Neurooncol 1992;13:63–72.
24. Marchese MJ, Chang CH. Malignant astrocytic gliomas in children. Cancer 1990;65:2771–2778.
25. Hochberg FH, Parker LM, Takvorian T et al. High-dose BCNU with autologous bone marrow rescue for recurrent glioblastoma multiforme. J Neurosurg 1981;54:455–460.
26. Phillips GL, Wolff SN, Fay JW et al. Intensive 1,3-bis (2-chloroethyl)-1-nitrosourea (BCNU) mono-chemotherapy and autologous marrow transplantation for malignant glioma. J Clin Oncol 1986;4:639–645.

27. Johnson DB, Thompson JM, Corwin JA et al. Prolongation of survival for high-grade malignant gliomas with adjuvant high-dose BCNU and autologous bone marrow transplantation. J Clin Oncol 1987;5:783–789.

28. Heideman RL, Douglass EC, Krance RA et al. High-dose chemotherapy and autologous bone marrow rescue followed by interstitial and external-beam radiotherapy in newly diagnosed pediatric malignant gliomas. J Clin Oncol 1993;11:1458–1465.

29. Kedar A, Mari BL, Graham-Pole J et al. High-dose chemotherapy with marrow reinfusion and hyperfractionated irradiation for children with high-risk brain tumors. Med Pediatr Oncol 1994;23:428–436.

30. Bouffet E, Motolese C, Jouvet A et al. Etoposide and thiotepa followed by ABMT (autologous bone marrow transplantation) in children and young adults with high-grade gliomas. Eur J Cancer 1997;33:91–95.

31. Finlay JL, Goldman S, Wong MC et al. Pilot study of high-dose thiotepa and etoposide with autologous bone marrow rescue in children and young adults with recurrent CNS tumors. J Clin Oncol 1996;14:2495–2503.

32. Papadakis V, Dunkel IJ, Cramer LD et al. High-dose carmustine, thiotepa and etoposide followed by autologous bone marrow rescue for the treatment of high risk central nervous system tumors. Bone Marrow Transplant 2000;26:153–160.

33. Grovas AC, Boyett JM, Lindsley K et al. Regimen-related toxicity of myeloablative chemotherapy with BCNU, thiotepa, and etoposide followed by autologous stem cell rescue for children with newly diagnosed glioblastoma multiforme: report from the Children's Cancer Group. Med Pediatr Oncol 1999;33:83–87.

34. Farwell JR, Dohrmann GJ, Flannery JT. Central nervous system tumors in children. Cancer 1977;40:3123–3132.

35. Packer RJ, Vezina G. Pediatric glial neoplasms including brain-stem gliomas. Semin Oncol 1994;21:260–272.

36. Freeman CR, Krischer JP, Sanford RA et al. Final results of a study of escalating doses of hyperfractionated radiotherapy in brain stem tumors in children: a pediatric oncology group study. Int J Radiat Oncol Biol Phys 1993;27:197–206.

37. Packer RJ, Boyett JM, Zimmerman RA et al. Outcome of children with brain stem gliomas after treatment with 7800 cGy of hyperfractionated radiotherapy: a Childrens Cancer Group Phase I/II trial. Cancer 1994;74:1827–1834.

38. Dunkel IJ, Garvin JH, Goldman S et al. High dose chemotherapy with autologous bone marrow rescue for children with diffuse pontine brain stem tumors. J Neurooncol 1998;37:67–73.

39. Bouffet E, Raquin M, Doz F et al. Radiotherapy followed by high dose busulfan and thiotepa: a prospective assessment of high dose chemotherapy in children with diffuse pontine gliomas. Cancer 2000;88:685–692.

40. Evans AE, Anderson JR, Lefkoweitz-Boudreaux IB, Finlay JL. Adjuvant chemotherapy of childhood posterior fossa ependymomas: craniospinal irradiation with or without adjuvant CCNU, vincristine, and prednisone: A Children's Cancer Group study. Med Pediatr Oncol 1996;27:8–14.

41. Perilongo G, Massimino M, Sotti G et al. Analyses of prognostic factors in a retrospective review of 92 children with ependymoma: Italian Pediatric Ceuro-oncology Group. Med Pediatr Oncol 1997;29:79–85.

42. Mason WP, Goldman S, Yates AJ et al. Survival following intensive chemotherapy with bone marrow reconstitution for children with recurrent intracranial ependymoma. J Neurooncol 1998;37:135–143.

43. Grill J, Kalifa C, Doz F et al. A high-dose busulfan-thiotepa combination followed by autologous bone marrow transplantation in childhood recurrent ependymoma. Pediatr Neurosurg 1996;25:7–12.

44. Shirato H, Nishi, M, Sawamura Y et al. Analysis of long-term treatment of intracranial germinoma. Int J Radiat Oncol Biol Phys 1997;37:511–515.

45. Buckner JC, Peethambaram PP, Smithson WA et al. Phase II trial of primary chemotherapy followed by reduced-dose radiation for CNS germ cell tumors. J Clin Oncol 1999;17:933–940.

46. Bouffet E, Baranzelli MC, Patte C et al. Combined treatment modality for intracranial germinomas: results of a multicentre SFOP experience. Societe Francaise d'Oncologie Pediatrique. Br J Cancer 1999;79:1199–1204.

47. Baranzelli MC, Pichon F, Patte C et al. High dose etoposide and thiotepa for recurrent intracranial germ cell tumours (IGCT). Med Pediatr Oncol 1998;31:256.

48. Bouffet E, Baranzelli MC, Patte C et al. on behalf of the Societe Francaise d'Oncologie Pediatrique(SFOP). High dose etoposide and thiotepa for refractory and recurrent malignant intracranial germ cell tumours (CNS-GCT). Neurooncol 2000;2(Suppl 2):S72.

49. Modak S, Gardner S, Dunkel I et al. High dose chemotherapy with autologous stem cell rescue in patients with recurrent CNS germ cell tumors. Childhood Cancer into the 21st Century, Birmingham, United Kingdom, April 23-25, 1997.

50. Tada T, Takizawa T, Nakazato F et al. Treatment of intracranial nongerminomatous germ-cell tumor by high-dose chemotherapy and autologous stem-cell rescue. J Neurooncol 1999;44:71–76.

51. Duffner PK, Cohen ME, Myers MH, Heise HW. Survival of children with brain tumors: SEER Program, 1973–1980. Neurology 1986;36:597–601.

52. Farwell JR, Dohrmann GJ, Flannery JT. Intracranial neoplasms in infants. Arch Neurol 1978;35:533–537.

53. Fessard C. Cerebral tumors in infancy. Am J Dis Child 1968;115:302–308.

54. Dupuis-Girod S, Hartmann O, Benhamou E et al. Will high dose chemotherapy followed by autologous bone marrow transplantation supplant cranio-spinal irradiation in young children treated for medulloblastoma? J Neurooncol 1996;27: 87–98.
55. Gururangan S, Dunkel IJ, Goldman S et al. Myeloablative chemotherapy with autologous bone marrow rescue in young children with recurrent malignant brain tumors. J Clin Oncol 1998;16:2486–2493.
56. Mason WP, Govas A, Halpern S et al. Intensive chemotherapy and bone marrow rescue for young children with newly diagnosed malignant brain tumors. J Clin Oncol 1998;16:210–221.
57. Korbling M. Autologous and allogeneic blood stem cell transplantation: potential advantage of blood-over marrow-derived stem cell grafts. Cancer Invest 1997;15:127–137.
58. Faulkner LB, Lindsley KL, Kher U et al. High-dose chemotherapy with autologous marrow rescue for malignant brain tumors: analysis of the impact of prior chemotherapy and craniospinal irradiation on hematopoietic recovery. Bone Marrow Transplant 1996;17:389–394.
59. Wolff SN, Herzig RH, Fay JW et al. High-dose N, N′,N″–triethylenethiophosphoramide (thiotepa) with autologous bone marrow transplantation: phase I study. Semin Oncol 1990;17:2–6.

# CHAPTER *XII*

# Acute Lymphoblastic Leukemia

ERIC SANDLER AND MICHAEL JOYCE

Acute lymphoblastic leukemia (ALL) is the most common cancer in children. In the United States, the incidence of leukemia in children is 4 per 100,000 children less than 15-years-old. Two thousand cases of ALL are diagnosed annually, accounting for 75% of the cases of leukemia in children, and the peak incidence is between 2 and 10 years of age. Three distinct subtypes of ALL are seen in children. B cell ALL is the leukemic presentation of Burkitt lymphoma. Pre-B ALL is the most common form of ALL in children. T cell ALL usually occurs in adolescents and presents with a mediastinal mass in over one-half of the cases.

The treatment of childhood acute lymphocytic leukemia (ALL) is one of the foremost success stories of pediatric oncology. Forty years ago, ALL was almost uniformly fatal with survival limited to only a few months. Through basic science and clinical research, substantial advances have been made in our understanding of the biology of ALL and in the treatment of this disorder. Today, 70% of all children diagnosed with ALL are cured and most children are cured with chemotherapy alone.[1]

Despite the advances in front line therapy for the treatment of ALL, relapse occurs in approximately 25% of cases.

Children with relapsed ALL or those who are found to be very high risk may require stem cell transplantation for cure of their disease. This chapter examines the role of hematopoietic stem cell transplantation in the treatment of ALL in children.

## ALL RISK GROUPS

Extensive clinical and laboratory investigation into the biology of childhood ALL over the last three decades has resulted in the determination of prognostic risk groups, which require different therapies. Treatment protocols for ALL are determined by the risk group assignment. Age and initial white blood cell (WBC) count at diagnosis have been identified as the most important prognostic factors for children with this disease. The Children's Oncology Group currently classifies children into low risk, standard risk, or high risk ALL based on age, WBC count, and cytogenetics of the leukemic cells. Children who are between the ages of 2 and 10 and with a WBC count of less than 50,000 are considered standard risk. Children who are greater than 10 years of age regardless of WBC count or less than 10 years of age with a WBC greater than 50,000 are considered high risk. Children who are standard risk by age and WBC are treated with a three-drug induction therapy (vincristine, prednisone, L-asparaginase), while those in the high risk group receive a four-drug induction therapy (vincristine, prednisone, L-asparaginase, and daunomycin). Children assigned to the standard risk group by age and WBC count and whose leukemic cells are found to contain trisomy of chromosomes 4 and 10 or TEL/AML are assigned to a low risk group as they appear to require a less intensive consolidation/intensification treatment for their disease. Patients with Philadelphia chromosome, or MLL gene rearrangement, ALL, and those who do not achieve remission by day 29, are considered very high risk. Since the presence of certain chromosomal translocations have a significant impact on risk group classification and treatment, it is essential that all new patients be evaluated for cytogenetic abnormalities in their leukemic cells. Standard karyotyping is performed on all patients at diagnosis. Patients with a DNA index >1.0 should have fluorescent in situ hybridization (FISH) probes or polymerase chain reaction (PCR) performed for trisomy of chromosomes 4 and 10 and for the TEL/AML rearrangement. Patients are also screened for the presence of the Philadelphia chromosome or bcr/abl rearrangement by FISH probes or PCR. Children who present at less than one year of age are classified as infant ALL and are treated on a more intensive protocol. These infants often have an MLL gene rearrangement and have a worse prognosis.

## SOURCES OF STEM CELLS

Patients who are candidates for allogeneic transplantation have several potential stem cell sources. Human lymphocyte antigen (HLA)-identical siblings, or a closely matched (6/6, 5/6) family member, is considered to be the best stem cell source. For patients without a suitable HLA-matched family member, options include HLA-matched unrelated adult donors (URD), an umbilical cord donor (UCD), or a mismatched related donor (MRD). The National Marrow Donor Program (NMDP) now has several million registered adult donors. Over the past 10 years, the NMDP has significantly shortened the time it takes to identify a donor. In the past, donor identification may have taken four to six months, but now it may take less than 12 weeks to identify most donors. Once a volunteer donor is identified, the donor's stem cells can be harvested by bone marrow or peripheral blood stem cell harvesting. The donor is primed with granuloctye colony stimulating factor prior to peripheral stem cell harvest. The peripheral blood stem cells are then frozen until needed. Peripheral blood stem cell harvesting can be done through peripheral IV access and the donor does not have to undergo the risk of anesthesia or the discomfort associated with a bone marrow harvest. Unrelated umbilical cord blood donor units, which are cryopreserved at the time of delivery of a child, also can be used as a suitable source of hematopoietic cells for most pediatric patients. They are being used with increasing success as a donor source for adult patients as well. There are numerous cord blood banks in the United States and Europe that can provide a preliminary search in a short period of time. Preliminary data suggest that one and two antigen mismatches are well tolerated in umbilical cord transplantation, and thus there is a 90% or greater chance of finding a suitable cord blood donor. However, low cell doses may result in delayed or poor engraftment. In a few centers, a partially matched family member (haploidentical) may be used. Stem cells harvested from a partially matched family member will need to undergo T-cell depletion to prevent severe graft-versus-host disease.

| TABLE 12.1 | Conditioning Regimens for Bone Marrow Transplantation in Acute Lymphoblastic Lymphoma |
|---|---|
| **Regimen** | **Details** |
| TBI/Cytoxan | Total Body Radiation (1200 cGy total, fractionated as 200 cGy BID × 3 days or 150 cGy BID × 4 days) and cyclophosphemide 60 mg/kg × 2 doses |
| Hyperfractionated TBI/Cytoxan | Total Body Radiation (1320 cGy total, fractionated as 120 cGy TID for 11 fractions) and cyclophosphemide 60 mg/kg × 2 doses |
| TBI/VP16/Cytoxan | Total Body Radiation (1200 cGy), etoposide (30 mg/kg), and cytoxan 60 mg/kg × 2 doses |
| TBI/VP16 | Total Body Radiation (1200 cGy) and etoposide (60 mg/kg) |
| TBI/ARA-C | Total Body Radiation (1200 cGy) and cytarabine (3 g/m²/dose × 12 doses) |
| TBI/Melphalan | Total Body Radiation (1350 cGy) and melphalan (45 mg/m² × 3 doses) |
| Bu/Melphalan | Busulfan (16 mg/kg) and melphalan (45 mg/m²) |
| Bu/Cytoxan | Busulfan (16 mg/kg) and cyclophosphemide (50 mg/kg × 4) |

The role of autologous transplantation in ALL remains highly controversial and requires further investigation. In the autologous setting, stem cells may be obtained by bone marrow or peripheral blood stem cell harvesting. Peripheral blood stem cell collection requires mobilization of the stem cells with high dose G-CSF, often in conjunction with chemotherapy.

## CONDITIONING REGIMENS FOR TRANSPLANTATION

A number of different conditioning regimens are used for transplantation in children with ALL (▲ Table 12.1). In the treatment of leukemia, the conditioning regimen is designed for two purposes. The first is to provide adequate immunosuppression for engraftment of the donor hematopoietic cells and the second is to provide adequate treatment of the patient to eliminate the leukemic clone. Conditioning regimens for allogeneic or autologous transplantation can be divided into those that contain radiation and those that do not. The radiation-containing regimen combines total body irradiation (TBI) with chemotherapeutic agents, whereas the non-radiation regimens use multiple chemotherapeutic agents without TBI.

An initial study in the dog model revealed that 950 cGy of TBI resulted in complete chimeras. When cyclophosphamide alone was used for conditioning in the dog model, the result was mixed chimeras (donor and host cells were present). Preparative regimens using cyclophosphamide alone for patients with acute leukemia resulted in early relapses.[2–4] Researchers in Seattle have studied the combination of cyclophosphamide and total body irradiation extensively, and found that this combination resulted in engraftment in 99% of the cases and patients experienced a lower relapse rate when compared to cyclophosphamide or radiation alone. Initially, TBI was administered as a single fraction. Today, the

TBI dose is fractionated (4–9 fractions over 2–4 days) at lower dose rates. The total dose of TBI may vary in different centers and with different conditioning regimens; the total dose may range between 750 and 1400 cGy. Fractionation or hyperfractionation of TBI reduces toxicity to normal tissues, without reducing the antileukemic effect of the radiation.

The regimen of TBI and cyclophosphamide has been the most extensively studied conditioning regimen. In earlier studies the cyclophosphamide was administered prior to the TBI; most regimens in use today administer the TBI prior to the cyclophosphamide. The TBI dose varies between 1200 cGy to 1350 cGy, while the radiation is usually delivered in fractions ranging from 120 cGy to 200 cGy. For a fractionated regimen with a total dose of 1200 cGy, the radiation may be given at 200 cGy twice a day for three days, or may be given in fractions of 150 cGy twice a day for a total of four days. Hyperfractionated TBI delivers a lower fraction dose three times a day. The hyperfractionated regimen pioneered at Memorial Sloan-Kettering is the one that is commonly used, where the TBI is administered in 120 cGy fractions delivered three times a day for a total radiation dose of 1320 cGy. Following TBI, cyclophosphamide is administered at a dose of 60 mg/kg/day for two days. Conditioning with fractionated TBI and cyclophosphamide results in an overall survival of approximately 50% in patients transplanted for ALL.[5]

Other chemotherapeutic agents are often added to the combination of TBI and cyclophosphamide in the hope of reducing relapse. These include TBI, cytosine; TBI, arabinoside, etoposide; TBI, melphalan; TBI, VP16, cyclophsphamide, etc. The combination of etoposide, cyclophosphamide, and TBI is a commonly used and effective regimen for the treatment of hematologic malignancies.[6,7] Stomatitis is seen with this regimen due to the TBI and etoposide, but is manageable in most cases. Survival in a series of 41 pediatric patients who received a matched sibling donor or alternative donor transplant was 68% for patients without advanced disease and 17% for patients with advanced disease.[1] This conditioning regimen also has been used with success in infants with ALL.[2] Similarly, this conditioning regimen has been used with success in patients with Philadelphia chromosome positive ALL as well.[8] For such patients in first complete remission who underwent an allogeneic transplant, the estimated disease-free survival (DFS) at three years was 46% and patients under 30 years of age had a more favorable prognosis at three years of 61%.

The use of high dose etoposide with total body radiation has been investigated as a conditioning regimen for transplantation in children and adults with leukemia. TBI (1320 cGy) and etoposide (60 mg/kg) have been successful treatments for patients with high risk leukemia in first remission. The disease-free survival for ALL was 64% at three years and risk of relapse was only 12% in this study.[9] Etoposide is known to be associated with secondary malignancy and long-term follow-up is needed to ascertain the long-term risks associated with this conditioning regimen.

High-dose cytosine arabinoside with total body radiation therapy also has been used effectively in a number of centers. TBI is given twice a day in 200 cGy fractions for a total dose of 1200 cGy followed by cytosine arabinoside (3 g/m$^2$/dose) every 12 hours for a total of 12 doses. Kamani et al.[10] reported on 20 patients with acute leukemia who underwent transplantation with HLA identical sibling donors: 14 of those patients had ALL, 4 had AML, and 2 had mixed lineage leukemia. Thirteen of the patients remained in remission with a median follow-up of 68 months. Severe skin reactions (Grade III–IV) were noted in 20% of the patients and severe mucositis (Grade III–IV) was seen in 15% of the patients.

A retrospective multicenter report on the use of cytosine arabinoside followed by TBI in patients with ALL was associated with a DFS at three years of 54% for patients transplanted in CR1, 41% for CR2 or more, and 19% for patients in relapse.[11] Toxic deaths were more common in older patients. High dose cytarabine and fractionated total body radiation has been shown to be well tolerated in ALL patients with Down's syndrome who need to undergo transplantation.[12]

There have been few randomized prospective studies comparing conditioning regimens. Investigators at the University of Minnesota have reported on their experience using different preparative regimens for transplantation for ALL with matched sibling donors: cyclophosphamide plus single fraction TBI, cyclophosphamide and fractionated TBI, TBI and high dose cytarabine, and hyperfractionated TBI plus cyclophosphamide. The disease-free survival for all regimens was 29 ± 8%. A higher incidence of treatment-related mortality was noted in the TBI plus high dose cytarabine regimen. Leukemic relapse was the most common cause of treatment failure.[13] A similar study involving multiple institutions compared the following regimens: cyclophosphamide/TBI/VP16, cyclophosphamide/cytarabine/TBI, and TBI/cytarabine/melphalan. There was no significant difference in outcome for the different preparative regimens; however, it was noted that the TBI, cytarabine, and melphalan regimen had a lower relapse rate.[14]

In pediatrics there has been concern regarding the use of total body irradiation therapy in children due to the late effects associated with this therapy. These include the formation of cataracts, growth failure, and hormonal deficiency. Neuropsychological dysfunction is a serious concern, particularly in young children. Secondary malignancies have been associated with radiation therapy and are a concern for children undergoing transplant for curative intent. A number of non-radiation-containing regimens have been developed over the years for use in allogeneic or autologous transplantation. Busulfan (16 mg/kg total dose) has been substituted for TBI and combined with cyclophosphamide (200 mg/kg) as a conditioning regimen for children and adults with lymphocytic leukemia. In this series some patients also received etoposide, along with busulfan and cytoxan. The overall DFS was 43%, but the children did much better than the adults (DFS 63% vs. 30%).[15]

A randomized study compared TBI and cyclophosphamide to busulfan and cyclophosphamide in adults and children with leukemia. Busulfan and cyclophosphamide were associated with a greater incidence of venoocclusive disease of the liver and hemorrhagic cystitis. The disease-free survival for patients receiving the TBI regimen was 50% compared to 36% in the busulfan regimen, but this difference did not reach statistical significance.[16]

The International Bone Marrow Transplant Registry (IBMTR) recently reported on a retrospective review of their experience with cyclophosphamide/TBI and busulfan/cyclophosphamide as preparative regimens for HLA-identical sibling donor transplantation for children with ALL. The estimated three-year survival was 55% with cyclophosphamide/TBI versus 40% for busulfan/cyclophosphamide. This difference was statistically significant. The risk of relapse was not significantly different for these two preparative regimens; however, treatment-related mortality was much higher in the busulfan/cyclophosphamide group, which accounted for the difference in survival.[17] Based on these studies, there appears to be an advantage in using TBI/cyclophosphamide over busulfan/cyclophosphamide in children with ALL.

Long-term follow-up is important in evaluating conditioning regimens. Late effects of various regimens may have a significant impact on the quality of life of patients. For example, both radiation and etoposide have been associated with secondary malignancies. In summary, there are a variety of regimens that have been shown to be effective for transplantation in ALL. No one regimen has been found to be clearly superior. The choice of which regimen to use for a given patient must consider the curative potential, risk of relapse, risk of toxicity, and the late effects of the regimen.

## RESULTS OF TRANSPLANTATION IN ALL

### Chemotherapy Versus Allogeneic MSD Transplantation in CR2

Many investigators have attempted to compare the outcomes of allogeneic transplantation to the results obtained with chemotherapy in CR2 ALL. Most such studies have found that transplantation offers a significantly improved survival when compared to the use of chemotherapy in this setting. This is especially true for patients with a short CR1, that is, a first remission lasting <36 months, where the success of chemotherapy in this setting has not improved substantially. Although the transplant arms are usually associated with a higher transplant related mortality (TRM) secondary to infection and graft-versus-host disease (GVHD), chemotherapy series are usually associated with a much higher relapse rate.[3]

The largest such series is that by Barrett et al. who compared 376 children with CR2 ALL undergoing transplant, and reported to the IBMTR, to 540 children undergoing chemotherapy treatment on protocols of the Pediatric Oncology Group. As one would expect, they found a significant difference in the relapse rate, favoring transplanted patients (45% vs. 80%, $P$ <0.0001), while TRM was greater in the transplant group (27% vs. 14%, $P$ <0.001). Overall five-year DFS was 40% in transplanted patients versus 17% in chemotherapy-treated patients ($P$ <0.001). In the children with a CR1 <36 months, five-year DFS was 35% versus 10% and for children with a CR1 >36 months, five-year DFS was 53% versus 32% for transplant versus chemotherapy, respectively. Although a matched pair analysis was used, it should be noted that these data were retrospective registry data; thus, transplant patient selection was a confounding variable.[18] In addition, the chemotherapy protocols administered were less intensive and supportive care practices were different from those in current use. Other studies such as those published by investigators from Spain, the Netherlands, Memorial Sloan-Kettering Cancer Center (MSKCC), and the Children's Cancer Group have had similar findings.[19–21]

In these studies, the advantage of MSD transplantation persisted regardless of risk group assignment in CR1, duration of CR1, or intensity of initial therapy. Several more recent studies have continued to demonstrate a significant difference in outcomes for CR1 <36 months, but have not been able to show such a difference for long-term CR1 patients getting more contemporary chemotherapy protocols.

To date, patients with early relapse of ALL have clearly benefited from transplant in CR2, if they were fortunate enough to have a MSD. Whether this is true for all patients with late relapses remains to be determined. As front-line chemotherapy treatments improve, the group of relapsing children may present with much more refractory disease. Future studies must be done comparing similar groups of patients (▶ Table 12.2).

| TABLE 12.2 | Disease-Free Survival After Chemotherapy Versus Matched Sibling Donor Transplantation for Acute Lymphoblastic Leukemia in Second Complete Remission |
|---|---|

| BMT | Chemotherapy | Reference |
|---|---|---|
| 47% | 9% | Torres et al.[19] |
| 37% | 18% | Feig et al.[20] |
| 62% | 26% | Boulad et al.[21] |
| 48% (CR < 24 mo) 9% (CR < 24 mo) | | |
| 81% (CR > 24 mo) 37% (CR > 24 mo) | | |
| 40% | 17% | Barrett et al.[18] |
| 35% if CR < 36 mo | 10% if CR < 36 mo | |
| 53% if CR > 36 mo | 32% if CR > 36 mo | |

## Matched Sibling Donor Transplantation in CR1

The role of allogeneic transplantation in children with first remission ALL remains controversial. Patients who have the Philadelphia chromosome or bcr/abl transcript, the MLL gene rearrangement, or patients who have failed induction therapy are at very high risk for treatment failure with conventional chemotherapy. A number of reports have evaluated the use of allogeneic transplantation in high risk patients with ALL early in the treatment of their disease. Although there is a trend toward improved survival with BMT, those results have not been statistically significant.

The best reported results come from investigators in France who reported on 32 patients undergoing allogeneic transplantation in first remission. Children with a WBC of >100,000/μL, chromosomal abnormalities, or who had failed induction therapy were considered for transplantation if they had an HLA identical sibling. Conditioning consisted of TBI and cyclophosphamide. Nine patients presented with a WBC >100,000/μL and eleven patients presented with a WBC >250,000/μL. Ten out of fifteen children who had cytogenetics performed at diagnosis had an abnormal karyotype including t(8;14):5, t(4;11):1, t(9;22):2, Xp+:1, t(7;12):1. The DFS at five years was estimated to be 84%. The estimated relapse rate was only 3.5%. There were four deaths in the transplant group due to TRM. Only one patient in this group developed a relapse, which occurred four months posttransplant.[22]

However, several randomized studies of MSD transplant in CR1 have failed to show an advantage. The Medical Research Council Working Party on Childhood Leukemia reported their results in children with high risk ALL in CR1. Children who presented with a WBC > 100 × 10⁹/L were eligible for transplantation if they had a matched sibling donor. Children who did not have an HLA matched donor were treated with chemotherapy and cranial radiation. One hundred ninety-eight children presented with a WBC >100 × 10⁹. One hundred eighty-three of these children achieved complete remission. In 41 cases an HLA matched donor was identified and 34 proceeded to transplantation at a median of

| TABLE 12.3 | Allogeneic Transplantation for ALL with Matched Sibling Donor in Advanced Disease | |
|---|---|---|
| Disease Status | Disease-Free Survival | Reference |
| CR3 | 42% (MSD) | Brochstein et al.[5] |
| CR4 or relapse | 23% (MSD) | |
| CR3 | 49% | Borgmann et al.[25] |

17 weeks from diagnosis. Event-free survival (EFS) was 69% for the transplant group and 52.5% for the chemotherapy group. This difference was not significant. The relapse rate was 41% in the chemotherapy arm and 12% in the bone marrow transplant (BMT) arm ($P = 0.001$). The decreased relapse rate for the transplant group was offset by the increase in treatment-related mortality in the transplant arm.[23]

Uderzo et al. also reported a multiinstitutional study comparing the outcome for children treated with allogeneic BMT in first remission versus chemotherapy for high risk ALL. Their criteria for high risk ALL were: t(9:22), t(4:11), day 7 steroid dependence, T-immunophenotype, WBC >100 × 10$^9$/L, or failure to achieve CR by day 42. Their results were similar; the DFS was 58% in the BMT group and 47% in the chemotherapy group. The difference was not statistically significant ($P = 0.34$). The relapse rate was 48% at four years in the chemotherapy arm. In the BMT cohort, the relapse rate was 31%. This study showed that patients with high risk ALL had no survival advantage with allogeneic transplant versus chemotherapy.[24]

Although there is clearly a role for transplant in some children in first remission of ALL, other than induction failures, it is unclear which patients will truly benefit from this approach and further studies are needed.

## MSD Transplantation in CR3 or Greater or Refractory ALL

In most transplant centers, a child with relapsed ALL who has a matched sibling donor is transplanted in CR2. Thus, there are a limited number of studies that have evaluated the results of MSD transplant in CR3.

Borgmann et al. compared the results of matched sibling donor transplants on 169 patients from the BFM relapse study registry.[25] One hundred thirty-six patients were transplanted in CR2 and 33 patients in CR3. The majority of the patients received conditioning with FTBI 12 Gy with VP16 and/or cytoxan. The EFS at six years was 49% for the 136 children transplanted in CR2 and 48% for the 33 patients transplanted in CR3. A study from Memorial Sloan-Kettering showed similar results in CR3 with an EFS of 42% (▲ Table 12.3).[5]

Based on these results, a child with a matched sibling donor who has had a long first remission may opt to be treated with chemotherapy, which would result in a disease-free survival rate of 40%–50% compared to a DFS of 40%–60% reported for matched sibling donor transplantation in CR2. If relapse does occur, MSD transplantation could be performed in CR3. MSD transplantation is a viable option for patients in CR3 who have not undergone transplantation in CR2.

Patients who have advanced disease, CR4 or greater, or who are in relapse at the time of their transplant have a significantly worse outcome, with a disease-free survival at five years of 10%–25%.

## Unrelated Donor Transplantation in ALL

Unfortunately, only 20%–30% of children with leukemia requiring stem cell transplantation have available HLA-identical sibling donors.[26] Thus, for the majority of patients who do not have such a donor, alternative donors must be sought. Options include volunteer unrelated donors (URD), unrelated umbilical stem cell donors, or mismatched family member donors.[27] As all alternative donor sources offer donor cells that are at best phenotypically matched rather than genotypically matched, alternative donor procedures are associated with a higher risk of complications, including non-engraftment, acute and chronic GVHD, and greater transplant related mortality than that seen with MSD procedures. The most commonly utilized alternative stem cell source is the URD. Thanks to the emergence of large registries volunteers who are HLA typed and willing to donate their stem cells for patients who need them, throughout the world it is now possible to identify donors for a significant number of patients.[28] The largest such registry is the National Marrow Donor Program (NMDP). The NMDP began registering donors in 1986 and currently the registry contains HLA typing on 4.8 million volunteer unrelated donors. In addition, many of the worldwide registries now share their database information so that patients have access to a large pool of prospective donors. Limitations of these registries have historically been lower resolution HLA typing on donors, a long delay from the time of initiating a search to actual transplantation, and donor dropout due to a number of factors. Many patients with recurrent disease unfortunately will relapse while waiting for a donor to be identified. With the tremendous growth of the registries as well as funding support for higher resolution HLA typing of donors, these problems have dramatically improved. In 2000, the NMDP reported on 5246 patients transplanted between August 1991 and June 1999. The percentage of Caucasian patients for whom at least one donor was identified (HLA A, B, and DRB1 matched) has increased substantially between 1988 and 1997, while the time from initiation of search to transplantation decreased substantially during this same time period. Unfortunately, this improvement has not been as positive for some minority groups, due in part to fewer volunteer donors as well as greater potential heterogeneity in HLA types (personal communication from NMDP46).

Historically, URD transplants have been associated with a significantly higher incidence of GVHD and infections (especially fungal infections), which has resulted in a transplant-related mortality rate of 30%–50% in some series. Thus, overall outcomes were significantly worse than those from MSD transplants.[29–32] Interestingly, the relapse rates have been considerably less than what could be expected from MSD transplants, suggesting a role for a graft-versus-leukemia effect.[33] However, due in large part to increasing experience with MUD transplants, improvements in HLA typing strategies, improvements in the prevention and treatment of GVHD, and better supportive care of transplant recipients, more recent studies have shown that in many cases outcomes (DFS and survival) are approaching those seen with MSD transplants.[34–36]

Several recent reviews of the NMDP experience as well as single institution experience for children with ALL have identified a number of prognostic risk factors.[37–41] These studies have identified better outcomes associated with younger age of the recipient, less advanced disease, better donor recipient HLA matching, negative serology for CMV, male donor, and higher cell dose. In patients with CR2 ALL, duration of CR1 was an important prognostic factor, as in the MRD setting. In these series the overall survival ranged from 31%–70%, with the incidence of acute GVHD ranging from 30%–83%, with Grade III–IV in 29%–49%, chronic GVHD 11%–68%, TRM from 20%–50%, and relapse rates from 10%–50%.

In all of these studies, the occurrence of acute GVHD was strongly associated with TRM. As a result, several investigators have looked at T-cell depletion of grafts in an attempt to reduce the risk of GVHD.[42,43] In general, these trials have resulted in a lower incidence of GVHD but higher rates of non-engraftment and relapse. To overcome the engraftment problem, some investigators have significantly increased the intensity of the conditioning regimen with a resultant improvement in engraftment but at the expense of an increased incidence of TRM.

Several recent studies have compared URD and MSD transplants.[44–46] For example, Saarinen-Pihkala et al.[47] looked specifically at children in second remission of ALL. They compared the use of matched sibling donors, when available, with transplants done with URD donors from 1990 to 1997. In this series, MSD patients had a five-year EFS of 39% versus 54% for URD donors ($P = 0.4$), with relapse rates of 76% versus 40% (NS), respectively, and toxic death rates of 19 versus 11% (NS). They did find a significantly increased risk of Grade II–IV acute GVHD and chronic GVHD in the URD patients. Another study done at St Jude's Children's Research Hospital looked at outcomes for 103 consecutive patients undergoing transplantation with MSD or URD donors.[46] Stem cells from unrelated donors were partially T cell depleted using anti–T cell antibodies and complement. The authors found no significant difference in outcomes between these groups, with an 81% survival in the MSD group versus 73% in the URD group for low risk patients and a 31% vs. 32% survival in high risk patients.

Recently, several studies have examined the use of URD peripheral blood stem cells (PBSC) versus marrow stem cells. The advantages of PBSC include shorter engraftment times and ease in harvesting cells. Early results suggest that overall survival is similar. There does not seem to be a significant increase in the risk of acute GVHD and this has prompted the NMDP to allow donor choice in donation of bone marrow versus PBSC.[48]

As with other types of alternative donor transplants, increasing experience with URD transplants has resulted in improved outcomes. Newer therapies to prevent and treat GVHD will be essential to further improvements in outcome. In addition, patient and donor selection continues to be a challenge. Patients transplanted earlier in their disease process and those with better matched donors are likely to have better outcomes than those transplanted with resistant disease, significant organ toxicity, underlying infection, or mismatched donors. Better refinements in identifying those patients likely to need transplant at an earlier stage of disease will result in more successful outcomes.

## Unrelated Cord Blood Transplantation in ALL

Matched sibling donor transplantation is associated with higher cure rates in many children with relapsed ALL. Unfortunately, most patients (70%–80%) will not have a matched sibling donor. Individuals with relapsed ALL who require an allogeneic transplantation will need either an unrelated adult donor, unrelated cord blood donor, or partially matched family member as the source of their allogeneic stem cells. In the last fifteen years, unrelated umbilical cord blood has been shown to be a viable source of hematopoietic stem cells for pediatric and selected adult patients. Today there are several cord blood banks worldwide supplying umbilical cord blood units for these patients. Several studies have shown that unrelated umbilical cord blood is a reliable source of hematopoietic stem cells.[49–51]

The rates of engraftment of cord blood has varied between 90% and 100% in these studies, but is often slower than that seen with other donor sources. Engraftment is successful for fully HLA-matched unrelated cord blood donor units as well as units with a one, two, or three antigen mismatch. The incidence of acute GVHD has been reported to be 20% to 50% and chronic GVHD in 10% to 25%. There are a few potential advantages for unrelated cord blood transplantation over unrelated adult donor transplantation. First, the cord blood donor banks have a greater degree of ethnic diversity, which is helpful in identifying donors for patients who are members of minority groups that may have unique HLA antigens. Second, a perfect HLA match is not required as one to three antigen mismatched cord blood units can be suitable donors, and the probability of finding a donor is 90% or greater for most patients. Third, the time for finding a donor is much shorter for cord blood than for an unrelated donor transplant.

Several investigators[27,51,52] have reported on the outcome of unrelated cord blood transplantation in ALL. Kurtzberg et al.[51] reported on 12 patients with ALL in a series of 25 patients undergoing unrelated cord blood transplantation. Survival was 41% (5 of 12) at the time of the report. The majority of the patients (9 of 12) were in CR2, two were in relapse and one was an infant ALL in CR1. The incidence of acute GVHD (Grade II–IV) was 44% in this series of 25 patients. Barker et al.[52] reported on patients with a variety of diagnoses who underwent umbilical cord blood transplantation or unrelated adult bone marrow transplantation. They used matched pair analysis to compare the outcome of umbilical cord blood transplantation (UCB) to unrelated adult bone marrow transplantation (URD) and also did a matched pair analysis to compare UCB to T-cell depleted URD. Thirty-six out of 114 patients had ALL. The majority of the patients undergoing cord blood transplantation received TBI and cyclophosphamide (120 mg/kg). Patients who could not receive TBI were conditioned with busulfan 16 mg/kg and cyclophosphamide (200 mg/kg). GVHD prophylaxis was cyclosporine and prednisone. The two-year survival for patients receiving UCB (53%) compared favorably to patients receiving URD (41%). When UCB was compared to T-cell depleted URD, the survival was similar: 52% versus 56%. The incidence of acute GVHD (Grade II–IV) also was similar (42% vs. 35%). Chronic GVHD was much lower in the UCB (5%) compared to the URD (20%) group, and TRM at day 100 was 22% versus 15%, respectively.

Rocha et al.[27] reported similar results in the Eurocord experience: EFS of 31% versus 43% versus 37% for UCB versus URD versus T-cell depleted URD. The treatment related mortality was 39% for UCB versus 19% for URD and 14% for T-cell depleted URD. The incidence of acute GVHD (Grade II–IV) was 33%, 30%, and 8%, respectively, and chronic GVHD in this series was 25%, 46%, and 12%.

Overall, these studies show that umbilical cord blood transplantation is a viable alternative for patients with relapsed or very high risk ALL who require allogeneic transplantation for treatment of their disease. As demonstrated earlier, the survival rates are similar between cord blood transplantation and unrelated adult donor transplantation. The incidence of acute GVHD is comparable as well. UCB transplantation has a much lower risk of chronic GVHD than seen in URD. As the field of cord blood transplantation advances, it is anticipated that the treatment-related mortality rate will improve as we have seen in the field of unrelated donor transplantation.

## Partially Matched Family Member Transplantation in ALL

The use of mismatched related donors (MRT) is another donor option for children with high risk ALL.[53-64] It is especially important to consider MRT in cases where no MSD is available and either no URD or UCB is available. The advantage of MRT is the easy accessibility of a donor for all patients. However, there is a significantly increased risk of graft failure, GVHD, and TRM in this setting when compared to MSD transplantation.[54,55] There also has been a substantial incidence of prolonged immune dysregulation, late opportunistic infections, and lymphoproliferative disorders. Most patients have required higher intensity conditioning and immunosuppression to allow for engraftment as well as T-cell depletion to prevent severe GVHD. Many studies have shown that related one-antigen mismatched donors, particularly of class I antigens, have outcomes similar to MSD.[56] However, because of the unique requirements and complications of these transplant procedures, historically only selected centers have done transplants of recipient-donor pairs with greater than a one-antigen mismatch. In the selection of a donor, mismatched sibling donors tend to result in better outcomes than mismatched parental donors.[57] Limited data also suggest that those who are mismatched at the maternal haplotype may have superior outcomes to those mismatched at the paternal haplotype. The available literature on MRT is limited, and often reports on a very high risk group of patients. One of the largest series to date is from Henslee-Downey et al.[54] In their series of 72 consecutive patients undergoing MRT from haploidentical family donors, conditioning included TBI, etoposide, cytosine arabinoside, cyclophosphamide, and high dose prednisolone. GVHD prophylaxis included cyclosporine, antithymocyte globulin, and T cell depletion of the graft with T10B9 antibodies. Overall survival was 35% at two years, with low risk patients at 55% versus 27% for high risk patients. Although GVHD incidence was quite low, TRM risk was 43% and relapse rate was 32%. Interestingly, neither incidence of GVHD or survival was correlated with degree of mismatch. Non-engraftment risk was associated with degree of mismatch.

The roles of URD, mismatched URD, or haploidentical family donors in a single institution were recently compared. The investigators[64] found that outcomes were better in HLA identical URD versus mismatched URD or MRT (58% vs. 34% vs. 21%) and recommended that a phenotypically matched URD was a better choice than either a mismatched URD or MRT.

Until there is more experience with successful MRT, such transplants should be best performed at experienced centers and as part of clinical trials.

## Autologous Stem Cell Transplantation

Use of autologous stem cells for transplantation in children with ALL clearly offers some unique advantages to the use of alternative donor sources.[65] TRM is significantly reduced in the autologous setting as there is no risk of GVHD and complete immunosuppression is not required. In addition, donors are immediately available for all patients and the costs associated with autologous procedures are less. However, the use of autologous procedures is associated with a much higher risk of relapse secondary to potential residual leukemia in the transplanted product or in the patient, and to the lack of a graft-versus-leukemia (GVL) effect. Several investigators[66–75] have attempted to overcome this disadvantage by purging of the harvested product using chemotherapy agents, immunotoxins, monoclonal antibodies, and complement or immunomagnetic procedures to reduce the risk of tumor contamination. Other investigators[69–76,77] have attempted to induce an immunologic reaction similar to GVHD/GVL in an attempt to reduce the risk of relapse. Published reports[77–80] of autologous procedures for patients with ALL report a survival of 20%–50%, TRM of <10% and a 30%–70% rate of relapse. To date, no purging technique or immunologic intervention has been shown to offer a significant advantage.

Multiple retrospective reviews[81,82] have tried to compare outcomes for ABMT versus chemotherapy or other transplant procedures. To date, none have demonstrated an improved outcome over chemotherapy alone or other alternative donor procedures. More recently, there have been attempts to perform randomized studies comparing ABMT procedures to chemotherapy or other transplant modalities. None has been able to successfully complete a randomized trial due to significant bias by parents and investigators. In one recent attempt by the MRC[83] to look at a randomized trial of ABMT versus alternative donor transplant versus chemotherapy for patients in CR2 ALL, who did not have a matched sibling donor, only 9% of eligible patients were actually randomized. In this study, outcomes by actual treatment received did not differ significantly from those who received chemotherapy, autologous, MSD, or alternative donor procedures.[83]

Some authors have advocated a role for ABMT in specific subgroups of patients with ALL. For example, a study by Messina et al.[84] reported a five-year DFS for children with isolated CNS relapse of 56%, which they compare to a concurrent group of children treated with chemotherapy showing a 12.6% five-year DFS. Similarly, a study by Billett et al.[85] examined immunotoxin purging and found a DFS of 53% for patients with late relapses, defined as a CR1 >36 months. However, their group of patients would have very favorable outcomes with chemotherapy alone. More recently, several investigators have attempted to examine the use of autologous PBSC procedures as an intensification to be followed by additional chemotherapy. In this setting, Powles et al.[86] treated 50 adults and children with ALL in CR1. Patients received standard induction and chemotherapy intensification followed by melphalan and TBI, and autologous bone marrow infusion. Then they continued chemotherapy with methotrexate and 6MP for two years. The authors found a five-year DFS of 53%, which compared favorably to a similar group of patients receiving chemotherapy.[86]

At the time of this writing, the role of autologous procedures in children with ALL is unclear. Although it does offer some unique advantages over other types of transplants, the high relapse rates are concerning. As better methods of detection for minimal residual disease and a better understanding of the mechanism of the GVL effect are developed, it is possible that the very high risk of relapse after autologous procedures may decrease. At present, further clinical trials are necessary to define its role, and ABMT should only be performed within the context of clinical trials.

## Transplantation for Philadelphia Chromosome-Positive ALL

Philadelphia chromosome, t(9:22), positive ALL occurs in approximately 3%–5% of children with ALL. The translocation t(9:22) can result in a fusion protein of 210 kd when the *abl* protooncogene moves from chromosome 9 to the major breakpoint cluster region on chromosome 22. This fusion protein is seen most commonly in CML and is occasionally seen in Philadelphia-positive ALL. The *abl* gene also translocates to the minor breakpoint cluster region on chromosome 22, resulting in a 190 kd fusion protein that occurs exclusively in ALL. More than 90% of children with Philadelphia-positive ALL have this subtype of t(9:22). The presence of the Philadelphia chromosome is a poor prognostic feature.

Several recent publications have evaluated the outcome of transplantation for Philadelphia-positive ALL.[87–90] In the largest series, Aricò et al.[87] looked retrospectively at 326 patients with Philadelphia-positive ALL from multiple centers. One hundred twenty patients underwent transplant from a variety of stem cell sources including MSD, URD, MRT, and autologous stem cells, and 147 were treated with intensive chemotherapy. The five-year EFS was 28% for the group as a whole. Patients undergoing MSD transplant had a significantly improved EFS as compared to chemotherapy (65% vs. 25%); however, those with other donor sources showed no benefit over chemotherapy.

Currently, the Children's Oncology Group is planning a study of intensified chemotherapy for these very high risk patients, with the addition of Gleevac, a tyrosine kinase inhibitor that has been shown to be very effective in patients with CML. Transplant is recommended in CR1 for children with an MSD. Although there are currently no data to suggest a significant benefit to alternative donor transplant in this setting, for patients not eligible for specific very high risk chemotherapy studies, alternative donor transplant should be considered.

## Transplantation for Down's Syndrome Patients with ALL

Children with Down syndrome have a 15- to 20-fold increased risk of developing leukemia. The Children's Cancer Study Group[91] found 115 (2.1%) patients with Down syndrome out of a total of 5406 cases of ALL. The children with Down syndrome had a significantly lower remission rate (81% vs. 94%), a higher mortality rate during induction therapy (14% vs. 3%), and a poorer overall survival at five years (50% vs. 65%). If an initial CR was achieved, there was no significant difference in the remission duration, survival, or disease-free survival.

Transplantation in Down syndrome was initially felt to be associated with increased toxicity. More recent studies have shown that results of transplantation for Down syndrome are comparable to results seen in children without Down syndrome. Rubin et al.[92] reported on the largest series of children transplanted with Down syndrome. This report reviewed the results of 27 patients with Down syndrome who had undergone transplantation for the treatment of acute leukemia. Fourteen of the children had ALL and 13 had AML. Five children underwent autologous transplant and 22 had an allogeneic transplant. Sixteen patients had matched-sibling donor transplants, two had partially matched family member donors, and four had unrelated donors. Nine of the patients with ALL were transplanted in CR2 and five were in CR3. The conditioning regimen most commonly used was TBI and cytoxan. At three years, the relapse-free survival was 44% and overall survival was

48%. For the patients with ALL, 5 of 14 survive at the time of this report. The risk of death due to a non-leukemic cause was 39% at three years. A high frequency of airway and lung problems was noted in these patients. There was no statistically significant correlation between methotrexate and toxicity, but the authors[92] do suggest avoidance of methotrexate for GVHD prophylaxis in these patients.

In summary, the results for allogeneic transplant for Down syndrome children with ALL are not statistically different from results seen in non-Down syndrome children.

## Relapse After Allogeneic Transplantation: The Role of a Second Allogeneic Transplant

For children who undergo allogeneic transplantation, relapse of leukemia is a common cause of treatment failure. Patients who relapse posttransplant are at an extremely high risk of dying of their disease. A number of patients will enter a subsequent CR with chemotherapy, but the remissions will be of short duration. The International Bone Marrow Transplant Registry reviewed their experience with second transplants for leukemia. In their report, 114 patients who had an HLA-matched sibling donor transplant and relapsed underwent a second matched-sibling donor transplant. Twenty-nine patients had ALL, 46 had acute myeloid leukemia, and 39 chronic myelogenous leukemia. Treatment-related mortality was high, with an incidence of 41% at two years. Interstitial pneumonia and hepatic venoocclusive disease were much higher following a second transplant. The leukemia-free survival for all patients was 21% and the relapse rate was 65%. For patients who relapsed less than six months after their first transplant, leukemia-free survival was only 7% and treatment related mortality was 69%. For patients who relapsed more than six months posttransplant, the leukemia-free survival was 28%, with a relapse rate of 59%, and a treatment-related mortality of 30%. The best results were seen in patients who had a long remission after the first transplant and who were in remission at the time of the second transplant.[92]

Investigators at Johns Hopkins[94] reported on a series of 23 patients who underwent a second allogeneic transplant for treatment of relapsed leukemia. Four patients had ALL, 7 had AML, and 12 had chronic myelogenous leukemia. All patients had a matched-sibling donor transplant. The event-free survival at 26 months was 38% with a survival of 47%. One of the four children with ALL was a long-term survivor.

For patients who relapse after allo-BMT, a second allogeneic transplant can be considered if the patient is more than six months from the first transplant for pediatrics and more than one year for adults. The leukemia-free survival is 20%–30% in most series.

An alternative is the use of donor leukocyte infusions post-allogeneic transplantation to induce a remission in some patients with leukemia.[95] Although the majority of the patients who responded have had CML, one study saw a response in 4 of 13 patients with ALL.

Further work in this field may help us better understand the mechanisms by which donor leukocytes are able to induce remissions in patients with relapsed ALL post-BMT.

## SELECTION OF PATIENTS WITH ALL FOR TRANSPLANTATION

Treatment for pediatric ALL has continued to improve over the past decade and survival for all patients presenting with ALL now approaches 75%–80% long-term disease-free survival.

**TABLE 12.4**   Indications for Stem Cell Transplantation for ALL in Children

| Disease Status | Matched Sibling Donor | Unrelated Marrow or Cord Blood Donor |
|---|---|---|
| CR1, t(9;22) | Recommended, results with chemotherapy are poor | Controversial, treat with Gleevac or consider unrelated donor transplant if patient relapses or fails to enter cytogenetic remission |
| CR1, induction failure (>28 days to achieve remission) | Recommended, very high risk of relapse | Transplant in CR1 if suitable donor can be identified |
| CR2, with CR1 <36 months | Recommend transplantation, results are superior to chemotherapy | Recommend transplantation if suitable donor can be identified |
| CR2, with CR1 >36 months | Transplantation with matched sibling donor is superior to chemotherapy | Transplant may be considered, but, chemotherapy offers equivocal DFS with less toxicity |
| CR3 or > | Transplantation is recommended | Transplantation is recommended |
| Refractory disease | May consider transplantation, DFS is low | May consider transplantation if donor identified, DFS is low |

DFS = disease free survival.

Thus, most patients with ALL will not be candidates for transplantation. There is, however, a small subset of patients with very high risk ALL who should be considered for transplantation early in the course of their disease. These include children who have Philadelphia chromosome [t(9;22)]-positive ALL, or those patients with hypodiploidy (<44 chromosomes or DNA index <0.81) and children with ALL who fail to enter complete remission after induction therapy (▲ Table 12.4).

The majority of patients with ALL will only be candidates for transplantation if they relapse with their ALL. For patients with a short first remission, allogeneic transplantation is superior to chemotherapy and should be recommended to the patient and family. Children with a long first remission (>36 months) may not need a transplant in order to be cured. Analysis of data on patients treated with intensive chemotherapy in second remission who had a CR >36 months, has shown a survival of 40%–50% long term, which compares favorably with most studies on allogeneic transplantation. If a patient who had a long first remission has an HLA identical sibling, transplantation may be considered. In this situation, a frank discussion of the risks and benefits of transplantation versus chemotherapy should occur with the family. Whether alternate donor transplantation for a patient with a long first remission ALL is associated with improved long-term survival compared to chemotherapy alone is unclear. All patients with a second relapse need to be considered for allogeneic transplantation regardless of length of first or second remission.

Isolated extramedullary relapse (CNS or testicular) is not an automatic indication for transplant. Excellent results with intensive chemotherapy and delayed cranial radiation for CNS relapse have been achieved with a DFS of 67% at three years. Similarly, excellent results have been achieved in testicular relapse with chemotherapy and radiation therapy to the testes. If CNS relapse occurs early in the course of therapy and an HLA identical sibling is available, then transplantation should be considered in selected cases.

# REFERENCES

1. Poplack D. Acute lymphocytic leukemia. In: Pizzo PA, Poplack D (eds). Principles and Practice of Pediatric Oncology (2nd ed). New York: Lippincott, 1993;431–481.
2. Thomas ED, Storb R, Clift RA et al. Bone marrow transplantation (first of two parts). N Engl J Med 1975;292:832–843.
3. Graw RG, Yankee RA, Rogentine GN et al. Bone marrow transplantation from HLA-matched donors to patients with leukemia: toxicity and antileukemic effects. Transplantation 1972;14:79–90.
4. Santos GW, Sensenbrenner LL, Burke PJ et al. Marrow transplantation in man following cyclophosphamide Transplant Proc 1971;3:400–404.
5. Brochstein JA, Kernan NA, Groshen S et al. Allogeneic bone marrow transplantation after hyperfractionated total-body irradiation and cyclophosphamide in children with acute leukemia. N Engl J Med 1987;317:1618–1624.
6. Cole CA, Rogers PCJ, Davis JE et al. Intensive conditioning regimen for bone marrow transplantation in children with high risk hematological disorders. Med Pediatr Oncol 1994;23:464–469.
7. Moussalem M, Bourdeau H, Devergie A et al. Allogeneic bone marrow transplantation for childhood acute lymphocytic leukemia in second remission: factors predictive of survival, relapse and graft versus host disease. Bone Marrow Transplant 1995;15:943–947.
8. Duerst RE, Horan JT, Liesveld JL et al. Allogeneic bone marrow transplantation for children with acute leukemia: cytoreduction with fractionated total body radiation, high-dose etoposide and cyclophosphamide. Bone Marrow Transplant 2000;25:489–494.
9. Pirich L, Haut P, Morgan E et al. Total body irradiation, cyclophosphamide, and etoposide with stem cell transplant as treatment for infants with acute lymphocytic leukemia. Med Pediatr Oncol 1999;32:1–6.
10. Kamani N, Bayever E, August C et al. Fractionated total-body irradiation preceding high-dose cytosine arabinoside as a preparative regimen for bone marrow transplantation in children with acute leukemia. Med Pediatr Oncol 1995;25:179–184.
11. Weyman C, Graham-Pole J, Emerson S et al. Use of cytosine arabinoside and total body irradiation as conditioning for allogeneic marrow transplantation in patients with acute lymphoblastic leukemia: a multicenter survey. Bone Marrow Transplant 1993;11:43–50.
12. Conter V, D'Angelo P, Rizzari C et al. High dose cytosine arabinoside and fractionated total body irradiation as a preparative regimen for the treatment of children with acute lymphoblastic leukemia and Down syndrome by allogeneic bone marrow transplantation. Bone Marrow Transplant 1996;17:287–289.
13. Weisdorf DJ, Woods WG, Nesbit ME et al. Allogeneic bone marrow transplantation for childhood acute lymphoblastic leukemia: risk factors and clinical outcome. Br J Haematol 1994;86:62–69.
14. Mousssalem M, Esperou Bourdeau H, Devergie A et al. Allogeneic bone marrow transplantation for childhood acute lymphocytic leukemia in second remission: factors predictive of survival, relapse and graft-versus-host disease. Bone Marrow Transplant 1995;15:943–947.
15. Von Bueltzingsloewen A, Belanger R, Perreault C et al. Allogeneic bone marrow transplantation following busulfan-cyclophosphamide with or without etoposide conditioning regimen for patients with acute lymphocytic leukemia. Br J Hematol 1993;85:706–713.
16. Ringden O, Ruutu T, Remberger M et al. A randomized trial comparing busulfan with total body irradiation as conditioning in allogeneic marrow transplant recipients with leukemia: A report from the Nordic Bone Marrow Transplant Group. Blood 1995;83:2723–2730.
17. Davies SM, Ramsay NKC, Klein JP et al. Comparison of preparative regimens in transplants for children with acute lymphoblastic leukemia. J Clin Oncol 2000;18:340–347.
18. Barrett J, Horowitz M, Pollack BH et al. Bone marrow transplants from HLA-identical siblings as compared with chemotherapy for children with acute lymphocytic leukemia in a second remission. N Engl J Med 1994;331:1253–1258.
19. Torres A, Martinez F, Gomez P et al. Allogeneic bone marrow transplantation versus chemotherapy in the treatment of childhood acute lymphocytic leukemia in second remission. Bone Marrow Transplant 1989;4:609–612.
20. Feig S, Harris R, Sather HN. Bone marrow transplantation versus chemotherapy for maintenance of second remission of childhood acute lymphocytic leukemia: a study of the Children's Cancer Group (CCG-1884). Med Pediatr Oncol 1997;29:534–540.
21. Boulad F, Steinhertz P, Reyes B et al. Allogeneic bone marrow transplantation versus chemotherapy for the treatment of childhood acute lymphocytic leukemia in second remission: a single institution study. J Clin Oncol 1999;17:197–207.
22. Bordigoni P, Vernant JP, Souillet G et al. Allogeneic bone marrow transplantation for children with acute lymphocytic leukemia in first remission: a cooperative study of the Groupe d'Etude de la Greffe de Moiele Osseuse. J Clin Oncol 1989;7:747–753.
23. Chessels JM, Bailey J, Wheeler K et al. Bone marrow transplantation for high-risk childhood lymphoblastic leukemia in first remission: experience in MRC UKALL X. Lancet 1992;340:565–568.

24. Uderzo C, Vasecchi MG, Balduzzi A et al. Allogeneic bone marrow transplantation versus chemotherapy in high-risk childhood acute lymphoblastic leukemia in first remission. Associazion Italiana de Ematologia ed Oncologia Pediatrica (AIEOP) and the Gruppo Italiano Trapianto de Midollo Osseo (GITMO). Br J Haematol 1997;96:387–394.

25. Borgmann A, Baumgarten E, Schmid H et al. Allogeneic bone marrow transplantation for a subset of children with acute lymphocytic leukemia in third remission: a conceivable alternative? Bone Marrow Transplant 1997;20:939–944.

26. Davies SM, Wagner JE, Shu XO et al. Unrelated donor bone marrow transplantation for children with acute leukemia. J Clin Oncol 1997;15:557–565.

27. Rocha V, Cornish J, Sievers EL et al. Comparison of outcomes of unrelated bone marrow and umbilical cord blood transplants in children with acute leukemia. Blood 2001;97:2962–2971.

28. Balduzzi A, Gooley T, Anasetti C et al. Unrelated donor marrow transplantation in children. Blood 1995;86:3247–3256.

29. Geller RB, Devine SM, O'Toole K et al. Allogeneic bone marrow transplantation with matched unrelated donor for patients with hematologic malignancies using a preparative regimen of high-dose cyclophosphamide and fractioned total body irradiation. Bone Marrow Transplant 1997;20:219–225.

30. A consensus statement on unrelated donor bone marrow transplantation from Consensus Panel chaired by ED Gordon Smith. Bone Marrow Transplant 1997;19:959–962.

31. Beatty PG, Hansen JA, Longton GM et al. Marrow transplantation from HLA-matched unrelated donors for treatment of hematologic malignancies. Transplantation 1991;51:443–447.

32. Anasetti C, Howe C, Petersdorf EW et al. Marrow transplants from HLA matched unrelated donors: an NMDP update and the Seattle experience. Bone Marrow Transplant 1994;13:693–695.

33. Bunin N, Carston M, Wall D et al. Unrelated marrow transplantation for children with acute lymphoblastic leukemia in second remission. Blood 2002;99:3151–3157.

34. Woolfrey AE, Anasetti C, Storer B et al. Factors associated with outcome after unrelated marrow transplantation for treatment of acute lymphoblastic leukemia in children. Blood 2002;99:2002–2008.

35. Cornelissen JJ, Carston M, Kollman C et al. Unrelated marrow transplantation for adult patients with poor-risk acute lymphoblastic leukemia: strong graft-versus-leukemia effect and risk factors determining outcome. Blood 2001;97:1572–1577.

36. Dini G, Lanino E, Lamparelli T et al. Unrelated donor marrow transplantation: initial experience of the Italian Bone Marrow Transplant Group (GITMO). Bone Marrow Transplant 1996;17:55–62.

37. Downie TR, Hows JM, Gore SM et al. A survey of use of unrelated volunteer donor bone marrow transplantation at 46 centres worldwide, 1989–93. Bone Marrow Transplant 1995;15:499–503.

38. Uderzo C, Dini G, Locatelli F et al. Treatment of childhood acute lymphoblastic leukemia after the first relapse: curative strategies. Haematologica 2000;85(Suppl. 11):47–53.

39. Kollman C, Howe CWS, Anasetti C et al. Donor characteristics as risk factors in recipients after transplantation of bone marrow from unrelated donors: the effect of donor age. Blood 2001;98:2043–2051.

40. Davies SM, Shu XO, Blazar BR et al. Unrelated donor bone marrow transplantation: Influence of HLA A and B incompatibility on outcome. Blood 1995;86:1636–1642.

41. Sasazuki T, Juji T, Morishima Y et al. Effect of matching of Class I HLA alleles on clinical outcome after transplantation of hematopoietic stem cells from an unrelated donor. N Engl J Med 1998;339:1177–1185.

42. Davies SM, Kollman C, Anasetti C et al. Engraftment and survival after unrelated-donor bone marrow transplantation: a report from the National Marrow Donor Program. Blood 2000;96:4096–4102.

43. Sierra J, Storer B, Hansen JA et al. Transplantation of marrow cells from unrelated donors for treatment of high-risk acute leukemia: The effect of leukemic burden, donor HLA-matching, and marrow cell dose. Blood 1997;89:4226–4235.

44. Casper J, Camitta B, Truitt R et al. Unrelated bone marrow donor transplants for children with leukemia or myelodysplasia. Blood 1995;85:2354–2363.

45. Petersdorf EW, Gooley TA, Anasetti C et al. Optimizing outcome after unrelated marrow transplantation by comprehensive matching of HLA class I and II alleles in the donor and recipient. Blood 1998;92:3515–3520.

46. Hongeng S, Krance RA, Bowman LC et al. Outcomes of transplantation with matched-sibling and unrelated-donor bone marrow in children with leukemia. Lancet 1997;350:767–771.

47. Saarinen-Pihkala UM, Goran G, Ringden O et al. No disadvantage in outcome of using matched unrelated donors as compared with matched sibling donors for bone marrow transplantation in children with acute lymphoblastic leukemia in second remission. J Clin Oncol 2001;19:3406–3414.

48. Remberger M, Ringden O, Blau I-W et al. No difference in graft-versus-host disease, relapse, and survival comparing peripheral stem cells to bone marrow using unrelated donors. Blood 2001;98:1739–1745.

49. Wagner J, Rosenthal J, Sweetman R et al. Successful transplantation of HLA-matched and HLA-mismatched umbilical cord blood from unrelated donors: analysis of engraftment and acute graft-versus-host-disease. Blood 1996;88:795–802.

50. Rubenstein P, Carrier C, Scaradavou A et al. Outcomes among 562 recipients of placental blood transplants from unrelated donors. N Engl J Med 1998;339:1565–1577.

51. Kurtzberg J, Laughlin M, Graham M et al. Placental blood as a source of hematopoietic stem cells for transplantation into unrelated recipients. N Engl J Med 1996;335:157–166.
52. Barker J, Davies S, DeFor T et al. Survival after transplantation of unrelated donor umbilical chord blood is comparable to that of human leukocyte antigen-matched unrelated donor bone marrow: results of a matched-pair antigen. Blood 2001;97:2957–2961.
53. Beelen DW, Ottinger HD, Elmaagacli A et al. Transplantation of filgrastim-mobilized peripheral blood stem cells from HLA-identical sibling or alternative family donors in patients with hematologic malignancies: A prospective comparison on clinical outcome, immune reconstitution, and hematopoietic chimerism. Blood 1997;90:4725–4735.
54. Henslee-Downey PJ, Abhyankar SH, Parrish RS et al. Use of partially mismatched related donors extends access to allogeneic marrow transplant. Blood 1997;89:3864–3872.
55. Munn RK, Henslee-Downey PJ, Romond EH et al. Treatment of leukemia with partially matched related bone marrow transplantation. Bone Marrow Transplant 1997;19:421–427.
56. Fleming DR, Henslee-Downey PJ, Romond EH et al. Allogeneic bone marrow transplantation with T cell-depleted partially matched related donors for advanced acute lymphoblastic leukemia in children and adults: a comparative matched cohort study. Bone Marrow Transplant 1996;17:917–922.
57. Aversa F, Tabilio A, Velardi A et al. Treatment of high-risk acute leukemia with T-cell-depleted stem cells from related donors with one fully mismatched HLA haplotype. N Engl J Med 1998;339:1186–1193.
58. Green A, Clarke E, Hunt L et al. Children with acute lymphoblastic leukemia who receive T-cell-depleted HLA mismatched marrow allografts from unrelated donors have an increased incidence of primary graft failure but a similar overall transplant outcome. Blood 1999;94:2236–2246.
59. Ash RC, Horowitz MM, Gale RP et al. Bone marrow transplantation from related donors other than HLA-identical siblings: effect of T cell depletion. Bone Marrow Transplant 1991;7:443–452.
60. Szydlo R, Goldman JM, Klein JP et al. Results of allogeneic bone marrow transplants for leukemia using donors other than HLA-identical siblings. J Clin Oncol 1997;15:1767–1777.
61. Beatty PG, Clift RA, Mickelson EM et al. Marrow transplantation from related donors other than HLA-identical siblings. N Engl J Med 1985;313:765–771.
62. Van Rood JJ, Loberiza MJZ Jr, Oudshoorn M et al. Effect of tolerance to noninherited maternal antigens on the occurrence of graft-versus-host disease after bone marrow transplantation from a parent or an HLA-haploidentical sibling. Blood 2002;99:1572–1577.
63. Godder KT, Hazlett LJ, Abhyankar SH et al. Partially mismatched related-donor bone marrow transplantation for pediatric patients with acute leukemia: Younger donors and absence of peripheral blasts improve outcome. J Clin Oncol 2000;18:1856–1866.
64. Drobyski WR, Klein J, Flomenberg N et al. Superior survival associated with transplantation of matched unrelated versus one-antigen–mismatched unrelated or highly human leukocyte antigen-disparate haploidentical family donor marrow grafts for the treatment of hematologic malignancies: establishing a treatment algorithm for recipients of alternative donor grafts. Blood 2002;99:806–814.
65. The Medical Advisory Panel of the Blue Cross and Blue Shield Association Technology Evaluation Center. High-dose chemotherapy with autologous stem-cell support for treatment of adult acute lymphoblastic leukemia. Cancer Therapeutics 1998;1:244–254.
66. Canals C, Torrico C, Picon M et al. Immunomagnetic bone marrow purging in children with acute lymphoblastic leukemia. J Hematother 1997;6:261–268.
67. Gonzalez-Chambers R, Przepiorka D, Shadduck RK et al. Autologous bone marrow transplantation with 4-hydroperoxycyclophosphamide-purged marrow for acute lymphoblastic leukemia. Med Pediatr Oncol 1991;19:160–164.
68. Verdonck LF, Witteveen EO, van Heugten HG et al. Selective killing of malignant cells from leukemic patients by alkyl-lysophospholipid. Cancer Res 1990;50:4020–4025.
69. Preijers FWMB, DeWitte T, Wessels JMC et al. Autologous transplantation of bone marrow purged in vitro with Anti-CD7-(WT1-) Ricin A immunotoxin in T-cell lymphoblastic leukemia and lymphoma. Blood 1989;74:1152–1158.
70. Rowley SD, Miller CB, Piantadosi S et al. Phase I study of combination drug purging for autologous bone marrow transplantation. J Clin Oncol 1991;9:2210–2218.
71. Stoppa AM, Hirn J, Blaise D et al. Autologous bone marrow transplantation for B cell malignancies after in vitro purging with floating immunobeads. Bone Marrow Transplant 1190;6:301–307.
72. Morishima Y, Miyamura K, Kojima S et al. Autologous BMT in high risk patients with CALLA-positive ALL: possible efficacy of ex vivo marrow leukemia cell purging with monoclonal antibodies and complement. Bone Marrow Transplant 1993;11:255–259.
73. Gress RE. Purged autologous bone marrow transplantation in the treatment of acute leukemia. Oncology 1990;4:35–40.
74. Gilmore MJML, Hamon MD, Prentice HG et al. Failure of purged autologous bone marrow transplantation in high risk acute lymphoblastic leukemia in first complete remission. Bone Marrow Transplant 1991;8:19–26.

75. Freedman AS, Nadler LM: Developments in purging in autotransplantation. Autologous bone marrow transplantation. Hematol Oncol Clin North Am 1993;7:687–715.
76. Lopez-Jimenez J, Perez-Oteyza J, Munoz A et al. Subcutaneous versus intravenous low-dose IL-2 therapy after autologous transplantation: results of a prospective, non-randomized study. Bone Marrow Transplant 1997;19:429–434.
77. Robinson N, Benyunes MC, Thompson JA et al. Interleukin-2 after autologous stem cell transplantation for hematologic malignancy: a phase I/II study. Bone Marrow Transplant 1997;19:435–442.
78. Sierra J, Granena A, Garcia J et al. Autologous bone marrow transplantation for acute leukemia: results and prognostic factors in 90 consecutive patients. Bone Marrow Transplant 1993;12:517–523.
79. Sallan SE, Niemeyer CM, Billett AL et al. Autologous bone marrow transplantation for acute lymphoblastic leukemia. J Clin Oncol 1989;7:1594–1601.
80. Ringden O, Labopin M, Gluckman E et al. Donor search or autografting in patients with acute leukemia who lack an HLA-identical sibling? A matched-pair analysis. Acute Leukaemia Working Party of the European Cooperative Group for Blood and Marrow Transplantation (EBMT) and the International Marrow Unrelated Search and Transplantation (IMUST) Study. Bone Marrow Transplant 1997;19:963–968.
81. Weisdorf D, Bishop M, Dharan B et al. Autologous versus allogeneic unrelated donor transplantation for acute lymphoblastic leukemia: comparative toxicity and outcomes. Biol Blood Marrow Transplant 2002;8:213–220.
82. Herve P, Labopin M, Plouvier E et al. Autologous bone marrow transplantation for childhood acute lymphoblastic leukemia—a European survey. Bone Marrow Transplant 1991;8(Suppl 1):72–75.
83. Lawson SE, Harrison G, Richards S et al. The UK experience in treating relapsed childhood acute lymphoblastic leukaemia: a report on the Medical Research Council UKALLR1 study. Br J Haematol 2000;108:531–543.
84. Messina C, Valsecchi MG, Aricò M et al. Autologous bone marrow transplantation for treatment of isolated central nervous system relapse of childhood acute lymphoblastic leukemia. Bone Marrow Transplant 1998;21:9–14.
85. Billett AL, Kornmehl E, Tarbell NJ et al. Autologous bone marrow transplantation after a long first remission for children with recurrent acute lymphoblastic leukemia. Blood 1993;81:1651–1657.
86. Powles R, Mehta J, Singhal S et al. Autologous bone marrow or peripheral blood stem cell transplantation followed by maintenance chemotherapy for adult acute lymphoblastic leukemia in first remission: 50 cases from a single center. Bone Marrow Transplant 1995;16:241–247.
87. Aricò M, Valsecchi MG, Camitta B et al. Outcome of treatment in children with Philadelphia chromosome-positive acute lymphoblastic leukemia. N Engl J Med 2000;342:998–1006.
88. Mori T, Manabe A, Masahiro T et al. Allogeneic bone marrow transplantation in first remission rescues children with Philadelphia chromosome-positive acute lymphoblastic leukemia: Tokyo Children's Cancer Study Group (TCCSG) Studies L89-12 and L92-13. Med Pediatr Oncol 2001;37:426–431.
89. Sierra J, Radich J, Hansen JA et al. Marrow transplantation from unrelated donors for treatment of Philadelphia chromosome-positive acute lymphoblastic leukemia. Blood 1997;90:1410–1414.
90. Marks DI, Bird JM, Cornish JM et al. Unrelated donor bone marrow transplantation for children and adolescents with Philadelphia-positive acute lymphoblastic leukemia. J Clin Oncol 1998;16:931–936.
91. Robison LL, Nesbit ME, Sather HN et al. Down syndrome and acute leukemia in children: a 10-year retrospective survey from Children's Cancer Study Group. J Pediatr 1984;105:235–242.
92. Rubin CM, Mick R, Johnson FL. Bone marrow transplantation for the treatment of haematological disorders in Down's syndrome: toxicity and outcome. Bone Marrow Transplant 1996;18:533–540.
93. Mrsic M, Horowitz MM, Atkinson JC et al. Second HLA-identical sibling transplants for leukemia recurrence. Bone Marrow Transplant 1992;9:269–275.
94. Wagner JE, Vogelsang GB, Zehnbauer BA et al. Relapse of leukemia after bone marrow transplantation: effect of second myeloablative therapy. Bone Marrow Transplant 1992;9:205–209.
95. Giralt SA, Champlin RE. Leukemia relapse after allogeneic bone marrow transplantation: a review. Blood 1994;84:3603–3612.

# CHAPTER *XIII*

# Stem Cell Transplantation for Patients with Acute Myelogenous Leukemia

SUNEETHA CHALLAGUNDLA AND PAULETTE MEHTA

## ACUTE MYELOGENOUS LEUKEMIA

Acute myelogenous leukemia is one of the more uncommon and challenging childhood cancers. Bone marrow transplantation has been used to treat children with acute myelogenous leukemia since the 1970s when physicians experimented with allogeneic, and then autologous, stem cell transplantation for patients with acute myelogenous leukemia.[1–10] Numerous studies have shown the benefits of early stem cell transplantation for acute myelogenous leukemia; this remains the treatment of choice for most children with acute myelogenous leukemia who are fortunate enough to have a matched sibling donor.

Meanwhile, improvements in supportive care have been made such that children who receive chemotherapy may have results that are as good as those with a matched sibling receiving allogeneic stem cell transplantation, and significantly better than those without a sibling matched donor. Autologous stem cell transplantation, once of great interest in patients without sibling donors, has lost favor as supportive care has improved, thereby improving results with chemotherapy alone. It has also lost favor as alternate donors (especially umbilical cord blood donors) have become more available and results have improved, as purging has shown itself to be less effective than initially thought and, as our understanding of graft-versus-leukemia has evolved from one of high-dose killing to one of immunotherapy from ablative dose chemotherapy.[11] All of these factors now make allogeneic transplantation more attractive than autologous transplantation in the proper settings. This chapter will discuss the steps in the evolution of these ideas, conclusions of trials, and future directions.

## DIFFICULTIES IN THE INTERPRETATION OF STUDIES

Interpretation of studies of allogeneic and of autologous bone marrow transplantation in children with acute myelogenous leukemia is fraught with difficulties. First, acute myelogenous leukemia is a heterogeneous disease; yet the heterogeneities have not been well enough understood to separate out the diseases within acute myelogenous leukemia.[12–21] Thus, although stem cell transplantation may be preferable for some types of acute myelogenous leukemia, it may not be preferable for all types of acute myelogenous leukemia. In particular, some good prognosis types of acute myelogenous leukemia have been identified, and patients with these types of acute myelogenous leukemia do well with conventional chemotherapy. Patients with M4-eos do particularly well with conventional therapy, and patients with acute promyelocytic leukemia (APML) do better with retinoic acid-based therapy. Other heterogeneities include patients who develop acute myelogenous leukemia in association with Down syndrome (whether homozygous or mosaic); these patients have a better outcome with chemotherapy than do other patients because of their exquisite sensitivity to chemotherapy.[18,22] In contrast, patients with treatment-related acute myelogenous leukemia have a dismal prognosis regardless of therapy.[23]

An important way in which prognosis can be predicted is by the day-14 and day-28 bone marrow response to treatment.[24] Those patients who respond quickly to therapy have a distinctly good prognosis and these may be the ones preferentially selected for stem cell transplantation, thus biasing results away from non-stem cell transplantation arms.

## Impact of an Induction and Conditioning Regimen Prior to the Bone Marrow Transplant

Another important difficulty in evaluating data is that even before the stem cell transplantation begins and before patients have been transferred to a stem cell transplantation center, the induction therapy and consolidation therapy are variable. It may be the induction therapy that is more important than subsequent therapy in the final outcome of the patient.

### Induction Therapy

A confounding factor in all of the stem cell transplantation studies is that the induction therapies may be variable, and in acute myelogenous leukemia induction therapy may be as important or more important than consolidation or maintenance therapy. Woods et al.[25] showed evidence that, regardless of the stem cell transplantation regimen used, induction therapy remained the most important factor in ultimate outcome of patients. In CCG 2891 study, patients were randomized at diagnosis to one of two induction approaches involving a four day cycle of five active chemotherapy drugs, with the second cycle administered either ten days after the first (regardless of counts, i.e., "intensive timing" regimen) compared to receiving the second and subsequent cycles 14 days or later depending on the bone marrow status (i.e., "standard timing regimen"). All of the patients were then allocated to allogeneic stem cell transplantation if there was a matched family donor, or to aggressive chemotherapy followed by autologous purged stem cell transplantation rescue if not. There was a marked improvement in outcome for patients randomized to the intensive timing arm with an actuarial event-free survival of three years of 42% versus 27% for those on the standard timing arm. This improvement in results for patients treated on the intensively timed arm remained similar regardless of whether they received a subsequent allogeneic or autologous stem cell transplantation.

### Conditioning Regimen

Another theoretical reason for the differences could be the conditioning regimen, although this has received less attention than would be expected. The original regimen developed by the group at the Fred Hutchinson Cancer Center has proven to be at least as effective as every successor-conditioning regimen studied, although some of the successors may offer lower long-term toxicities than the original protocol.[5,7,26–28] The rationale for these regimens was based on "ablating" bone marrow disease through myeloablative therapy combined with immunosuppressive therapy to "make room for new marrow," allow graft cells to engraft, and prevent the graft from overtaking the host (graft-versus-host disease).

A second generation of conditioning regimens has developed in order to decrease long-term toxicities from the original high-dose myeloablative–total body irradiation effects.[29–31] Newer regimens have tended to have less, or fractionated, radiation therapy containing regimens compared to the earlier ones. Fractionation and hyperfractionation of radiation therapy have resulted in the use of higher doses than otherwise possible, with less toxicity. Increasing the intervals of radiation therapy allows for recovery of normal cells, thereby lowering the long-term effects. In this sense, hyperfractionation may allow for better outcomes in some of the stem cell transplantation regimens, although this has been mentioned only rarely as a variable in conditioning regimens.

One of the major changes in the second generation conditioning regimens has been the substitution of total body irradiation for busulfan.[27,32–35] Busulfan, however, is difficult to use because in its oral form it is not always well tolerated. Moreover, it is subject to variations in absorption, distribution and metabolism. Very young patients have a higher metabolic clearance of busulfan and require higher doses than do older children or adults. Measurements of serum busulfan concentrations are not always possible.[34] The availability of an intravenous form of busulfan has greatly improved the ability to use busulfan as a substitute for total body irradiation, although monitoring of levels is still recommended. Individualized dose adjustment is critical, especially for younger children, since high concentrations predispose to venoocclusive disease and low concentrations to nonengraftment. The early toxicity of seizures after busulfan can be largely averted through the use of prophylactic anticonvulsant therapy.

A newer, third generation of conditioning regimens has been conceived based on the modern paradigm of stem cell transplantation as immunological therapy rather than myeloablative therapy.[11,36] This paradigm exploits graft-versus-host (and thereby graft-versus-leukemia) by decreasing the amount of graft-versus-host disease prophylaxis and by immunological, rather than myeloablative, conditioning. These regimens are generally better tolerated and can be used more easily in the patient who may not tolerate myeloablative doses of chemotherapy, or in otherwise frail patients. Whether these nonmyeloablative regimens will offer the same long-term results as the myeloablative regimens is not yet known.

## Randomization by Biology

A final potential difficulty in interpretation is that no patient is randomized purely by chance to either the stem cell transplantation or non-stem cell transplantation arm. Rather, the concept of biological randomization has become standard practice in stem cell transplantation studies. Thus, patients having a sibling donor are preferentially randomized to stem cell transplantation, whereas those without sibling donors are randomized to non-stem cell or to autologous transplantation. There is no reason to believe that this intrinsic bias in randomization results in any bias in interpretation of studies, and there appears to be no ethical way around this type of randomization.

## IMPACT OF THE STEM CELL CENTER

An interesting factor in determining prognosis of patients is the actual center in which the transplant is being performed. Frassoni et al.[37] studied outcome of allogeneic bone marrow transplantation patients treated at different European centers. Patients who did worse were characterized by the following associations: over 45 years of age; time from first diagnosis to first complete remission longer than 54 days; and specific center at which bone marrow transplantation was being done ($P < .013$). Thus, the outcome of bone marrow transplantation for acute myeloid leukemia in complete remission is influenced more by the center in which the procedure is done, than by most other factors.[37] The greater the number of patients treated in a particular center, the more expertise develops in that center. Moreover, the longer the group has been together, the better the expertise.

## ALLOGENIC BONE MARROW TRANSPLANTATION STUDIES FOR CHILDREN WITH ACUTE MYELOGENOUS LEUKEMIA

### Early Studies

The first stem cell transplantation studies of patients with acute myelogenous leukemia and high dose chemotherapy were done at the University of Washington and showed complete remission rates of up to 86%.[4-7,10,32] An updated report in 1977 indicated that six of the early patients remained alive and disease-free for up to four to six years later. Subsequently, these same investigators reported on 34 patients with refractory leukemia who had received stem cell transplantations from identical twins. Seventy percent of these patients achieved a complete remission and 24% were alive and disease-free 80 months after stem cell transplantation.

### Randomized Controlled Trials and Meta-Analysis

Recently, Bleakley et al. evaluated all of the reported studies on allogeneic stem cell transplantation and performed a meta-analysis for those studies that met the following criteria: performed during 1985 through 2000; patients under 21 years of age; studies including an intent-to-treat analysis; and studies including sufficient data to determine the quality of study.[38] Using these criteria, the investigators evaluated six studies (▶ Figure 13.1).

In each of these studies, patients treated on the stem cell transplantation arms did better than those who were treated with chemotherapy alone. The study done by the Pediatric Oncology Group (POG 8821) showed a statistically significant lower rate of relapses for patients undergoing stem cell transplantation. In the Medical Research Council study, (MRC AML 10), patients who underwent stem cell transplantation had improved disease free survival; similarly, in the study by the Children's Cancer Group (CCG213/22) overall survival was higher in patients who underwent stem cell transplantation compared to those who did not.

The single best predictor for those who will do well after bone marrow transplantation is the length of duration of the prior remission. In the MRC AML 10 trial, the length of first remission was shown to be the most important factor affecting response rates. Children with a first remission of less than one year did poorly whereas those with longer first remissions did better.[21] Another predictor for patients who do well compared to those who do

**Comparison:** 01 Relapse
**Outcome:** 01 event = relapse

| Study | Treatment n/N | Control/ n/N | RR (95% CI Random) | Weight % | RR (95% CI Random) |
|---|---|---|---|---|---|
| AEIOP LAM 87 (9) | 11 / 24 | 71 / 103 | | 20.3 | 0.66 (0.42, 1.05) |
| CCG 2891 (11, 12) | 32 / 181 | 128 / 356 | | 35.4 | 0.49 (0.35, 0.69) |
| LAME 89/91 (24) | 9 / 33 | 55 / 116 | | 12.0 | 0.58 (0.32, 1.04) |
| MRC AML 10 (13) | 22 / 74 | 96 / 214 | | 28.8 | 0.66 (0.45, 0.97) |
| RAHC (23) | 3 / 10 | 8 / 21 | | 3.5 | 0.79 (0.26, 2.35) |
| Total (95% CI) | 77 / 322 | 358 / 810 | | 100.0 | 0.59 (0.48, 0.72) |

Test for heterogeneity chi square = 2.02, df = 4, $P$ = 73
Test for overall effect z = –5.06, $P$ = 0.00001

0.1   0.2           1           5   10
Favors treatment        Favors control

**Comparison:** 02 Relapse or death
**Outcome:** 01 event = death or relapse

| Study | MSD n/N | No donor n/N | RR (95% CI Random) | Weight % | RR (95% CI Random) |
|---|---|---|---|---|---|
| AEIOP LAM 87 (9) | 12 / 24 | 75 / 103 | | 14.5 | 0.69 (0.45, 1.04) |
| CCG 213 (22) | 61 /113 | 185 / 298 | | 28.5 | 0.87 (0.72, 1.05) |
| CCG 2891 (11, 12) | 42 / 140 | 171 / 310 | | 22.6 | 0.54 (0.41, 0.71) |
| LAME 89/91 (24) | 9 / 33 | 60 / 116 | | 9.1 | 0.53 (0.29, 0.95) |
| MRC AML 10 (13) | 33 / 85 | 114 / 230 | | 20.9 | 0.78 (0.58, 1.05) |
| RAHC (23) | 4 / 11 | 10 / 23 | | 4.3 | 0.84 (0.34, 2.08) |
| Total (95% CI) | 161 / 406 | 615 / 1080 | | 100.0 | 0.71 (0.58, 0.86) |

Test for heterogeneity chi square = 9.66, df = 5, $P$ = 0.085
Test for overall effect z = –3.40, $P$ = 0.00007

0.1   0.2           1           5   10
Favors treatment        Favors control

**Comparison:** 03 Death
**Outcome:** 01 event = death

| Study | MSD n/N | Donor n/N | RR (95% CI Random) | Weight % | RR (95% CI Random) |
|---|---|---|---|---|---|
| CCG 213 (22) | 54 / 113 | 161 / 298 | | 35.6 | 0.88 (0.71, 1.10) |
| CCG 2891 (11, 12) | 34 / 140 | 150 / 310 | | 30.8 | 0.50 (0.37, 0.69) |
| MRC AML 10 (13) | 25 / 85 | 91 / 230 | | 28.1 | 0.74 (0.52, 1.07) |
| RAHC (23) | 2 / 11 | 10 / 23 | | 5.6 | 0.42 (0.11, 1.59) |
| Total (95% CI) | 115 / 349 | 412 / 861 | | 100.0 | 0.71 (0.58, 0.95) |

Test for heterogeneity chi square = 9.51, df = 5, $P$ = 0.023
Test for overall effect z = –2.24, $P$ = 0.02

0.1   0.2           1           5   10
Favors treatment        Favors control

**Comparison:** 04 Treatment-related morbidity
**Outcome:** 01 event = rreatment-related death

| Study | MSD n/N | No donor n/N | RR (95% CI Random) | Weight % | RR (95% CI Random) |
|---|---|---|---|---|---|
| AEIOP LAM 87 (9) | 0 / 24 | 9 / 103 | | 9.0 | 0.22 (0.01, 3.64) |
| CCG 2891 (11, 12) | 0 / 181 | 3 / 356 | | 8.2 | 0.28 (0.01, 5.40) |
| LAME 89/91 (24) | 1 / 33 | 8 / 116 | | 15.6 | 0.44 (0.06, 3.39) |
| MRC AML 10 (13) | 11 / 74 | 16 / 230 | | 54.3 | 1.86 (0.90, 3.85) |
| RAHC (23) | 1 / 11 | 2 / 23 | | 12.9 | 1.05 (0.11, 10.33) |
| Total (95% CI) | 13 / 334 | 38 / 828 | | 100.0 | 0.97 (0.40, 2.38) |

Test for heterogeneity chi square = 5.05, df = 5, $P$ = 0.28
Test for overall effect z = –0.06, $P$ = 1

0.1   0.2           1           5   10
Favors treatment        Favors control

Abbreviations: AEIOP LAM 87 5 Associazione Italiana Ematologia Ed Oncologia Pediatrica/Leucemia Acuta Mieloide #87;[39] CCG 2891 5 Children's Cancer Group protocol #2891;[22,40,41] LAME 89/91 5 Leucamie Aique Myeloide Enfant 89/91 study;[42] MRC 5 Medical Research Council study on acute myelogenous leukemia (AML) 10;[43] CCG 213/22 5 Children's Cancer Group protocol #213/22;[45] BMT 5 bone marrow transplantation; RR 5 relative risk; CI 5 confidence interval; df 5 degrees of freedom. Reproduced with permission from Nature Publishing Group-NPG and Bleakley et al.[38]

**FIGURE 13.1** Meta-analysis of selected allogeneic bone marrow transplantation studies in children with acute myelogenous leukemia.

not is the presence of cytogenetic findings. Patients with FLT-3 internal tandem duplication had higher risks of leukocytosis, lower complete remission rates, higher induction failure rates, increased relapse rates, and lower event free and overall survivals.[17]

# AUTOLOGOUS BONE MARROW TRANSPLANTATION

## Early Studies

The research team at the Fred Hutchinson Cancer Research Center performed autologous bone marrow transplantation initially for those patients who did not have matched sibling donors and who had a poor prognosis with chemotherapy alone.[2,3,6,10,46,47] As the results of trials using allogeneic stem cell transplantation improved, it became logical to use autologous stem cell transplantation for those patients for whom matched donors were not available. These studies were problematic, however, since bone marrows of these patients, from whom and to whom they would be given, were never completely clear of leukemic cells.

The best review on the effectiveness of autologous bone marrow transplantation in patients with AML is from Bleakley et al. (▼ Figure 13.2).[38] This group identified studies that met criteria for adequate statistical analysis and interpretation. They evaluated studies from the Associazione Italiana Ematologia Ed Oncologia Pediatrica/Leucemia Acuta Mieloide (AEIOP-LAM 87), Children's Cancer Group study (CCG 2891), Medical Research Council (MRC AML 10), and Pediatric Oncology Group (POG 8821). In three of the studies, patients were randomized to receive further therapy after induction therapy,[39,45,49] while in one, patients were randomized to receive further chemotherapy after induction of remission.[43] In one of the studies,[49] bone marrow cells were purged, while in the other studies, bone marrow cells were not purged. These studies[49] showed a lower risk of relapse with bone marrow transplantation (BMT; 41% vs. 58%). This was also the only study to have purged bone marrow cells for reinfusion, and to have a significantly higher treatment-related mortality than controls. Thus, the improvement in relapse rate was in part offset by

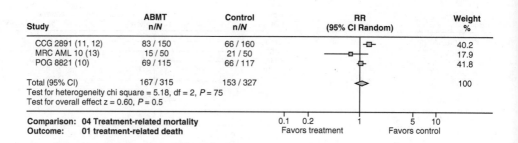

| Study | ABMT n/N | Control n/N | RR (95% CI Random) | Weight % |
|---|---|---|---|---|
| CCG 2891 (11, 12) | 83 / 150 | 66 / 160 | | 40.2 |
| MRC AML 10 (13) | 15 / 50 | 21 / 50 | | 17.9 |
| POG 8821 (10) | 69 / 115 | 66 / 117 | | 41.8 |
| Total (95% CI) | 167 / 315 | 153 / 327 | | 100 |

Test for heterogeneity chi square = 5.18, df = 2, P = 75
Test for overall effect z = 0.60, P = 0.5

Comparison:  04 Treatment-related mortality
Outcome:        01 treatment-related death

0.1   0.2                1           5   10
Favors treatment              Favors control

Abbreviations: CCG 2891 = Children's Cancer Group protocol #2891;[55,56] MRC AML 10 = Medical Research Council protocol on Acute Myelogenous Leukemia #10;[46,59] POG 8821 = Pediatric Oncology Group protocol #8821;[44] RR = relative risk; CI = confidence interval. Reproduced with permission from Nature Publishing Group-NPG and Bleakley et al.[38]

**FIGURE 13.2** Meta-analysis of selected allogeneic bone marrow transplantation studies in children with acute myelogenous leukemia.

the increase in toxicity. Only one study showed a significant increase in disease-free survival,[43] while one study showed a significant decrease in disease-free survival.[45] The two others showed no significant difference between autologous BMT and chemotherapy alone. These survival differences are shown in Figure 13.2. The composite results of these studies suggest that the benefit of autologous bone marrow transplantation is equivocal and should not automatically be used as front-line therapy in the first remission of AML.

## Purging Techniques

Many groups experimented with different types of purging regimens in order to cleanse autologous bone marrow to make it safe enough to return to patients after high-dose ablative chemotherapy. These methods and studies are listed in ▼ Table 13.1.[53,54,59–62] In general, the results were indeterminate because purging was often not complete, and because removal of protective T-lymphocyte populations rendered these patients at high risk for fatal fungal and other infections.

Several major problems with autologous bone marrow transplantation have been noted, including the observation that they are often not superior to chemotherapy in outcome measurements. Another problem with autologous bone marrow transplantation is the risk of tumor cell contamination upon reinfusion despite careful purging. In this regard, Brenner et al.[41] showed that relapse after autologous transplantation in patients with acute myeloid leukemia (and neuroblastoma), back-tracked by the NeoR marker, often originated from purged cells returned to patients. This observation has greatly dampened enthusiasm for autologous transplantation, even when cells can be apparently purged.

| TABLE 13.1 | Methods of Purging Bone Marrow for Autologous Stem Cell Transplantation | |
|---|---|---|
| **Reference** | **Method** | **Outcome** |
| Lemoli et al.[53] | 4-Hydroperoxycyclophosphamide, etoposide | 57% disease-free survival in recipients of purged marrows vs. 32% in recipients of unpurged marrows. |
| Miller et al.[54] | 4-Hydroperoxycyclophosphamide | Higher leukemia-free survival in recipients of purged marrow cells. |
| Chao et al.[59] | Mafosfamide + amifostine | Mafosfamide and amifostine purging of autologous peripheral blood stem cells in patients with AML is feasible. |
| Fauth et al.[60] | Nitrogen mustard, etoposide, mafosfamide | Effective for purging leukemia cells in vitro. |
| Motta et al.[61] | Mafosfamide or interleukin-2 and consolidation with high dose melphalan | Purging is feasible; event-free survival and overall survival similar to that of recipients with unpurged marrows. |
| Cesaro et al.[62] | Nitrogen mustard + VP16 | Purging of leukemic cells is feasible. |

Autologous stem cell transplantation also began to lose favor as a new mechanism of stem cell transplantation became apparent. Using the paradigm of stem cell transplantation as immunotherapy in which the graft delivers an antileukemia effect, the value of allogeneic stem cell transplantation became increasingly important. Not only does allogeneic stem cell transplantation allow for graft-versus-leukemia effects, it also allows for donor lymphocyte infusions (DLIs) subsequently to treat relapses if and whenever they occur after the initial stem cell transplantation.

The increasing number of donors available through umbilical cord donor programs also has decreased enthusiasm for autologous bone marrow transplantation. Although unrelated matches remain extremely problematic for adult patients, the availability of cord blood cell transplantation lowers this dilemma for the young patient. Cord blood cell transplantation allows for a graft-versus-leukemia effect and for engraftment of new cells with lower risk of fatal graft-versus-host disease and with greater tolerance for diversity of human lymphocyte antigen (HLA) type between host and donor than non-cord matched unrelated donor stem cell transplantation. It also offers no chance of tumor cell contamination. A disadvantage of cord blood stem cell transplantation over bone marrow or peripheral blood stem cell transplantation is that additional cells for subsequent donor lymphocyte reinfusions cannot be obtained.

# UMBILICAL CORD BLOOD TRANSPLANTATION FOR PATIENTS WITH ACUTE MYELOGENOUS LEUKEMIA

Umbilical cord blood stem cells have become a valuable source of donor cells with which to transplant patients with acute myelogenous leukemia. The stem cell source of choice is always a matched related sibling, but this fortunate situation only occurs in 25% of patient's situations. When a matched related sibling source is not available, the choice remains between unrelated bone marrow transplant or unrelated cord blood stem cell transplant. The latter has many advantages including easy availability and a greater chance of finding matches for minority populations due to the establishment of several large-scale umbilical cord blood banks. This development has made more than 30,000 cord blood units available for transplantation and has facilitated more than 1,200 unrelated umbilical cord blood transplants for children as well as adults. However, it suffers from several disadvantages as well. First, there is less experience and there is still not enough information to know how durable these grafts will be in the future. Secondly, the number of cells is often limited, thereby permitting only partial engraftment in some patients, in particular those who are older and heavier. Third, there is no ability to go back to the donor for additional cells in case this may be necessary for donor lymphocyte infusions, such as for relapse of leukemia.

Despite these limitations, umbilical blood stem cells remains an appropriate choice for patients with acute myelogenous leukemia for whom there is no sibling match available, especially in the case of relapse after chemotherapy or in the case of high-risk disease (i.e., Philadelphia chromosome positive AML or AML secondary to chemotherapy).

Rocha et al. recently reviewed the outcomes of patients who were registered within the EuroCord Blood Transplant Group (CBTG). A total of 262 children with acute leukemia underwent umbilical stem cell transplantation. These patients were compared to similar patients receiving unmanipulated or T cell-depleted bone marrow stem cell transplants: 18 to 59% of patients in each of the groups were in first remission (especially those undergoing unmanipulated bone marrow transplantation), 39 to 50% in second remission, and 14 to 49% in third or later remission. In total, poor risk patients (defined as those having advanced disease and in third or later remission) constituted between 9 and 20% of patients of the umbilical cord stem cell transplant patients.

Patients who received an umbilical cord blood transplantation had a greater number of HLA mismatches (92%) compared to those who received unmanipulated or manipulated bone marrow stem cell transplants. Despite this fact, the two-year survival and two-year event-free survival rates were similar (49% and 43%) compared to that of patients receiving bone marrow stem cell transplants.

Engraftment was slower in patients who received cord blood transplantation compared to those who received bone marrow transplants. Because of this delay, the 100 day transplant-related mortality was higher in the cord blood transplant group. Graft-versus-host disease was less, however, although it is not clear if this was associated with decreased graft-versus-leukemia effects. Patients who received T cell-depleted bone marrow transplants had less acute graft-versus-host disease, but greater risk of relapse. The differences in survival evened out after day 100 following transplant. Patients with T cell-depleted bone marrow transplants and with umbilical cord blood transplant had less graft-versus-host disease than those who received regular bone marrow transplant. The overall mortality was higher in the groups of patients who received T cell-depleted bone marrow transplantation.

These and other results suggest that umbilical bone marrow transplantation and umbilical cord blood transplantation for patients who do not have matched siblings are adequate. Much work needs to be done to increase the number of units available, to expand these cells in vitro, and to match them with greater sensitivity.

## WHEN TO TRANSPLANT AND WHEN NOT TO TRANSPLANT

Certain patients should not be transplanted either because of particularly good prognoses with chemotherapy or because of particularly bad prognoses with stem cell transplantation.

Chen and his coinvestigators recently addressed the controversy as to which patients should be treated with bone marrow transplantation.[56] In reviewing the literature, they noted that all studies demonstrate fewer relapses in patients intended to receive allogeneic bone marrow transplantation and a superior disease-free survival in patients assigned to allogeneic bone marrow transplantation, despite the higher toxicity rates. The evidence therefore favors consolidation therapy with allogeneic bone marrow transplantation as more likely to be curative than either autologous bone marrow transplantation or chemotherapy. In fact, autologous bone marrow transplantation has not been found to be advantageous compared to chemotherapy in a variety of studies.[43,49,57] In evaluating overall survival, perhaps a better endpoint, allogeneic bone marrow transplantation gives superior results compared to chemotherapy. In all five pediatric cooperative group studies, long-term survival was better for patients assigned to allogeneic bone marrow transplantation.

A risk adapted approach to therapy may be best. Patients who have favorable features with AML might be deferred for consideration for bone marrow transplantation, while those with high-risk features may be offered bone marrow transplantation early on. This may become more relevant as results with less intensive regimens improve due to better supportive care. Chromosomes should be considered in the risk assessment, such that patients with trisomy 15, 17 should be treated with ATRA-based regimens, and patients with trisomy 21 should be considered for chemotherapy alone. Patients with nonavailability of matched sibling donor and high risk features could be considered for alternative allogeneic bone marrow transplant with cord blood donors if possible, or otherwise, with nonrelated matched donors.[58]

# REFERENCES

1. Bernasconi C, Lazzarino M, Canevari A et al. Allogeneic versus autologous bone marrow transplantation versus intensive post-remission chemotherapy in acute leukaemias. Bone Marrow Transplant 1989;4(Suppl 4):73–76.
2. Burnett AK. Autologous bone marrow transplant in the treatment of acute leukaemia. Baillieres Clin Haematol 1991;4:751–773.
3. Carella AM, Frassoni F, van Lint MT et al. Autologous and allogeneic bone marrow transplantation in acute myeloid leukemia in first complete remission: an update of the Genoa experience with 159 patients. Ann Hematol 1992;64:128–131.
4. Clift RA, Buckner CD, Appelbaum FR et al. Allogeneic marrow transplantation during untreated first relapse of acute myeloid leukemia. J Clin Oncol 1992;10:1723–1729.
5. Geller RB, Saral R, Piantadosi S et al. Allogeneic bone marrow transplantation after high-dose busulfan and cyclophosphamide in patients with acute nonlymphocytic leukemia. Blood 1989;73:2209–2218.
6. Geller RB, Vogelsang GB, Wingard JR. Successful marrow transplantation for acute myelocytic leukemia following therapy for Hodgkin's disease. J Clin Oncol 1988;6:1558–1561.
7. Petersen FB, Buckner CD, Appelbaum FR et al. Busulfan, cyclophosphamide and fractionated total body irradiation as a preparatory regimen for marrow transplantation in patients with advanced hematological malignancies: a phase I study. Bone Marrow Transplant 1989;4:617–623.
8. Prentice HG. New developments in post-induction therapy for acute myeloblastic leukaemia. Bone Marrow Transplant 1989;4(Suppl 3):2–5.
9. Sheridan WP, Boyd AW, Green MD et al. High-dose chemotherapy with busulphan and cyclophosphamide and bone-marrow transplantation for drug-sensitive malignancies in adults: a preliminary report. Med J Aust 1989;151:379–386.
10. Trigg ME. Bone marrow transplantation for treatment of leukemia in children. Pediatr Clin North Am 1988;35:933–948.
11. Champlin R, Khouri I, Kornblau S et al. Allogeneic hematopoietic transplantation as adoptive immunotherapy. Induction of graft-versus-malignancy as primary therapy. Hematol Oncol Clin North Am 1999;13:1041–1057, vii–viii.
12. Baranger L, Baruchel A, Leverger G et al. Monosomy-7 in childhood hemopoietic disorders. Leukemia 1990;4:345–349.
13. Boayue KB, Gu L, Yeager AM et al. Pediatric acute myelogenous leukemia cells express IL-6 receptors and are sensitive to a recombinant IL6-pseudomonas exotoxin. Leukemia 1998;12:182–191.
14. Grimwade D, Walker H, Oliver F et al. What happens subsequently in AML when cytogenetic abnormalities persist at bone marrow harvest? Results of the 10th UK MRC AML trial. Medical Research Council Leukaemia Working Parties. Bone Marrow Transplant 1997;19:1117–1123.
15. Grimwade D, Walker H, Oliver F et al. The importance of diagnostic cytogenetics on outcome in AML: analysis of 1,612 patients entered into the MRC AML 10 trial. The Medical Research Council Adult and Children's Leukaemia Working Parties. Blood 1998;92:2322–2333.
16. Imrie KR, Dube I, Prince HM et al. New clonal karyotypic abnormalities acquired following autologous bone marrow transplantation for acute myeloid leukemia do not appear to confer an adverse prognosis. Bone Marrow Transplant 1998;21:395–399.
17. Kottaridis PD, Gale RE, Frew ME et al. The presence of a FLT3 internal tandem duplication in patients with acute myeloid leukemia (AML) adds important prognostic information to cytogenetic risk group and response to the first cycle of chemotherapy: analysis of 854 patients from the United Kingdom Medical Research Council AML 10 and 12 trials. Blood 2001;98:1752–1759.
18. Leblanc T, Berger R. Molecular cytogenetics of childhood acute myelogenous leukaemias. Eur J Haematol 1997;59:1–13.
19. Lo Coco F, Pisegna S, Diverio D. The AML1 gene: a transcription factor involved in the pathogenesis of myeloid and lymphoid leukemias. Haematologica 1997;82:364–370.
20. McGrattan P, Alexander HD, Humphreys MW et al. Tetrasomy 13 as the sole cytogenetic abnormality in acute myeloid leukemia M1 without maturation. Cancer Genet Cytogenet 2002;135:192–195.
21. Webb DK, Harrison G, Stevens RF et al. Relationships between age at diagnosis, clinical features, and outcome of therapy in children treated in the Medical Research Council AML 10 and 12 trials for acute myeloid leukemia. Blood 2001;98:1714–1720.
22. Abella E, Ravindranath Y. Therapy for childhood acute myeloid leukemia: role of allogeneic bone marrow transplantation. Curr Oncol Rep 2000;2:529–538.
23. Shearer P, Kapoor G, Beckwith JB et al. Secondary acute myelogenous leukemia in patients previously treated for childhood renal tumors: a report from the National Wilms Tumor Study Group. J Pediatr Hematol Oncol 2001;23:109–111.

24. Wells R, Arthur DC, Srivastava A et al. Prognostic variables in newly diagnosed children and adolescents with acute myeloid leukemia. Leukemia 2002;16:601–607.
25. Woods WG, Neudorf S, Gold S et al. A comparison of allogeneic bone marrow transplantation, autologous bone marrow transplantation, and aggressive chemotherapy in children with acute myeloid leukemia in remission. Blood 2001;97:56–62.
26. Dohy H, Kyo T. [Progress in the treatment of acute myelogenous leukemia]. Gan To Kagaku Ryoho 1989;16:1976–1981.
27. Geller RB, Myers S, Devine S et al. Phase I study of busulfan, cyclophosphamide, and timed sequential escalating doses of cytarabine followed by bone marrow transplantation. Bone Marrow Transplant 1992;9:41–47.
28. Hurwitz CA, Mounce KG, Grier HE. Treatment of patients with acute myelogenous leukemia: review of clinical trials of the past decade. J Pediatr Hematol Oncol 1995;17:185–197.
29. Appelbaum FR. Is there a best transplant conditioning regimen for acute myeloid leukemia? Leukemia 2000;14:497–501.
30. Aurer I, Gale RP. Are new conditioning regimens for transplants in acute myelogenous leukemia better? Bone Marrow Transplant 1991;7:255–261.
31. Wang C, Qiao Z, Yang L et al. The combination of melphalan, cyclophosphamide and cytosine arabinoside as a conditioning regimen for autologous bone marrow transplantation for acute leukemia. Chin Med J (Engl) 1996;109:304–307.
32. Bensinger WI, Buckner CD, Clift RA et al. Phase I study of busulfan and cyclophosphamide in preparation for allogeneic marrow transplant for patients with multiple myeloma. J Clin Oncol 1992;10:1491–1497.
33. Buggia I, Locatelli F, Regazzi MB, Zecca M. Busulfan. Ann Pharmacother 1994;28:1055–1062.
34. Dix SP, Wingard JR, Mullins RE et al. Association of busulfan area under the curve with veno-occlusive disease following BMT. Bone Marrow Transplant 1996;17:225–230.
35. Van der Jagt RH, Appelbaum FR, Petersen FB et al. Busulfan and cyclophosphamide as a preparative regimen for bone marrow transplantation in patients with prior chest radiotherapy. Bone Marrow Transplant 1991;8:211–215.
36. Visani G, Lemoli RM, Isidori A et al. Double reinforcement with fludarabine/high-dose cytarabine enhances the impact of autologous stem cell transplantation in acute myeloid leukemia patients. Bone Marrow Transplant 2001;27:829–835.
37. Frassoni F, Labopin M, Powles R. Effect of centre on outcome of bone-marrow transplantation for acute myeloid leukaemia. Acute Leukaemia Working Party of the European Group for Blood and Marrow Transplantation. Lancet 2000;355:1393–1398.
38. Bleakley M, Lau L, Shaw PJ et al. Bone marrow transplantation for pediatric AML in first remission: a systematic review and meta-analysis. Bone Marrow Transplant 2002;29:843–852.
39. Amadori S, Testi AM, Arico M et al. Prospective comparative study of bone marrow transplantation and post-remission chemotherapy for childhood acute myelogenous leukemia. The Associazione Italiana Ematologia ed Oncologia Pediatrica Cooperative Group. J Clin Oncol 1993;11:1046–1054.
40. Woods WG, Kobrinsky N, Buckley JD et al. Timed-sequential induction therapy improves postremission outcome in acute myeloid leukemia: a report from the Children's Cancer Group. Blood 1996;87:4979–4989.
41. Brenner MK, Rill DR, Moen RC et al. Gene marking and autologous bone marrow transplantation. Ann N Y Acad Sci 1994;716:204–214; discussion 214–215, 225–227.
42. Michel G, Leverger G, Leblanc T et al. Allogeneic bone marrow transplantation vs aggressive post-remission chemotherapy for children with acute myeloid leukemia in first complete remission. A prospective study from the French Society of Pediatric Hematology and Immunology (SHIP). Bone Marrow Transplant 1996;17:191–196.
43. Stevens RF, Hann IM, Wheatley K et al. Marked improvements in outcome with chemotherapy alone in paediatric acute myeloid leukaemia: results of the United Kingdom Medical Research Council's 10th AML trial. MRC Childhood Leukaemia Working Party. Br J Haematol 1998;101:130–140.
44. Shaw PJ, Bergin ME, Burgess MA et al. Childhood acute myeloid leukemia; outcome in a single centre using chemotherapy and consolidation with busulphan/cyclophosphamide for bone marrow transplantation. J Clin Oncol 1994;12:2138–2145.
45. Wells RJ, Woods WG, Buckley JD et al. Treatment of newly diagnosed children and adolescents with acute myeloid leukemia: a Children's Cancer Group study. J Clin Oncol 1994;12:2367–2377.
46. Mills LE, Cornwell GG 3rd, Ball ED. Autologous bone marrow transplantation in the treatment of acute myeloid leukemia: the Dartmouth experience and a review of literature. Cancer Invest 1990;8:181–190.
47. Gorin NC. [Autografts and acute leukemia: 15 years later]. Presse Med 1994;23:1710–1716.
48. Burnett AK, Goldstone AH, Stevens RM et al. Randomised comparison of addition of autologous bone-marrow transplantation to intensive chemotherapy for acute myeloid leukaemia in first remission: results of MRC AML 10 trial. UK Medical Research Council Adult and Children's Leukaemia Working Parties. Lancet 1998;351:700–708.

49. Ravindranath Y, Yeager AM, Chang MN et al. Autologous bone marrow transplantation versus intensive consolidation chemotherapy for acute myeloid leukemia in childhood. N Engl J Med 1996;334:1428–1434.

50. Brown RA, Wolff SN, Fay JW et al. High-dose etoposide, cyclophosphamide and total body irradiation with allogeneic bone marrow transplantation for resistant acute myeloid leukemia: a study by the North American Marrow Transplant Group. Leuk Lymphoma 1996;22:271–277.

51. Lenarsky C, Weinberg K, Petersen J et al. Autologous bone marrow transplantation with 4-hydroperoxy-cyclophosphamide purged marrows for children with acute non-lymphoblastic leukemia in second remission. Bone Marrow Transplant 1990;6:425–429.

52. Linker CA, Ries CA, Damon LE et al. Autologous bone marrow transplantation for acute myeloid leukemia using 4-hydroperoxycyclophosphamide-purged bone marrow and the busulfan/etoposide preparative regimen: a follow-up report. Bone Marrow Transplant 1998;22:865–872.

53. Lemoli RM, Visani G, Leopardi G et al. Autologous transplantation of chemotherapy-purged PBSC collections from high-risk leukemia patients: a pilot study. Bone Marrow Transplant 1999;23:235–241.

54. Miller CB, Rowlings PA, Zhang MJ et al. The effect of graft purging with 4-hydroperoxycyclophospha mide in autologous bone marrow transplantation for acute myelogenous leukemia. Exp Hematol 2001;29:1336–1346.

55. Smith BD, Jones RJ, Lee SM et al. Autologous bone marrow transplantation with 4-hydroperoxycyclophosphamide purging for acute myeloid leukaemia beyond first remission: a 10-year experience. Br J Haematol 2002;117:907–913.

56. Chen AR, Alonzo TA, Woods WG et al. Current controversies: which patients with acute myeloid leukaemia should receive a bone marrow transplantation? An American view. Br J Haematol 2002;118:378–384.

57. Ferrero D, De Fabritiis P, Amadori S et al. Autologous bone marrow transplantation in acute myeloid leukemia after in-vitro purging with an anti-lacto-N-fucopentaose III antibody and rabbit complement. Leuk Res 1987;11:265–272.

58. Dinndorf P, Bunin N. Bone marrow transplantation for children with acute myelogenous leukemia. J Pediatr Hematol Oncol 1995;17:211–224.

59. Chao NJ, Stein AS, Long GD et al. Busulfan/etoposide—initial experience with a new preparatory regimen for autologous bone marrow transplantation in patients with acute nonlymphoblastic leukemia. Blood 1993;81:319–323.

60. Fauth F, Martin H, Sonnhoff S et al. Purging of G-CSF-mobilized peripheral autografts in acute leukemia with mafosfamide and amifostine to protect normal progenitor cells. Bone Marrow Transplant 2000;25:831–836.

61. Motta MR, Mangianti S, Rizzi S et al. Pharmacological purging of minimal residual disease from peripheral blood stem cell collections of acute myeloblastic leukemia patients: preclinical studies. Exp Hematol 1997;25:1261–1269.

62. Cesaro S, Meloni G, Messina C et al. High-dose melphalan with autologous hematopoietic stem cell transplantation for acute myeloid leukemia: results of a retrospective analysis of the Italian Pediatric Group for Bone Marrow Transplantation. Bone Marrow Transplant 2001;28:131–136.

# CHAPTER XIV

# Myelodysplastic Disorders and Related Diseases

MICHAEL L. NIEDER AND VICKI L. FISHER

Myelodysplastic and myelodysplastic/myeloproliferative disorders constitute less than 10% of the hematologic malignancies in children. However, the successful treatment of these disorders has been challenging. Although new therapies with imatinib mesylate show promise, hematopoietic stem cell transplantation is the only known curative therapy survival for this group of illnesses. Unfortunately, even for those patients fortunate enough to identify a donor, the long-term survival has been less than 50%.

## JUVENILE MYELOMONOCYTIC LEUKEMIA

The International Myelomonocytic Leukemia Working Group has determined that juvenile myelomonocytic leukemia [JMML; formerly juvenile chronic myelocytic leukemia (JCML)] is a distinct entity and should no longer be classified as a myelodysplastic syndrome.[1] It is almost exclusively seen in children under the age of five years (mean age is two years) and is twice as common in boys.[2]

### Diagnostic Criteria

JMML should be considered only when the white blood count (WBC) $> 13 \times 10^9$/L, the absolute monocyte count is $> 1 \times 10^9$/L, the peripheral blood smear demonstrates immature myeloid elements, the bone marrow has fewer than 30% blasts and there is no cytogenetic evidence of either t(9;22)(q34;q21) or rearrangement of BCR/ABL.[1] In addition, the majority of patients will have evidence of hepatosplenomegaly. Other common presenting signs may include bruising, rash, elevated hemoglobin F levels and infection. As many as 10% of patients will have neurofibromatosis type 1.[3] Though not mandated, bone marrow culture with colony assays and sensitivity to granulocyte-macrophage colony-stimulating factor (GM-CSF) should be performed on all patients with this suspected diagnosis.

### Therapeutic Considerations

Most nonablative approaches to the therapy of JMML have either been ineffective (low dose chemotherapy[4]) or temporarily effective (intensive therapy,[5] retinoic acid,[6] alpha-interferon[7]). To date, only allogeneic stem cell transplantation is potentially curative. The role of splenectomy prior to transplantation has not been studied in any randomized fashion. However, many oncologists believe that a significantly enlarged spleen should be removed prior to ablative therapy.

In 2000, Matthes-Martin et al.[8] reviewed the published data on stem cell transplantation for JMML. The overall relapse rate was 47%. In 11 of the 24 patients who relapsed, additional curative therapy was attempted. Of five patients whose immunosuppression was withdrawn, three achieved a second remission. Donor lymphocyte infusions induced a second remission in one of two children. Six children underwent a second stem cell transplant and three achieved remission. Overall, the transplant-related mortality was 27.5%. In this series, graft-versus-host disease did not seem to play a role in preventing relapse. Though not statistically significant, patients who received total body irradiation faired worse than those who did not.

In contrast to Matthes-Martin and associates' review, Orchard and colleagues[9] reported on a young girl with JMML who relapsed early after an unrelated donor transplant. Her immunosuppression was withdrawn and she manifested signs of graft-versus-host disease. When graft-versus-host disease occurred, blasts in the peripheral blood disappeared, the proportion of donor cells in the marrow increased and her skin rash resolved.

MacMillan et al.[10] reported on the Minnesota's experience with seven children (1984–1998) with JMML who were transplanted with allogeneic related or unrelated bone marrow or umbilical cord blood. The children underwent a conditioning regimen of cyclophosphamide and total body irradiation ± busulfan. One patient failed to engraft and subsequently underwent two additional transplant procedures. One other patient underwent a second procedure following relapse. Only one patient remained free of disease and one additional patient achieved a second remission after cyclosporine A was withdrawn.

There are several reports of alternative donor transplantation for JMML. One experience was reported by Bunin and colleagues in 1999.[11] Twelve patients with JMML received marrow from unrelated donors ($N = 9$) or a mismatched family member ($N = 3$). Four different conditioning regimens were used: busulfan/cytarabine/cyclophosphamide/ total body irradiation (TBI) ($N = 7$); etoposide/TBI ($N = 1$); busulfan/cyclophosphamide ($N = 1$); cyclophosphamide/etoposide/TBI ($N = 3$). Eight of the patients were alive and in remission 11–56 months at the time of the report. Six of the eight patients had performance scores of 100%, but two of the children remained debilitated.

Locatelli et al.[12] described the outcome of 43 patients with JMML, 20 of whom had either a mismatched related, matched unrelated or mismatched unrelated transplant. Various preparative regimens were used and the disease-free survival was approximately 20%.

The Seattle experience[13] was reported in 1994 with 17 mismatched related or matched unrelated donors. The majority of patients received at TBI-containing regimen. Overall survival for this group of children was less than 20%, and the majority of failures were secondary to relapse.

Relapse after stem cell transplantation is a common event in patients with JMML. One novel approach to salvaging patients was reported by Ohta et al.[14] In 1998, a five-year-old boy with JMML underwent a bone marrow transplant after receiving conditioning with cyclophosphamide and TBI. The patient relapsed six months later and a previously undetected monosomy[7] was noted. Immunosuppression was discontinued but remission did not occur. The patient was started on interferon-alpha and achieved cytogenetic remission within two to four months.

In conclusion, hematopoietic stem cell transplantation remains the only curative option for patients with JMML. Unfortunately, the substantial relapse rates after transplantation suggest that alternative and adjuvant therapies need to be explored. Multicenter, randomized trials using novel transplant approaches, retinoic acid, GM-CSF receptor blockade and other biologics are necessary in order to improve the prognosis for the majority of these children.

# MYELODYSPLASTIC SYNDROMES

Myelodysplastic syndromes (MDS) are considered to be a heterogeneous collection of acquired, clonal bone marrow stem cell disorders. They are invariably diagnosed when both ineffective erythropoiesis and marrow dysplasias of one or more marrow cell lines are present. MDS are somewhat rare in children (incidence < 3.4/1,000,000 children).[15] Children with MDS almost always have advanced disease (RAEB-1 and RAEB-2), may be difficult to differentiate from children with acute myelogenous leukemia, and progress to leukemia more often than adults.[16] Of note, chronic myelomonocytic leukemia (CMML) is now placed in a new category of diseases called "myelodysplastic/myeloproliferative disorders."

## Diagnostic Criteria

▼ Table 14.1 outlines the newest diagnostic categories for classifying myelodysplastic syndromes. The International MDS Risk Analysis Workshop developed an International Prognostic Scoring System (IPSS) for assigning risk to patients with MDS.[17] The risk scores assigned are dependent on the following variables: bone marrow blast percentage, number of cytopenias and cytogenetic subgroup. To date, the usefulness of this scoring system for assigning risk to young children has not been determined.

## Therapeutic Considerations

Almost no children with MDS can be in the "low risk" group. Although 10 to 20% of adults with low or intermediate MDS become less anemic with erythropoietin, this is not a definitive approach to the disease and will not be helpful in the management of most children. In adult patients with low or intermediate risk MDS, previous and ongoing clinical trials have compared the efficacy of supportive therapy with or without novel drug therapy. While some of these agents can reduce need for transfusions and enhance quality of life, none are curative.[18] To date, erythropoietin, thrombopoietin, antithymocyte globulin, cyclosporine A, anti-tumor necrosis factor, anti-CD33 calicheamicin, thalidomide, amifostine and all-*trans*-retinoic acid have yielded mixed results. These agents have not been proven to be very helpful in children, who almost always have higher risk MDS. High risk MDS patients treated with standard acute myelogenous leukemia-type chemotherapy have very poor long-term outcomes.[19]

Several authors have described stem cell transplantation as curative therapy for MDS. Utilizing matched sibling donors as the stem cell source, Runde et al.[20] reported the outcomes of 131 patients with MDS who underwent transplantation without prior remission induction chemotherapy. Various conditioning regimens were used. The five-year disease-free survival for patients under the age of 20 years was 45%.

| TABLE 14.1   Classification of Myelodysplastic Syndromes | |
|---|---|
| **Disease** | **Bone Marrow Findings** |
| Refractory anemia (RA) | ▪ Erythroid dysplasia<br>▪ <5% blasts<br>▪ <15% ringed sideroblasts |
| Refractory anemia with ringed sideroblasts (RARS) | ▪ 15% ringed sideroblasts<br>▪ Erythroid dysplasia<br>▪ <5% blasts |
| Refractory cytopenia with multilineage dysplasia (RCMD) | ▪ Dysplasia in ≥10% of cells in two or more myeloid cell lines<br>▪ <5% blasts in marrow<br>▪ No Auer rods<br>▪ <15% ringed sideroblasts |
| Refractory cytopenia with multilineage dysplasia and ringed sideroblasts (RCMD-RS) | ▪ Dysplasia in ≥10% of cells in two or more myeloid cell lines<br>▪ <5% blasts in marrow<br>▪ No Auer rods<br>▪ ≥15% ringed sideroblasts |
| Refractory anemia with excess blasts-1 (RAEB-1) | ▪ Unilineage or multilineage dysplasia<br>▪ 5-9% blasts<br>▪ No Auer rods |
| Refractory anemia with excess blasts-2 (RAEB-2) | ▪ Unilineage or multilineage dysplasia<br>▪ 10-19% blasts<br>▪ ±Auer rods |
| Myelodysplastic syndrome-unclassified (MDS-U) | ▪ Unilineage dysplasia of one myeloid cell line<br>▪ <5% blasts<br>▪ No Auer rods |
| Myelodysplastic syndrome with isolated del(5q) | ▪ Normal or increased megakaryocytes with hypolobated nuclei<br>▪ <5% blasts<br>▪ Isolated del(5q) in marrow cells<br>▪ No Auer rods |

Drs. Appelbaum and Anderson[21] reported that 60% of patients with MDS, who were under the age of 20 years at the time of transplantation, survived more than 10 years. These patients were conditioned with either busulfan + cyclophosphamide or cyclophosphamide + TBI. Nearly 60% of the donors were matched siblings; alternative donors included incompletely matched family members or matched unrelated donors.

A large review of 510 patients with MDS who underwent matched unrelated marrow transplantation was published in 2002.[22] Many different conditioning regimens were utilized. The incidence of graft failure was 8%. The overall two-year event-free survival was

29%. Several different strategies were used to provide graft-versus-host disease (GVHD) prophylaxis. Grade II-IV GVHD developed in 47% of the patients, while chronic GVHD was noted in 27% of the recipients.

In 1997, Locatelli et al.[23] compared the outcomes of children with chronic myelomonocytic leukemia (formerly considered to be MDS) who were treated with chemotherapy alone or bone marrow transplantation. Only 6% of the children treated with chemotherapy were alive 10 years later. Of those patients who underwent transplantation, 39% were alive 10 years later.

Although the timing of bone marrow transplantation for adults with MDS is not straightforward,[24] most children should be transplanted relatively promptly. Children often have more than 5% myeloblasts in their marrow, have monosomy[7] or have other high risk characteristics. Unless leukemic transformation has occurred, taking the time to identify the optimal donor while providing supportive care is probably the most prudent approach to take in these younger patients. For patients with MDS, no studies have compared immediate transplantation to a two-stage protocol of induction chemotherapy followed by transplantation as consolidation (as one would treat acute myelogenous leukemia). Although one might consider this approach for a child with more than 15%–20% blasts in the marrow, there are no data that identify such a threshold value. In contrast to this, some groups are now investigating non-ablative therapies for patients with MDS.

The stem cell source of choice is not known at this time. There remains controversy as to whether peripheral blood, bone marrow, or umbilical cord blood stem cells provide superior engraftment, improved disease-free survival, less GVHD and improved quality of life.

Reduced-intensity conditioning regimens prior to stem cell transplantation are now being utilized for some patients with MDS. Although outcome data for children do not yet exist, the regimens are tolerable. Very limited data are available for adult patients; one description of 12 patients reported a two-year disease-free survival of only 12%.[25]

Understanding the biology of MDS will likely result in novel therapies in the years to come. Although it is not known if inhibition of tumor necrosis factor-alpha (TNF-α) production (pentoxifylline + ciprofloxacin + dexamethasone) or if agents like farnesyl transferase can result in long-term remissions, newer biologic therapies may eventually become the mainstay of therapy for these disorders.[26]

## SECONDARY MYELODYSPLASTIC SYNDROMES

As more children are cured of cancer, the number of cases of secondary MDS is rising. Secondary MDS is also a late complication of stem cell transplantation.

### Diagnostic Criteria

Since patients with secondary MDS almost always progress rapidly to leukemia, the classification system for de novo MDS is neither helpful nor prognostic.[27] Many patients who have undergone autologous stem cell transplantation and who do not have MDS, do have dysplastic features in their marrow. Therefore, it is important to identify cytogenetic abnormalities in the bone marrow or peripheral blood. It is understood that all patients with secondary MDS are considered to be high risk.

## Therapeutic Considerations

Secondary MDS is often a rapidly fatal disease, but there are reports of long-term survival for some patients who are treated with stem cell transplantation. In 1997, Ballen and colleagues[28] reported on 18 patients (mostly adults) with therapy-related MDS (median interval from primary diagnosis to secondary MDS was 66 months) who underwent an allogeneic transplant. Three different conditioning regimens were used and only one patient had received pre-transplant induction chemotherapy. The actuarial disease free survival was 24% with a median follow-up of three years.

In 1999, Leahy and colleagues described the outcomes for 11 children with secondary MDS (median time from primary diagnosis to secondary MDS was 33 months).[29] The four patients with RAEB did not receive pre-transplant induction chemotherapy. The other patients had progressed to leukemia and were all induced into remission with chemotherapy prior to the transplant. Four conditioning regimens were used: five patients received busulfan + cyclophosphamide; four received busulfan + cyclophosphamide + ATG; one received busulfan + cyclophosphamide + etoposide; one received cyclophosphamide + cytarabine + TBI. Three patients remained free of disease for a two-year actuarial survival of 24%.

Hale and colleagues[30] reported their experience with secondary MDS from St. Jude Children's Research Hospital. Acute myelogenous leukemia developed in 21 patients who had previously been treated for acute lymphoblastic leukemia. Pretransplant induction chemotherapy was given to 13 patients. All patients were conditioned with cytarabine, cyclophosphamide and TBI. Eleven patients received unmanipulated marrow from matched sibling donors. Eight children received T-cell depleted marrow from matched unrelated donors. Two patients received marrow from their haploidentical family members. The three-year disease-free survival was 19%.

In one representative adult series,[31] the survival after transplantation for MDS was as low as 9%. Without transplantation, few if any patients with secondary MDS can expect to survive more than two years. Allogeneic stem cell transplantation offers the hope of cure for only a small number of patients. Because of poor survival and small numbers of reported patients, there are not enough data to suggest that either stem cell source or choice of conditioning regimen will significantly alter the outcome for these patients.

## CHRONIC MYELOGENOUS LEUKEMIA

Chronic myelogenous leukemia (CML) accounts for less than 5% of all leukemia cases in childhood and for nearly 20% of newly diagnosed cases in adults. The disease is considered to have three phases. The chronic phase can last for up to ten years, but this indolent phase transitions to the more aggressive and much briefer accelerated phase and finally to blast crisis. The vast majority of patients have the reciprocal chromosomal translocation t(9;22), which is called the Philadelphia chromosome.[32] The resulting BCR-ABL gene product is a protein kinase that has been shown to regulate cell growth.[33]

## Diagnostic Criteria

Patients with CML often present with fever, splenomegaly and elevated white blood cell counts. The platelet count and hemoglobin may be normal or decreased. The peripheral blood smear often has many immature elements including nucleated red blood cells, early granulocyte precursors and even blasts. Cytogenetic analysis reveals the t(9;22) abnormality in 95% of patients, while an additional 2.5% have the BCR-ABL gene identified with polymerase chain reaction.

## Therapeutic Considerations

Currently, there are at least five treatment options available to patients with CML in chronic phase: hydroxyurea, interferon-alpha, busulfan, imatinib mesylate or allogeneic stem cell transplantation. Neither hydroxyurea nor interferon alpha is considered to be curative, but both drugs can effect a clinical and cytogenetic remission in patients who present in chronic phase. The newest available therapy, imatinib mesylate, selectively inhibits the BCR-ABL tyrosine kinase. In 2002, Kantarjian et al.[34] published the results from a multi-institutional study of imatinib, which was given to 532 patients with late chronic CML who had failed to respond to interferon-alpha. The overall rate of major cytogenetic response was 64%, with 49% of patients having a complete response. The estimated rate of progression-free survival at 24 months was 84%. It is not clear that treatment with imatinib is curative; to date, only allogeneic stem cell transplant has been proven to cure some patients with this disease.

The timing of allogeneic transplant has been debated. In 1998, Gale and colleagues[35] compared the survival of patients with CML who had been treated either with stem cell transplantation, hydroxyurea, or interferon-alpha. They analyzed the International Bone Marrow Transplant Registry database and found 548 patients who had undergone an HLA-identical sibling transplant. In the first 18 months after diagnosis, survival was higher in the nontransplant cohort of 196 patients. From 18–56 months, survival was similar in both groups. After 56 months, survival was greater in the transplanted group. Seven years after diagnosis, 58% of patients in the transplanted group were still alive, while only 32% of patients taking either interferon or hydroxyurea survived. Gale further reported that patients transplanted in the first year after diagnosis fared better than those transplanted later. Since this report was an analysis of worldwide data, transplant conditioning regimens, supportive care and GVH prophylaxis were quite varied.

Somewhat different results were reported in the following year by Hehlmann et al.[36] The results of the German CML-Study Group showed similar survival at five years in the transplant and drug-therapy groups ($\sim$ 58%). When interferon therapy was stopped at least 90 days prior to transplant, no adverse effect on outcome was noted. Survival also was similar in related and unrelated transplants. Most patients received TBI in the conditioning regimen, but 28% received busulfan-based therapy. A small number of patients received antithymocyte globulin as part of the GVH prophylaxis. Eight percent of patients received marrows that were depleted of T cells.

Unrelated donor stem cell transplants might be an option for some of the 70% of patients with CML who have no sibling donor. In 1998, Hansen et al.[37] reported that 57% of 196 patients with CML who underwent unrelated donor transplants were alive five years later. In this study, all patients received cyclophosphamide (60 mg/kg for two days) and 1200 or 1320 cGy of total body irradiation. Donor marrow was not T cell-depleted, and all patients initially received cyclosporine and methotrexate for GVH prophylaxis. Patients fared worse if they were transplanted one year or more from the time of initial diagnosis,

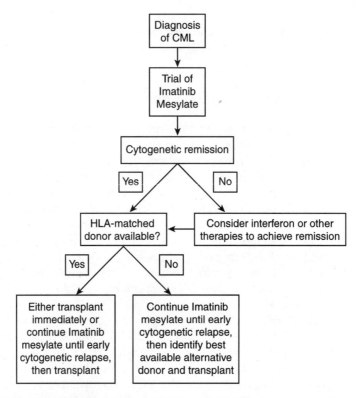

**FIGURE 14.1** Decision tree for children with chronic myelogenous leukemia.

if they were older than 50 years of age, if there was a donor-recipient mismatch at the HLA-DRB1 locus or if the patient had a high body-weight index. In fact, the five-year survival for patients who were younger than 50 years and who received an HLA-matched donor transplant within one year after diagnosis was 74%.

In 2001, Goldman and Druker[38] proposed two treatment schemas for patients with CML. Since the long-term survival for patients treated with imatinib is not known, they recommended that two options be considered. One option was that all patients receive a trial of imatinib and continue taking this drug if they achieve a remission. Once cytogenetic remission is obtained with imatinib, we currently do not know if immediate transplantation for children with an HLA-matched sibling donor will indeed be superior to continued or indefinite use of imatinib (▲ Figure 14.1). Although most centers use cyclophosphamide and TBI for conditioning, there are no randomized trials to support the superiority of a TBI-based regimen over one that uses busulfan. Questions about the ideal stem cell source remain unanswered at this time.

# REFERENCES

1. Haas OA, Gadner H. Pathogenesis, biology and management of myelodysplastic syndromes in children. Semin Hematol 1196;33:225–235.
2. Niemeyer CM, Arico M, Biondi A et al. Chronic myelomonocytic leukemia in childhood: A retrospective analysis of 110 cases. Blood 1997;89:3534–3543.
3. Stiller CA, Chessells JM, Fitchett M. Neurofibromatosis and childhood leukemia/lymphoma: A population-based UKCCSG study. Br J Cancer 1994;70:969–972.
4. Castro-Malaspina H, Schaison G, Passe S et al. Subacute and chronic myelomonocytic leukemia in children (juvenile CML). Cancer 1984;54:675–686.
5. Chan HS, Estrov Z, Weitzman S et al. The value of intensive combination chemotherapy for juvenile chronic myelogenous leukemia (JCML). Leukemia 1987;5:1960–1967.
6. Castleberry RP, Chang M, Maybee D et al. A phase II study of 13-cis-retinoic acid in juvenile myelomonocytic leukemia. A Pediatric Oncology Group Study (Abstr). Blood 1997;90:346a.
7. Mutz ID, Zoubek A. Transient response to alpha-interferon in juvenile chronic myelomonocytic leukemia. Pediatr Hematol Oncol 1988;5:71–75.
8. Matthes-Martin S, Mann G, Peters C et al. Allogeneic bone marrow transplantation for juvenile myelomonocytic leukemia: a single center experience and review of the literature. Bone Marrow Transplant 2000;26: 377–382.
9. Orchard PJ, Miller JS, McGlennen R et al. Graft-versus-leukemia is sufficient to induce remission in juvenile myelomonocytic leukemia. Bone Marrow Transplant 1998;22:201–203.
10. MacMillan ML, Davies SM, Orchard PJ et al. Haematopoietic cell transplantation in children with juvenile myelomonocytic leukemia. Br J Haematol 1998;103:552–558.
11. Bunin N, Saunders F, Leahey A et al. Alternative donor bone marrow transplantation for children with juvenile myelomonocytic leukemia. J Pediatr Hematol Oncol 1999;21:479–485.
12. Locatelli F, Niemeyer CM, Angelucci E et al. Allogeneic bone marrow transplantation for chronic myelomonocytic leukemia in childhood. J Clin Oncol 1997;15:566–573.
13. Smith FO, Sanders J, Robertson KA et al. Allogeneic marrow transplantation (BMT) for children with juvenile chronic myelogenous leukemia (JCML) (Abstr). Blood 1994;84:201a.
14. Ohta H, Kawai M, Sawada A et al. Juvenile myelomonocytic leukemia relapsing after allogeneic bone marrow transplantation successfully treated with interferon-alpha. Bone Marrow Transplant 2000;26:681–683.
15. Hasle H, Jacobsen BB, Pederson NT. Myelodysplastic syndromes in childhood: a population-based study of nine cases. Br J Haematol 1992;81:495–498.
16. Vallespi T, Imbert M, Mecucci C et al. Diagnosis, classification and cytogenetics of myelodysplastic syndromes. Haematologica 1998;83:258–275.
17. Greenberg P, Cox C, LeBeau M et al. International scoring system for evaluating prognosis in myelodysplastic syndromes. Blood 1997;89:2079–2088.
18. Verbeek W, Ganser A. Evolving treatment options of myelodysplastic syndromes. Ann Hematol 2001;80: 499–509.
19. Beran M. Intensive chemotherapy for patients with high risk myelodysplastic syndrome. Int J Hematol 2000;72:139–150.
20. Runde V, de Witte T, Arnold R et al. Bone marrow transplantation from HLA-identical siblings as first-line therapy in patients with myelodysplastic syndromes: early transplantation is associated with improved outcome. Bone Marrow Transplant 1998;21:255–261.
21. Appelbaum F, Anderson J. Bone marrow transplantation for myelodysplasia in adults and children: when and who? Leuk Res 1998;22(Suppl):S35–S39
22. Castro-Malaspina HC, Harris RE, Gajewski J et al. Unrelated donor marrow transplantation for myelodysplastic syndromes: outcome analysis of 510 transplants facilitated by the National Marrow Donor Program. Blood 2002;99:1943–1951.
23. Locatelli F, Niemeyer C, Angelucci E et al. Allogeneic bone marrow transplantation for chronic myelomonocytic leukemia in childhood: a report from the European Working Group on myelodysplastic syndromes in childhood. J Clin Oncol 1997;15:566–570.
24. Sutton L, Leblond V, Ribaud P et al. Indications and timing of allogeneic bone marrow transplantation in myelodysplastic syndromes. Leuk Lymphoma 1997;27:475–485.
25. Kröger N, Schetelig J, Zabelina T et al. A fludarabine-based dose-reduced conditioning regimen followed by allogeneic stem cell transplantation from related or unrelated donors in patients with myelodysplastic syndrome. Bone Marrow Transplant 2001;28:643–647.
26. Preisler H. The treatment of myelodysplastic syndromes. Cancer 1999;86:1893–1899.
27. Amigo ML, del Canizo MC, Rios A et al. Diagnosis of secondary myelodysplastic syndromes (MDS) following autologous transplantation should not be based on morphological criteria used for diagnosis of de novo MDS. Bone Marrow Transplant 1999;23:997–1002.

28. Ballen KK, Gilliland DG, Guinan E et al. Bone marrow transplantation for therapy-related myelodysplasia: comparison with primary myelodysplasia. Bone Marrow Transplant 1997;20:737–743.
29. Leahy AM, Friedman DL, Bunin NJ. Bone marrow transplantation in pediatric patients with therapy-related myelodysplasia and leukemia. Bone Marrow Transplant 1999;23:21–25.
30. Hale GA, Heslop HE, Bowman LC et al. Bone marrow transplantation for therapy-induced acute myeloid leukemia with previous lymphoid malignancies. Bone Marrow Transplant 1999;24:735–739.
31. Park S, Brice P, Noguerra ME et al. Myelodysplasias and leukemias after autologous stem cell transplantation for lymphoid malignancies. Bone Marrow Transplant 2000;26:321–326.
32. Rowley JD. A new consistent chromosomal abnormality in chronic myelogenous leukemia identified by quinacrine fluorescence and Giemsa staining. Nature 1973;243:290–293.
33. Sawyer CL. Chronic myeloid leukemia. N Engl J Med 1999;340:1330–1340.
34. Kantarjian H, Sawyers C, Hochhaus A et al. Hematologic and cytogenetic responses to imatinib mesylate in chronic myelogenous leukemia. N Engl J Med 2002;346:645–652.
35. Gale RP, Hehlmann R, Zhang MJ et al. Survival with bone marrow transplantation versus hydroxyurea or interferon for chronic myelogenous leukemia. Blood 1998;91:1810–1819.
36. Hehlmann R, Hochhaus A, Kolb HJ et al. Interferon alpha before allogeneic bone marrow transplantation in chronic myelogenous leukemia does not affect outcome adversely, provided it is discontinued at least 90 days before the procedure. Blood 1999;94:3668–3677.
37. Hansen JA, Gooley AT, Martin PJ et al. Bone marrow transplants from unrelated donors for patients with chronic myeloid leukemia. N Engl J Med 1998;338:962–968.
38. Goldman J, Druker B. Chronic myeloid leukemia: current treatment options. Blood 2001;98:2039–2042.

# CHAPTER XV

# Metabolic Diseases

CHARLES PETERS

The metabolic diseases are a diverse group that includes mucopolysaccharidoses, leukodystrophies, and disorders of glycoprotein metabolism. Typically, an enzyme deficiency results in failure to hydrolyze specific substrate. Due to substrate accumulation, organelle dysfunction occurs and cell destruction ensues. While disease phenotypes vary widely, they can be identified by the presence of abnormal cellular metabolites due to the specific enzyme deficiency. Hematopoietic cell transplantation (HCT) is either the only therapy or the most effective long-term treatment for selected metabolic diseases.[1] This chapter focuses on a subset of these lysosomal and peroxisomal storage diseases as well as on osteopetrosis (▼ Table 15.1). Metabolic diseases that are effectively treated by HCT include: Hurler (MPS I),[2–11] Maroteaux-Lamy (MPS VI),[12,13] and Sly (MPS VII) syndromes; cerebral X-linked adrenoleukodystrophy (CALD),[14–19] globoid-cell leukodystrophy (GLD),[17,20,21] and metachromatic leukodystrophy (MLD);[1,15,17,20,22–33] and α-mannosidosis[34] and aspartylglucosaminuria.[1,35] There are additional diseases for which HCT is probably effective, such as fucosidosis and Gaucher, types 1 and 3[36–39] as well as diseases for which HCT is possibly effective such as Farber lipogranulomatosis, galactosialidosis, GM1 gangliosidosis, mucolipidosis II (I-cell disease),[29,40–43] multiple sulfatase deficiency, Niemann-Pick types B and C[44] neuronal ceroid lipofuscinosis, sialidosis, and Wolman. Finally, as currently performed, HCT has been ineffective for three mucopolysaccharidoses: Hunter (MPS II),[20] Sanfilippo (MPS III),[45] and Morquio (MPS IV) syndromes.[46]

Objectives of HCT for these progressive, fatal diseases are: 1) to prolong survival; 2) to improve somatic and, when appropriate, neuropsychologic development; and 3) to enhance quality of life. The International Storage Disease Collaborative Study Group was formed to promote these objectives through three goals: 1) to establish an international disease-specific database; 2) to facilitate communication among health care professionals, patients, and families; and 3) to support international collaborative basic, translational, and clinical research.

With successful engraftment of allogeneic hematopoietic cells, the recipient acquires a leukocyte enzyme level equal to that of the donor. Indications for and benefits from HCT vary greatly. This chapter analyzes each group of diseases by presenting the available information including an overview, transplant indications, and transplant outcomes.

| TABLE 15.1 | Inborn Errors of Metabolism: Lysosomal and Peroxisomal Storage Diseases and Indications for Hematopoietic Cell Transplantation (HCT) | |

| Disease | HCT Indicated? | Comments |
| --- | --- | --- |
| **Mucopolysaccharidoses (MPS)** | | |
| Hurler syndrome (MPS I) | Yes | Preservation of intelligence and improved cardiopulmonary status, skeletal deformities persist |
| Hunter syndrome (MPS II) | No | Intelligence and somatic status continue to deteriorate despite HCT for severe MPS II |
| Sanfilippo syndrome (MPS III) | No | Intelligence continues to deteriorate despite HCT |
| Morquio syndrome (MPS IV) | No | Skeletal deformities persist despite HCT |
| Maroteaux-Lamy syndrome (MPS VI) | Yes | Significant somatic improvement especially cardiopulmonary |
| Sly syndrome (MPS VII) | Yes | Effective in two cases |
| **Leukodystrophies** | | |
| Childhood onset cerebral X-adrenoleukodystrophy (COCALD) | Yes | Neuropsychologic and neurologic function can be preserved after HCT |
| Globoid-cell leukodystrophy (GLD) | Yes | Dramatic improvements in neurologic, neuropsychologic, and neurophysiologic function have been noted after HCT, including cases of infantile onset |
| Metachromatic leukodystrophy (MLD) | Yes | Stabilization of CNS in juvenile and adult onset cases; however, PNS disease typically progresses especially in late infantile cases |
| Multiple sulfatase deficiency | Possibly | HCT experience in 1 case |

# MUCOPOLYSACCHARIDOSES

The mucopolysaccharidoses (MPS) are a family of heritable disorders caused by deficiency of lysosomal enzymes needed to degrade glycosaminoglycans. The diseases include Hurler and its attenuated variants Hurler-Scheie and Scheie (MPS I), Hunter (MPS II), Sanfilippo (MPS III), Morquio (MPS IV), Maroteaux-Lamy (MPS VI), and Sly (MPS VII) syndromes. Except for MPS II, all are inherited in an autosomal recessive manner. To date, transplant successes have been limited to Hurler, Maroteaux-Lamy, and Sly syndromes. The shortcomings of transplantation for Hunter, Sanfilippo, and Morquio syndromes are presented.

| TABLE 15.1 | Inborn Errors of Metabolism: Lysosomal and Peroxisomal Storage Diseases and Indications for Hematopoietic Cell Transplantation (HCT)—cont'd | |
|---|---|---|
| **Disease** | **HCT Indicated?** | **Comments** |
| *Glycoprotein Disorders* | | |
| α-mannosidosis | Yes | Significant improvement in somatic aspects including bones after HCT |
| Fucosidosis | Probably | Experience still limited; however, HCT appears to stabilize CNS |
| Aspartylglucosaminuria (AGU) | Yes | HCT very effective in small number of cases |
| *Other Lysosomal Disorders* | | |
| Glycogen storage disease, type II (Pompe disease) | No | Enzyme replacement trials in progress |
| Mucolipidosis II (I-cell disease) | Possibly | Limited HCT primarily in patients with end-stage disease |
| Wolman disease | Possibly | 1 survivor of HCT |
| Farber lipogranulomatosis (ceramidase deficiency) | Possibly | Limited HCT experience |
| Niemann-Pick | Possibly | HCT not effective for type A, can be effective for type B, possibly effective for type C |
| Gaucher | Possibly | HCT can ameliorate the somatic disease in type 1 though primary therapy is enzyme replacement; is not indicated for type 2; probably effective in type 3 |
| Fabry | No | Enzyme replacement trials in progress |
| Neuronal ceroid lipofuscinosis (NCL 1: palmitoyl protein thioesterase deficiency and NCL 2: transpeptidase deficiency) | Possibly | Limited HCT experience for infantile (NCL 1) and late infantile (NCL) 2 forms |
| $G_{M1}$ gangliosidosis | Possibly | |
| Galactosialidosis | Possibly | |
| $G_{M2}$ gangliosidoses | No | |

## Hurler Syndrome

Hurler syndrome (MPS IH) leads to premature death usually by five years of age. It is the most severe form of MPS I and is distinguishable clinically from the attenuated forms of MPS I, namely, Hurler-Scheie (MPS IH/S) and Scheie (MPS IS) syndromes. Deficiency of leukocyte α-L-iduronidase enzyme activity and the consequent accumulation of heparan sulfate and dermatan sulfate substrates contribute to the characteristic facial features, hepatosplenomegaly, cardiac disease, severe skeletal abnormalities or dysostosis multiplex, hydrocephalus, and progressive mental retardation.[47] Recently, the history of HCT for Hurler syndrome and the neuropsychological outcomes following transplant were reviewed.[4,11]

## Transplant Indications

The best Hurler syndrome candidates for HCT have stable, normal cardiopulmonary function and normal intelligence. These characteristics are more likely to be present in a child who is less than or equal to two years of age at the time of transplant.[2,3] HCT is not recommended for children with significant cardiopulmonary dysfunction and/or moderate to severe developmental delay. In the former instance, the risks of regimen-related toxicity such as pulmonary hemorrhage and/or heart failure are markedly increased. In children with marked developmental delay, the likelihood of achieving independence later in life is greatly reduced.

## Transplant Outcomes

Guidelines for HCT in Hurler children focus on six areas. Timely diagnosis is critical. The progressive developmental delay associated with Hurler syndrome can lead to an insurmountable barrier to successful outcomes. For most affected children, the diagnosis of Hurler syndrome is made during the second year of life, often due to one of the following clinical features or problems: pneumonia, cardiac failure or murmur, frequent upper respiratory tract or ear infections, characteristic somatic abnormalities, and developmental delay.

Timing of HCT is highly dependent upon the identification and selection of the optimal stem cell donor. The lowest risk of HCT-related morbidity and mortality has been associated with HLA-identical sibling donors.[3] However, few Hurler syndrome children will have such a matched, unaffected sibling to donate stem cells. Consequently, an expeditious search for an unrelated donor of bone marrow, peripheral blood, or umbilical cord blood is necessary. Delay in donor identification and processing can decrease the ultimate effectiveness of HCT due to the progression of Hurler syndrome and the associated developmental delay. While most of the clinical HCT experience has been with marrow stem cells, umbilical cord and peripheral blood stem cells are being using with increasing frequency. When successful, all stem cell sources correct the enzyme deficiency.

Preparation for HCT and long-term follow-up of a child with Hurler syndrome requires multidisciplinary team expertise. This team should consist of health care professionals in the following areas: bone marrow transplant;[2–5,48] neuropsychology;[20,49] neurology;[49] radiation therapy;[50–53] pulmonary; cardiology;[54–56] audiology;[57,58] endocrinology; ophthalmology;[59,60] physical, occupational, and speech therapy; orthopedic surgery;[61–63] otolaryngology; anesthesia;[64] nursing; as well as chaplains; social workers; and volunteer staff. The logistics of care coordination are considerable. Specialists should assess for disease involvement, potential sources of transplanted-related morbidity, and provide expert advice and support to patients and families. Furthermore, these patients should be evaluated annually after HCT since enhanced survival for these children necessitates addressing medical concerns not alleviated by HCT.

In the setting of a "timely" HCT, transplant morbidity and mortality should be minimized while maximizing the benefit of donor engraftment. Preparation for the transplant must be sufficiently immunosuppressive and myeloablative to enhance the likelihood of donor cell engraftment while minimizing the chance of rejection. Failure to achieve stable engraftment in Hurler patients has been a concern following both related and unrelated donor bone marrow transplantation (BMT).[2,3,5] A consensus regarding optimal myeloablative and immunosuppressive preparation for BMT in Hurler syndrome awaits future study as suggested by Peters and Guffon and other investigators.[2,3,10] Preliminary work suggests that the Hurler hematopoietic microenvironment may be relatively inhospitable to the support of normal hematopoiesis and Hurler stem cells may be more resistant to myeloablative therapy (Verfaillie C and Gupta P, personal communication). These areas require further laboratory and clinical investigation. In addition, toxicity to fragile organ systems such as the brain, lungs, and heart should be minimized. It is clear that Hurler children who undergo HCT are at increased risk for regimen-related complications such as pulmonary hemorrhage and pneumonitis.[65] The etiology of pulmonary hemorrhage remains obscure, but may be due, in part, to the effect of radiation and/or chemotherapy on lung parenchyma that contains glycosaminoglycan storage material and activated macrophages. Other important peri- and posttransplant issues include choosing a stem cell source, matching, and optimizing cell dose, as well as preventing graft-versus-host disease (GVHD), which has been observed at an increased frequency and severity in transplanted Hurler patients.[2,3] GVHD is of no clinical benefit to these patients; in fact, Hurler syndrome children who develop grade II or worse acute GVHD following HCT have significantly poorer cognitive outcomes. However, with improved technology in the area of immunophenotyping and matching, the likelihood of correctly identifying a matched unrelated donor has been enhanced.

Long-term neurodevelopment of a Hurler child is dependent upon the baseline level of function prior to HCT, the beneficial effects of donor-derived α-L-iduronidase enzyme activity, and the recommendations and individual education programs which stem from detailed annual neuropsychologic evaluations after HCT.[2,3,15,49,66] HCT can lead to stabilization of intellectual function over 6 to 12 months after HCT. Importantly, donor-derived monocytes can provide a level of enzyme equal to that of the donor; central nervous system microglia arise from monocytes. The ultimate enzyme level achieved appears to correlate with long-term neuropsychologic function.[3]

As more Hurler children become long-term survivors of HCT, the concept of "favorable outcome" will evolve from engrafted survival with continuing cognitive development to include the concept of independence in activities of daily living as well as a positive quality-of-life. Mobility, cognitive competence, preservation of sensory ability, independence in daily activities, and the absence of pain are factors that contribute to a positive quality-of-life outcome.[4]

Outcomes following HCT in Hurler patients can and should be assessed from a variety of perspectives. The Hurler transplant experience of the North American Storage Disease Collaborative Study Group has been reported for 40 patients undergoing unrelated donor transplant and for 54 patients transplanted from related donors.[2,3] Briefly, these two reports describe the patient characteristics for the largest groups of Hurler patients transplanted in the world. Regimen-related complications included significant acute and chronic GVHD as well as mortality. Likelihood of survival with donor-derived engraftment was 73% for related donor transplants and 33% for unrelated donor transplants. The reports concluded that Hurler patients, particularly those less than 24 months of age with a baseline Mental Developmental Index greater than 70, could achieve a favorable long-term outcome with continuing cognitive development and prolonged survival after successful transplant. The ultimate enzyme activity level achieved did influence neuropsychologic outcome. Current protocols are addressing the high risk of graft rejection or failure and the impact of GVHD in this patient population.

Engraftment after HCT leads to reduction of substrate in liver, tonsils, conjunctiva, cerebrospinal fluid (CSF), and urine.[5,59,64,67,68] With respect to the brain, successful HCT can prevent the development of hydrocephalus.[6,20] In Hurler syndrome, the pathology of the brain shows accumulation of mucopolysaccharide material around the blood vessels in the brain. This is visualized by brain magnetic resonance imaging (MRI). Subsequent to transplantation, these areas are significantly reduced. Opening CSF pressure as determined by lumbar puncture normalizes after successful engraftment.

The effect of donor enzyme status on neuropsychological outcome in Hurler children who had a Mental Developmental Index (MDI) over 70 before HCT has been studied. The correlation of normalized α-L-iduronidase enzyme activity levels with the latest MDI scores for these children was significant.[3] Normalized α-L-iduronidase enzyme activity levels correlated with the latest MDI scores for these children. No child whose ultimate enzyme activity level was low due to either a heterozygous carrier donor or partial engraftment from a homozygous normal donor had normal mental functioning at follow-up. Children who retained fully normal intelligence were all completely engrafted from a homozygous enzymatically-normal donor.

Hearing has normalized in 30% of transplanted patients, in contrast to the natural progressive loss of hearing in untransplanted patients.[17] Careful follow-up is indicated. If a significant hearing deficit persists, appropriate intervention such as fitting for hearing aids should be performed. In most instances, sleep apnea resolves after HCT and tonsillectomy and adenoidectomy are not required. While otitis media is usually reduced; in many instances, myringotomy with placement of tympanostomy tubes are still needed.

Cardiac failure due to narrowed epicardial coronary arteries and myocardial glycosaminoglycan (GAG) accumulation has been common in untransplanted Hurler children.[54,55] The grave consequences secondary to cardiac problems have been obviated in those engrafted for one to two years after HCT. Myocardial muscle function is stabilized or improved and epicardial coronary artery patency has been documented up to 14 years after HCT.[56] The sensitivity of pulse Doppler during echocardiography has allowed an evaluation of the cardiac valves. Murmurs related to mitral and tricuspid insufficiency have been noted, along with increased thickening of the respective valves. The relative amount of changes in valves is considerably less than in the untransplanted child; however, in long-term survivors significant deposition of GAG has been observed, necessitating long-term cardiology follow-up. To date, after more than 19 years, no transplanted Hurler patient from the University of Minnesota has required cardiac valve replacement.

Survival of engrafted Hurler syndrome patients is radically changed from that of untransplanted patients.[7] Long-term survival data indicate that the life span will be extended many decades. This remarkable improvement is directly attributable to persistence of leukocyte α-L-iduronidase enzyme activity. Permanent enzyme expression is due to adoptive transfer of the donor hematopoietic system that includes a new monocyte-phagocyte system.

Although engraftment provides resolution of the lysosomal lesions in most organs of the body after transplantation, generally this does not occur in the skeletal system. The mucopolysaccharide collection in the lysosomes of the chondrocytes persists after engraftment.[61] Direct cell-to-cell contact between the chondrocytes of the recipient and the monocyte-macrophage of the hematopoietic system is limited. Transplanted Hurler patients will likely require orthopedic surgery for carpal tunnel syndrome and trigger digits,[62] genu valgum,[63] hip acetabular dysplasia, and possibly for kyphoscoliosis.[48] In contrast, odontoid hypoplasia corrects by eight to ten years of age following successfully engrafted transplants.[69] This is important since ondontoid hypoplasia can be associated with C1-C2 vertebral instability, displacement, and consequent paraplegia. Future transplantation of mesenchymal stem cells could decrease this need for orthopedic interventions.[70,71] In vitro, human mesenchymal stem cells provide progenitors for osteoblasts and chondrocytes. Such differentiated progeny are not supplied by hematopoietic stem cells.

Further study of factors and procedures that lead to a better quality of life for Hurler patients is needed, as the outcomes of quality of life assessments based upon the perspectives of the parent, child, and physician may differ.[4] Quality of life with respect to health outcomes in long-term engrafted Hurler patients ranges from restricted to near normal from the physician's point of view. While we believe that improved quality of life after HCT will occur as a result of earlier diagnosis and transplant preferably during the first year of life, additional study is needed.

Particular attention has been given to genotypic analysis and the ability to predict disease severity or phenotype. Although many mutations have been found that result in a spectrum of severity, two mutations, W402X and Q70X, as well as others result in the severe form of the disease.[2,3,6,8–10,72–76] Over 40 children with phenotypically severe Hurler syndrome from the University of Minnesota had mutation analysis performed by Dr. John Hopwood at Adelaide Children's Hospital, Australia. All children had the following evaluations at baseline: MDI, head circumference, height, weight, vision, hearing, skeletal abnormalities, echocardiograms, computerized axial tomographic volumetric studies of liver and spleen ($N = 12$), and scan of the brain and upper cervical spine. Enzyme level at baseline for all children was $<0.1$ nm/mg of protein/h. Based on these data, we concluded that mutations other than W402X and Q70X did not allow prediction of a severe phenotype for patients with Hurler syndrome.

The indication for HCT is less clear in the attenuated phenotypes of MPS I due to the much slower disease course.[47] Central nervous system (CNS) deterioration can be insidious; for MPS IS, life expectancy can extend into the fourth and fifth decades. It seems likely that enzyme replacement therapy (ERT)[77] will become the mainstay of therapy for these children, since lack of CNS penetration of administered enzyme is presumably less crucial than in MPS IH. However, this may change if transplantation technology improves substantially, especially with the use of reduced intensity conditioning regimens.

## Hunter, Sanfilippo, and Morquio Syndromes

Hunter syndrome comprises two recognized clinical entities, severe and attenuated, arising from deficiency of lysosomal iduronate sulfatase enzyme activity. The severe form of Hunter syndrome has features similar to those of Hurler syndrome, except for the lack of corneal clouding and slower progression of somatic and central nervous system involvement. Coarse facial features, short stature, skeletal deformities, joint stiffness, and mental retardation characterize the severe form of Hunter syndrome with onset between two and four years of age. The attenuated form is somewhat analogous to MPS IS, with a prolonged life span, minimal to no CNS involvement, and a slow progression of somatic deterioration. An X-linked recessive pattern of inheritance is found in both forms of Hunter syndrome.[47]

Sanfilippo syndrome is comprised of four biochemically diverse but clinically similar groups (type A: heparan N-sulfatase; type B: α-N-acetylglucosaminidase; type C: acetyl

CoA:α-glucosaminide acetyltransferase; and type D: N-acetylglucosamine 6-sulfatase). The four enzymes are required for the degradation of heparan sulfate. Sanfilippo syndrome is characterized by severe CNS degeneration yet with only mild somatic disease. Onset of clinical features usually occurs between two and six years in a child who previously appeared normal. Presenting features can include hyperactivity with aggressive behavior, delayed development, coarse, hirsutism, sleep disorders, and mild hepatosplenomegaly. Skeletal involvement is minimal, with only mild dysostosis multiplex, usually normal stature, and mild joint stiffness, that rarely causes loss of function. Recurrent and sometimes severe diarrhea is unexplained but usually improves in older children. Speech development is often delayed, with poor articulation and content. Severe hearing impairment is common. Seizures can occur in the older patient. Severe neurologic degeneration occurs in most patients by six to ten years of age, accompanied by rapid deterioration of social and adaptive skills.[47]

Morquio syndrome is caused by defective degradation of keratan sulfate due to deficiency in either N-acetylgalactosamine 6-sulfatase (MPS IVA) or β-galactosidase (MPS IVB). Both types of Morquio syndrome are characterized by short trunk dwarfism, corneal clouding, a skeletal (spondyloepiphyseal) dysplasia distinct from that seen in the other MPS disorders, and preservation of intelligence. The predominant clinical features of Morquio syndrome are those related to the skeleton and its effects on the CNS. Patients with Morquio syndrome appear normal at birth. The appearance of genu valgum, kyphosis, growth retardation with short trunk and neck, and waddling gait with a tendency to fall are early symptoms of the syndrome. Odontoid hypoplasia is a universal clinical finding with grave medical consequences. Instability of the hypoplastic odontoid process with ligamentous laxity can result in life-threatening atlantoaxial subluxation. Patients with the severe form of Morquio syndrome can develop cervical myelopathy early in life; consequently, they may not survive beyond the third or fourth decades. Paralysis from the myelopathy, restrictive chest wall movement, and valvular heart disease all contribute to their shortened life spans.[47]

### Transplant Indications

It had been hoped that HCT would achieve similar benefits in severe Hunter syndrome to those observed in Hurler patients. Unfortunately, HCT in boys with severe Hunter has failed to alter the disease course favorably and significantly.[20] Furthermore, at this time, the risk attendant with HCT appears to be greater than any possible benefits in MPS IIB. For MPS III, Sanfilippo syndrome, the cumulative, long-term follow-up experience of HCT also has been very disappointing from a neuropsychologic standpoint.[45] Clearly, this is an area that merits additional study. Finally, HCT does not ameliorate the severe skeletal deformities that are associated with Morquio syndrome.[20]

### Transplant Outcomes

HCT is not recommended for either severe or attenuated Hunter syndrome as it fails to stabilize intellectual function in the former case and is not justifiable in the latter; it also fails to stabilize intellectual function in children with Sanfilippo syndrome. Unfortunately, HCT is not currently recommended for Morquio disease as well.[20,45] However, with the development of mesenchymal stem cell transplant, these and other disorders may become amenable to transplantation.

## Maroteaux-Lamy Syndrome

Maroteaux-Lamy syndrome is due to deficiency of leukocyte arylsulfatase B enzyme activity. Patients with Maroteaux-Lamy syndrome usually exhibit normal mental development, though physical and visual impairments may impede psychomotor performance. The somatic involvement in the severe form of Maroteaux-Lamy syndrome is similar to that in Hurler syndrome. An enlarged head and a deformed chest may be present at birth. Obvious corneal clouding develops in some patients and can result in visual impairment. Hepatomegaly and umbilical or inguinal hernias are common. The skeletal changes are similar to those seen in the dysostosis multiplex of Hurler syndrome. Spinal cord compression from thickening of the dura in the upper cervical spinal canal with resultant myelopathy is frequent in the milder forms of MPS VI.[47] Short stature is the rule. Claw-hand deformities develop and carpal tunnel syndrome can occur. Restriction of joint movement (knee, hip, and elbow) develops in the first years of life, and the children assume a crouched stance. Cardiac abnormalities characterized by thickening and stenosis of the aortic and mitral valves have been observed. Current methodology examining urinary excretion of glycosaminoglycans is indicative of disease severity.

### Transplant Indications

Patients should be comprehensively examined to ensure stable cardiopulmonary function and to establish baseline neuropsychological function. Particular care must be taken if a patient with advanced stage disease is to be transplanted. Catastrophic pulmonary complications including hemorrhage have been observed in a significant percentage of MPS VI transplants. For many patients with MPS VI, ERT will be an alternative therapy to transplant.

### Transplant Outcomes

Reports of the benefits of bone marrow transplantation in Maroteaux-Lamy have been published.[12,13] Following successful engraftment, arylsulfatase B enzyme activity levels have normalized, hepatosplenomegaly has decreased, and visual acuity and joint mobility were improved.

## Sly Syndrome

Sly syndrome is characterized by deficiency of leukocyte β-glucuronidase enzyme activity.

### Transplant Indications

Assessments of cardiopulmonary and neuropsychologic function at baseline are recommended.

### Transplant Outcomes

In mice deficient in β-glucuronidase enzyme activity, HCT reverses the pathology of the cochlea, tympanic membranes, and inner ear, as well as the hearing capacity.[78] In two patients with MPS VII, HCT appeared to be a potentially beneficial therapy. Longer follow-up and careful selection of cases for HCT are needed.

# LEUKODYSTROPHIES

The leukodystrophies are a group of progressive degenerative disorders involving myelin of the central and peripheral nervous systems. The principle diseases to be considered are cerebral X-linked adrenoleukodystrophy (CALD), globoid-cell leukodystrophy (GLD), and metachromatic leukodystrophy (MLD).

## Cerebral X-linked Adrenoleukodystrophy

X-linked adrenoleukodystrophy is a disorder that affects the white matter of the nervous system, adrenal cortex, and testes. Its minimum incidence is estimated to be 1:20,000. While clinical manifestations are most severe in males, approximately 20% of female carriers have mild to moderate disability. At least six distinct phenotypes have been described. They range in severity from the rapidly progressive childhood cerebral form, more slowly progressive adult forms that affect the spinal cord mainly, to rarer forms in which the nervous system remains intact. The various phenotypes co-occur frequently within the same family or kindred. The illness does not manifest clinically before the age of three years. Biochemical or genetic studies can diagnose it in the newborn period and also prenatally; however, these tests do not permit prediction of the phenotype. The principal biochemical abnormality is the accumulation of saturated very long chain fatty acids (VLCFA), due to the impaired capacity to degrade these substances in the peroxisome. The defective gene has been mapped to Xq28 and codes for a peroxisomal membrane protein that is a member of the adenosine 5'-triphosphate (ATP) binding cassette transporter family, and appears to be required for the transport of VLCFA into the peroxisome. The adrenal insufficiency can be readily managed by glucocorticoid and mineralocorticoid replacement therapy. The testicular dysfunction is relatively rare. However, central nervous system involvement is frequent, progressive, and fatal.[79] The only effective therapy for CALD is HCT.[14,18,19]

The cerebral form of X-linked adrenoleukodystrophy (ALD) is a demyelinating disorder of the central nervous system that leads to a vegetative state and death. The symptoms include a variety of neuropsychologic and neurologic manifestations due to demyelination located preferentially in parieto-occipital white matter and pyramidal tracts within the brain stem, and less frequently in frontal white matter or the internal capsules.[80,81] The disease can progress for one to three years; at this stage, patients may have either no neurologic signs or minor changes and subtle neurocognitive defects (visual spatial deficits in the occipital forms, execution and attention deficits in the frontal form). Then, demyelination accelerates, leading to a vegetative state or death within three years.[80] This advanced stage corresponds to the onset of inflammatory lesions with accumulation of macrophages and mononuclear cells within the active edge of demyelinating lesions. At this stage, MRI shows marked progression of demyelination and focal disruption of the blood-brain barrier.[80,81] Allogeneic HCT had been unsuccessful when performed at an advanced stage of cerebral disease.[82-84] An early report raised hope that HCT performed at an earlier stage of disease could stabilize and even reverse demyelination, thus supporting further evaluation of this therapeutic approach.[14]

### Transplant Indications

The mechanisms by which functional bone marrow cells exert favorable effects on cerebral demyelination in ALD remain unclear. Recent observations have raised the possibility of normalization of VLCFA in ALD patients by pharmacological approaches.[85,86] However, over the past decade, HCT remains the only therapeutic approach of proven benefit in the cerebral form of ALD. It is hoped that better selection of human lymphocyte antigen (HLA)-matched donors may decrease the risk of the procedure.

The clinical experience with HCT for CALD and the natural history of X-linked ALD raise two important questions. First, given the wide phenotypic variation in X-linked ALD, which patients with the biochemical defect of X-linked ALD are likely to develop cerebral demyelination and therefore would be recommended to have HCT? Second, which factors immediately prior to transplant predict the outcome of HCT? Because HCT carries significant risks, these questions are not trivial.

No correlation has been found between the nature of the ALD gene mutation,[87] the biochemical defect,[80] and the clinical phenotype.[88] Consequently, diagnosis of cerebral ALD is difficult in the early stages. As no definitive biological marker has been found, careful monitoring with MRI and neuropsychologic tests demonstrate the onset and progression of early cerebral demyelination in boys for whom HCT is recommended and prognosis is favorable. Initial identification of these boys occurs as a result of documenting elevated VLCFA levels (identified during family screening) or is due to isolated adrenal insufficiency. All boys diagnosed before 10 years of age with adrenal insufficiency should be tested for X-linked ALD.

MRI site and extent of demyelination, neuropsychologic test results, and rate of progression prior to HCT are the only predictors of beneficial outcome.[19,66,89,90] From experience at the University of Minnesota, we have learned that MRI severity score predicts the likelihood of survival after HCT and also accurately identifies the early onset of disease. Furthermore, the performance IQ component of the neuropsychologic profile predicts the degree of disability in survivors and identifies patients at high risk for poor outcomes. Determining the rate of disease progression before BMT is also crucial, particularly in patients less than eight years of age who can have a very rapid progression of demyelination. Evaluation of MRI and neuropsychological decline at intervals of three to four months before BMT will provide an estimate of the rate of disease progression. This is important given the usual progression of demyelinating lesions during the six months following HCT and the relatively narrow window of opportunity that patients with advanced disease may have before rapid decline. Clearly, biological markers are urgently needed to help with this decision. A proton magnetic resonance spectroscopy (MRS) study demonstrated a correlation between the neuropsychological scores and the abnormal choline/creatine and N-acetylaspartate/creatinine ratios in white matter from ALD patients.[88,91] Longitudinal studies are needed to determine if these MRS abnormalities are useful markers of disease evolution.

## Transplant Outcomes

The following transplant guidelines for boys and men with cerebral X-linked ALD are provided. Timing of HCT is critically important. Patients, biochemically diagnosed who are still without signs of the disease by neuropsychologic and/or neurologic evaluation, require serial monitoring to identify the onset of cerebral disease.[66] MRI of the brain with determination of the Loes severity score is also very informative.[90,91] In the cases of patients diagnosed with CALD on the basis of clinical neuropsychologic and/or neurologic abnormalities, if HCT is to be performed, it must occur as soon as possible. Historically, we recommended that patients receive dietary therapy and Lorenzo's oil for at least one month prior to HCT to achieve normalization of plasma VLCFA. There had been clinical experience suggesting that this reduced the risk of certain life-threatening hemorrhagic complications during and after the transplant. It is now unclear whether there is any benefit from Lorenzo's oil and a restricted diet before or after HCT.

The optimal stem cell source for these patients is not known. Successes have occurred following both bone marrow and umbilical cord blood transplants. The significance of using a donor who is a carrier for X-linked ALD is not clear. The transplant process should be designed to minimize neurotoxicity. For example, busulfan is neurotoxic and can cause seizures.[92] Total body irradiation has typically been delivered to the entire brain. A novel total body irradiation technique has led to sparing of the brain. At some institutions, intravenous intralipid nutrition and benzodiazepines have been avoided on the basis of either adverse clinical events or other considerations. Long-term follow-up should include assessments of neuropsychological function, neurologic status, and MRI of the brain. It is recognized that many patients with cerebral disease will have long-term disabilities requiring additional supportive services.[49]

The outcomes following HCT for cerebral X-linked ALD have been highly variable depending upon disease status at transplant as well as transplant-related complications. Shapiro et al. reported that BMT can halt the progressive demyelination and neurological deterioration.[18] Twelve engrafted patients with childhood onset of cerebral ALD have been followed for five to ten years after bone marrow transplantation. Magnetic resonance imaging, neurological, neuropsychological, electrophysiological, and plasma VLCFA measurements were used to evaluate the effect of this treatment. Magnetic resonance imaging showed complete reversal in two patients and improvement in one. One patient showed no change from baseline to last follow-up. All eight patients who showed an initial period of continued demyelination stabilized and remained unchanged thereafter. Motor function remained normal or improved after transplant in ten patients. Verbal intelligence remained within the normal range for eleven patients. Performance (nonverbal) abilities were improved or were stable in seven patients. Decline followed by stability occurred in five patients. Plasma VLCFA levels decreased by 55% and remained slightly above the upper limits of normal. Five- to ten-year follow-up of twelve patients with childhood cerebral adrenoleukodystrophy demonstrated the long-term beneficial effect of bone marrow transplantation when the procedure was performed at an early stage of the disease.[18]

From 1981 to 1999, 126 consecutive males with cerebral X-linked ALD with a wide range of disease severity underwent transplants using HLA-identical matched sibling donors, partially-matched related donor, or unrelated donors. Stem cell sources included bone marrow and umbilical cord blood. Ninety percent of patients engrafted with donor cells. The five-year survival was 58%. The leading causes of death were progressive ALD, pulmonary complications, and GVHD. Preliminary results indicate that stabilization of neurologic and neuropsychologic status did occur following engraftment in a large proportion of evaluable, engrafted survivors. Severity of disease, as measured by the pre-transplant performance IQ, was the most sensitive indicator of prognosis.[93] Performance IQ evaluates visual perception, spatial, motor, and reasoning abilities.

HCT in severely involved patients with cerebral X-ALD presents a significant challenge. One marker of marked disease severity, a Performance IQ less than 80 (average range = 85 to 115) has proven to be a reliable predictor of failure. Patients in this group showed rapid rates of disease progression and mortality, despite treatment with HCT. Unrelated donors were used to treat most of these severely involved patients, due to a lack of unaffected HLA matched sibling donors. Engraftment has been a complicating factor as well. To enhance engraftment, several preparative regimen protocols were compared. Many severely affected patients who received total body irradiation and/or busulfan as part of their preparative regimen experienced rapid neurologic and neuropsychologic deterioration. Busulfan is neurotoxic;[92] furthermore, it was hypothesized that radiation-induced demyelination was contributing to rapid disease progression immediately following HCT.[94] Despite favorable rates of engraftment with total body irradiation, significant CNS deterioration and death often followed. A novel approach using immunosuppression is being evaluated in boys with advanced stage cerebral disease who are not candidates for transplant.

## Globoid Cell Leukodystrophy

Globoid cell leukodystrophy is an autosomal recessive disease due to greatly diminished or absent activity of the lysosomal enzyme galactocerebrosidase. The disease is characterized by progressive loss of central and peripheral myelin, and spasticity, dementia, and peripheral neuropathy. It ends in a chronic vegetative state and early death. The more common form begins in early infancy during the first six months of life with nonspecific symptoms such as irritability or hypersensitivity to external stimuli, but soon progresses rapidly, often leading to death by two years of age. The late onset form of the disease has a more insidious onset from childhood to adulthood and progresses over a period of several years to a decade to death.[95–97]

### Transplant Indications

The indications and contraindications for HCT will be enumerated. HCT has been used to treat more than 34 patients with GLD around the world. In some cases, the anticipated progression of signs and symptoms were arrested after engraftment, supporting the hypothesis that allogeneic HCT can be effective in GLD. In a recent report, five patients with GLD (one with early onset type, four with late onset type) were treated by allogeneic HCT.[99] Evaluations including leukocyte galactocerebrosidase levels, neurological examinations, neuropsychological tests, magnetic resonance imaging of central nervous system, cerebrospinal fluid protein assays, and neurophysiologic measurements were performed before and after transplant with follow-up from one to nine years. Engraftment of donor derived hematopoietic cells occurred in all patients and was followed by restoration of leukocyte galactocerebrosidase. In the four patients with late onset disease the central nervous system deterioration was reversed, while in the patient with the infantile form anticipated signs and symptoms have not appeared. Magnetic resonance imaging has shown a decrease in signal intensity in the three late onset patients who were assessed before and after transplantation. Cerebrospinal fluid total protein abnormalities were corrected in three late onset disease patients and significantly reduced in the patient with the infantile form. Central nervous system manifestations of GLD can be reversed by allogeneic HCT.[99]

The GLD patients most likely to benefit from HCT are those with late onset disease, since the rate of disease progression is slower and the severity of disease is generally less than that encountered in an infant with early onset GLD. When HCT has failed, it has been due to either progression of disease in early onset cases or a transplant-related complication such as GVHD in an adolescent or adult with late onset GLD.[99]

## Transplant Outcomes

Guidelines for performing HCT for both early and late onset GLD patients are as follows:

First, the extent, severity of disease, and its rate of progression should be carefully studied prior to HCT using neurologic, neuropsychologic, neuroradiologic, and neurophysiologic examinations. A lumbar puncture with determination of CSF protein and opening pressure can be informative.

Second, the natural history of the disease should be considered together with the time needed to stabilize the disease process. This period includes: a) time to perform HLA typing, b) donor search, c) preparative therapy and HCT, and d) the six to twelve month period following HCT, which is needed to stabilize the GLD through the delivery of donor-derived enzyme-producing cells to the nervous system.

Generally, it has been difficult to arrest the disease course satisfactorily in the early onset form of GLD. To date, if Krabbe disease is diagnosed antenatally, it can only be ameliorated if HCT is performed in the neonatal period;[99,100] however, for cases of late onset disease, it has been possible to achieve stability or even improvement in some cases. The limited number of HCT cases makes generalization difficult.

## Metachromatic Leukodystrophy

Metachromatic leukodystrophy (MLD) is an autosomal recessive inherited disorder of myelin metabolism characterized by accumulation of cerebroside sulfate in white matter of the central nervous system and in peripheral nerves. MLD is one of the more common lysosomal storage disorders.[100,101] The estimated incidence has ranged from 1 in 25,000 to 1 in 40,000 with a gene frequency of 0.5%. Documentation of deficiency of arylsulfatase A enzyme activity is necessary but not sufficient to diagnose the disease. The reason is that the arylsulfatase A pseudodeficiency allele is common in the general population; nearly 30% of the general population are carriers. In MLD kindreds, up to 15% of family members are heterozygous for the arylsulfatase A pseudodeficiency allele. Patients with MLD also demonstrate excessive amounts of sulfatides in the urine. MLD may appear at any age. The late infantile form is first recognized in the second year of life and is fatal within a few years. Juvenile forms present between the ages of 4 and 12 years, while the adult form may begin from the mid-teenage years to the seventh decade. In each type, gait disturbance, mental regression, and urinary incontinence are among the earliest signs. Other common signs in the childhood forms include blindness, loss of speech, quadriparesis, peripheral neuropathy, and seizures. In the adult with MLD, behavioral disturbances and dementia are the major presenting signs that are often mistakenly attributed to a psychiatric disorder. The adult form of MLD may progress slowly over decades.

Diagnostic testing should include at least leukocyte arylsulfatase A enzyme activity and measurement of urinary sulfatides. Other evaluations typically include neurologic, neuroradiologic, neuropsychologic, and neurophysiologic examinations as well as a lumbar puncture. A skin biopsy may be performed to conduct radiolabeled sulfatide loading studies on fibroblasts. Sural nerve biopsy is sometimes performed.[100,101]

## Transplant Indications

HCT is an effective method of providing normal arylsulfatase A enzyme activity to patients with MLD. With long-term engraftment, many patients have had amelioration of disease signs and symptoms and prolongation of survival. These patients were treated after a clinical diagnosis was made and supported by biochemical abnormalities. The selection of an appropriate candidate for HCT must take into account an array of factors.

First, symptomatic patients with late infantile MLD have been relatively poor candidates for HCT because of the propensity for the disease to progress rapidly prior to the time when stabilization can be accomplished by HCT.[1,24,30,31] Furthermore, the peripheral nervous system disability is relatively refractory to the beneficial effects of HCT, which are primarily to the central nervous system. In the cases of juvenile and adult onset cases, careful neurologic, neuropsychologic, neuroradiologic, and neurophysiologic assessments will assist the transplant team in determining the likelihood that a particular patient will derive significant benefit from transplant.[24,28,30,31]

Second, the world's HCT experience remains limited to less than 100 cases. Opportunities to intervene with HCT before the appearance of clinical disease have been few. The advantages include, most importantly, the prevention of clinical symptoms. Due to a diagnosis of MLD in an older sibling, the patient can be treated by HCT prior to the onset of clinical signs. A small cohort of patients with MLD have been evaluated and transplanted prior to development of clinical signs.[30] Several caveats apply. In order to maximize the effectiveness of the transplant therapy, the donor should have homozygous normal arylsulfatase A enzyme activity. Where this has not been the case, the results have been less encouraging. Effective GVHD prophylaxis is essential in order to minimize central nervous system deterioration secondary to damage by activated microglia. Time of transplantation relative to disease onset in the prior affected sibling is critical. As a general rule, at least one year should separate the age at which the older sibling developed clinical signs and the age at transplant of the younger pre-symptomatic, biochemically diagnosed patient.

Finally, there are plans for several centers to collaborate in an infant screening program for MLD. By examining urinary sulfatides, it may be possible to identify affected children before onset of symptoms. These clinically unaffected infants could be considered as potential candidates for HCT. This approach could herald the beginning of a new era in clinical care and management for MLD.

## Transplant Outcomes

The extent, severity of disease, and its rate of progression should be carefully studied prior to HCT using neurologic, neuropsychologic, neuroradiologic, and neurophysiologic examinations. A lumbar puncture with determination of CSF protein and opening pressure can be informative. The natural history of the disease should be considered together with the time needed to stabilize the disease process. This period includes: a) time to perform HLA typing, b) donor search, c) preparative therapy and HCT, and d) the six to twelve month period following HCT, which is needed to stabilize the MLD through the delivery of donor-derived enzyme-producing cells to the nervous system.

Generally, it has been difficult to arrest the disease course satisfactorily in the late infantile form of MLD; however, for cases of juvenile and adult onset disease, it has been possible to achieve stability in the central nervous system in some cases. Pre-symptomatic, biochemically diagnosed patients with MLD appear to derive the greatest benefit from HCT. The limited number of HCT cases can make generalization difficult.[24,28,30,31]

## Gaucher Disease

Gaucher disease is a lysosomal glycolipid storage disorder characterized by the accumulation of glucosylceramide (glucocerebroside) due to a deficiency of glucocerebrosidase enzyme activity.[102] Three types of Gaucher disease have been described. Type 1, the most common with a prevalence of 1:40,000, is distinguished from types 2 and 3 disease by the lack of primary central nervous system involvement. Type 2, the acute neuronopathic form of Gaucher disease, has an early onset with severe CNS involvement and death usually within the first two years of life. Type 3, subacute neuronopathic Gaucher disease, has neurologic symptoms with a later onset and a more chronic course than that observed in type 2 disease. Hepatosplenomegaly, bone lesions, and occasionally involvement of lungs and other organs occur in all forms of Gaucher disease. The quality of life of Gaucher patients can be im-proved by a variety of medical and surgical procedures such as joint replacement and splenectomy. The accumulation of glucosylceramide and associated clinical manifestations can be reversed by repeated infusions of modified acid beta-glucosidase (alglucerase). ERT has been used extensively and effectively in type 1 disease and to a lesser extent and with much less efficacy for type 2 and 3 patients. Issues of intravenous access and associated complications, patient comfort and lifestyle, as well as resources have led to a critical review of the risks and benefits of ERT enzyme replacement therapy. Furthermore, evidence is accumulating that some organs or tissues such as lungs, lymphoid tissue, and the nervous system may derive little benefit from ERT. In fact, progressive dementia and myoclonic encephalopathy have been observed in type 3 patients who were so treated.[103]

### Transplant Indications

The indications for HCT are less clearly defined for Gaucher disease than for other lysosomal storage diseases. The therapeutic successes of ERT for type 1 Gaucher disease have led to a general reluctance to intervene with a treatment modality with significant morbidity and mortality. However, with persistence or progression of severe bone pain (type 1) (Grabowski G. personal communication), the expense of ERT,[104–106] and the progression of neurologic disease (type 3),[103] more careful and critical consideration is being given to the use of HCT for these disease types and circumstances.

### Transplant Outcomes

The HCT experience is limited in Gaucher disease due, in part, to the enthusiasm for enzyme replacement therapy. However, cure of type 3 and severe type 1 disease can be achieved by HCT.[1,20,36,37,39,107] The hematologic and visceral effects of HCT on the disease have been excellent. The transplanted children have experienced catch-up in growth and no further neurological or mental deterioration.

## Mannosidosis

Alpha-mannosidosis is an autosomal-recessive inherited lysosomal storage disease caused by deficiency of alpha-mannosidase enzyme activity.[108] This defect in degradation of glycoproteins leads to excretion of mannose-rich oligosaccharides in the urine and accumulation of oligosaccharides in various tissues, including central nervous system, liver, and bone marrow.[108] Type I (infantile) alpha-mannosidosis, a more severe form, closely resembles Hurler syndrome. The onset of symptoms occurs before age 12 months, with macrocephaly, coarse facial features, hepatosplenomegaly, dysostosis multiplex, loss of previously acquired developmental skills, mental retardation, and recurrent infections. There is progressive deterioration, with death typically occurring between 3 and 12 years of age. Walkley et al.[109] demonstrated that HCT is effective in the feline model of mannosidosis. They showed that α-mannosidase could be detected in the brain of transplanted animals.

### Transplant Indications

Wall and colleagues[34] have described successful HCT for a 19-month-old child with alpha-mannosidosis leading to complete resolution of the recurrent sinopulmonary disease and organomegaly, improvement in the bony disease, and stabilization of neurocognitive function. Since this report at least three additional patients with α-mannosidosis have received HCT. At this time, four of five patients transplanted are long-term engrafted survivors and have derived significant benefits from HCT. It should be noted that several patients have experienced significant pulmonary complications from 10 to 20 weeks after transplant. No infectious etiology could be identified. Storage disease patients appear to be at increased risk for pulmonary complications including hemorrhage and/or bronchiolitis obliterans organizing pneumonitis.

### Transplant Outcomes

Thorough clinical assessment is indicated for patients with α-mannosidosis prior to HCT. Generally, patients transplanted early in their disease course prior to the onset of significant disease-related complications are the best candidates.

## Aspartylglucosaminuria

Aspartylglucosaminuria (AGU) is caused by deficiency of aspartylglucosaminidase (AGA) leading to interruption of the ordered breakdown of glycoproteins in lysosomes.[108] As a consequence of the disturbed glycoprotein catabolism, patients with AGU exhibit severe cell dysfunction especially in the CNS. The uniform phenotype observed in these patients would make effective evaluation of treatment trials feasible in the future. The medical center in Helsinki has experience with HCT for three patients with AGU transplanted at 1.5, 2, and 2.6 years of age.[35] With follow-up ranging from 1 to 5.6 years, serial MRI, biochemical, and clinical examinations were performed. The MR images of six healthy children and five untransplanted AGU children served as controls. The MRIs of the two transplanted patients with at least two years of follow-up showed nearly normal gray-white matter relationships. Improvement in neuropsychological function also appears to have occurred.

## Fucosidosis

Fucosidosis is an autosomal recessive disorder resulting from a deficiency of the lysosomal hydrolase, alpha-fucosidase.[108] The enzyme defect results in the accumulation and excretion of a variety of glycoproteins, glycolipids, and oligosaccharides containing fucoside moieties.

While at least two phenotypes have been described in this disorder, recent experience suggests that the disease may reflect a continuum of severity. The more severely affected patients have, within the first year of life, the onset of psychomotor retardation, coarse facies, growth retardation, dysostosis multiplex, neurologic retardation, and increase in sweat sodium chloride. Detailed studies of springer spaniels have revealed that this canine demonstrates a valid animal model for human fucosidosis, and correction of the fucosidase enzyme activity deficiency by allogeneic BMT following total lymphoid irradiation was demonstrated by using this animal model.[110] There is very limited experience in three children with HCT. Due to disease variability, a definitive conclusion regarding the benefits cannot be reached at this time.

## Niemann-Pick Disease

Niemann-Pick disease types A and B are lysosomal storage disorders resulting from deficient activity of acid sphingomyelinase.[111] Type A is a fatal disorder of infancy characterized by failure to thrive, hepatosplenomegaly, a rapidly progressive neurodegenerative course culminating in death by two to three years of age. HCT has been shown not to be effective in preventing the inexorable neurodevelopmental decline.[44] Type B is a phenotypically variable disorder that is usually diagnosed in childhood due to the presence of marked hepatosplenomegaly. Typically there is no neurologic involvement and the life span can extend into adulthood. HCT does appear to effectively treat the somatic manifestations of type B Niemann-Pick disease.

Niemann-Pick disease, type C, is an autosomal recessive lipidosis resulting from a unique error in cellular trafficking of exogenous cholesterol and is associated with lysosomal accumulation of unesterified cholesterol.[112] Type C is biochemically distinct from the primary sphingomyelin lipidoses, types A and B. Most patients with type C disease have progressive neurologic disease, although hepatic injury is prominent in some cases. There is a single case report of a child with Niemann-Pick disease, type C, undergoing HCT. At this time, the value of HCT is unclear.

## $G_{M2}$ Gangliosidoses: Tay-Sachs, Sandhoff, and $G_{M2}$ Activator Deficiency Diseases

The $G_{M2}$ gangliosidoses are a group of inherited disorders caused by excessive accumulation of ganglioside $G_{M2}$ and related glycolipids in lysosomes, particularly in neuronal cells.[113] There are three forms: 1) Tay-Sachs disease and variants, resulting from mutations of the hexosaminidase A gene and associated with deficient activity of hexosaminidase A but normal hexosaminidase B activity; 2) Sandhoff disease and variants, resulting from mutations of the hexosaminidase B gene and associated with deficient activity of both hexosaminidase A and hexosaminidase B; and 3) $G_{M2}$ activator deficiency. Clinical phenotypes in the $G_{M2}$ gangliosidoses vary widely, ranging from infantile-onset, rapidly progressive neurodegenerative disease that ends in death by age four years (classic Tay-Sachs disease, Sandhoff disease, and $G_{M2}$ activator deficiency) to later-onset, subacute or chronic forms with more slowly progressive neurologic conditions compatible with survival into childhood or adolescence or with long-term survival. HCT does not appear to successfully treat the $G_{M2}$ gangliosidoses; however, future therapy that combines a direct CNS intervention with systemic therapy such as HCT ultimately may prove beneficial in these disorders.[20,113]

## Mucolipidosis II (I-cell Disease)

I-cell disease shows many of the clinical and radiographic features of Hurler syndrome, but usually presents earlier and does not demonstrate mucopolysacchariduria.[114] There is severe progressive psychomotor retardation, and death usually occurs in the first decade of life. The deficient enzyme in I-cell disease is a phosphotransferase, which contains a catalytic component as well as a special recognition site for lysosomal enzymes. The experience using HCT for I-cell disease has been limited, in large part, to patients with advanced stage disease.[29,40–43] Assessment of benefit from transplant has been difficult.

## Wolman Disease

The autosomal-recessive inborn error due to deficient activity of lysosomal acid lipase resulting in massive accumulation of cholesteryl esters and triglycerides in most body tissues is called Wolman disease.[115] In 1956, Abramov, Schorr, and Wolman described an infant with abdominal distention, hepatosplenomegaly, and massive calcification of the adrenal glands. The disease occurs in infancy and is nearly always fatal by the first birthday. HCT has been performed in a small number of patients with Wolman disease. A patient, who is engrafted six years following an unrelated donor bone marrow transplant at the University of Minnesota, is one of the few HCT survivors with Wolman disease.

## Malignant Infantile Osteopetrosis (MIOP)

Absence or defective function of osteoclasts causes this disease of bone sclerosis.[116] There are many animal models, both spontaneously occurring and created by gene knockouts, although few seem to have overlap with human disease.[117–119] It is becoming apparent that there are also multiple causes in humans.[118,120,121] The most common is mutation of a gene encoding a vacuolar proton pump, which is responsible for approximately 50% of human cases.[121,122] All of the described genetic causes of osteopetrosis are defects in acidification and are not abnormalities of osteoclast differentiation. However, the phenotypic variation of the disease suggests that additional gene defects will be defined.

Some other forms of MIOP are metabolic diseases with a neurological component. These include carbonic anhydrase II deficiency (renal tubular acidosis and cerebral calcification)[123] and a severe disease characterized by early onset of spasticity and death with eosinophilic inclusion bodies seen on CNS pathological examination (here termed "neuronopathic" osteopetrosis, since it mimics neuronal ceroid lipofuscinosis).[124,125] In both diseases HCT abolishes bone sclerosis. However, it has no impact on neurodegenerative disease in the latter form[124,126] and CNS amelioration in CAII deficiency seems unlikely.[123,127] Therefore, these issues must be considered as transplantation is discussed in affected children.

Distinguishing children with neuronopathic osteopetrosis from those with the conventional disease is difficult, especially since these children are often irritable. This can be due to occult hypocalcemia in the first two months,[128] multiple fractures, hydrocephalus, or raised intracranial venous pressure (due to bony encroachment on the jugular foramen). There should be strong suspicion of primary neurological disease if irritability does not respond to correction of hypocalcemia and analgesia. Finding cerebral atrophy on computed tomography (CT) scan, retinopathy (as distinct from optic atrophy) may provide other clues on ophthalmic examination and abnormal electroencephalograph (EEG). Mutation analysis of the OC116 and CLCN7 genes should be considered in children who do not have CA II deficiency.[121]

Successful allogeneic HCT is currently, the only therapy capable of producing long-term benefit in children.[129–133] This results in bone remodeling, restoration of growth, and reconstitution of normal hematopoiesis and neutrophil function. Early HCT offers the best possibility for limiting neurosensory defects and impaired growth. Serious risks include high frequencies of graft rejection, venoocclusive disease, and the newly recognized problem of severe pulmonary hypertension. The latter is easy to mistake for pneumonitis but affects up to 25% of transplanted patients (CG Steward et al., manuscript submitted for publication). Results using alternative donors have typically yielded poor results, but megadose stem cell transplants from family donors matching at least one haplotype are now giving more promising results.[134]

## NEW APPROACHES: MESENCHYMAL STEM CELL THERAPY

Bone marrow contains both hematopoietic and mesenchymal stem cells. Conventional HCT has used the former cells for considerable therapeutic benefit including in patients with selected lysosomal and peroxisomal storage diseases. Mesenchymal stem cells can give rise to mesenchymal tissues such as bone, cartilage, muscle, ligaments and tendons, endothelium, and marrow stroma.[69,135–140] Harnessing these cells for therapeutic benefit in a transplant setting could greatly extend the efficacy of transplant by facilitating engraftment as well as through disease-specific outcomes, e.g., skeletal abnormalities, peripheral neuropathies.[1]

## SUMMARY AND CONCLUSIONS

Two decades of clinical experience with HCT shows that it effectively treats some but not all cases of Hurler, Maroteaux-Lamy, and Sly syndromes, childhood onset cerebral X-linked adrenoleukodystrophy, globoid-cell leukodystrophy, metachromatic leukodystrophy, alpha-mannosidosis, and aspartylglucosaminuria. HCT is probably effective for such diseases as fucosidosis and Gaucher, types 1 and 3. HCT is possibly effective in cases of Farber lipogranulomatosis, galactosialidosis, $G_{M1}$ gangliosidosis, mucolipidosis II (I-cell disease), multiple sulfatase deficiency, Niemann-Pick, neuronal ceroid lipofuscinosis, sialidosis, and Wolman disease. As currently performed, HCT has been ineffective in preventing neurocognitive decline for Hunter and Sanfilippo syndromes and in treating the severe dysostosis multiplex in Morquio syndrome. HCT has been most effective when applied early in the disease process or when the patient has been biochemically diagnosed but is still asymptomatic. Disease manifestations, such as the skeletal deformities of the MPS disorders and the peripheral neuropathies of the leukodystrophies, have been relatively refractory to the beneficial effects of HCT. To overcome these obstacles, novel approaches may be needed. Mesenchymal stem cells, other cellular therapeutic interventions as well as enzyme replacement therapy may play an evolving role in the short- and long-term management of these patients with complex, progressive, fatal diseases. Decisions regarding these therapies including HCT will continue to require a team of knowledgeable clinical investigators who use state-of-the-art laboratory and clinical resources.

# REFERENCES

1. Peters C, Steward CG. Hematopoietic cell transplantation for inherited metabolic diseases: an overview of outcomes and practice guidelines. Bone Marrow Transplant 2003;31:229–239.
2. Peters C, Balthazor M, Shapiro EG et al. Outcome of unrelated donor bone marrow transplantation in 40 children with Hurler syndrome. Blood 1996;87:4894–4902.
3. Peters C, Shapiro EG, Anderson J et al. Hurler syndrome: II. Outcome of HLA-genotypically identical sibling and HLA-haploidentical related donor bone marrow transplantation in fifty-four children. Blood 1998;91: 2601–2608.
4. Peters C, Shapiro EG, Krivit W. Hurler syndrome: Past, present, and future. J Pediatr 1998;133:7–9.
5. Hobbs J, Hugh-Jones K, Barrett A et al. Reversal of clinical features of Hurler's disease and biochemical improvement after treatment by bone marrow transplantation. Lancet 1981;2:709–712.
6. Whitley C, Belani K, Chang P et al. Long-term outcome of Hurler syndrome following bone marrow transplantation. Am J Med Genet 1993;46:209–218.
7. Krivit W, Henslee-Downey J, Klemperer M et al. Survival in Hurler's disease following bone marrow transplantation in 84 patients. Bone Marrow Transplant 1995;15(Suppl 1):S182–S185.
8. Hoogerbrugge PM, Brouwer OF, Bordigoni P et al. Allogeneic bone marrow transplantation for lysosomal storage diseases. The European Group for Bone Marrow Transplantation. Lancet 1995;345:1398–1402.
9. Vellodi A, Young E, Cooper A et al. Bone marrow transplantation for mucopolysaccharidosis type I: experience of two British centres. Arch Dis Child 1997;76:92–99.
10. Guffon N, Souillet G, Maire I et al. Follow-up of patients with Hurler syndrome after bone marrow transplantation. J Pediatr 1998;133:119–125.
11. Peters C, Shapiro EG, Krivit W. Neuropsychological development in children with Hurler syndrome following hematopoietic cell transplantation. Pediatr Transplant 1998;9:250–254.
12. Krivit W, Pierpont M, Ayaz K et al. Bone marrow transplantation in the Maroteaux-Lamy syndrome (mucopolysaccharidosis type VI). N Engl J Med 1984;311:1606–1611.
13. Krivit W. Maroteaux-Lamy syndrome (Mucopolysaccharidosis Type VI): Treatment by allogeneic bone marrow transplantation in 6 patients and potential for autotransplantation bone marrow gene insertion. Int Pediatr 1992;7:47–52.
14. Aubourg P, Blanche S, Jamabaque I et al. Reversal of early neurologic and neuroradiologic manifestations of X-linked adrenoleukodystrophy by bone marrow transplantation. N Engl J Med 1990;332:1860–1866.
15. Krivit W, Shapiro E, Lockman L et al. Bone marrow transplantation treatment for globoid cell leukodystrophy, metachromatic leukodystrophy, adrenoleukodystrophy, and Hurler syndrome. In: Moser H, ed. Neurodystrophies and Neurolipidoses (vol 22), Handbook of Clinical Neurology. Amsterdam: Elsevier Science, 1996;87–106.
16. Krivit W, Lockman LA, Shapiro EG: Childhood onset of cerebral adrenoleukodystrophy: Effective treatment by bone marrow transplantation. In: Steward CG, Hobbs JR (eds). Correction of Genetic Diseases by Transplantation, III. London: The COGENT Press, 1995;48–56.
17. Krivit W, Lockman LA, Watkins PA et al. The future for treatment by bone marrow transplantation for adrenoleukodystrophy, metachromatic leukodystrophy, globoid cell leukodystrophy and Hurler syndrome. J Inherit Metab Dis 1995;18:398–412.
18. Shapiro EG, Krivit W, Lockman L et al. Long-term effect of bone-marrow transplantation for childhood-onset of cerebral X-linked adrenoleukodystrophy. Lancet 2000;356:713–718.
20. Krivit W, Sung JH, Lockman LA et al. Bone marrow transplantation for treatment of lysosomal and peroxisomal storage diseases: Focus on central nervous system reconstitution. In: Rich RR, Fleisher TA, Schwartz BD et al. (eds). Principles of Clinical Immunology (vol 2). St. Louis: Mosby Yearbook Press, 1995;1852–1864.
21. Arvidsson J, Hagberg B, Mansson JE et al. Late onset globoid cell leukodystrophy (Krabbe's disease)—Swedish case with 15 years of follow-up (Review). Acta Paediatr 1995;84:218–221.
22. Stillman AE, Krivit W, Shapiro EG et al. Serial MRI after bone marrow transplantation in two patients with MLD. AJNR Am J Neuroradiol 1994;15:1929–1932.
23. Pridjian G, Humbert J, Willis J et al. Presymptomatic late-infantile MLD treated with bone marrow transplantation. J Pediatr 1994;125:755–758.
24. Fasth A, Oskarsdottir S, Tulinius M et al. Bone marrow transplantation in metachromatic leukodystrophy (MLD): disease progress in a boy despite transplantation two years before expected onset of symptoms. In: Ringden O, Hobbs JR, Steward CG (eds). Correction of Genetic Diseases by Transplantation IV. Middlesex: The COGENT Press, 1997;24–27.
25. Krivit W, Lockman L, Shapiro E. Metachromatic leukodystrophy. In: Steward C, Hobbs J (eds). Correction of Genetic Diseases by Transplantation III. Middlesex: The COGENT Press, 1995;41–47.
26. Krivit W, Shapiro E, Kennedy W et al. Treatment of late infantile metachromatic leukodystrophy by bone marrow transplantation. N Engl J Med 1990;322:28–32.

27. Navarro C, Dominguez C, Fernandez JM et al. Case report: four-year follow-up of bone-marrow transplantation in late juvenile metachromatic leukodystrophy. J Inherit Metabol Dis 1995;18:157–158.
28. Malm G, Ringden O, Winiarski J et al. Clinical outcome in four children with metachromatic leukodystrophy treated by bone marrow transplantation. Bone Marrow Transplant 1996;17:1003–1008.
29. Imaizumi M, Gushi K, Kurobane I et al. Long-term effects of bone marrow transplantation for inborn errors of metabolism: a study of four patients with lysosomal storage diseases. Acta Paediatr Jpn 1994;36:30–36.
30. Peters C, Waye JS, Vellodi A et al. Hematopoietic cell transplantation for metachromatic leukodystrophy prior to onset of clinical signs and symptoms. In: Ringden O, Hobbs JR, Steward CG (eds). Correction of Genetic Diseases by Transplantation IV. London: The COGENT Press, 1997;34–48.
31. Solders G, Celsing G, Hagenfeldt L et al. Bone marrow transplantation for adult metachromatic leukodystrophy. In: Ringden O, Hobbs JR, Steward CG (eds). Correction of Genetic Diseases by Transplantation IV. Middlesex: The COGENT Press, 1997;323.
32. Bayever E, Ladish S, Phioppart M et al. Bone-marrow transplantation for metachromatic leukodystrophy. Lancet 1985;2:471–473.
33. Dhuna A, Toro C, Torres F et al. Longitudinal neuropsychological studies in a patient with metachromatic leukodystrophy following bone marrow transplantation. Arch Neurol 1992;49:1082–1092.
34. Wall DA, Grange DK, Goulding P et al. Bone marrow transplantation for the treatment of alpha-mannosidosis. J Pediatr 1998;133:282–285.
35. Autti T, Santavuori P, Raininko R et al. Bone marrow transplantation in aspartylglucosaminuria: MRI of the brain suggests normalizing myelination. In: Ringden O, Hobbs JR, Steward CG (eds). Correction of Genetic Diseases by Transplantation. London: The COGENT Press, 1997;92.
36. Rappeport JM, Ginns EI. Bone-marrow transplantation in severe Gaucher disease. N Engl J Med 1984;311:84–88.
37. Ringden O, Groth C, Erikson A et al. Long-term results of bone marrow transplantation for Gaucher disease. In: Steward C, Hobbs J (eds). Correction of Genetic Diseases by Transplantation III. Middlesex: The COGENT Press, 1995;57–63.
38. Ringden O, Groth CG, Winiarski J et al. Bone marrow transplantation for Gaucher disease. In: Ringden O, Hobbs JR, Steward CG (eds). Correction of Genetic Diseases by Transplantation IV. Middlesex: The COGENT Press, 1997;80–86.
39. Hobbs J. Juvenile Gauchers: 8 patients 5.6 - 11.2 years postgraft. In: Steward C, Hobbs J (eds). Correction of Genetic Diseases by Transplantation III. Middlesex: The COGENT Press, 1995;64–70.
40. Kurobane I, Inoue S, Gotoh Y et al. Biochemical improvement after treatment by bone marrow transplantation in I-cell disease. Tohoku J Exp Med 1986;150:63–68.
41. Kurobane I, Aikawa J-I, Narisawa K et al. Bone marrow transplantation in I-cell disease. In: Hobbs JR, ed. Correction of certain genetic diseases by transplantation. London: The COGENT Press, 1989;132–136.
42. Yamaguchi K, Hayasaka S, Hara S et al. Improvement of tear lysosomal enzyme levels after treatment with bone marrow transplantation in a patient with I-cell disease. Ophthalmic Res 1989;21:226–229.
43. Tang X, Hinohara T, Kato S et al. I-cell disease: report of an autopsy case. Tokai J Exp Clin Med 1995;20:109–120.
44. Bayever E, August CS, Kamani N et al. Allogeneic bone marrow transplantation for Niemann-Pick disease (Type IA). Bone Marrow Transplant 1992;10(Suppl 1):85–86.
45. Klein KA, Krivit W, Whitley CB et al. Poor cognitive outcome of eleven children with Sanfilippo syndrome after bone marrow transplantation and successful engraftment. Bone Marrow Transplant 1995;15(Suppl 1):S176–181.
46. Krivit W, Shapiro E. Bone marrow transplantation for storage diseases. In: Desnick R, ed. Treatment of Genetic Diseases. New York: Churchill-Livingstone, 1991;203.
47. Neufeld E, Muenzer J. The mucopolysaccharidoses. In: Scriver C, Beaudet A, Sly W et al. (eds). The Metabolic and Molecular Bases of Inherited Disease (vol 3, 8th ed). New York: McGraw-Hill, 2001;3421–3452.
48. Krivit W, Shapiro E, Balthazor M et al. Hurler syndrome: Outcomes and planning following bone marrow transplantation. In: Steward C, Hobbs J (eds). Correction of Genetic Diseases by Transplantation, III. London: The COGENT Press, 1995;25–40.
49. Shapiro EG, Lockman LA, Balthazor M et al. Neuropsychological outcomes of several storage diseases with and without bone marrow transplantation. J Inherit Metabol Dis 1995;18:413–429.
50. Kramer J, Crittenden M, Halberg F et al. A prospective study of cognitive functioning following low-dose cranial irradiation for bone marrow transplantation. Pediatrics 1992;90:447–450.
51. Kaleita T, Shields W, Tesler A et al. Normal neurodevelopment in four young children treated with bone marrow transplantation for acute leukemia or aplastic anemia. Pediatrics 1989;83:753–757.
52. Smedler A, Bergman H, Holme P. Neuropsychological functioning in children treated with bone marrow transplantation. J Clin Exp Neuropsychol 1988;10:325.
53. Dusenbery KD, Gerbi BJ. Total body irradiation in conditioning regimens for bone marrow transplantation. In: Levitt J, Tapley (eds). Levitt and Tapley's Technological Basis of Radiation Therapy (3rd ed). Philadelphia: Lippincott Williams & Wilkins, 1999;499.

54. Braunlin EA, Hunter DW, Krivit W. Evaluation of coronary artery disease in the Hurler syndrome. Am J Cardiol 1992;62:1487–1489.
55. duCret RP, Weinberg EJ, Jackson CA et al. Resting Tl-201 scintigraphy in the evaluation of coronary artery disease in children with Hurler syndrome. Clin Nucl Med 1994;19:975–978.
56. Braunlin EA, Rose AG, Hopwood JJ et al. Coronary artery patency following long-term successful engraftment 14 years after bone marrow transplantation in the Hurler syndrome. Am J Cardiol 2001;88:1075–1077.
57. Schachern P, Shea D, Paparella M. Mucopolysaccharidosis I-H (Hurler's syndrome) and human temporal bone histopathology. Ann Otol Rhinol Laryngol 1984;93(1 Pt 1):65–69.
58. Krivit W, Lockman LA, Watkins PA et al. The future for treatment by bone marrow transplantation for adrenoleukodystrophy, metachromatic leukodystrophy, globoid cell leukodystrophy and Hurler syndrome (Review). J Inherit Metabol Dis 1995;18:398–412.
59. Summers CG, Purple RL, Krivit W et al. Ocular changes in the mucopolysaccharidoses after bone marrow transplantation. Ophthalmology 1989;96:977–984.
60. Gullingsrud E, Krivit W, Summers C. Ocular abnormalities in the mucopolysaccharidoses following bone marrow transplantation: longer follow-up. Ophthalmology 1997;105:1099–1105.
61. Field RE, Buchanan JAF, Copplemans MGJ et al. Bone marrow transplantation in Hurler syndrome. Effect on skeletal development. J Bone Joint Surg 1994;76–B:975–981.
62. Van Heest A, House J, Krivit W et al. Surgical treatment of carpal tunnel syndrome and trigger digits in children with mucopolysaccharide storage diseases. J Hand Surg 1997;23:236–243.
63. Odunusi E, Peters C, Krivit W et al. Genu valgum deformity in Hurler syndrome after hematopoietic cell transplantation: Correction by surgical intervention. J Pediatr Orthop 1999;19:270–274.
64. Belani KG, Krivit W, Carpenter BL et al. Children with mucopolysaccharidosis: perioperative care, morbidity, mortality, and new findings. J Pediatr Surg 1993;28:403–408.
65. Woodard P, Wagner JE, DeFor T et al. Effect of two hematopoietic stem cell transplant (HCT) preparative regimens on outcomes in patients with inborn errors of metabolism (IEOM). Blood 1998;92:516a.
66. Shapiro E, Lockman L, Balthazor M et al. Neuropsychological and neurological function and quality-of-life before and after bone marrow transplantation for adrenoleukodystrophy. In: Ringden O, Hobbs JR, Steward CG (eds). Correction of Genetic Diseases by Transplantation IV. London: The COGENT Press, 1997;52–62.
67. Resnick JM, Krivit W, Snover DC et al. Pathology of the liver in mucopolysaccharidosis: light and electron microscopic assessment before and after bone marrow transplantation. Bone Marrow Transplant 1992;10:273–280.
68. Resnick JM, Whitley CB, Leonard AS et al. Light and electron microscopic features of the liver in mucopolysaccharidosis. Hum Pathol 1994;25:276–286.
69. Hite SH, Peters C, Krivit W. Correction of odontoid dysplasia following bone-marrow transplantation and engraftment (in Hurler syndrome MPS 1H). Pediatr Radiol 2000;30:464–470.
70. Prockop DJ: Marrow stromal cells as stem cells for nonhematopoietic tissues. Science 1997;276:71–74.
71. Pittenger MF, Mackay AM, Beck SC et al. Multilineage potential of adult human mesenchymal stem cells. Science 1999;284:143–147.
72. Whitley C, Krivit W, Ramsay N et al. Mutation analysis and clinical outcome of patients with Hurler syndrome (mucopolysaccharidosis type I-H) undergoing bone marrow transplantation. Am J Hum Genet 1993;53:101a.
73. Scott H, Litjens T, Hopwood J et al. A common mutation for mucopolysaccharidosis Type I associated with a severe Hurler syndrome phenotype. Hum Mutat 1992;1:103–108.
74. Moskowitz S, Tieu P, Neufeld E. A deletion/insertion mutation in the IDUA gene in a Libyan Jewish patient with Hurler syndrome (mucopolysaccharidosis I). Hum Mutat 1993;2:71–73.
75. Bach G, Moskowitz S, Tieu P et al. Molecular analysis of Hurler syndrome in Druze and Muslim Arab patients in Israel: Multiple allelic mutations of the IDUA gene in a small geographic area. Am J Hum Genet 1993;53:330–338.
76. Scott H, Litjens T, Nelson P et al. Identification of mutations in the alpha-L-iduronidase gene (IDUA) that cause Hurler and Scheie syndromes. Am J Hum Genet 1993;53:973–986.
77. Kakkis ED, Muenzer J, Tiller GE et al. Enzyme-replacement therapy in mucopolysaccharidosis I. N Engl J Med 2001;344:182–188.
78. Sands MS, Erway LC, Vogler C et al. Syngeneic bone marrow transplantation reduces the hearing loss associated with murine mucopolysaccharidosis type VII. Blood 1995;86:2033–2040.
79. Moser HW, Smith KD, Watkins PA. X-linked adrenoleukodystrophy. In: Scriver CR, Beaudet AL, Sly WS et al. (eds). The Metabolic and Molecular Bases of Inherited Disease (vol 3, 8th ed.). New York: McGraw-Hill, 2001;3257–3302.
80. Moser HW. Adrenoleukodystrophy: phenotype, genetics, pathogenesis and therapy. (Review). Brain 1997;120:1485–1508.
81. Aubourg P. X-linked adrenoleukodystrophy. In: Vinken PJ, Bruyn GW, Moser HW (eds). Handbook of Clinical Neurology: Neurodystrophies and Neurolipidoses. Amsterdam: Elsevier, 1997;447–483.

82. Moser HW, Borel J. Dietary management of X-linked adrenoleukodystrophy (Review). Ann Rev Nutr 1995; 15:379–397.
83. Moser HW. Komrower Lecture. Adrenoleukodystrophy: natural history, treatment and outcome (Review). J Inherit Metabol Dis 1995;18:435–447.
84. Moser HW. Adrenoleukodystrophy (Review). Curr Opin Neurol 1995;8:221–226.
85. Kemp S, Wei H-M, Lu J-F. Gene redundancy and pharmacological implications for X-linked adrenoleukodystrophy. Nat Med 1998;4:1261–1268.
86. Singh I, Pahan K, Khan M. Lovastatin and sodium phenylacetate normalize the levels of very long chain fatty acids in skin fibroblasts of X-adrenoleukodystrophy. FEBS Lett 1998;426:342–346.
87. Mosser J, Douar AM, Sarde CO et al. Putative X-linked adrenoleukodystrophy gene shares unexpected homology with ABC transporters. Nature 1993;361:726–730.
88. Rajanayagam V, Balthazor M, Shapiro EG et al. Proton MR spectroscopy and neuropsychological testing in adrenoleukodystrophy. AJNR Am J Neuroradiol 1997;18:1909–1914.
89. Loes DJ, Hite S, Moser H et al. Adrenoleukodystrophy: A scoring method for brain MR observations. AJNR Am J Neuroradiol 1994;15:1761–1766.
90. Loes DJ, Hite SW, Stillman AE et al. Childhood cerebral form of adrenoleukodystrophy: short-term effect of bone marrow transplantation on brain MRI observations. AJNR Am J Neuroradiol 1994;15:1767–1771.
91. Rajanayagam V, Grad J, Krivit W et al. Proton MR spectroscopy of childhood adrenoleukodystrophy. AJNR Am J Neuroradiol 1996;17:1013–1024.
92. Vassal G, Deroussent A, Hartman O et al. Dose dependent neurotoxicity of high-dose busulfan in children: a clinical pharmacological study. Cancer Res 1990;50:6203–6207.
93. Peters C, Anderson JR, Lockman LA et al. Treatment of high risk childhood onset cerebral adrenoleukodystrophy (COCALD) with modified hematopoietic cell transplantation (HCT) (Abstr). Pediatr Res 1998; 43:323a.
94. Peterson K, Rosenblum MK, Powers JM et al. Effect of brain irradiation on demyelinating lesions. Neurology 1993;43:2105–2112.
95. Wenger DA, Suzuki K, Suzuki Y et al. Galactosylceramide lipidosis: Globoid-cell leukodystrophy (Krabbe disease). In: Scriver CR, Beaudet AL, Sly WS et al. (eds). The Metabolic and Molecular Bases of Inherited Disease (vol 3, 8th ed.). New York: McGraw-Hill, 2001;3669–3694.
96. Kolodny EH. Globoid leukodystrophy. In: Moser HW (ed). Handbook of Clinical Neurology: Neurodystrophies and Neurolipidoses (vol 66). Amsterdam: Elsevier, 1996;187–210.
97. Wenger DA, Rafi MA, Luzi P. Molecular genetics of Krabbe disease (globoid cell leukodystrophy): diagnostic and clinical implications (Review). Hum Mutat 1997;10:268–279.
98. Krivit W, Shapiro EG, Peters C et al. Hematopoietic stem-cell transplantation in globoid-cell leukodystrophy. N Engl J Med 1998;338:1119–1126.
99. Kurtzberg J, Richards K, Wenger D et al. Correction of Krabbe disease with neonatal hematopoietic stem cell transplantation (Abstr #130). Biol Blood Marrow Transplant 2002;8:97.
100. Von Figura K, Gieselmann V, Jaeken J. Metachromatic leukodystrophy. In: Scriver CR, Beaudet AL, Sly WS et al. (eds). The Metabolic and Molecular Bases of Inherited Disease (vol 3, 8th ed.). New York: McGraw-Hill, 2001;3695–3724.
101. Kolodny EH. Metachromatic leukodystrophy and multiple sulfatase deficiency: sulfatide lipidosis. In: Rosenberg RN, Prusiner SB, DiMauro S et al. (eds). The Molecular and Genetic Bases of Neurological Diseases (vol 1). Boston: Butterworth-Heinemann, 1996;433–442.
102. Beutler E, Grabowski GA. Gaucher disease. In: Scriver CR, Beaudet AL, Sly WS et al. (eds). The Metabolic and Molecular Bases of Inherited Disease (vol 3, 8th ed.). New York: McGraw-Hill, 2001;3635–3668.
103. Schiffmann R, Heyes MP, Aerts JM et al. Prospective study of neurological responses to treatment with macrophage-targeted glucocerebrosidase in patients with type 3 Gaucher's disease. Annal Neurol 1997;42: 613–621.
104. Beutler E. Gaucher disease: New molecular approaches to diagnosis and treatment. Science 1992;256: 794–799.
105. Figueroa ML, Rosenbloom BE, Kay A et al. A less costly regimen of alglucerase to treat Gaucher's disease. N Engl J Med 1992;327:1632–6.
106. Brady RO, Barton NW. Enzyme replacement and gene therapy for Gaucher's disease. Lipids 1996;(31 Suppl):S137–139.
107. Erikson A, Mansson J-E. Enzyme infusion therapy of Gaucher disease. In: Ringden O, Hobbs JR, Steward CG (eds). Correction of Genetic Diseases by Transplantation. London: The COGENT Press, 1997;87–90.
108. Thomas GH. Disorders of glycoprotein degradation: alpha-mannosidosis, beta-mannosidosis, fucosidosis, and sialidosis. In: Scriver CR, Beaudet AL, Sly WS et al., (eds). The Metabolic and Molecular Bases of Inherited Disease (vol 3, 8th ed.). New York: McGraw-Hill, 2001;3507–3533.
109. Walkley S, Thrall M, Dobrenis K et al. Bone marrow transplantation corrects the enzyme defect in neurons of the central nervous system in a lysosomal storage disease. Proc Natl Acad Sci USA 1994;91:2970–2974.

110. Taylor RM, Farrow BRH, Stewart GJ et al. Enzyme replacement in nervous tissue after allogenic bone-marrow transplantation for fucosidosis in dogs. Lancet 1986;2:772–774.

111. Schuchman EH, Desnick RJ. Niemann-Pick disease types A and B: Acid sphingomyelinase deficiencies. In: Scriver CR, Beaudet AL, Sly WS et al. (eds). The Metabolic and Molecular Bases of Inherited Disease (vol 3, 8th ed.). New York: McGraw-Hill, 2001;3589–3610.

112. Patterson MC, Vanier MT, Suzuki K et al. Niemann-Pick disease type C: A lipid trafficking disorder. In: Scriver CR, Beaudet AL, Sly WS et al. (eds). The Metabolic and Molecular Bases of Inherited Disease (vol 3, 8th ed.). New York: McGraw-Hill, 2001;3611–3633.

113. Gravel RA, Kaback MM, Proia RL et al. The $G_{M2}$ gangliosidoses. In: Scriver CR, Beaudet AL, Sly WS et al. (eds). The Metabolic and Molecular Bases of Inherited Disease (vol 3, 8th ed.). New York: McGraw-Hill, 2001;3827–3876.

114. Kornfeld S, Sly WS. I-cell disease and pseudo-Hurler polydystrophy: Disorders of lysosomal enzyme phosphorylation and localization. In: Scriver CR, Beaudet AL, Sly WS et al. (eds). The Metabolic and Molecular Bases of Inherited Disease (vol 3, 8th ed.). New York: McGraw-Hill, 2001;3469–3482.

115. Assmann G, Seedorf U: Acid lipase deficiency: Wolman disease and cholesteryl ester storage disease. In: Scriver CR, Beaudet AL, Sly WS et al. (eds). The Metabolic and Molecular Bases of Inherited Disease (vol 3, 8th ed.). New York: McGraw-Hill, 2001;3551–3572.

116. Coccia PF. Cells that resorb bone. N Engl J Med 1984;310:456–458.

117. Popoff SN, Marks SC Jr. The heterogeneity of the osteopetroses reflects the diversity of cellular influences during skeletal development. Bone 1995;17:437–445.

118. Felix R, Hofstetter W, Cecchini MG. Recent developments in the understanding of the pathophysiology of osteopetrosis. Eur J Endocrinol 1996;134:143–156.

119. Seifert MF, Popoff SN, Jackson ME et al. Experimental studies of osteopetrosis in laboratory animals. Clin Orthop 1993;294:23–33.

120. Kornak U, Kasper D, Bosl MR et al. Loss of the ClC-7 chloride channel leads to osteopetrosis in mice and man. Cell 2001;104:205–215.

121. Kornak U, Schulz A, Friedrich W et al. Mutations in the a 3 subunit of the vacuolar H(+)-ATPase cause infantile malignant osteopetrosis. Hum Mol Genet 2000;9:2059–2063.

122. Frattini A, Orchard PJ, Sobacchi C et al. Defects in TCIRG1 subunit of the vacuolar proton pump are responsible for a subset of human autosomal recessive osteopetrosis. Nat Genet 2000;25:343–346.

123. Sly WS, Whyte MP, Sundaram V et al. Carbonic anhydrase II deficiency in 12 families with the autosomal recessive syndrome of osteopetrosis with renal tubular acidosis and cerebral calcification. N Engl J Med 1985;313:139–145.

124. Gerritsen EJ, Vossen JM, van Loo IH et al. Autosomal recessive osteopetrosis: variability of findings at diagnosis and during the natural course. Pediatrics 1994;93:247–253.

125. Jagadha V, Halliday WC, Becker LE et al. The association of infantile osteopetrosis and neuronal storage disease in two brothers. Acta Neuropathol (Berl) 1988;75:233–240.

126. Gerritsen EJ, Vossen JM, Fasth A et al. Bone marrow transplantation for autosomal recessive osteopetrosis. A report from the Working Party on Inborn Errors of the European Bone Marrow Transplantation Group. J Pediatr 1994;125:896–902.

127. McMahon C, Will A, Hu P et al. Bone marrow transplantation corrects osteopetrosis in the carbonic anhydrase II deficiency syndrome. Blood 2001;97:1947–1950.

128. Srinivasan M, Abinun M, Cant AJ et al. Malignant infantile osteopetrosis presenting with neonatal hypocalcaemia. Arch Dis Child Fetal Neonatal Ed 2000;83:F21–F23.

129. Eapen M, Davies SM, Ramsay NK et al. Hematopoietic cell transplantation for infantile osteopetrosis. Bone Marrow Transplant 1998;22:941–946.

130. Sieff CA, Chessells JM, Levinsky RJ et al. Allogeneic bone-marrow transplantation in infantile malignant osteopetrosis. Lancet 1983;1:437–441.

131. Fischer A, Griscelli C, Friedrich W et al. Bone-marrow transplantation for immunodeficiencies and osteopetrosis: European survey, 1968–1985. Lancet 1986;2:1080–1084.

132. Coccia PF, Krivit W, Cervenka J et al. Successful bone-marrow transplantation for infantile malignant osteopetrosis. N Engl J Med 1980;302:701–708.

133. Cheow HK, Steward CG, Grier DJ. Imaging of malignant infantile osteopetrosis before and after bone marrow transplantation. Pediatr Radiol 2001;31:869–875.

134. Schulz AS, Classen CF, Mihatsch WA et al. HLA-haploidentical blood progenitor cell transplantation in osteopetrosis. Blood 2002;99:3458–3460.

135. Bruder SP, Fink DJ, Caplan AI. Mesenchymal stem cells in bone development, bone repair, and skeletal regeneration therapy. J Cell Biochem 1994;56:283–294.

136. Jaiswal N, Haynesworth SE, Caplan AI et al. Osteogenic differentiation of purified, culture-expanded human mesenchymal stem cells in vitro. J Cell Biochem 1997;64:295–312.

137. Mackay AM, Beck SC, Murphy JM et al. Chondrogenic differentiation of cultured human mesenchymal stem cells from marrow. Tissue Eng 1998;4:415–428.

138. Kadiyala S, Young RG, Thiede MA et al. Culture expanded canine mesenchymal stem cells possess osteo-chondrogenic potential in vivo and in vitro. Cell Transplant 1997;6:125–134.

139. Cassiede P, Dennis JE, Ma F et al. Osteochondrogenic potential of marrow mesenchymal progenitor cells exposed to TGF-beta 1 or PDGF-BB as assayed in vivo and in vitro. J Bone Miner Res 1996;11:1264–1273.

140. Bruder SP, Jaiswal N, Ricalton NS et al. Mesenchymal stem cells in osteobiology and applied bone regeneration. Clin Orthoped 1998;(355 Suppl):S247–256.

# CHAPTER XVI

# Hematopoietic Stem Cell Transplantation For Hemoglobinopathies

LAKSHMANAN KRISHNAMURTI

## HSCT FOR SICKLE CELL DISEASE

In 1960, sickle cell disease (SCD) was a disease of children with few patients surviving into adulthood.[1] In the last 30 years there have been many advances in the health care of children with SCD. Important among these include newborn screening, early introduction of penicillin, the pneumococcal vaccines and comprehensive care.[1-3] These and other advances have resulted in a marked improvement in the life expectancy of patients with SCD. Yet, this disease continues to be associated with considerable morbidity and mortality, particularly as patients reach adult age. Stroke, organ failure, acute chest syndrome, and recurrent pain crises are major complications that shorten life expectancy and impair overall health-related quality of life (HRQOL). While hydroxyurea (HU) and chronic transfusion regimens can ameliorate several of the complications of SCD, allogeneic hematopoietic stem cell transplantation (HSCT) is the only curative treatment option.

### Pathogenesis of Sickle Cell Complications

SCD is an autosomal recessively inherited disorder resulting from an amino acid substitution of valine for glutamic acid at the sixth position of the β-globin chain, due to a single nucleotide substitution, GAG→GTG in codon 6 of the β-globin gene on chromosome 11p15.5. Deoxygenation causes the polymerization of Hemoglobins S (Hb S). The rigid polymers deform red cells causing vasoocclusion in the small vessels. Adherence of sickle cells to vascular endothelium results in intimal hyperplasia in larger vessels and causes slowed blood flow.[4] The high white blood cell count found in most patients with SCD results in the production of injurious cytokines.[5] Individual patients may have other genetically controlled factors that increase thrombotic tendencies by mechanisms distinct from those that are due to sickle cells. In addition, known and unknown environmental factors can precipitate vasoocclusion.[6] Acidosis in the muscle or body fluids, dehydration, cold temperatures, and infections are known precipitants. Genetic modifiers also may play pivotal roles in determining SCD phenotype.[7] These include: interaction with other β-globin gene mutations, genetic elements linked to the β-globin gene cluster, XmnI polymorphism upstream of the γ globin gene,[8] β-globin gene haplotype[9] or other genes that lead to increased fetal globin production[10] coinheritance of α thalassemia,[11] erythroid enzymopathies, membrane protein abnormalities, or genetic loci of the globin gene cluster of as yet undetermined clinical significance. The effect of genetic loci that modulate erythrocyte-endothelial cell adhesion,[4] stroke susceptibility,[5,12] neutrophil activation,[13,14] and erythrocyte dehydration[15] on sickle cell phenotype are the subjects of active investigation.

## Clinical Features

### Variability of Phenotype and Prediction of Severity

The clinical manifestations of Hb S homozygotes are extremely variable. Approximately 10% to 20% of SCD patients develop strokes that may result in serious disabilities. In a prospective study, most SCD patients had zero to one painful episode per year, and 5% to 10% of patients had three or more painful crises per year. The occurrence of more than three painful crises per year was found to be a risk factor for early mortality in adults with SCD.[16] Of the 392 infants in a cohort followed by the Cooperative Study on SCD (CSSCD)[17] for more than 10 years, 70 (18%) subsequently had an adverse outcome, defined as death (26%), stroke (36%), frequent pain (24%), or recurrent acute chest syndrome (18%). Three manifestations of SCD that may appear in the first two years of life (dactylitis, severe anemia, and leukocytosis) predicted the possibility of these SCD related adverse outcomes.

### Cerebral Vasculopathy

The problem of stroke in SCD has been known for more than 75 years.[18] Recent insights into the pathophysiology, clinical manifestations, and prediction of stroke have led to the development of novel prevention and treatment strategies. The CSSCD included a cohort of 4,082 SCD patients followed from 1978 to 1988.[19] Patients were followed for an average of 5.2 ± 2.0 years. Age-specific prevalence and incidence rates of cerebrovascular accident (CVA) in patients with the common genotypes of SCD were determined, and the effects of hematological and clinical events on the risk of CVA were analyzed.[20] An age-adjusted prevalence of stroke was 4.96% in patients with homozygous SCD. The chances of having a first CVA by 20 years of age, 30 years of age, and 45 years of age were estimated at 11%, 15%, and 24%, respectively, for Hb S homozygotes. Children enrolled in the CSSCD were evaluated also with brain magnetic resonance imaging (MRI) and neuropsychological evaluation. Central nervous system (CNS) abnormalities were identified on the MRI in 22.2% of children with HbSS21. The addition of positron emission tomography (PET) to MRI identified a much greater proportion of children with SCD with neuroimaging abnormalities, particularly in those who had no history of overt neurologic events.[22] Lower than average full-scale intelligence quotient (FSIQ) was associated with either overt CVA or silent ischemic lesions. Silent infarct identified at age 6 years or older is associated with increased stroke risk.[23] Thus, the burden of cerebral vasculopathy in SCD is substantial and is more extensive than that indicated by clinical CVA alone.

### Pulmonary Disease

Although the episodic and unpredictable vasoocclusive crisis (VOC) or pain crisis is the hallmark of SCD, acute chest syndrome (ACS) is the second most common cause of hospitalization in patients with SCD and is responsible for up to 25% of deaths.[24] Clinically,

ACS is often a self-limited acute pulmonary illness, but may rapidly progress to life-threatening respiratory insufficiency. Repeated events have been associated with an increased risk of chronic lung disease and early death.[24] Multiple infectious and noninfectious etiologic factors underlie this syndrome including community-acquired pneumonia, infarction, hypoventilation (after surgery, rib infarcts, or narcotic administration), and pulmonary fat embolism from infarcted bone marrow.[25] ACS is the leading cause of death in SCD, and many patients suffer from multiple, severe episodes. Age has a striking effect on the clinical course and outcome of ACS, with children having milder disease that often is infectious. Adults may have severe disease often with pulmonary fat embolism in severe cases. Among older patients and those with neurologic symptoms, the syndrome often progresses to respiratory failure.

*Pain*

Acute episodes of pain are the principal symptom of SCD, but little is known about the epidemiologic features or the risk factors for these episodes. Thirty-nine percent of patients with SCD had no episodes of pain, and 1% had more than six episodes per year.[16] Among sickle cell patients who are more than 20 years old, those with high rates of pain episodes (>3 episodes a year) tend to die earlier than those with low rates.[16]

## Morbidity and Costs of Care for SCD

On average there are an estimated 75,000 hospitalizations per year of children and adults with SCD. In the United States the total direct cost for hospitalization (in 1996 dollars) is $475 million per year.[26] In 66% of hospital discharge records, government programs were listed as the expected principal source of payment. Thus, despite advances in care and treatment of SCD, this disease is associated with disproportionate morbidity, mortality, and individual and societal costs.

## Survival

The CSSCD demonstrated that the mean age of death for patients with SCD is 42 years for males and 48 years for females.[1] This constitutes a 25–30 year loss of life expectancy compared to African Americans in general. Fifty percent of patients with SCD survive beyond the fifth decade. Of patients with sickle cell-hemoglobin C disease, the median age at death is 60 years for males and 68 years for females. Among adults with SCD, 18% of the deaths occur in patients with overt organ failure, predominantly renal. Thirty-three percent were clinically free of organ failure but died during an acute sickle crisis.

## Indications for HSCT

Indications for HSCT have been empirically determined from prognostic factors derived from studies of natural history of SCD. ▼ Table 16.1 describes criteria for transplantation used in the recently concluded national collaborative study of HSCT for SCD.[27] Prognostic factors that predicted outcome were first described in a study of life expectancy of patients with SCD in the United States during the 1980s.[1] Fetal hemoglobin level, renal insufficiency, acute chest syndrome, seizures, and white cell count were significant risk factors. Interest has

---

**TABLE 16.1**    Indications for HSCT in SCD

*Patients with SCD 16 years of age or less years with an HLA-identical sibling bone marrow donor with one or more of the following:*

- Stroke, CNS hemorrhage or a neurologic event lasting longer than 24 hours, or abnormal cerebral MRI or cerebral arteriogram or MRI angiographic study and impaired neuropsychological testing,
- Acute chest syndrome with a history of recurrent hospitalizations or exchange transfusions,
- Recurrent vasoocclusive pain three or more episodes per year for three years or more or recurrent priapism,
- Impaired neuropsychological function and abnormal cerebral MRI scan,
- Stage I or II sickle lung disease,
- Sickle nephropathy (moderate or severe proteinuria or a glomerular filtration rate (GFR) 30%–50% of the predicted normal value),
- Bilateral proliferative retinopathy and major visual impairment in at least one eye,
- Osteonecrosis of multiple joints with documented destructive changes,
- Requirement for chronic transfusions but with RBC alloimmunization > 2 antibodies during long term transfusion therapy.

Modified from Walters et al., 1996.[27]

---

been raised in the potential use of the prognostic model proposed by Miller et al.[17] to predict risk of adverse outcome in determining selection criteria for HSCT. In this model dactylitis, a steady-state hemoglobin level of less than 7 g per deciliter, and leukocytosis in the absence of infection at an early age correlated significantly with probability of severe disease later in childhood that was 36% or greater (i.e., at least twice that in the general population of children with SCD). The use of this classification would have a low rate of false positive results (1%). However, it would result in the identification of only 20% of patients with severe disease. Further studies are indicated to determine how to use this or other models to identify or exclude patients for HSCT. With the advent of decreased intensity conditioning regimens and improved outcomes for HSCT, the risk/benefit ratio of HSCT versus conventional treatment is likely to change.

## Results

Allogeneic HSCT after myeloablative therapy has been performed in approximately 190 young patients (< 16 years of age) with SCD (▼ Table 16.2). The backbone of the preparative regimens utilized have consisted of busulfan (BU) 14–16 mg/kg and cyclophosphamide (CY) 200 mg/kg. Additional immunosuppressive agents in use include: antithymocyte globulin (ATG), rabbit ATG (rATG),[30] antilymphocyte globulin (ALG),[34] or total lymphoid irradiation (TLI).[35] Cyclosporine A (CsA) alone or in combination with methylprednisolone (MP) or methotrexate (MTX) has been utilized for posttransplant graft-versus-host disease (GVHD) prophylaxis.

The event-free survival (EFS) is 85% with less than 10% dying from therapy related complications.[28,29,32–34,36–47] Stabilization or reversal of organ damage from SCD has been documented after HSCT.[28] Among 22 of 26 patients who had stable donor engraftment, complications related to SCD were resolved, and none experienced further episodes of pain, stroke, or acute chest syndrome. All 10 engrafted patients with a prior history of stroke had stable or improved cerebral MRI results. Updated results on 55 patients revealed that SCD patients who are successfully allografted do not experience sickle-related CNS complications and have evidence of stabilization of CNS disease by cerebral MRI.[48] Pulmonary function tests were stable in 22 of 26 patients, worse in two, and not studied in two. Seven of eight patients transplanted for recurrent acute chest syndrome had stable pulmonary function. Linear growth measured by median height standard deviation score improved from -0.7 before transplantation to -0.2 after transplantation. An adverse effect of busulfan conditioning on ovarian function was demonstrated in five of seven evaluable females who are currently at least 13 years of age. None of the four males tested had elevated serum gonadotropin levels.[28] Four patients who received allogeneic bone marrow transplantation were compared to seven patients who received other therapy and to 13 untreated patients.[49] Quantitative analysis revealed a 10% increase in the measured diameter of 64 vessels ($P = .001$) following any treatment. Patients who had undergone allogeneic bone marrow transplantation exhibited a 12% increase in the lumen of 22 vessels ($P = .041$), whereas patients treated with chronic transfusion or hydroxyurea exhibited an 8% increase in 42 vessels ($P = .016$). In two patients with severe stenosis, the artery normalized after transplantation, and the blood flow rate was reduced in all patients who underwent transplantation. In untreated patients, there was a trend for the size of the arterial lumen to decrease, which is consistent with disease progression.[49] These results suggest that treatment can reverse progression of vasculopathy. However, worsening of large vessel vasculopathy[50,51] and stroke[52] has been reported following successful engraftment. A patient who had osteonecrosis of the humeral head secondary to SCD had clinical and radiological improvement of the humeral head following a successful HSCT.[53] Correction of the splenic reticuloendothelial dysfunction has been reported after successful HSCT.[29,54]

# HSCT FOR THALASSEMIA

## Pathogenesis of Thalassemia Complications

Thalassemia results from mutations in the globin gene or other regulatory elements that result in the decreased or absent synthesis of α- or β-globins. Nearly 200 different mutations have been described in patients with β thalassemia and related disorders.[55] All the mutations result in either the absence of the synthesis ($\beta^0$) or reduction in synthesis ($\beta^+$) of β-globin chains. β thalassemia is marked by ineffective erythropoiesis, which is the result of the deleterious effects of the relative excess of α-globin chains. This relative excess interferes with most stages of normal erythroid maturation. In severe untreated β thalassemia, erythropoiesis may be increased by a factor of up to 10, more than 95% of which may be ineffective. α thalassemia is caused by mutations of the α-globin genes, leading to decreased or absent α-globin chain production from the affected genes. Because α-globin chains normally are produced throughout gestation, fetuses without α-globin genes suffer from severe anemia, and develop hypoxia, heart failure, and hydrops fetalis.[56]

**TABLE 16.2    Results of HSCT for SCD**

| Reference | Preparative Regimen | GVHD Prophylaxis | N | Median Age (Range) | Overall Survival | Event-free Survival/ Follow-up | Complications |
|---|---|---|---|---|---|---|---|
| Walters et al.[28] | BU 14 mg/kg CY 200 mg/kg ATG 90 mg/kg | CsA CsA + MP CsA + MTX | 50 | 9.9 years (3.3–15.9) | 94% | 84% 2.2 years (0.1–5.6) | Rejection ($N = 4$) GVHD ($N = 1$) ICH ($N = 1$) |
| Vermylen et al.[29] | BU 14–16 mg/kg CY 200 mg/kg ATG/TLI | CsA alone ($N = 25$) CsA + MTX ($N = 25$) | 50 | 9.5 years (0.9–23.0) | 96% | 85% 3.1 years (0.3–6.5) | Rejection ($N = 3$) GVHD ($N = 1$) |
| Bernaudin et al.[30,31] | BU 14–22 mg/kg CY 200–260 mg/kg + rATG | CsA alone ($N = 13$) CsA + MTX ($N = 47$) | 60 | 8.8 years (2.2–22) | 90% | 82% 62 months (16–138) | Rejection ($N = 1$) ICH ($N = 1$) Fatal GVHD ($N = 4$) Fatal Sepsis ($N = 1$) |
| Giardini et al.[32] | BU 14–16 mg/kg CY 120–200 mg/kg ALG | Not described | 8 | 8.0 years (4.0–26.0) | 5/8 | 5/8 | GVHD ($N = 2$) ARDS ($N = 1$) |
| Abboud et al.[33] | BU 14 mg/kg CY 200 mg/kg | CsA + MTX ($N = 8$) CsA + MP ($N = 2$) | 10 | 12.4 years (3.8–19.3) | 9/10 | 9/10 | Infection ($N = 1$) |
| Ferster et al.[34] | BU 14 mg/kg CY 50 mg/kg ALG (in 6 pts) | CsA + MTX | 9 | 8 (2–11) | 9/9 | 6/9 | Rejection ($N = 3$) |

Abbreviations: GVHD = graft-versus-host disease; BU = busulfan; CY = cyclophosphamide; ATG = antithymocyte globulin; CsA = cyclosporine A; MP = methylprednisolone; MTX = methotrexate; ICH = Intracranial Hemorrhage; TLI = total lymphoid irradiation; rATG = rabbit antithymocyte globulin; ALG = antilymphocyte globulin; ARDS = Acute respiratory distress syndrome.

## Clinical Features

Severe ineffective erythropoiesis results in massive erythroid marrow expansion. Marrow expansion results in characteristic deformities of the skull and face as well as osteopenia and focal defects in bone mineralization. Increased erythropoietic drive also results in the formation of extramedullary erythropoietic tissue, primarily in the thorax and paraspinal region. The expanded erythron leads to increased iron absorption and progressive deposition of iron in tissues. Deletion of all four α-globin genes leads to hydrops fetalis, a severe form of α thalassemia, with ominous prognosis for the affected fetus. Advances in antenatal diagnosis, intrauterine intervention, and postnatal treatments have resulted in a few long-term survivors of this usually fatal condition.[57]

## Relationship between Genotype and Phenotype

Several genetic factors may ameliorate the severity of β thalassemia.[58,59] Underlying mutations vary widely in their effect on the synthesis of β-globin chains. Co-inheritance of α thalassemia may reduce the severity of the globin-chain imbalance.[60] Interactions of β thalassemia with structural hemoglobin variants such as hemoglobin S and hemoglobin E result in a complex series of clinical phenotypes. If hemoglobin S is inherited with β[0] thalassemia or severe β[+] thalassemia, the resulting clinical disorder may be indistinguishable from SCD. By contrast, interactions with mild β[+] thalassemia alleles produce a milder sickling disorder. Hemoglobin E/β thalassemia is probably the most common serious hemoglobinopathy worldwide.[61] The interaction of hemoglobin E and β thalassemia results in a wide spectrum of clinical disorders. Some of these disorders are indistinguishable from thalassemia major, while others are much milder and not transfusion-dependent. Acquired and environmental factors, including progressive splenomegaly, exposure to infections, socioeconomic factors, and the availability of medical care, also may modify the severity of the disease.[59]

## Iron Overload

The prognosis of patients with transfusion-dependent homozygous β thalassemia (thalassemia major) has been improved by regular transfusion and iron chelation therapy. Before the introduction of therapy with desferrioxamine, an iron-chelating agent, iron overload from transfusions was a frequent cause of morbidity and mortality in these patients. Extensive iron deposits are associated with cardiac hypertrophy and dilatation, degeneration of myocardial fibers, and, in rare cases, fibrosis.[62] In patients noncompliant with iron chelation, symptomatic cardiac disease has been reported within 10 years after the start of transfusions[63] and may be aggravated by myocarditis[64] and pulmonary hypertension.[65,66] The survival of patients with β thalassemia is determined by the magnitude of iron loading within the heart.[67,68] Iron-induced liver disease is a common cause of death in older patients[69] and may be aggravated by infection with hepatitis C virus (HCV). In the absence of chelation therapy, cirrhosis may develop in the first decade of life.[59]

## Survival

The prospect of improved survival without cardiac disease in patients with thalassemia major has greatly increased, especially for children with thalassemia born since the current treatment became widely available.[68,70] Nonetheless, there are still cases of iron-related illness and death, even in patients who apparently complied with desferrioxamine therapy. A sustained reduction in iron, as measured by the proportion of serum ferritin measurements that did not exceed 2500 ng/mL, is the most consistent predictive factor of survival without cardiac disease.[70] The estimated EFS after 15 years of chelation therapy is 91% among patients in whom fewer than one third of ferritin measurements exceeded 2500 ng/mL, 48% for patients in whom 33% to 67% of ferritin measurements exceeded 2500 ng/mL, and 18% for patients in whom more than 67% of ferritin measurements exceeded 2500 ng/mL. Since desferrioxamine treatment is very cumbersome, disruptive, and expensive, compliance is a major obstacle especially in adolescence and young adulthood.[71,72] Thus, for a large number of adolescent and young adult patients, chelation therapy would be unavailable, toxic, or unacceptable.

## Indications for HSCT

Patients with β thalassemia major who are transfusion dependent have been offered HSCT. Selected patients with severe forms of thalassemia intermedia such as E/β thalassemia also have been considered candidates for HSCT. Aggressive intrauterine and perinatal management has led to the improved survival of patients with hydrops fetalis due to the deletion of all four α-globin genes. A few such patients have now received HSCT.[73]

## Results

Allogeneic HSCT after myeloablative therapy has been performed in more than 1040 patients. (▼ Table 16.3) BU 14–16 mg/kg and CY 200 mg/kg with or without ATG is the backbone of preparative regimens used, although CY/TBI regimens have been used.[78] CsA alone or in combination with MP or MTX has been utilized for posttransplant GVHD prophylaxis. The Pesaro risk stratification system classifies patients with thalassemia undergoing HSCT into risk groups I through III on the basis of the presence of hepatomegaly, portal fibrosis, or adequacy of chelation (class 1 has no risk factor, class II has 2 risk factors, and class III has all 3).[83] The outcome of HSCT in over 800 patients with thalassemia is excellent especially in those who are young and do not have advanced disease.[85] The overall survival (OS) and EFS are 95% and 90% for Pesaro class I patients, 87% and 84% for class II patients, 79% and 58% for class III patients, and 66 % and 62% for adult patients, respectively. Recent modification of the conditioning regimen for young patients with class III disease has improved outcomes in these patients.[85] These patients received HU 30 mg/kg and azathioprine (AZA) 3 mg/kg given daily day -45 to day -11, fludarabine (FLU) 20 mg/m²/day, from day -17 to day -11, and BU 14 mg/kg. Class III patients aged less than 17 years received CY 160 mg/kg, while patients 17 years or older received CY 90 mg/kg. In this group of 31 Class III young thalassemic patients, OS and EFS were 97% and 90%, respectively.

Following HSCT, 40% of patients attained puberty normally despite clinical and hormonal evidence of gonadal dysfunction in most of them.[86] Hormonal dysfunction could be attributed to the cytotoxic effects of the preparative transplant regimen with alkylating agents, although in some patients it could be attributed to gonadotrophin insufficiency, secondary to previous iron overload. Iron overload and HCV infection are independent risk factors for liver fibrosis progression, and their concomitant presence results in a striking increase in risk.[87] In 41 patients treated with phlebotomy after successful HSCT, liver iron concentration decreased from 20.8 (15.5–28.1) to 3 (0.9–14.6) mg/g dry weight ($P <$ .0001), suggesting that phlebotomy is a safe and effective method to decrease iron overload in the "ex-thalassemic."[88] Six patients who developed liver cirrhosis before or after their thalassemia was cured by bone marrow transplantation received iron depletion and antiviral therapies. Follow-up biopsies showed regression of incomplete or definite cirrhosis in all patients.[89] Transplanted thalassemia patients with subclinical left ventricular diastolic dysfunction and impaired left ventricular contractility may reverse these processes with an effective regimen of iron reduction such as phlebotomy.[90] Short stature is present in a significant percentage of transplanted thalassemic children.[91] While there is a close effect of the age at time of transplant (before or after 7 years) on subsequent growth rate, the growth impairment in these subjects is probably multifactorial.

# NOVEL APPROACHES TO HSCT FOR HEMOGLOBINOPATHIES

Despite the potential for cure, few patients have considered allogeneic HSCT because of the paucity of suitable donors, restrictions in eligibility requirements, and risk of early death from regimen-related side effects. Moreover, "conventional" myeloablative therapy is potentially associated with the risk of late effects, including sterility and cancer. Novel approaches are needed to further improve the safety and applicability of HSCT for hemoglobinopathy patients.

## Nonmyeloablative HSCT

Myeloablation for the eradication of host hematopoiesis and host immunosuppression has been considered necessary to "create space" in the host marrow microenvironment and the prevention of immunologic rejection of the graft, respectively. However, the observation that in the immunosuppressed host, the allogeneic marrow graft itself can create its own "space" by means of a local graft-versus-host reaction has opened up a whole new area of investigation of HSCT following nonmyeloablative preparative regimen.[92–106] Several patients who developed persistent mixed hematopoietic chimerism after HSCT following a myeloablative conditioning regimen experienced a significant amelioration of their clinical phenotype.[107,108] Thus, nonmyeloablative HSCT with the elimination or reduction of myelotoxic therapies and the establishment of partial or complete donor chimerism is an attractive alternative for patients with hemoglobinopathies. A number of regimens have been proposed to reduce the toxicity associated with allogeneic HSCT. A truly nonmyeloablative regimen would not eradicate host hematopoiesis and would allow hematopoietic recovery even without donor stem cell infusion. Regimens that produce some myeloablation and require donor marrow infusion for hematopoietic recovery are termed reduced intensity conditioning.[103] Fludarabine, a purine analog is the backbone of most of the nonmyeloablative preparative regimens used. ▼ Table 16.4 describes the current results of nonmyeloablative HSCT for hemoglobinopathies. Duration of myelosuppression in both approaches has been comparable. While initial engraftment has been achieved in most patients using

**TABLE 16.3    Results of HSCT for Thalassemia**

| Reference | Preparative Regimen | GVHD Prophylaxis | N | Median Age (Range) | Overall Survival | Event-free Survival/Follow-up | Cause of death |
|---|---|---|---|---|---|---|---|
| Mentzer and Cowan[74] | BU 14 mg/kg CY 200 mg/kg ATG 90 mg/kg | CsA + MTX | 17 | 9.9 years (3.3–15.3) | 94% | 71% 2.2 years (0.1–5.6) | Rejection (N = 4) GVHD (N = 1) ICH (N = 1) |
| Lucarelli et al.[75–77] | BU 14–16 mg/kg CY 200 mg/kg | CsA + MTX | 886 | 9.5 years (1–23.0) | Class I 93% Class II 87% Class III 79% Adult 66 % | Class I 91% Class II 83% Class III 58% Adult 62 % 3.1 years (0.3–6.5) | Rejection (N = 3) GVHD (N = 1) |
| | BU 16 + CY 160 + FLU, AZA, HU (Class III) | | | | | | |
| | BU 16 + CY 90 + FLU, AZA, HU (Adult) | | | | | | |
| Boulad et al.[78,79] | CY 120+TBI or BU 14–16 mg/kg + CY 200 mg/kg or BU 14 mg/kg FLU 150 mg/m² ATG | MTX CsA+MP CsA + MTX | 17 | | 94% | 76% 5.5 years (1–8) | Grade IV GVHD (N = 1) |

**TABLE 16.3** Results of HSCT for Thalassemia—cont'd

| Reference | Preparative Regimen | GVHD Prophylaxis | N | Median Age (Range) | Overall Survival | Event-free Survival/ Follow-up | Cause of death |
|---|---|---|---|---|---|---|---|
| Chandy et al.[80] | BU 14–22 mg/kg CY 200–260 mg/kg | CsA + MTX | 106 | 8.6 years (2.2–14.8) | Class I 66% Class II 90% Class III 67% | Class I 66% Class II 90% Class III 55% 26 months (2–87) | Grade IV GVHD (N = 8) VOD (N = 6) IP (N = 6) Other (N = 7) |
| Lee et al.[81] | BU 14–16 mg/kg CY 120–200 mg/kg ALG | Not described | 8 | 8.0 years (4.0–26.0) | 5/8 | 5/8 | GVHD (N = 2) ARDS (N = 1) |
| Khojasteh et al.[82] | BU 14 mg/kg CY 200 mg/kg | CsA + MTX (N = 8) CsA + MP (N = 2) | 10 | 12.4 years (3.8–19.3) | 9/10 | 9/10 | Infection (N = 1) |

Abbreviations: AZA = azathioprine; FLU = fludarabine; VOD = venocclusive disease; IP = interstitial pneumonitis; GVHD = graft-versus-host disease; BU = busulfan; CY = cyclophosphamide; ATG = antithymocyte globulin; CsA = cyclosporine A; MP = methylprednisolone; MTX = methotrexate; ICH = Intracranial Hemorrhage; TLI = total lymphoid irradiation; rATG = rabbit antithymocyte globulin; ALG = antilymphocyte globulin; ARDS = Acute respiratory distress syndrome.

**TABLE 16.4   Results of Nonmyeloablative HSCT for Hemoglobinopathies**

| Reference | Preparative Regimen | GVHD Prophylaxis | N | Age in Years (Range) | Initial Chimerism | Deaths | Disease-free Survival/ Follow-up (Range) | AGVHD/ Comments |
|---|---|---|---|---|---|---|---|---|
| Krishnamurti et al.[109,110] | BU 8 mg/kg<br>FLU 175 mg/m²<br>ATG 90 mg/kg<br>TLI 500 cGy | CsA + MMF | 3 | 9.9 (3–15) | 3/3 | 0/2 | 2/3 (24–36 months) | grade II (N = 1) |
| Van Besien et al.[111] | FLU 14–16 mg/kg<br>MEL 200 mg/kg<br>ATG 200 mg/kg | CsA + MMF | 2 | 9.5 (1–23) | 2/2 | 2/2 severe GVHD | 0/2 | grade IV (N = 2) |
| Slavin et al.[112] | BU 8 mg/kg<br>FLU 180 mg/m²<br>ATG 40 mg/kg | CsA + MMF | 1 | 16 | 1/1 | 0/1 | 1/1 | |
| Schleuning et al.[113] | FLU 120 mg/m²<br>CY 120 mg/kg | CsA + MMF | 1 | 22 | 1/1 | 0/1 | 1/1 | Note: PBSCT |
| Hongeng et al.[114] | BU 8 mg/kg<br>CY 1050 mg/m²<br>FLU 90 mg/m²<br>ATG 90 mg/kg<br>TLI 500 cGy | CsA + MMF | 1 | 8.0 (4–26) | 1/1 | 0/1 | 1/1 | |
| Gomez-Almaguer et al.[115] | BU 8 mg/kg<br>FLU 175 mg/kg | CsA + MMF | 1 | | 1/1 | 0/1 | 1/1 | Note: PBSCT |

## TABLE 16.4   Results of Nonmyeloablative HSCT for Hemoglobinopathies—cont'd

| Reference | Preparative Regimen | GVHD Prophylaxis | N | Age in Years (Range) | Initial Chimerism | Deaths | Disease-free Survival/ Follow-up (Range) | AGVHD/ Comments |
|---|---|---|---|---|---|---|---|---|
| Iannone et al.[116–118] | FLU 90–150 mg/kg TBI 200 cGy ATG 90 mg/kg | CsA or Tacrolimus + MMF | 7 | 9 (3–20) | 7/7 | 0/7 | 0/7 | grade II (N = 1) |
| Horan et al.[52] Walters et al.[119] | FLU 125 mg/m² TBI 200 cGy rATG 19 mg/kg | CsA + MMF | 3 | 25 (9–30) | 4/4 | 0/4 | 3/4 6 months (1–6) | CVA (N = 1) 3 patients on immunosuppression |
| Van Besien et al.[120,121] | FLU 120 mg/m² MEL 140 mg/m² Campath 1H 20 mg × 1 or Campath 1H 20 mg × 5 | Tacrolimus + MMF | 2 | 21 (19–24) | 2/2 | 0/2 | 1/2 (still on immunosuppression) 68 days | 1 patient on immunosuppression |
| Isola et al.[122] | Campath 1H 20 mg/d × 5 + FLU + CY | Campath 1H 20 mg in bag + MMF | 3 | 23 (20–45) | 2/3 | 0/3 | 0/3 | |

Abbreviations: MMF = mycophenolate mofetil; PBSCT = peripheral blood stem cell transplantation; CVA = cerebrovascular accident; MEL = Melphalan; GVHD = graft-versus-host disease; BU = busulfan; CY = cyclophosphamide; ATG = antithymocyte globulin; CsA = cyclosporine A; MP = methylprednisolone; MTX = methotrexate; ICH = Intracranial Hemorrhage; TLI = total lymphoid irradiation; rATG = rabbit antithymocyte globulin; ALG = antilymphocyte globulin; ARDS = Acute respiratory distress syndrome.

either approach, sustained engraftment has been achieved mainly using the reduced intensity conditioning regimens that have included the use of reduced doses of myelosuppressive medications such as BU, CY, or MEL (Melphalan). However, preliminary results suggest that increased immunosuppression with rabbit ATG[52] or Campath 1H[120] can result in sustained engraftment using truly nonmyeloablative regimens. Because of prior chemotherapy, patients with hematological malignancies may have varying degrees of immunosuppression as well as decreased marrow reserve prior to HSCT. In contrast, patients with hemoglobinopathies have received no prior immunosuppressive therapies and may actually have significant marrow hyperplasia. Moreover, they also may be allosensitized due to repeated blood transfusion. These factors may be responsible for the 10%–30% risk of graft rejection after HSCT in hemoglobinopathy patients.[28,76,123] Thus, rejection of donor marrow is likely to be a challenge in nonmyeloablative HSCT for hemoglobinopathies.

## Matched Umbilical Cord Blood from Sibling as Stem Cell Source for HSCT

Recently, 44 patients with hemoglobinopathies (33 thalassemia, 11 SCD) received an umbilical cord blood (UCB) transplantation from a sibling.[47] Forty-one umbilical cord blood (UCB) donors were human leukocyte antigen (HLA) matched, and three had one HLA-A difference. Median recipient age was five years (range 1–20) and median follow-up was 27 months (range 1–85). The two year OS and EFS were 100% and 81%, respectively. In patients with thalassemia, addition of thiotepa (THIO) to the combination of BU/CY or BU/FLU was associated with a better outcome, DFS of patients who did or did not receive THIO being 94% versus 62%, respectively ($P < .05$).[47] Remote-site collection and directed-donor banking of UCB for sibling recipients with malignancy, SCD, thalassemia major, non-malignant hematological conditions, and metabolic errors have been accomplished with a high success rate. Sixteen of 17 UCB allograft recipients had stable engraftment of donor cells.[124] ▶ Table 16.5 describes the experience with UCB transplantation for hemoglobinopathies.

## HSCT from Unrelated Donors

While young patients without advanced disease who have received HSCT from a matched sibling have an excellent outcome, the applicability of HSCT for these conditions is limited by the fact that fewer than one third of these patients will find a suitable HLA matched related or family donor.[130] In the past, HSCT from unrelated donors (URD) has not been offered to patients with hemoglobinopathies. Since these diseases may be associated with prolonged survival, the increased regimen related toxicity (RRT) of URD HSCT was considered unacceptable. The worldwide number of alternative donor transplants for hemoglobinopathies remains limited to date.[41,125–127,131,132] The National Marrow Donor Program® (NMDP) has facilitated HSCT in three SCD and 15 thalassemia patients.[133] The advent of novel strategies for reduction of RRT, including the use of nonmyeloablative preparative regimens[109,113] and the improvement in outcomes of URD HSCT,[134] has sparked fresh interest in the consideration of URD HSCT for patients with hemoglobinopathies. ▶ Table 16.5 describes the outcomes of URD HSCT for hemoglobinopathies. With improvement in supportive care, the

**TABLE 16.5   Results of Alternative Donor HSCT for Hemoglobinopathies**

| Reference | Preparative Regimen | GVHD Prophylaxis | N | Median Age (Range) | Overall Survival | Event-free Survival/ Follow-up | Complications/ Comments |
|---|---|---|---|---|---|---|---|
| La Nasa et al.[125] | BU 14 mg/kg CY 120–200 mg/kg TT 10 mg/kg | CsA + MTX | 32 | 9.9 years (3.3–15.3) | 79% | 66% 30 months (7–109) | Improved outcome with extended haplotype match |
| Contu et al.[126] | BU 14 mg/kg CY 160 mg/kg | Not described | 1 | 16 years | 1/1 | 1/1 7 months | |
| Gaziev et al.[127] | BU 14–16 mg/kg CY 120–200 mg/kg ALG/TLI/TBI | NA | 23 | 8.0 years (4.0–26.0) | 65% | 21% 7.5 years (0.6–17) | Related HLA mismatched donor |
| Locatelli et al.[47] | BU 14 mg/kg CY 200 mg/kg | CsA + MTX (N = 8) CsA + MP (N = 2) | 44 | 12.4 years (3.8–19.3) | 100% | 81% | Sibling donor UCB |
| Krishnamurti et al.[128] | BU 14 CY 200 mg/kg | Not described | 1 | 4.0 | 1/1 | 1/1 5 years | Sibling donor UCB |
| Gore et al.[44] | BU CY 200 mg/kg | Not described | 1 | 8.0 | 1/1 | 1/1 | Sibling donor UCB |
| Brichard et al.[45] | BU 16 mg/kg CY 200 mg/kg ATG 30 mg/kg | Not described | 1 | | 1/1 | 1/1 | Sibling donor UCB |
| Werner et al.[46] | CY 6 g/m$^2$ VP 16 1.8 g/m$^2$ TBI 1200 cGy | Not described | 1 | 19.0 | 1/1 | 1/1 | Unrelated donor UCB for SCD with AML |
| Yeager et al.[129] | BU 16 mg/kg CY 200 mg/kg ATG 90 mg/kg | CsA | 2 | 6 years, 12 years | 2/2 | 2/2 (2 years & 4 years) | 1 extensive CGVHD unrelated donor UCB for SCD |

Abbreviations: TT = Thiotepa; HLA = human lymphocyte antigen; UCB = umbilical cord blood; TBI = total body irradiation; GVHD = graft-versus-host disease; BU = busulfan; CY = cyclophosphamide; ATG = antithymocyte globulin; CsA = cyclosporine A; MP = methylprednisolone; MTX = methotrexate; ICH = Intracranial Hemorrhage; TLI = total lymphoid irradiation; rATG = rabbit antithymocyte globulin; ALG = antilymphocyte globulin; ARDS = Acute respiratory distress syndrome.

outcomes of HSCT for this group of disease also have improved. However, the overall survival of 81% in one series of thalassemia patients must be compared with the survival of 90% to age 20 years in transfusion dependent patients who receive optimal chelation. Thus, while the progress is encouraging, the role of URD HSCT for hemoglobinopathies is as yet unclear and must only be undertaken in the context of controlled clinical trials.

## FUTURE DIRECTIONS

Development of less toxic nonmyeloablative conditioning regimens have the potential to reduce procedure-related mortality to even lower levels and improve applicability of HSCT to patients to whom it is currently unavailable. Improvement in the risk benefit ratio also would impact on the indications for HSCT, particularly for SCD. There may be differences in recommendations of health care providers and risk accepted by patients or parents.[135] The majority of parents and patients are willing to accept some risk of mortality. Further studies are indicated to study the effect of parental beliefs and preferences on selection of patients for HSCT. Selection criteria currently in use were empirically derived and require the patient to manifest features of severe disease or involvement of target organ. The risk prediction model[17] potentially offers objective criteria for the selection of patients with SCD for HSCT. Additional studies are required in the use of this or similar models for this purpose. A better understanding of the effect of HSCT on the natural history of vasculopathy and organ damage would impact on selection of patients for HSCT. Expansion of the donor pool by use of unrelated matched donors awaits further improvement in outcomes of unrelated donor HSCT. The representation of minorities in donor registries and the availability of potential HLA matched donors for hemoglobinopathy patients has improved.[136] However, there remain several limitations to the possibility of finding fully HLA-matched donors for patients with hemoglobinopathies. Implementation of strategies for improved minority donor registration and retention are critical to the development of this therapeutic option for patients with hemoglobinopathies. UCB offers the possibility of reduced complications such as severe GVHD. Ex vivo expansion of UCB cells[137] or the use of multiple UCB units[138] also offers the possibility of this source of stem cells for adult hemoglobinopathy patients.

## ACKNOWLEDGMENT

I am grateful to Dr. Andrew M. Yeager for reviewing this manuscript and for his helpful comments and revisions.

# REFERENCES

1. Platt OS, Brambilla DJ, Rosse WF et al. Mortality in sickle cell disease. Life expectancy and risk factors for early death (see comments). N Engl J Med 1994;330:1639–1644.
2. Leikin SL, Gallagher D, Kinney TR et al. Mortality in children and adolescents with sickle cell disease. Cooperative Study of Sickle Cell Disease. Pediatrics 1989;84:500–508.
3. Serjeant GR. Natural history and determinants of clinical severity of sickle cell disease. Curr Opin Hematol 1995;2:103–108.
4. Hebbel RP. Adhesive interactions of sickle erythrocytes with endothelium. J Clin Invest 1997;100(Suppl 11): S83–S86.
5. Taylor VI JG, Tang DC, Savage SA et al. Variants in the VCAM1 gene and risk for symptomatic stroke in sickle cell disease. Blood 2002;100:4303–4309.
6. Wethers DL. Sickle cell disease in childhood: Part I. Laboratory diagnosis, pathophysiology and health maintenance. Am Fam Physician 2000;62:1013–1020, 1027–1018.
7. Chui DH, Dover GJ. Sickle cell disease: no longer a single gene disorder. Curr Opin Pediatr 2001;13:22–27.
8. Craig JE, Rochette J, Fisher CA et al. Dissecting the loci controlling fetal haemoglobin production on chromosomes 11p and 6q by the regressive approach. Nat Genet 1996;12:58–64.
9. Nagel RL. Severity, pathobiology, epistatic effects, and genetic markers in sickle cell anemia. Semin Hematol 1991;28:180–201.
10. Chang YP, Maier-Redelsperger M, Smith KD et al. The relative importance of the X-linked FCP locus and beta-globin haplotypes in determining haemoglobin F levels: a study of SS patients homozygous for beta S haplotypes. Br J Haematol 1997;96:806–814.
11. Steinberg MH. Modulation of the phenotypic diversity of sickle cell anemia. Hemoglobin 1996;20:1–19.
12. Styles LA, Hoppe C, Klitz W et al. Evidence for HLA-related susceptibility for stroke in children with sickle cell disease. Blood 2000;95:3562–3567.
13. Garner C, Tatu T, Reittie JE et al. Genetic influences on F cells and other hematologic variables: a twin heritability study. Blood 2000;95:342–346.
14. Romana M, Muralitharan S, Ramasawmy R et al. Thrombosis-associated gene variants in sickle cell anemia. Thromb Haemost. 2002;87:356–358.
15. Bookchin RM, Lew VL. Sickle red cell dehydration: mechanisms and interventions. Curr Opin Hematol 2002;9:107–110.
16. Platt OS, Thorington BD, Brambilla DJ et al. Pain in sickle cell disease. Rates and risk factors. N Engl J Med 1991;325:11–16.
17. Miller ST, Sleeper LA, Pegelow CH et al. Prediction of adverse outcomes in children with sickle cell disease. N Engl J Med 2000;342:83–89.
18. Bridges W. Cerebral vascular disease accompanying sickle cell anemia. Am J Pathol 1939;15:353–360.
19. Gaston M, Smith J, Gallagher D et al. Recruitment in the Cooperative Study of Sickle Cell Disease (CSSCD). Control Clin Trials 1987;8:131S–140S.
20. Ohene-Frempong K, Weiner SJ, Sleeper LA et al. Cerebrovascular accidents in sickle cell disease: rates and risk factors. Blood 1998;91:288–294.
21. Armstrong FD, Thompson RJ Jr., Wang W et al. Cognitive functioning and brain magnetic resonance imaging in children with sickle cell disease. Neuropsychology Committee of the Cooperative Study of Sickle Cell Disease. Pediatrics 1996;97:864–870.
22. Powars DR, Conti PS, Wong WY et al. Cerebral vasculopathy in sickle cell anemia: diagnostic contribution of positron emission tomography. Blood 1999;93:71–79.
23. Miller ST, Macklin EA, Pegelow CH et al. Silent infarction as a risk factor for overt stroke in children with sickle cell anemia: a report from the Cooperative Study of Sickle Cell Disease. J Pediatr 2001;139:385–390.
24. Vichinsky EP, Neumayr LD, Earles AN et al. Causes and outcomes of the acute chest syndrome in sickle cell disease. National Acute Chest Syndrome Study Group. N Engl J Med 2000;342:1855–1865.
25. Golden C, Styles L, Vichinsky E. Acute chest syndrome and sickle cell disease. Curr Opin Hematol 1998; 5:89–92.
26. Davis H, Moore RM Jr., Gergen PJ. Cost of hospitalizations associated with sickle cell disease in the United States. Public Health Rep 1997;112:40–43.
27. Walters MC, Patience M, Leisenring W et al. Bone marrow transplantation for sickle cell disease. N Engl J Med 1996;335:369–376.
28. Walters MC, Storb R, Patience M et al. Impact of bone marrow transplantation for symptomatic sickle cell disease: an interim report. Multicenter investigation of bone marrow transplantation for sickle cell disease. Blood 2000;95:1918–1924.
29. Vermylen C, Cornu G, Ferster A et al. Haematopoietic stem cell transplantation for sickle cell anaemia: the first 50 patients transplanted in Belgium. Bone Marrow Transplant 1998;22:1–6.
30. Bernaudin F, Vernant JP, Vilmer E et al. Results of allogeneic stem cell transplant for severe sickle cell disease (SCD) in France and consideration about conditioning regimen and indications in 2002. Washington, DC:

30th Anniversary of the National Sickle Cell Disease Program National Heart, Lung, and Blood Institute, National Institutes of Health, and the Sickle Cell Disease Association of America, Inc. (Abstr #33) 2002;33.

31. Bernaudin F, Souillet G, Vannier JP et al. Bone marrow transplantation (BMT) in 14 children with severe sickle cell disease (SCD): the French experience. GEGMO. Bone Marrow Transplant 1993;12(Suppl 1): 118–121.

32. Giardini C, Galimberti M, Lucarelli G et al. Bone marrow transplantation in sickle-cell anemia in Pesaro. Bone Marrow Transplant 1993;12(Suppl 1):122–123.

33. Abboud M, Kletzel M, Miller S et al. Bone marrow transplantation for sickle cell disease (Abstr #1010). Blood 1997;90(Suppl 1):228a.

34. Ferster A, Corazza F, Vertongen F et al. Transplanted sickle-cell disease patients with autologous bone marrow recovery after graft failure develop increased levels of fetal haemoglobin which corrects disease severity. Br J Haematol 1995;90:804–808.

35. Vermylen C, Fernandez Robles E, Ninane J et al. Bone marrow transplantation in five children with sickle cell anaemia. Lancet 1988;1:1427–1428.

36. Hoppe CC, Walters MC. Bone marrow transplantation in sickle cell anemia. Curr Opin Oncol 2001;13: 85–90.

37. Vermylen C, Cornu G. Bone marrow transplantation for sickle cell anemia. Curr Opin Hematol 1996;3: 163–166.

38. Bernaudin F, Souillet G, Vannier JP et al. Bone marrow transplantation (BMT) in 14 children with severe sickle cell disease (SCD): the French experience. GEGMO. Bone Marrow Transplant 1993;12(Suppl 1): 118–121.

39. Abboud MR, Jackson SM, Barredo J et al. Bone marrow transplantation for sickle cell anemia. Am J Pediatr Hematol Oncol 1994;16:86–89.

40. Brichard B, Vermylen C, Ninane J et al. Persistence of fetal hemoglobin production after successful transplantation of cord blood stem cells in a patient with sickle cell anemia. J Pediatr 1996;128:241–243.

41. Golden F. The sickle-cell kid. An experimental transplant succeeds, giving a brave little boy the best Christmas present he can imagine. Time 1999;154:92.

42. Bernaudin F. [Results and current indications of bone marrow allograft in sickle cell disease]. Pathol Biol (Paris) 1999;47:59–64.

43. Platt OS, Brambilla DJ, Rosse WF et al. Mortality in sickle cell disease. Life expectancy and risk factors for early death. N Engl J Med 1994;330:1639–1644.

44. Gore L, Lane PA, Giller RH. Successful cord blood stem cell transplantation for sickle cell anemia from an HLA-identical sibling (Abstr #4492). Blood 1997;90(Suppl 1):388b.

45. Brichard B, Vermylen C, Ninane J et al. Persistence of fetal hemoglobin production after successful transplantation of cord blood stem cells in a patient with sickle cell anemia (see comments). J Pediatr 1996;128: 241–243.

46. Werner E, Yanovich S, Rubinstein P et al. Unrelated placental cord blood transplantation in a patient with sickle cell disease and acute non-lymphocytic leukemia (Abstr #4942). Blood 1997;90(Suppl 1):399b.

47. Locatelli F, Rocha V, Reed W et al. Related cord blood transplant in patients with thalassemia and sickle cell disease (Abstr #1736). Blood 2001;98:413a.

48. Walters MC, Patience M, Leisenring W et al. Updated results of bone marrow transplantation (BMT) for sickle cell disease (SCD): Impact on CNS disease (Abstr #160). Blood 2002;100:46a.

49. Steen RG, Helton KJ, Horwitz EM et al. Improved cerebrovascular patency following therapy in patients with sickle cell disease: initial results in 4 patients who received HLA-identical hematopoietic stem cell allografts. Ann Neurol 2001;49:222–229.

50. Kalinyak KA, Morris C, Ball WS et al. Bone marrow transplantation in a young child with sickle cell anemia. Am J Hematol 1995;48:256–261.

51. Adamkiewicz T, Chiang KY, Haight A et al. Significant progression of large central nervous system (CNS) vessel disease following full matched sibling marrow engraftment in a child with hemoglobin SS. Washington, DC: 30th Anniversary of the National Sickle Cell Disease Program National Heart, Lung, and Blood Institute, National Institutes of Health, and the Sickle Cell Disease Association of America, Inc. (Abstr #1) 2002;1.

52. Horan J, Liesveld J, Fenton P et al. Hematopoietic stem cell transplantation for sickle cell disease and thalassemia after low dose TBI, fludarabine and rabbit ATG. Washington, DC: 30th Anniversary of the National Sickle Cell Disease Program National Heart, Lung, and Blood Institute, National Institutes of Health, and the Sickle Cell Disease Association of America, Inc. (Abstr #34) 2002;34.

53. Hernigou P, Bernaudin F, Reinert P et al. Bone-marrow transplantation in sickle-cell disease. Effect on osteonecrosis: a case report with a four-year follow-up. J Bone Joint Surg Am 1997;79:1726–1730.

54. Ferster A, Bujan W, Corazza F et al. Bone marrow transplantation corrects the splenic reticuloendothelial dysfunction in sickle cell anemia. Blood 1993;81:1102–1105.

55. Weatherall DJ. Thalassemia in the next millennium. Keynote address. Ann N Y Acad Sci 1998;850:1–9.

56. Chui DH, Waye JS. Hydrops fetalis caused by alpha-thalassemia: an emerging health care problem. Blood 1998;91:2213–2222.
57. Singer ST, Styles L, Bojanowski J et al. Changing outcome of homozygous alpha-thalassemia: cautious optimism. J Pediatr Hematol Oncol 2000;22:539–542.
58. Weatherall DJ. Phenotype-genotype relationships in monogenic disease: lessons from the thalassaemias. Nat Rev Genet 2001;2:245–255.
59. Olivieri NF. The beta-thalassemias. N Engl J Med 1999;341:99–109.
60. Krishnamurti L, Chui DH, Dallaire M et al. Coinheritance of alpha-thalassemia-1 and hemoglobin E/beta zero-thalassemia: practical implications for neonatal screening and genetic counseling. J Pediatr 1998;132:863–865.
61. Weatherall DJ. Introduction to the problem of hemoglobin E-beta thalassemia. J Pediatr Hematol Oncol 2000;22:551.
62. Buja LM, Roberts WC. Iron in the heart. Etiology and clinical significance. Am J Med 1971;51:209–221.
63. Wolfe L, Olivieri N, Sallan D et al. Prevention of cardiac disease by subcutaneous deferoxamine in patients with thalassemia major. N Engl J Med 1985;312:1600–1603.
64. Kremastinos DT, Tiniakos G, Theodorakis GN et al. Myocarditis in beta-thalassemia major. A cause of heart failure. Circulation 1995;91:66–71.
65. Du ZD, Roguin N, Milgram E et al. Pulmonary hypertension in patients with thalassemia major. Am Heart J 1997;134:532–537.
66. Aessopos A, Stamatelos G, Skoumas V et al. Pulmonary hypertension and right heart failure in patients with beta-thalassaemia intermedia. Chest 1995;107:50–53.
67. Olivieri NF, Nathan DG, MacMillan JH et al. Survival in medically treated patients with homozygous beta-thalassemia (see comments). N Engl J Med 1994;331:574–578.
68. Brittenham GM, Griffith PM, Nienhuis AW et al. Efficacy of deferoxamine in preventing complications of iron overload in patients with thalassemia major. N Engl J Med 1994;331:567–573.
69. Zurlo MG, De Stefano P, Borgna-Pignatti C et al. Survival and causes of death in thalassaemia major. Lancet 1989;2:27–30.
70. Olivieri NF, Nathan DG, MacMillan JH et al. Survival in medically treated patients with homozygous beta-thalassemia. N Engl J Med 1994;331:574–578.
71. Hoffbrand AV, AL-Refaie F, Davis B et al. Long-term trial of deferiprone in 51 transfusion-dependent iron overloaded patients. Blood 1998;91:295–300.
72. Hoffbrand AV. Iron chelation therapy. Curr Opin Hematol 1995;2:153–158.
73. Chik KW, Shing MM, Li CK et al. Treatment of hemoglobin Bart's hydrops with bone marrow transplantation. J Pediatr 1998;132:1039–1042.
74. Mentzer WC, Cowan MJ. Bone marrow transplantation for beta-thalassemia: the University of California San Francisco experience. J Pediatr Hematol Oncol 2000;22:598–601.
75. Giardini C, Lucarelli G. Bone marrow transplantation for beta-thalassemia. Hematol Oncol Clin North Am 1999;13:1059–1064, viii.
76. Lucarelli G, Andreani M, Angelucci E. The cure of thalassemia by bone marrow transplantation. Blood Rev 2002;16:81–85.
77. Lucarelli G, Clift RA, Galimberti M et al. Bone marrow transplantation in adult thalassemic patients. Blood 1999;93:1164–1167.
78. Boulad F, Giardina P, Gillio A et al. Bone marrow transplantation for homozygous beta-thalassemia. The Memorial Sloan-Kettering Cancer Center experience. Ann N Y Acad Sci 1998;850:498–502.
79. Boulad F, Giardina P, Small TN et al. Allogeneic bone marrow transplantation (BMT) for the treatment of homozygous beta thalassemia (HB-Thal) - The MSKCC experience (Abstr #891). Blood 2002;100:29b.
80. Chandy M, Srivastava A, Dennison D et al. Allogeneic bone marrow transplantation in the developing world: experience from a center in India. Bone Marrow Transplant 2001;27:785–790.
81. Lee YS, Kristovich KM, Ducore JM et al. Bone marrow transplant in thalassemia. A role for radiation? Ann N Y Acad Sci 1998;850:503–505.
82. Khojasteh NH, Zakernia M, Ramzi M et al. Bone marrow transplantation for hematological disorders—Shiraz experience. Indian J Pediatr 2002;69:31–32.
83. Lucarelli G, Galimberti M, Polchi P et al. Bone marrow transplantation in patients with thalassemia. N Engl J Med 1990;322:417–421.
84. Lucarelli G, Andreani M, Angelucci E. The cure of the thalassemia with bone marrow transplantation. Bone Marrow Transplant 2001;28(Suppl 1):S11–S13.
85. Sodani P, Gaziev D, Erer B et al. New preparative regimen for bone marrow transplantation in Class 3 young thalassemic patients (Abstr # 3314). Blood 2002;100:840a.
86. De Sanctis V, Galimberti M, Lucarelli G et al. Pubertal development in thalassaemic patients after allogenic bone marrow transplantation. Eur J Pediatr 1993;152:993–997.

87. Angelucci E, Muretto P, Nicolucci A et al. Effects of iron overload and hepatitis C virus positivity in determining progression of liver fibrosis in thalassemia following bone marrow transplantation. Blood 2002;100: 17–21.

88. Angelucci E, Muretto P, Lucarelli G et al. Treatment of iron overload in the "ex-thalassemic". Report from the phlebotomy program. Ann N Y Acad Sci 1998;850:288–293.

89. Muretto P, Angelucci E, Lucarelli G. Reversibility of cirrhosis in patients cured of thalassemia by bone marrow transplantation. Ann Intern Med 2002;136:667–672.

90. Mariotti E, Angelucci E, Agostini A et al. Evaluation of cardiac status in iron-loaded thalassaemia patients following bone marrow transplantation: improvement in cardiac function during reduction in body iron burden. Br J Haematol 1998;103:916–921.

91. De Simone M, Verrotti A, Iughetti L et al. Final height of thalassemic patients who underwent bone marrow transplantation during childhood. Bone Marrow Transplant 2001;28:201–205.

92. Storb R, Yu C, Zaucha JM et al. Stable mixed hematopoietic chimerism in dogs given donor antigen, CTLA4Ig, and 100 cGy total body irradiation before and pharmacologic immunosuppression after marrow transplant. Blood 1999;94:2523–2529.

93. Sachs DH. Mixed chimerism as an approach to transplantation tolerance. Clin Immunol 2000;95(Suppl 2):S63–S68.

94. Bornhauser M, Thiede C, Platzbecker U et al. Dose-reduced conditioning and allogeneic hematopoietic stem cell transplantation from unrelated donors in 42 patients. Clin Cancer Res 2001;7:2254–2262.

95. Burt RK, Barr W, Oyama Y et al. Future strategies in hematopoietic stem cell transplantation for rheumatoid arthritis. J Rheumatol 2001;28(Suppl 64):42–48.

96. Champlin R, Khouri I, Komblau S et al. Reinventing bone marrow transplantation. Nonmyeloablative preparative regimens and induction of graft-vs-malignancy effect. Oncology (Huntingt) 1999;13:621–628; discussion 631, 635–638, 641.

97. Champlin R, Khouri I, Anderlini P et al. Nonmyeloablative preparative regimens for allogeneic hematopoietic transplantation. Bone Marrow Transplant 2001;27(Suppl 2):S13–S22.

98. Childs RW. Nonmyeloablative blood stem cell transplantation as adoptive allogeneic immunotherapy for metastatic renal cell carcinoma. Crit Rev Immunol. 2001;21:191–203.

99. Craddock C. Nonmyeloablative stem cell transplants. Curr Opin Hematol 1999;6:383–387.

100. Feinstein L, Sandmaier B, Maloney D et al. Nonmyeloablative hematopoietic cell transplantation. Replacing high-dose cytotoxic therapy by the graft-versus-tumor effect. Ann N Y Acad Sci 2001;938:328–337; discussion 337–339.

101. McSweeney P. Nonmyeloablative allogeneic hematopoietic cell transplants: any role for rheumatoid arthritis? J Rheumatol 2001;28(Suppl 64):49–54.

102. Slavin S, Or R, Aker M et al. Nonmyeloablative stem cell transplantation for the treatment of cancer and life-threatening nonmalignant disorders: past accomplishments and future goals. Cancer Chemother Pharmacol 2001;48(Suppl 1):S79–S84.

103. Storb RF, Champlin R, Riddell SR et al. Non-myeloablative transplants for malignant disease. Hematology (Am Soc Hematol Educ Program) 2001:375–391.

104. Storb R, Yu C, Wagner JL et al. Stable mixed hematopoietic chimerism in DLA-identical littermate dogs given sublethal total body irradiation before and pharmacological immunosuppression after marrow transplantation. Blood 1997;89:3048–3054.

105. Storb R, Yu C, Deeg HJ et al. Current and future preparative regimens for bone marrow transplantation in thalassemia. Ann N Y Acad Sci 1998;850:276–287.

106. Slavin S, Nagler A, Naparstek E et al. Allogeneic nonmyeloablative stem cell transplantation and cell therapy as an emerging new modality for immunotherapy of hematologic malignancies and nonmalignant diseases (Abstr). Blood 1998;92:519a.

107. Walters MC, Patience M, Leisenring W et al. Stable mixed hematopoietic chimerism after bone marrow transplantation for sickle cell anemia. Biol Blood Marrow Transplant 2001;7:665–673.

108. Andreani M, Nesci S, Lucarelli G et al. Long-term survival of ex-thalassemic patients with persistent mixed chimerism after bone marrow transplantation. Bone Marrow Transplant 2000;25:401–404.

109. Krishnamurti L, Blazar BR, Wagner JE. Bone marrow transplantation without myeloablation for sickle cell disease. N Engl J Med 2001;344:1071–1078.

110. Krishnamurti L, Blazar BR, Grossi M et al. Successful use of non-myeloablative therapy in the treatment of severe hemoglobinopathies: Proof of principle (Abstr #3734). Blood 2000;96:18b.

111. van Besien K, Bartholomew A, Stock W et al. Fludarabine-based conditioning for allogeneic transplantation in adults with sickle cell disease. Bone Marrow Transplant 2000;26:445–449.

112. Slavin S, Nagler A, Naparstek E et al. Nonmyeloablative stem cell transplantation and cell therapy as an alternative to conventional bone marrow transplantation with lethal cytoreduction for the treatment of malignant and nonmalignant hematologic diseases. Blood 1998;91:756–763.

113. Schleuning M, Stoetzer O, Waterhouse C et al. Hematopoietic stem cell transplantation after reduced-intensity conditioning as treatment of sickle cell disease. Exp Hematol 2002;30:7–10.

114. Hongeng S, Chuansumrit A, Hathirat P et al. Full chimerism in nonmyeloablative stem cell transplantation in a beta-thalassemia major patient (class 3 Lucarelli). Bone Marrow Transplant 2002;30:409–410.

115. Gomez-Almaguer D, Ruiz-Arguelles GJ, Gonzalez-Llano O et al. [Peripheral blood hematopoietic cell transplant using immunosuppressive chemotherapy without bone marrow destruction: "minitransplant"]. Gac Med Mex 2002;138:235–239.

116. Iannone R, Chen AR, Casella JF. Commentary on "Summary of symposium: the future of stem cell transplantation for sickle cell disease." J Pediatr Hematol Oncol 2002;24:515–517.

117. Iannone R, Casella JF, Woolfrey A et al. Non-myeloablative hematopoietic cell transplantation (NST) for hemoglobinopathies. Washington, DC: 30th Anniversary of the National Sickle Cell Disease Program National Heart, Lung, and Blood Institute, National Institutes of Health, and the Sickle Cell Disease Association of America, Inc., 2002;35.

118. Iannone R, Casella JF, Fuchs EJ et al. Failure of a minimally toxic non-myeloablative regimen to establish stable donor engraftment after transplantation for sickle cell anemia and thalassemia (Abstr #161). Blood 2002; 100:46a.

119. Walters MC, Nienhuis A, Vichinsky E. Novel therapeutic approaches in sickle cell disease. Hematology (Am Soc Hematol Educ Program). 2002:10–34.

120. van Besien K, Smith S, Stock W et al. Allogeneic stem cell transplantation with fludarbine, melphalan and campath in adults with advanced sickle cell disease. Preliminary experience with a well tolerated regimen. Washington, DC: 30th Anniversary of the National Sickle Cell Disease Program National Heart, Lung, and Blood Institute, National Institutes of Health, and the Sickle Cell Disease Association of America, Inc. (Abstr #40), 2002;40.

121. van Besien K, Stock W, Smith S et al. Allogeneic stem cell transplantation with fludarabine, melphalan and campath conditioning for adults with advanced sickle cell disease (Abstr # 5398). Blood 2002;100:455b.

122. Isola LM, Chao NJ, Weinberg RS et al. Donor chimerism after T-cell depleted (TCD)-non-myeloablative allogeneic SCT (NST) in hemoglobinopathies (Abstr #5172). Blood 2002;100:401b.

123. Miniero R, Rocha V, Saracco P et al. Cord blood transplantation (CBT) in hemoglobinopathies. Eurocord. Bone Marrow Transplant 1998;22(Suppl 1):S78–S79.

124. Reed W, Smith R, Dekovic F et al. Comprehensive banking of sibling donor cord blood for children with malignant and nonmalignant disease. Blood 2003;101:351–357.

125. La Nasa G, Giardini C, Argiolu F et al. Unrelated donor bone marrow transplantation for thalassemia: the effect of extended haplotypes. Blood 2002;99:4350–4356.

126. Contu L, La Nasa G, Arras M et al. Successful unrelated bone marrow transplantation in beta-thalassaemia. Bone Marrow Transplant 1994;13:329–331.

127. Gaziev D, Galimberti M, Lucarelli G et al. Bone marrow transplantation from alternative donors for thalassemia: HLA-phenotypically identical relative and HLA-nonidentical sibling or parent transplants. Bone Marrow Transplant 2000;25:815–821.

128. Krishnamurti L, Perentesis JP, Wagner JE. Umbilical cord blood transplant from a sibling with hemoglobin E and a thalassemia into a patient with hemoglobin E/β⁰thalassemia: Implications for donor selection for stem cell transplant (Abstr #2850). Blood 1997;90.

129. Yeager AM, Mehta PS, Adamkiewicz TV et al. Unrelated placental/umbilical cord blood cell (UCBC) transplantation in children with high-risk sickle cell disease (SCD) (Abstr # 5336). Blood 2000;96:366b.

130. Walters MC, Patience M, Leisenring W et al. Barriers to bone marrow transplantation for sickle cell anemia. Biol Blood Marrow Transplant 1996;2:100–104.

131. Crespo Chozas D, Maldonado Regalado MS, Munoz Villa A. [Unrelated donor bone marrow transplantation in a girl with thalassemia major]. Med Clin (Barc) 2000;114:598–599.

132. Cheng CN, Lu CC, Sun HF et al. Successful matched-unrelated bone marrow transplantation in a patient with Beta-thalassemia major. J Pediatr Hematol Oncol 2002;24:579–581.

133. Krishnamurti L, Abel S, Maiers M, Flesch S. Availability of unrelated donors hematopoietic stem cell transplantation for hemoglobinopathies. Bone Marrow Transplant 2003;31:547–550.

134. Chakraverty R, Peggs K, Chopra R et al. Limiting transplantation-related mortality following unrelated donor stem cell transplantation by using a nonmyeloablative conditioning regimen. Blood 2002;99: 1071–1078.

135. Kodish E, Lantos J, Stocking C et al. Bone marrow transplantation for sickle cell disease. A study of parents' decisions. N Engl J Med 1991;325:1349–1353.

136. Krishnamurti L, Abel S, Maiers M et al. Availability of unrelated donors for hematopoietic stem cell transplantation for hemoglobinopathies. Bone Marrow Transplant 2003;31:547–550.

137. Shpall EJ, Quinones R, Giller R et al. Transplantation of ex vivo expanded cord blood. Biol Blood Marrow Transplant 2002;8:368–376.

138. Barker JN, Weisdorf DJ, Wagner JE. Creation of a double chimera after the transplantation of umbilical-cord blood from two partially matched unrelated donors. N Engl J Med 2001;344:1870–1871.

# Hematopoietic Stem Cell Transplantation for Inherited Bone Marrow Failure Syndromes

ADRIANNA VLACHOS AND JEFFREY MICHAEL LIPTON

The advent of in vivo and in vitro clonal assays for pluripotent stem cells and committed hematopoietic progenitors, as well as the characterization of lympho-hematopoietic cell surface antigens by flow cytometry, has resulted in the developmental model of hematopoiesis. The inherited bone marrow failure syndromes can be described in the context of this scheme in which the proliferation and differentiation of pluripotent stem cells give rise to progeny that can populate the entire immunologic and hematopoietic systems.[1] The immediate offspring of the stem cell are the committed progenitors of both the lymphoid and myeloid lineage. The multipotent myeloid progenitor, the CFU-GEMM, has the potential to give rise to committed progenitors. In turn, each of these progenitors possesses a unique biologic program of differentiation and replication that provides the recognizable precursors of the granulocyte, erythrocyte, monocyte/macrophage, megakaryocyte as well as eosinophil and basophil lineages. These progenitors appear as immature, undifferentiated mononuclear cells and are present in small numbers in the bone marrow. Thus, the identifiable precursors that constitute the bone marrow are often abnormal or absent in inherited bone marrow failure syndromes as the result of a more fundamental defect manifest in hematopoietic cells lacking distinguishing morphologic features. Furthermore, these abnormalities are not always restricted to hematopoiesis, accounting for the vast array of congenital anomalies and organ dysfunction associated with such disorders as Fanconi anemia (FA), dyskeratosis congenita (DC), Diamond Blackfan anemia (DBA), Shwachman Diamond syndrome (SDS) and others.

Cell culture and recombinant DNA technology have led to the identification and, in many cases, the cloning of the genes for a number of hematopoietic growth factors. These stimulatory as well as inhibitory factors influence the survival, differentiation, proliferation and function of hematopoietic cells. Thus, in addition to hematopoietic stem cells and progenitors, the bone marrow contains a complex array of support elements or stroma populated with accessory lymphocytes, macrophages, fibroblasts, endothelial cells and adipocytes as well as growth agonists and antagonists. These elements create a regulatory "niche", described by Williams as a "local area network."[2] Specific receptor-ligand relationships create a microenvironment consisting of local neighborhoods that support the proliferation and differentiation of specific cell types under the control of intrinsic transcriptional regulators.[3] These niches provide a scaffold on which blood forming cells, accessory cells and growth factors may interact at close range.

Stem cell "seeds" are anchored by receptor-ligand "roots" nurtured in stromal "soil" by specific and nonspecific growth factor "fertilizer" and "nutrients" to give rise to a complex and beautiful "hematopoietic garden."[4] Thus, the array of potential mechanisms for bone marrow failure includes faulty stem/progenitor cells (seeds), defective stroma and accessory cells (soil), immunologic "weeds", abnormal growth factors (fertilizer), or deficient non-specific nutrients. Clinical examples of every imaginable hematopoietic lesion[5] have not been identified, but the "hematopoietic garden" provides a framework for understanding defective hematopoiesis in the inherited bone marrow failure syndromes. The precise pathophysiology of the inherited single cell and multi-lineage cytopenias has not yet been elucidated, despite the identification of many of the genes mutated in these disorders (► Table 17.1). However, an intrinsic cellular defect, faulty "seeds" with a predilection to apoptosis, has been demonstrated in virtually all of the syndromes.[6–9] As mentioned earlier, the "failure" in the inherited bone marrow failure syndromes is usually not restricted to hematopoiesis. The pathology of many of these disorders includes congenital anomalies, multiorgan dysfunction and, in some cases, extreme susceptibility to the toxicity of transplantation conditioning regimens.[10–12] Therein lies the problem. To achieve "bone marrow success" through hematopoietic stem cell transplantation (HSCT) the transplanter must be aware of these confounding circumstances lest they lead to extreme toxicity when traditional conditioning regimens are utilized. The decision to perform a transplant must involve a careful risk versus benefit assessment. Transplanters who deal with rare bone marrow failure syndromes must have knowledge of the natural history and the available non-transplant options. These will be described for each disorder covered in this chapter. Furthermore, a detailed understanding of the clinical presentation and genetics may prevent transplant-related disasters. There is a transplant tale, perhaps apocryphal, that illustrates the problem. During a consultation, a noted transplanter was seeing a young woman with Fanconi anemia and her sister, the proposed human leukocyte antigen (HLA)-matched donor. The physician turned to the young woman possessing the obvious stigmata of FA, and asked, "When were you diagnosed?" Much to his surprise the reply was, "Oh no doctor—my sister has Fanconi anemia, and I am the donor." The moral of the story is obvious, but the identification of an unaffected HLA-matched related donor may not be. Classic serial transplant experiments in mice[13] have demonstrated the markedly reduced engraftment potential of "damaged" stem cells. It is obvious that an HSCT utilizing a donor with FA would at best result in no change in the hematologic status of the recipient. However, the more likely outcome would be nonengraftment. Indeed, the fact that a physical examination, complete blood count, and current diagnostic tests will reveal virtually all individuals with FA makes this scenario unlikely but not unreported.[14] Thus, the near absolute ascertainment of the absence of FA in the donor is a requirement, certain mosaics not withstanding. This is particularly so when the stem cell source is umbilical cord blood from an HLA-matched related newborn sibling who likely may be hematologically normal even in the presence of disorders such as Fanconi anemia or dyskeratosis congenita. There are other settings, however, where the diagnosis of a marrow failure syndrome may be less obvious and the sorting out of a donor with a "silent phenotype" may not be a simple matter.[15] These will be discussed later.

| TABLE 17.1 | Inherited Bone Marrow Failure Syndrome Genes, Known and Presumed |

| Disorder | Gene | Locus | Genetics | Gene Product |
|---|---|---|---|---|
| Fanconi anemia | | | Autosomal recessive | |
| | FANCA | 16q24.3 | | FANCA |
| | FANCB | 13q12.3 | | ? |
| | FANCC | 9q22.3 | | FANCC |
| | FANCD1 | 13q12.3 | | BRCA2 |
| | FANCD2 | 3p25.3 | | FANCD2 |
| | FANCE | 6p21.3 | | FANCE |
| | FANCF | 11p15 | | FANCF |
| | FANCG | 9p13 | | FANCG |
| | FANCH | ? | | ? |
| | FANCI | ? | | ? |
| Dyskeratosis congenita | DKC1 | Xq28 | X-linked recessive | Dyskerin |
| | hTR (DKC2) | 3q | Autosomal dominant | Telomerase RNA |
| | DKC3 | ? | Autosomal recessive | ? |
| Shwachman Diamond syndrome | SBDS | 7q11 | Autosomal recessive | SBDS |
| Diamond Blackfan anemia | RPS19 (DBA1) | 19q13.2 | Autosomal dominant | RPS19 |
| | DBA2 | 8p23.3-p22 | | ? |
| | DBA3 | ? | | ? |
| | ? | ? | Autosomal recessive | ? |
| Kostmann syndrome (SCN) | ELA2 | 19p13.3 | Autosomal dominant | Neutrophil elastase |
| | ? | ? | Autosomal recessive | ? |
| Amegakaryocytic thrombocytopenia | c-mpl | 1p34 | Autosomal recessive | Thrombopoietin |

Abbreviation: SCN = severe chronic neutropenia.

Traditionally, the inherited bone marrow failure syndromes have been divided into those resulting in pancytopenia (Fanconi anemia and dyskeratosis congenita) and those apparently restricted to a single hematopoietic lineage (Diamond Blackfan anemia, congenital neutropenia [Kostmann syndrome {KS}, cyclic neutropenia, Shwachman Diamond syndrome], congenital amegakaryocytic thrombocytopenia [CAT] and thrombocytopenia absent radii [TAR] syndrome). We will preserve this nosology; however, it has become evident that most of these "single cell cytopenias" may manifest abnormalities in other hematopoietic cell lines. Indeed, in some patients with Shwachman Diamond syndrome and CAT, for example, pancytopenia is fairly common.

Young and Alter's small masterpiece, *Aplastic Anemia Acquired and Inherited,*[16] is recommended to those readers desiring a more complete discussion of bone marrow failure. Although published in 1994 and somewhat outdated, Young and Alter describe the inherited bone marrow failure syndromes in exquisite detail. We will endeavor to provide a discussion of developments since 1994 relevant to the topic at hand. The extremely rare disorder reticular dysgenesis as well as thrombocytopenia absent radii syndrome and cyclic neutrope-nia, disorders for which HSCT is virtually never indicated, will be mentioned only in passing.

## THE SYNDROMES

### Pancytopenia

#### *Fanconi Anemia*

**Pathophysiology and Clinical Features.** Fanconi anemia, first described in 1927,[17] is a rare autosomal recessive inherited bone marrow failure syndrome characterized by abnormal skin pigmentation (café au lait and hypopigmented spots), short stature and congenital malformations. These malformations are most frequently skeletal (upper limb and classical thumb abnormalities) followed by renal anomalies. Other abnormalities, including cardiac and genital anomalies, have been catalogued in great detail.[16] However, it has been estimat-ed that as many as 40% of FA patients lack obvious physical abnormalities.[18]

The median age at hematologic presentation of patients reported to the International Fanconi Anemia Registry (IFAR) database is approximately seven years.[19] All racial and ethnic groups are affected. Hematologic dysfunction usually presents with thrombocy-topenia, often leading to progressive pancytopenia and severe aplastic anemia (SAA), fre-quently terminating in myelodysplastic syndrome (MDS) and/or acute myeloid leukemia (AML). Thrombocytopenia is usually preceded by macrocytosis. The actuarial risk of developing bone marrow failure, hematologic and nonhematologic neoplasms are 90%, 33%, and 28%, respectively, by 40 years of age.[20] When the cumulative incidence of non-hematologic cancer is estimated in the presence of competing risks, Rosenberg and col-leagues suggest that the risk of solid tumors ". . . may become even higher as death from aplastic anemia is reduced, and as post-HSCT patients survive longer."[21] These data must be considered in the context of HSCT, in particular when the risk of nonhematologic malignancy is likely to increase as a result of HSCT conditioning regimens and chronic graft-versus-host disease (GVHD).

Fanconi anemia cells are hypersensitive to chromosomal breaks induced by DNA cross-linking agents. This observation is the basis for the commonly used chromosome breakage test for FA. The clastogens diepoxybutane (DEB) and mitomycin C (MMC) are the agents most frequently used *in vitro* to induce chromosome breaks and radial forms.[22] Clastogens also induce cell cycle arrest in G2/M. The hypersensitivity of FA lymphocytes to G2/M arrest, detected using cell cycle analysis by flow cytometry, more recently has been exploited as a screening tool for FA.[23] Elevated serum alpha-fetoprotein levels have been described in FA patients independent of androgen use and liver disease and also may be a reliable screening tool when FA is suspected.[24]

The differential diagnosis of FA generally includes diverse disorders such as acquired aplastic anemia, TAR syndrome and vertebral, anorectal, tracheo-esophageal, radial, and renal (VATER) syndrome. Actually, FA may be easily distinguished from TAR syndrome. There is an intercalary defect in TAR, absent radii with normal thumbs, whereas in FA the defect is terminal, an abnormal radius always being associated with anomalies of the thumb. FA testing is warranted in any patient who presents with hematologic cytopenias, unexplained macrocytosis, aplastic anemia or AML, as well as representative congenital abnormalities or solid tumors typical of FA such as head and neck, esophageal or gyneco-logic tumors presenting at an early age.[25]

Somatic cell hybridization studies thus far have defined ten FA complementation groups[26] and of these, seven FA genes have been cloned.[26,27] The gene products of these seven genes have been shown to cooperate in a common pathway. Five of the FA proteins (FANCA, C, E, F, and G) assemble in a nuclear complex that is required to monoubiquinate and acti-vate FANCD2. Ubiquinated FANCD2 is translocated to a nuclear focus containing BRCA1.[28] Recently, FANCD1 has been identified as BRCA2.[29] The exact mechanism of FANCD2 monoubiquitination and the role of FANCD2, BRCA2 (FANCD1), and BCRA1 in DNA repair are yet to be unraveled.[30]

**Genetics.** Fanconi anemia is inherited as an autosomal recessive disorder and is the most frequently inherited aplastic anemia. As mentioned earlier, ten FA complementation groups have been described and seven genes cloned thus far (Table 17.1). Representing 70% of cases, FANCA is the most common complementation group. A recent analysis from the IFAR suggests an earlier onset of pancytopenia and shorter survival for patients with FANCC.[20] However, genotype-phenotype correlation is complex and probably relates as much to the nature of the gene product and other factors as to the specific complementa-tion group.[31,32]

**Front Line Therapy.** The art of FA patient management, in particular the diagnostic workup, treatment of growth failure and other endocrine abnormalities, detection, and management of cancer as well as medical and psychosocial support are beyond the scope of this chapter. Those who are interested should refer to the handbook, *Fanconi Anemia Standards for Clinical Care,*[33] based on recommendations from a similarly titled conference sponsored by the Fanconi Anemia Research Fund (FARF) and published in 1999. At the writing of this chapter a second conference is scheduled for late winter 2003. Devoutly to be wished but as yet unrealized, gene therapy ultimately may play an important role in the treatment of FA.

Treatment of bone marrow failure is considered for an absolute neutrophil count <500/mm,[3] hemoglobin <8 g/dL or a platelet count <30,000/ mm.[3] Hematologic mani-festations of FA can be improved in 50% to 75% of FA patients with the use of androgens and hematopoietic growth factors. For neutropenia alone, granulocyte colony-stimulating factor (G-CSF) or granulocyte-macrophage colony-stimulating factor (GM-CSF) is the first line of therapy. For anemia and thrombocytopenia, oxymetholone and G-CSF or GM-CSF are recommended.

**Hematopoietic Stem Cell Transplantation: Indications, Outcomes and the Approach to the Patient.** Historically, the majority of patients succumb to the complications of severe aplastic anemia, followed by leukemia and solid tumors. Recently, the median survival for FA has improved to approximately 30 years of age.[25]

Unquestionably, since the groundbreaking observations of Gluckman and colleagues,[10] marrow failure has been cured and the risk of leukemia in FA ameliorated by the use of allogeneic stem cell transplantation. Excellent results have been obtained with HLA-matched sibling donors. Thus, there is general agreement that otherwise healthy FA patients with significant cytopenias (absolute neutrophil count <1000/mm,[3] hemoglobin <8g/dL or a platelet count <40–50,000/ mm[3]) and an available HLA-matched sibling donor should undergo HSCT rather than proceed to androgen/growth factor therapy.[33] Beyond that, this rapidly moving field is fraught with conflicting approaches and passionate disagreement. Practitioners are implored to consult with experienced physicians and have patients participate in clinical trials whenever possible.

It is neither possible nor practical to review all the subsequent modifications in the HSCT approach to FA since Dr. Gluckman's earlier studies. Interested readers are referred to an excellent review by Harris.[33] Therefore, we hope that our choice of salient contributions in the development of successful HSCT for FA will not offend the authors of those important studies we fail to mention.

Fanconi anemia patients have an increased sensitivity to DNA cross-linking agents, in particular alkylating agents commonly used for HSCT conditioning such as cyclophosphamide as well as radiation therapy. Thus, toxicity to FA patients resulting from traditional transplant conditioning regimens was extreme. In particular, severe mucositis and gastrointestinal toxicity as well as severe cardiac, hepatic, and cutaneous complications led to frequent early death following transplantation. These observations ultimately resulted in a modified regimen proposed by Gluckman and colleagues that consisted of low-dose cyclophosphamide (5 mg/kg/day × 4 for a total 20 mg/kg, or one tenth the standard dose) and 500 cGy thoracoabdominal irradiation (TAI).[10,34] These reductions in dose resulted in diminished morbidity and mortality post-transplantation. From 1981 to 1996, 50 FA patients underwent transplant from HLA-identical sibling donors using this regimen.[35] The stem cell source was bone marrow in 46 and umbilical cord blood in four. Cyclosporine A (CsA) alone was used for graft-versus-host disease (GVHD) prophylaxis. Four patients had MDS and were given a higher dose of cyclophosphamide (10 mg/kg × 4). The five-year disease-free survival was 74 ± 6%. The only factor associated with a decreased survival was the number of transfusions prior to HSCT. Grade II or higher acute GVHD developed in half of the patients. Twenty patients developed chronic GVHD. A unique and significant late complication was the development of squamous cell carcinoma of the tongue in five patients. No cases of secondary MDS or AML were seen following HSCT. Other late complications reported were those known to occur following HSCT. The reduced toxicity of this regimen, however, was accompanied by a concomitant increase in graft failure. Further modifications, including the pretransplant and posttransplant administration of antithymocyte globulin (ATG) and a decrease in the dose of irradiation to 400 cGy, resulted in improved engraftment and a reduced incidence and severity of GVHD.[36] Sixteen of 17 patients engrafted and were alive, without any grade II to IV acute GVHD.

In a review of the results of 243 HLA-matched sibling HSCT done between 1974 and 1994 and reported to the Fanconi Anemia Transplant Registry,[37] there was an overall survival of 61%. Age at the time of transplant was a significant prognostic factor with a five-year survival of 80% for patients <10 years but only 50% for those >10 years of age. For those transplants done after 1990 the survival was 75%. In particular, those HSCTs done after 1990 and using a conditioning regimen of low-dose cyclophosphamide and limited field TAI with ATG had superior outcomes with overall survivals of ~ 94%. Liver dysfunction and graft rejection were noted in many patients who had been on long-term androgen therapy and/or had received >10 transfusions, leading to a poorer survival in those patients. The presence of MDS or AML was a significant adverse prognostic factor. Alternative donor transplants fared less well with patients undergoing a 6/6 serologically HLA-matched related nonsibling donor HSCT having a survival of only 48%. This was, however, much better than mismatched related transplants with a survival of 13%.

Transplants from unrelated 6/6 HLA-matched donors had a survival of 34% while there were too few 5/6 HLA-mismatched HSCT to evaluate (2 of 12 patients alive).

Unfortunately, most patients with Fanconi anemia do not have an HLA-matched, unaffected related donor. Unrelated donors show some promise as a stem cell source, however, the risk of complications is increased.

Significant morbidity and mortality has been associated with grade III-IV GVHD in FA patients undergoing HSCT using HLA-matched unrelated donors. Davies and colleagues reported the results from the University of Minnesota between 1990 and 1994 using cyclophosphamide 10 mg/kg/d × 4 with total body irradiation (TBI) 400 to 450 cGy without T cell-depletion.[38] Severe oropharyngeal mucositis was noted in all patients. Three of seven patients survived, one without GVHD and two with extensive chronic GVHD. Two patients succumbed to infection along with grade IV GVHD. There were two early deaths due to infection, one with concurrent venoocclusive disease.[38] The European Group for Blood and Marrow Transplantation analyzed the results of 69 patients with FA undergoing HSCT using an HLA-matched unrelated donor.[39] The overall actuarial survival at three years was 33%. The incidence of grade III-IV GVHD was dramatically reduced by T cell depletion. However, with the reduction in mortality from GVHD came a concomitant increase in primary and secondary graft failure resulting in no difference in survival for those patients receiving either the T cell depleted or nondepleted grafts. There was a statistically significant improvement in neutrophil recovery in those patients receiving $\geq 2 \times 10^6$ CD34+ cells/kg recipient body weight. The authors point out that molecular HLA-typing should improve upon these results.

The next major step was developed to exploit nonmyeloablative, highly immunosuppressive regimens in FA to prevent graft rejection. Kapelushnik and colleagues used a conditioning regimen consisting of fludarabine (30 mg/M² × 5), ATG (10 mg/kg × 4) and cyclophosphamide (10 mg/kg × 2) for HLA-matched related HSCT. They were able to obtain sustained engraftment and only Grade II mucositis, diarrhea, abdominal pain, and hyperbilirubinemia.[40] The use of fludarabine appears to facilitate the omission of radiation therapy from the conditioning regimen. This is of particular importance in diminishing immediate toxicity and may be of significance in reducing the incidence of second malignancies.

A review from the International Bone Marrow Transplantation Registry (IBMTR) reported a two-year probability of survival of 66% versus 29% using HLA-matched sibling donors compared to FA patients who underwent HSCT using bone marrow from unrelated donors or partially matched relatives as a stem cell source.[41] Good prognostic indicators included young age at HSCT, higher pretransplant platelet counts, use of low-dose cyclophosphamide along with ATG and CsA for GVHD prophylaxis.

The results reported from the EBMT were comparable using HLA-identical relatives and HLA-identical sibling donors, a finding not terribly unexpected in a rare autosomal recessive disorder. Unrelated donor HSCT was performed in 76 FA patients through the EBMT. The conditioning regimen for these unrelated HSCT used cyclophosphamide (20 or 40 mg/kg total) and TAI or TBI. Most patients received ATG, pre- and post-HSCT. The two-year event-free survival was 23 ± 5%. The main causes of death were GVHD and infections. A male donor and T cell depletion resulted in better outcomes. Unrelated donor patients undergoing transplants using unrelated donor cells did significantly better than those using an HLA-mismatched relative. Higher dose cyclophosphamide and the use of ATG did not improve the two-year event-free survival.[40]

The Italian Bone Marrow Donor Registry[42] reported 10 FA patients transplanted using unrelated donors. Only three patients had successful outcomes. They concluded that the fewer number of transfusions received prior to transplantation, the better the outcome. Their newest protocol in use for FA patients undergoing unrelated HSCT consists of cyclophosphamide (40 mg/kg), TBI (450 cGy) and ATG with a CD34+ selected graft.

As a final note, in a preliminary report Wagner and MacMillan[43] have described a dramatic improvement in outcome for both HLA-matched sibling as well as unrelated donor HSCT in FA. All seven patients with FA transplanted from allogeneic HLA-matched sibling donors using a fludarabine- and cyclophosphamide-based conditioning regimen with T cell-depleted CD34+ cells are alive and well. Furthermore, the actuarial survival for 25 selected, "standard risk" patients utilizing T cell-depleted CD34+ stem cells, who received a matched unrelated transplant is 81% at approximately two years. These investigators define "standard risk" as those patients with a 6/6 HLA-matched unrelated bone marrow or a 5/6 HLA-matched umbilical cord blood (UCB) donor who are <18 years of age, free of infection and have either SAA or early MDS only. The results of this study are promising.

In summary, serological HLA-A/B typing of the patient and family is recommended at the time of diagnosis. HSCT from an HLA-matched sibling donor is recommended for patients who develop significant cytopenias. Such patients should move on to HSCT prior to the institution of androgen therapy and/or blood product transfusions. Based on the above experience, the Minnesota team is advocating either HLA-matched sibling or "matched" unrelated HSCT for all "standard risk" patients prior, if possible, to any attempt at nontransplant medical management. This recommendation, based on their excellent preliminary results and reports of poor HSCT outcomes in androgen-treated and heavily transfused patients in the context of molecular typing for HLA-matched, nonrelated HSCT, is logical. They suggest that older and sicker patients and those without good donors should be transplanted when more conservative measures have failed. The results for patients with advanced MDS and AML are poor but no other options exist at this time. It has been suggested that any patient with an HLA-matched sibling donor be considered for HSCT in the context of a clinical research study. However, more data are required before preemptive HSCT for patients with FA and no significant cytopenias, particularly when an HLA-matched related sibling donor is not available, is considered the standard of care. It is quite likely that other risk factors will emerge that do support early HSCT in some patients. Besides overall survival, issues such as the potential for nonhematologic cancers as a result of the conditioning regimen and perhaps GVHD as well as hematopoietic malignancy as a consequence of mixed hematopoietic chimerism and residual host cells need to be explored.

**Hematopoietic Stem Cell Transplantation: Matched-Related Donor Evaluation.** The pretransplant donor evaluation should include a very careful physical exam and relevant hematologic laboratory evaluation. A chromosome breakage test for FA must be done and, perhaps in the future, mutation analysis may be performed to screen potential donors for "silent" homozygosity. To rule out FA mosaicism all potential donors should have chromosome breakage assays performed using skin fibroblasts. Obviously, the use of cells from an FA affected donor must be assiduously avoided.[14] Recently, the advent of preimplantation genetic diagnosis has provided the opportunity for FA and other inherited bone marrow failure syndrome families to conceive not only unaffected children, but also HLA-matched sibling umbilical cord stem cell donors. A short discussion of this emerging technology is provided in the final section of this chapter.

## Dyskeratosis Congenita

**Pathophysiology and Clinical Features.** Ectodermal dysplasia and hematopoietic failure characterize dyskeratosis congenita (DC). The classic triad of abnormal skin pigmentation, dystrophic nails and leukoplakia of mucous membranes defines DC. In addition to the classic triad there are a number of other somatic findings in DC. The most common of these are epiphora (tearing due to obstructed tear ducts), developmental delay, pulmonary disease, short stature, esophageal webs, dental carries, tooth loss, premature gray hair and hair loss. Other ocular, dental, skeletal, cutaneous, genitourinary, gastrointestinal, and central nervous system (CNS) abnormalities have been reported.[12,16]

The Dyskeratosis Congenita Registry (DCR), established in 1995, has provided valuable data regarding epidemiology, pathophysiology, genetics, and treatment of dyskeratosis congenita. As of a recently published report[12] there were 148 patients from 92 families emanating from 20 countries enrolled in the DCR. The median age for the onset of mucocutaneous abnormalities in patients enrolled in the DCR is six to eight years. Nail changes occur first. Pancytopenia is the hematologic hallmark of DC. The median age for the onset of pancytopenia is ten years. Approximately 50% of patients reported in the literature develop severe aplastic anemia[16] and greater than 90% of individuals reported in the DCR have developed at least a single cytopenia by 40 years of age.[12] In a number of cases, aplastic anemia preceded the onset of abnormal skin, dystrophic nails, or leukoplakia. As with FA it is the nonhematologic manifestations of DC that are of particular concern when hematopoietic stem cell transplantation for bone marrow failure is contemplated.

Recent evidence establishes dyskeratosis congenita to be the result of deficient telomerase activity.[44] Telomerase adds DNA sequence back to the ends of chromosomes that are eroded with each DNA replication. Telomerase activity is found only in tissues with rapid turnover such as the basal layer of the epidermis, squamous epithelium of the oral cavity, hematopoietic stem cells and progenitors and in other tissues affected in DC. The lack of telomerase activity also gives rise to chromosome instability, resulting in the high rate of premature cancer observed in these tissues. Epithelial malignancies develop at or beyond the third decade of life. About one in five patients will develop progressive pulmonary disease characterized by fibrosis, resulting in diminished diffusion capacity and/or restrictive lung disease. Of note, Type 2 alveolar epithelial cells express telomerase. It is likely that more pulmonary disease would be evident if patients did not succumb earlier to the complications of severe aplastic anemia and cancer. The failure of HSCT in DC has been due in large part to pulmonary complications. It is prudent to assume that all DC patients are at a high risk of interstitial pulmonary disease when undergoing HSCT. Unfortunately, there have been too few transplant survivors to determine whether an increase in the prevalence of cancer will follow as a consequence of HSCT. An immunoablative rather than a myeloablative approach may reduce the incremental risk of pulmonary toxicity as well as the hypothesized incremental nonhematologic cancer risk. Sixty-seven percent of the deaths in the DCR appear to be a consequence of bone marrow failure, while 9% died of lung disease with or without HSCT. Almost 9% (13 of 148) of patients developed cancer.

Of these, four patients had MDS, one had Hodgkin's disease and eight had carcinoma. The degree of predisposition to leukemia is yet to be clearly defined. The Registry has, somewhat surprisingly, revealed the presence of significant progressive immunodeficiency in DC. Indeed, the vast majority of patients (80%), with or without consequential neutropenia who died did so from infection, some opportunistic, usually before 30 years of age. With over half of the patients studied having a predominantly cellular immune defect it is reasonable to assume that immunodeficiency as well as neutropenia plays a significant role in infectious morbidity and mortality in DC.[12] Young and Alter's review of the literature reveals a median survival of approximately 35 years for both X-linked and autosomal recessive forms of DC.[16] There are too few autosomal dominant cases for such an analysis. Despite the immaturity of the DCR and the bias inherent in the literature, it is safe to say that the prognosis for patients with DC is poor.

**Genetics.** Dyskeratosis congenita is most commonly inherited as an X-linked recessive with 86% of patients in the Registry being male, although some of these represent autosomal dominant or recessive inheritance.[12] The gene responsible for the X-linked form was mapped to Xq28[45] and subsequently identified as DKC1.[46] DKC1 codes for dyskerin, a nucleolar protein associated with nucleolar RNAs. Dyskerin also is associated with the telomerase complex, and this latter function appears to be the one involved in the pathophysiology of DC,[44] as the dominant form has recently been mapped to a gene that encodes telomerase RNA (hTR).[47] Furthermore, the clinical heterogeneity of DC may be explained by different allelic mutations giving rise to differences in mutated proteins as well as by mutations leading to decreased amounts of normal protein. Autosomal recessive forms have been inferred from pedigrees, in particular those described with brother-sister pairs in consanguineous families.[12,16] There are many features in common to all three genetic subtypes; however, autosomal recessive patients appear to have a more severe phenotype.[12] As well, affected members within the same family may exhibit wide variability in clinical presentation suggesting the influence of modifying genes and environmental factors.

**Front Line Therapy.** Responses to androgens, G-CSF or GM-CSF, as well as erythropoietin have been documented (reviewed by Young and Alter[16]). However, for the most part these responses have been transient. Young and Alter report temporary responses to splenectomy. Supportive care with blood products, antibiotics and antifibrinolytics are similar to that used for idiopathic aplastic anemia. Once these measures are required, hematopoietic stem cell transplantation should be considered for those patients with an HLA-matched related donor or an acceptable alternative donor and no DC-related contraindications. Standard medical management of severe aplastic anemia using immunomodulatory therapy, as would be expected, was ineffective in a patient reported by Drachtman and Alter[48] and is not recommended.

**Hematopoietic Stem Cell Transplantation: Indications, Outcomes and the Approach to the Patient.** The vast majority of patients with DC succumb to the complications of pancytopenia and/or immune deficiency. Thus, it seems intuitive that hematopoietic stem cell transplantation be instituted at the earliest sign of significant hematopoietic or immunologic failure. Hematologic criteria such as those recommended for *intervention* in Fanconi anemia are reasonable.[33] These are an absolute neutrophil count <500/mm,[3] hemoglobin <8 g/dL and a platelet count <30,000/mm.[3] Patients meeting these criteria should be considered for HSCT, particularly if a DC-unaffected matched sibling donor is available. Unfortunately, the results of HSCT in DC to date have been abysmal, and indeed much worse than that for recent patients with FA undergoing HSCT. Patients without a matched sibling donor and those at high risk for transplant related organ failure should be observed and managed medically for as long as is reasonable. Young and Alter describe seven HSCT in patients with DC reported between 1982 and 1992.[16] All transplants for which the information is reported were from allogeneic HLA-matched relatives utilizing a variety of standard myeloablative conditioning regimens. Three HSCT were performed used a conditioning regimen of cyclophosphamide with total abdominal or total body irradiation. Four HSCT utilized chemotherapy only. Only two patients were alive at five and six years posttransplant. These patients received cyclophosphamide only and cyclophosphamide/TAI. Two patients died of complications of GVHD at 51 days and three months post-HSCT, respectively. One patient died from interstitial pneumonitis eight years posttransplant and two died from diffuse vasculitis, renal failure, and venoocclusive disease two and seven years, respectively, posttransplant. The two patients alive at the time of the report were the youngest, each two years of age at the time of transplant. The late deaths in this series indicate that those surviving patients remain at risk for serious complications related to HSCT. There have been no case control studies done to evaluate the impact of HSCT on the natural history of pulmonary disease, but the rapidity of the onset of pulmonary failure in some cases suggests an incremental relationship to HSCT.

A report from the DCR briefly described eight patients with DC who underwent HSCT. At the time of the report three of the matched allogeneic sibling and the one unrelated HSCT, of the seven new patients, were alive at four, five, seven and three years post HSCT, respectively. Three patients are dead. There are insufficient details to sort out the cause of death in these patients. Of the eight patients, Young and Alter[16] and Berthou et al.[49] had already reported one case. The patient died at six years posttransplant from renal failure and venoocclusive disease. ▼ Table 17.2 describes the reasonably well-documented cases reported in the literature.[50–60]

The largest available series, consisting of eight patients with aplastic anemia and DC, was reported by the group from the Fred Hutchinson Cancer Center.[56] Six HSCT utilized HLA-matched sibling donors and two were transplanted from unrelated alternative donors. Those who received an HLA-matched sibling transplant were conditioned with cyclophosphamide with or without ATG. Those receiving an alternative donor transplant were conditioned with cyclophosphamide and TBI. There were four early deaths; one patient died from refractory GVHD on day 44 posttransplant and three died of invasive fungal infection. Three of the four remaining patients developed pulmonary failure at 70 days, eight years and 20 years posttransplant, and one was alive at the time of the report but had developed Duke stage C rectal carcinoma. The three unique patients (2 previously reported by Young and Alter[16]) reported by Rocha et al.[52] also fared poorly. One patient succumbed to venoocclusive disease and hepatic failure at 17 years of age, six years posttransplant. One patient developed pulmonary fibrosis three years posttransplant and was alive at the time of the report. The remaining patient died secondary to immune deficiency and an invasive *Aspergillus* infection 19 months posttransplant. An isolated case, terminating in chronic restrictive pulmonary disease at age 9, seven years posttransplant from a partially matched sibling, conditioned with cyclophosphamide and TAI, has been reported.[59] Two more recent cases reported by Ghavamzadeh and colleagues[60] received a milder busulfan/ cyclophosphamide conditioning regimen and were alive and well at six and five years posttransplant, respectively.

| TABLE 17.2 | Summary of Published Stem Cell Transplants for Dyskeratosis Congenita | | | |

| Reference | Age/Sex | HLA Match | Conditioning Regimen | Outcome |
|---|---|---|---|---|
| Mahmoud et al.[50] Young and Alter[16] | 33/M | Sibling | Cy 200 mg/kg | Died (51 days) Liver failure |
| Conter et al.[51] Young and Alter[16] | 4/F | Sibling | Bu 8 mg/kg Cy 240 mg/kg | Died (3 months) GVHD/GI bleeding |
| Young and Alter[16] | 2/M | ? | Cy 200 mg/kg TAI 3 Gy | Alive (6 years) |
| Berthou et al.[49] Rocha et al.[52] Young and Alter[16] | 6/M | Sibling | Cy 120 mg/kg TBI 7 Gy | Died (6 years) VOD/Renal failure Pulmonary fibrosis |
| Berthou et al.[49] Rocha et al.[52] Young and Alter[16] | 11/M | Sibling | Cy 150 mg/kg TAI 6 Gy | Died (2 years) VOD/Renal failure Pulmonary fibrosis |
| Berthou et al.[49] | ?/? | ? | Cy 200 mg/kg | Alive (8 months) |
| Dokal et al.[53] | 29/M | URD | Cy 200 mg/kg | Rejection |
| Phillips et al.[54] Chessells and Harper[55] Young and Alter[16] | 2/M | Sibling | Cy 200 mg/kg | Alive (5 years) |
| Langston et al.[56] | 3/F | Sibling | Cy 200 mg/kg | Died (20 years) Pulmonary fibrosis |
| Langston et al.[56] Ling et al.[57] Young and Alter[16] | 11/F | Sibling | Cy 200 mg/kg | Died (8 years) Pulmonary fibrosis |
| Langston et al.[56] Storb et al.[58] | 8/M | Sibling | Cy 200 mg/kg | Died (7 days) *Aspergillosis* |

*Continued*

In summary, of the 22 reported cases of HSCT for DC, for whom there is adequate documentation, 15 are dead and seven alive. Six of the deaths are attributable to interstitial pulmonary disease, four patients had venoocclusive disease and liver failure (2 with concomitant pulmonary failure) and seven died from other transplant related causes. The median time to pulmonary death in these patients was 7.5 years posttransplant (range, 70 days to 20 years). Thus, many of the patients remained at risk for pulmonary disease at the time they were reported; indeed, one of the living patients had pulmonary fibrosis eight years posttransplant at the time of publication. A preliminary description of a recent series[61] describes five patients with DC who received HLA-matched sibling HSCT. All five were conditioned with cyclophosphamide 200 mg/kg and were alive at 20, 449, 1070, 1593, and 2949 days at the time of the abstract publication, respectively. It is too early to evaluate these patients for pulmonary and hepatic toxicity; however, less aggressive conditioning regimens may provide better results in the modern transplant era. The number of

| TABLE 17.2 | Summary of Published Stem Cell Transplants for Dyskeratosis Congenita—cont'd | | | |
|---|---|---|---|---|
| *Reference* | *Age/Sex* | *HLA Match* | *Conditioning Regimen* | *Outcome* |
| Langston et al.[56] | 26/M | Sibling | Cy 200 mg/kg | Died (70 days) Pulmonary fibrosis |
| Langston et al.[56] | 33/M | Sibling | Cy 140 mg/kg ATG 90 mg/kg | Alive (463 days) Rectal carcinoma |
| Langston et al.[56] | 22/M | Sibling | Cy 140 mg/kg ATG 90 mg/kg | Died (44 days) Acute GVHD |
| Langston et al.[56] | 23/M | URD | Cy 120 mg/kg TBI 12 Gy | Died (13 days) Candidiasis |
| Langston et al.[56] | 20/M | URD | Cy 120 mg/kg TBI 12 Gy | Died (14 days) Candidiasis |
| Yabe et al.[59] | 2/M | DP Mismatch | Cy 200 mg/kg TAI 3 Gy | Died (7 years) Pulmonary fibrosis |
| Rocha et al.[52] | 11/M | Sibling | ? | Died (4 years) VOD/liver failure |
| Rocha et al.[52] | ?/M | Sibling | ? | Alive (8 years) Pulmonary fibrosis |
| Rocha et al.[52] | ?/M | Sibling | ? | Died (19 months) GVHD/Invasive *aspergillosis*/CMV |
| Ghavamzadeh et al.[60] | 18/M | Sibling | Cy 80mg/kg Bu 0.8mg/kg | Alive (6 years) |
| Ghavamzadeh et al.[60] | 21/F | Sibling | Cy 80 mg/kg Bu 0.8 mg/kg | Alive (5 years) |

Table adapted from Yabe et al.[59] Abbreviations: Cy = cyclophosphamide; Bu = busulfan; GVHD = graft-versus-host disease; TAI = thoracoabdominal irradiation; TBI = total body irradiation; VOD = venoocclusive disease; ATG = antithymocyte globulin; URD = unrelated donor transplant.

documented cases is too few to determine the precise incremental risk of pulmonary and hepatic death as a consequence of HSCT.

In conclusion, HSCT does have the potential to cure aplastic anemia in DC and should be utilized in selected patients with significant marrow failure. However, the overall results have been sufficiently poor to date so as to warrant a study that would evaluate a potentially less toxic, immunoablative rather than a myeloablative conditioning regimen, similar to the approach taken with Fanconi anemia. The cloning of both the X-linked recessive and the autosomal dominant genes for DC may allow, in the future, a predictive genotype-phenotype correlation for predisposition to pulmonary or hepatic disease in DC. Eventually, tailor-made conditioning regimens based on specific mutation analysis and designed to reduce specific organ toxicities may become available. Currently, all patients with DC should undergo a thorough pretransplant evaluation. In addition to the standard pretransplant work-up, this must include cancer screening as well as pulmonary and hepatic function tests, including tissue biopsies when indicated. The presence of certain cancers and significant pulmonary or hepatic dysfunction may preclude transplantation using even non-myeloablative conditioning regimens.

**Hematopoietic Stem Cell Transplantation: Matched-Related Donor Evaluation.** We are unaware of any presymptomatic family members with DC being used as HSCT donors. However, in five of the families in the DCR, the diagnosis of DC was made only after seven male family members died from severe aplastic anemia, by the identification of another family member with SAA and the stigmata of DC. Furthermore, patients with SAA have been transplanted, only to make the diagnosis of DC after the fact.[52,55,57] Thus, we are less confident that a larger number of patients transplanted for SAA did not have unrecognized DC. The pretransplant donor evaluation should include a very careful physical and laboratory exam with a mutation analysis for either the X-linked recessive or autosomal dominant subtypes, particularly when the use of stem cells from a potentially presymptomatic newborn or young donor is contemplated.

## Single Cytopenias

### Diamond Blackfan Anemia

**Pathophysiology and Clinical Features.** Diamond Blackfan anemia (DBA) is a rare pure red cell aplasia predominantly of infancy and childhood,[62] resulting from an intrinsic hematopoietic cell defect[63,64] in which erythroid progenitors and precursors are highly sensitive to death by apoptosis.[6] Josephs described the first two cases in 1936.[65] A more detailed report of four cases by Diamond and Blackfan in 1938[66] and Dr. Diamond's life-long interest in the disorder earned it the appellation Diamond Blackfan anemia.[67,68]

The Diamond Blackfan Anemia Registry (DBAR) of North America, established in 1993,[69] has provided demographic, laboratory, and clinical data on DBA patients in the United States and Canada.[70] For the 354 patients reported to the DBAR, the median age at presentation of anemia is two months and the median age at diagnosis of DBA is three months; over 90% of the patients present during the first year of life. Physical anomalies, excluding short stature, were found in 47% of the patients in the DBAR. Of these, 50% were of the face and head, 38% upper limb and hand, 39% genitourinary, and 30% cardiac. Patients with multiple anomalies within each of the above four categories were considered as having a single anomaly within that category. Using this criterion more than one anomaly was found in 21% of the patients.

An elevated erythrocyte adenosine deaminase (eADA) activity found in approximately 85% of patients as well as macrocytosis and an elevated fetal hemoglobin are supportive but not diagnostic of DBA. These parameters have been helpful in distinguishing DBA from transient erythroblastopenia of childhood (TEC), a self-resolving hypoplastic anemia, thus avoiding unnecessary treatment. Furthermore, as described later in this chapter, these parameters may be useful in avoiding potential matched-related HSCT donors with genotypic DBA.

The recognition of DBA as a cancer predisposition syndrome further complicates management decisions. In a recent report there were 6 of 354 evaluable patients in the DBAR with malignancy: three patients had osteogenic sarcoma; one, myelodysplastic syndrome; one, colon carcinoma; and one, a soft tissue sarcoma.[71] A review of the literature revealed

23 additional cases of cancer. Among these were ten cases of AML/MDS, four lymphoid malignancies, two cases of osteosarcoma, two breast cancers, and five other cancers.[71] Furthermore, instances of significant cytopenias including aplastic anemia are emerging.[72]

**Genetics.** The first DBA gene, DBA1, has been cloned and is identified as RPS 19, a gene that codes for a ribosomal protein, located at chromosome 19q13.2.[73,74] Studies show that RPS 19 mutations account for only 20% to 25% of both sporadic and familial cases. The function of this protein is not fully understood. A second gene, DBA2, has been localized by linkage analysis to chromosome 8p22-23.[75] This second locus may account for 40% to 45% of patients. Almost 20% of families were inconsistent for linkage to either 19q or 8p, strongly suggesting further genetic heterogeneity. Approximately 10% of families have more than one affected individual. The majority of these cases appear to have been of dominant inheritance. Within these pedigrees considerable heterogeneity exists in the expression of the DBA phenotype.[70]

**Front Line Therapy.** Historically there have been two treatment options for patients with DBA. Since 1951, corticosteroids have been the mainstay of treatment[76] with red cell transfusions reserved for those patients who fail this modality as a consequence of either non-responsiveness or toxicity. Approximately 80% of DBA patients will respond initially to corticosteroid therapy. The remaining 20% require transfusion therapy. Patients usually are started on prednisone at doses of 2 to 4 mg/kg and weaned to the lowest dose at which the hemoglobin concentration is both clinically acceptable and stable. Corticosteroid use is fraught with myriad potential side effects. Patients with DBA on low-dose alternate-day therapy of long duration, starting in early infancy, may manifest significant steroid toxicity. Indeed, steroid-related side effects were observed in most patients, with 40%, 12%, and 6.8% manifesting cushingoid features, pathologic fractures, and cataracts, respectively. The major complication of transfusion therapy is iron overload, the consequences of which include diabetes mellitus, cardiac, and hepatic dysfunction, growth failure as well as other endocrine problems. Iron chelation with deferoxamine is therefore an essential component of a transfusion program; however, many patients find nearly daily subcutaneous chelation therapy onerous and compliance is often poor. Of note, the DBAR has documented the presence of sustained hematologic remissions defined as stable hemoglobin and no transfusion or steroid requirement for six months.[70] At the time of the last DBAR analysis, 44% of patients were receiving corticosteroids; 36% were on red cell transfusions; the remainder were on alternative treatments, had undergone HSCT or had died. In summary, both chronic corticosteroid therapy and chronic transfusion therapy may lead to a number of significant immediate and long-term complications, supporting a role for HSCT. The overall actuarial survival at approximately 40 years of age is $77.9 \pm 5.6\%$, 100% for those in sustained remission, $87.4\% \pm 6.9\%$ for corticosteroid-maintainable patients, and $57.5\% \pm 12.9\%$ for transfusion dependent patients.

**Hematopoietic Stem Cell Transplantation: Indications, Outcomes and the Approach to the Patient.** The first "successful" bone marrow transplant for DBA was performed by August and colleagues in 1976.[77] The patient died of interstitial pneumonitis on day +55, but hematopoietic engraftment from donor bone marrow confirmed DBA as a transplantable disease. Since the initial case, 50 additional transplants, virtually all from HLA-matched sibling donors, have appeared in the literature,[78-95] the majority done prior to 1993. Bone marrow was the most common stem cell source; however, matched-sibling donor HSCT as well as unrelated HSCT, using UCB as a stem cell source also have been reported.[92-94]

A series of 10 patients (8 of 10 from HLA-matched allogeneic siblings) has been reported to the IMBTR[90] with a two-year survival of 58% for all patients and 72% for sibling HSCT patients. The French registry has compiled another 13 transplants (11 of 13 from HLA-matched allogeneic siblings).[95] In 1998 a review of HSCT in DBA by Alter[96] included 35 of 37 cases from the literature. The projected actuarial survival for HSCT, done utilizing predominantly allogeneic HLA-matched related donor-derived stem cells (33 siblings, 1 mother and one unrelated donor transplant), was 66%.

The DBAR reported the results of 20 patients undergoing hematopoietic stem cell transplantation for DBA.[72] The median age at transplant for all patients was 6 years 2 months; 3 years 10 months versus 9 years 1 month for the 8 HLA-matched sibling and 12 alternative donor HSCT, respectively. While there was a trend towards alternative donor transplants being performed at an older age than matched allogeneic transplants, the difference in age was not statistically significant. Of the 12 alternative donor HSCT, two were from a mismatched relative and ten were from unrelated donors. The major indication for HSCT was transfusion dependence. However, two patients had developed severe aplastic anemia and one had significant thrombocytopenia. Of the eight HLA-matched allogeneic sibling transplants, seven were done using bone marrow and one using UCB as the stem cell source. Of the 12 alternative donor transplants, eight were done using bone marrow and four were done using UCB. All of the HLA-matched sibling HSCT were done using a non-irradiation-containing conditioning regimen, whereas the majority of alternative donor HSCT were performed using myeloablative chemotherapy and total body irradiation. The vast majority of patients received a cyclosporine-containing GVHD prophylaxis regimen. The actuarial survival for allogeneic HLA-matched sibling and alternative donor SCT were 87.5% ± 11.7% at 77.2 months and 14.1% ± 12.1% at 61.9 months ($P = .015$), respectively. If a death from osteogenic sarcoma is considered to be non-transplant related, then the survival for alternative donor SCT was 28.1% ± 13.7% ($P = .025$).

In general, favorable transplant outcomes are most likely if the patient is in good health at the time of HSCT and without complications of iron overload and allosensitization. Improvements in supportive care, GVHD prophylaxis, and infection control have resulted in a marked decrease in HLA-matched related HSCT transplant-related morbidity and mortality. Thus, sibling HSCT is recommended for young DBA patients prior to the development of significant allosensitization or iron overload, when there is an available HLA-matched related donor. The outcomes for alternative donor SCT are significantly inferior to those performed using HLA-matched sibling donors, supporting a more conservative approach.

With regard to treatment and response, concerns about the overuse of corticosteroids have been borne out, especially in light of the steroid-related side effects already mentioned. In addition, another confounding variable complicating the decision to perform HSCT is the observation that the actuarial likelihood that a DBA patient may enter a spontaneous remission by age 25 years is 20%, 77% doing so by their tenth birthday. Patients appear to have a similar chance of remitting from either transfusion or steroid therapy. The true incidence of aplastic anemia, myelodysplastic syndrome, and hematopoietic malignancy, and the predisposition to nonhematopoietic malignancy in DBA is being defined. These findings support a reappraisal of current clinical practices. In particular, transfusion therapy should be seriously considered in lieu of corticosteroids before significant growth retardation and/or other side effects ensue. Certainly there are few, if any circumstances for which corticosteroids are initiated in infancy and continued for decades. Furthermore, the preponderance of deaths in transfusion-dependent patients is attributable to HSCT-related complications, rather than the hemosiderosis. Thus, the decision to undergo a hematopoietic stem cell transplant in a patient with DBA must be based upon the availability of a suitable donor and an accurate assessment of the consequences of prolonged corticosteroid and transfusion therapy, as well as the natural history of DBA.

Dianzani et al.[97] point out the similarity between DBA and thalassemia major and suggest that similar criteria for HSCT should be applied in both. Indeed, the ideal thalassemia major HSCT candidate is a young patient who is minimally transfused or at least in good iron balance, with no evidence of significant hepatic damage, transplanted from an HLA-identical allogeneic sibling donor. The data support this observation with the caveat that the true incidence of severe aplastic anemia,[98] myelodysplasia, and leukemia[71] in DBA patients is unknown. Patients who develop other cytopenias, MDS, or leukemia should be evaluated for alternative donor transplants on a case-by-case basis.

**Hematopoietic Stem Cell Transplantation: Matched-Related Donor Evaluation.** Allogeneic sibling stem cell transplantation in young DBA patients without significant iron overload or organ dysfunction is a reasonable alternative to corticosteroid or transfusion therapy and, as well, obviates the risk of tri-lineage hematopoietic failure or hematologic malignancy. There must be a note of caution regarding allogeneic donor selection. Recently, a significant number of apparently hematologically normal family members of DBA patients have been found to have a silent DBA phenotype by virtue of macrocytosis, elevated fetal hemoglobin and/or erythrocyte adenosine deaminase activity.[99] An allogeneic HSCT inadvertently using one such donor, predictably, resulted in persistent red cell aplasia.[15] Allogeneic donor evaluations therefore should include assessment of eADA activity, mean corpuscular volume, fetal hemoglobin, along with a thorough genetic analysis to determine the presence of a known mutation.

In contrast to HLA-matched sibling HSCT alternative donor transplantation, especially in light of a reasonable likelihood of spontaneous remission, should be considered on a case-by-case basis when individual circumstances justify the risk. Improvements in the control of GVHD as well as more precise high resolution HLA typing and the availability of larger donor pools should lead to improved outcomes for transplants utilizing alternative donor sources. The risk of nonhematologic malignancy in patients with DBA[71] and the role of HSCT, particularly with radiation-based conditioning regimens,[100] need to be investigated. As such, alternative treatments and new approaches to achieving hematopoietic chimerism without aggressive myeloablation, keeping in mind the risk of AML/MDS, are being developed and should be explored in selected patients with Diamond Blackfan anemia.

**Alternative Therapy.** A number of treatments, including erythropoietin,[101] immunoglobulin,[102] megadose corticosteroids,[103] and androgens[16] have been utilized in DBA patients with little success. Some responses have been confirmed with other modalities. These include cyclosporine,[104] interleuken-3 (IL-3),[105] and most recently metoclopramide.[106] With the exception of metoclopramide, the toxicity seems unwarranted for most patients. A more extensive trial with metoclopramide is being planned. These agents should be explored on a case-by-case basis as an alternative to corticosteroids, transfusion or HSCT when the risk associated with these proven modalities warrants treatment.

## Kostmann Syndrome

**Pathophysiology and Clinical Features.** The Severe Chronic Neutropenia International Registry (SCNIR) defines severe chronic neutropenia as: three blood neutrophil counts of less than 500/μL obtained at least three months after birth within a six-month observation period; a typical pattern of recurrent fevers, chronic gingivitis, and infections at regular intervals; a bone marrow aspirate showing a "maturation arrest" at the promyelocyte or myelocyte stage; and a normal cytogenetic analysis.[107] In contrast to the single cell cytopenias, Diamond Blackfan anemia, and congenital amegakaryocytic thrombocytopenia, both of which may terminate in pancytopenia, the manifestations of Kostmann syndrome are virtually restricted to the granulocyte lineage. Classically, Kostmann syndrome was inferred when there was more than one affected child in a kindred, while congenital neutropenia was reserved for a single "sporadic" case in a family. The absolute neutrophil count (ANC) in KS is continuously less than 200/mm.³ Patients with Shwachman Diamond syndrome, described elsewhere in this chapter, are relatively easily distinguished on the basis of the clinical features of exocrine pancreatic insufficiency, malabsorption, and growth retardation, and are only rarely confused with the other syndromes. Autosomal dominant cyclic neutropenia is diagnosed when serial neutrophil counts reveal oscillations with a 21-day periodicity. Needless to say, there is considerable overlap between sporadic cases of congenital neutropenia and the autosomal recessive cases referred to as Kostmann syndrome. In this text Kostmann syndrome will continue to be used to refer to severe congenital neutropenia (SCN), the term preferred by some authors,[108] that is neither cyclic nor SDS, regardless of its mode of inheritance.

Recent advances in molecular genetics have resulted in clarification of the classification of these related disorders. Mutations of ELA2, the neutrophil elastase gene, predominate in both Kostmann syndrome and cyclic neutropenia.[109] Although the molecular defect in KS is defined for the majority of cases, the precise pathophysiology is still unclear. Furthermore, the etiology of Kostmann syndrome remains to be elucidated in those patients not demonstrating ELA2 gene mutations. However, as with the majority of the inherited bone marrow failure syndromes, the defect in ELA2 in this case results in accelerated apoptosis at the promyelocyte/myelocyte stage of neutrophil differentiation. Neutrophil elastase is synthesized and packaged in promyelocyte primary granules for release by neutrophils at sites of inflammation.[110] The rather restricted expression of ELA2 as compared to FANC (A-G), DKC1, hTR, and DBA1 appears to correlate with the limited hematologic and non-hematologic tissue involvement in KS and cyclic neutropenia as compared with the other inherited bone marrow failure syndromes. The severity and periodicity of neutropenia is a consequence of the location of the neutrophil elastase mutation and, perhaps to some degree, other genetic factors. As described by Dale and colleagues[109] the best mathematical model is one in which oscillations of the neutrophil count occur when there is reduced survival of neutrophil precursors and an intact feedback control with efficient neutrophil production. The degree to which production is rendered impaired and ineffective by highly accelerated apoptosis determines the severity and loss of periodicity of neutropenia. The severity of the defect, in large part, can be predicted by the specific position of the neutrophil elastase mutation. Cyclic neutropenia mutations, for the most part, cluster at the active site. In contrast, severe congenital neutropenia mutations largely present away from the active site, leading to conformational changes in the molecule, apparently resulting in more significant alterations in elastase function.

Prior to the availability of cytokine therapy the prognosis for patients with Kostmann syndrome was extremely poor. Only 30% of patients reported in Alter's review of the literature were predicted to survive beyond their twentieth birthday, with a median and mean age at death of seven months and two years, respectively. No patients developed aplastic anemia.[16] The clinical hallmark of KS is the early onset of severe bacterial infections. Omphalitis may present immediately after birth. The natural history without cytokine therapy included subsequent upper respiratory infections, otitis media, pneumonia, and abscesses of the skin and liver. In addition, these patients suffered from aphthous stomatitis, gingival hyperplasia, and consequent tooth loss.[111] The vast majority died from infection, in particular pneumonia or sepsis. Occasional cases of leukemia were reported, but the high early death rate precluded a true assessment of the risk of leukemia in KS.

**Genetics.** Kostmann syndrome was originally described in 1956 in an extended Swedish family as an autosomal recessively inherited disorder.[112] The majority of cases of Kostmann syndrome as well as cyclic neutropenia, however, are the result of dominant-acting mutations of the neutrophil elastase (ELA2) gene mapped to chromosome 19p13.3.[113] Furthermore, the specific mutations provide a reasonable genotype–phenotype correlation confirming cyclic neutropenia and Kostmann syndrome as distinct but overlapping disorders, with members of families with cyclic neutropenia having neutropenia without oscillations and, conversely, patients with autosomal dominant congenital neutropenia having periodicity in their neutrophil counts. Moreover, the majority of cases of congenital neutropenia are, like Diamond Blackfan anemia, autosomal dominant or new dominant-acting germline mutations.[109]

**Front Line Therapy.** Advances in our understanding of the regulation of granulopoiesis as well as the molecular etiology and pathophysiology of KS have been accompanied by improvements in clinical management. In particular, the antiapoptotic effect of G-CSF has been exploited as a treatment strategy with dramatic results. A randomized multicenter phase III trial of recombinant human G-CSF (rHuG-CSF) published in 1993 showed a 50% reduction in the incidence and duration of infection and a 70% reduction in antibiotic use.[114] Data from the SCNIR on more than 300 patients indicate that over 90% respond to G-CSF with an ANC of ≥1000/mm.[3][111] A recent review by Zeidler and colleagues[115] describes a consensus dosing scheme for rHuG-CSF, the goal being to find an acceptable dose that maintains an ANC of ≥ 1000/mm.[3] Nonresponders are those patients who do not have an increase in their neutrophil count sufficient to reduce infections at a rHuG-CSF dose of up to 120 μg/kg/day. Partial responders are defined as patients whose ANC reaches 500/mm³ but continue to have infections. Patients whose ANC exceeds 5000/mm³ may have their dose reduced to the lowest effective level or change to an every other day dosing schedule. Those 5% to 10% of patients who fail are considered candidates for HSCT when a matched-related or acceptable alternative donor exists. The use of HSCT in G-CSF-responders who have an HLA-matched sibling donor is controversial and must be considered in the context of the natural history of G-CSF-treated KS and the side effects of rHuG-CSF.

The major consequences of long-term G-CSF therapy are osteoporosis, vasculitis, splenomegaly and the appearance of leukemia/myelodysplasia.[111,115,116] Rare cases of thrombocytopenia, responding to G-CSF dose adjustment, and an apparent propensity to immune complex disease have been identified. There were abnormal results in about half of the 121 patients in the SCNIR for whom some determination of bone density was measured. The majority of patients were asymptomatic. Some patients with SCN had baseline osteoporosis/osteopenia. Thus, whether osteoporosis is a toxicity of G-CSF or represents the modified natural history of the disorder is not known. In contrast, the small percentage of patients who develop vasculitis will have resolution with the temporary cessation of G-CSF treatment. Splenomegaly is reported in approximately 20% of patients at diagnosis and in about one-third to one-half of patients over 10 years of treatment. The major recognized consequence of therapy has been the emergence of a cohort of patients who develop acute myeloblastic leukemia and/or myelodysplastic syndrome.[117] A cause and effect relationship between G-CSF and AML/MDS is felt to be unlikely. Clonal disease appears to be due, in large part, to the opportunity afforded by an extended life expectancy. However, some have suggested that a role for G-CSF in the pathogenesis of AML/MDS cannot be ruled out.[117] The most recent evaluation from the SCNIR reveals a crude rate for the development of AML/MDS of 9% with an actuarial risk of 13% (95% confidence interval, 8.4% to 18%) at eight years of rHuG-CSF treatment.[116] There are no survivors of AML treated with chemotherapy reported to the SCNIR.[117]

**Hematopoietic Stem Cell Transplantation: Indications, Outcomes and the Approach to the Patient.** Until 1993, when G-CSF was found to significantly increase the neutrophil count and ameliorate symptoms, hematopoietic stem cell transplantation was the only therapeutic modality for patients with KS.[118] Recombinant human G-CSF now has become front-line therapy. Indeed, an analysis of data from the SCNIR has resulted in the recommendation that HSCT be reserved for disease refractory to G-CSF.[111,115] These data are, however, open to another interpretation.

In the recently published transplant experience from the SCNIR,[119] 11 patients were transplanted for indications other than malignancy (rHuG-CSF partial or nonresponse, 8; neutropenia, 1; pancytopenia, 1; G-CSF receptor mutation, 1) between 1976 and 1998. Of the 11 patients, eight received an HLA-matched sibling donor HSCT. Of these eight, one received cyclophosphamide only as the conditioning regimen and rejected the graft. Five of the remaining seven are alive and well and apparently cured. The remaining two are "cured" but have significant sequelae of HSCT, severe chronic GVHD and severe hemorrhagic cystitis requiring a cystectomy, respectively. Two of the three patients transplanted from alternative donors died from transplant-related complications. The final patient suffers from extensive chronic GVHD.

In analyzing the decision to withhold HSCT from KS patients who have an HLA-matched related donor, three factors must be considered: first, the excellent outcome for HLA-matched sibling HSCT in the modern era; second, the actuarial risk of AML in G-CSF-treated patients with KS; and third, the predictability of the evolution to leukemia in G-CSF-treated patients.

The outcome of HSCT from an HLA-matched sibling donor is likely to be even better than that reported in the SCINR series that dates back to 1976. The actuarial risk of AML for G-CSF treated KS patients is 13% at eight years. Furthermore, AML in KS is likely incurable with the currently available therapeutic armamentarium. The results for HSCT in patients with KS and MDS/AML are, as expected, poor.[119] The SCINR has recorded 18 patients transplanted for leukemia, with only three surviving.[117,119] Only one of these patients had an HLA-matched sibling donor. Thus, the ability to reliably predict the emergence of AML and effectively intervene would allow for the highly selective use of HSCT in those patients at risk of malignant transformation. Mutations in the G-CSF receptor are found in the leukemic cells of the majority of patients who evolve to AML.[111,117,120] Most, but not all, patients acquire these mutations up to years prior to the development of overt leukemia.[121] However, it is unknown whether patients with G-CSF receptor mutations who undergo an HLA-matched sibling donor HSCT will have improved survival compared to those transplanted prior to the development of these mutations.

These data suggest the need for a careful prospective evaluation to determine the reliability of G-CSF mutation analysis as a predictive assay for the development of AML and the outcome of early transplant intervention. It is reasonable to consider patients with Kostmann syndrome who have an HLA-matched sibling donor as candidates for HSCT. Alternative donor transplants would be reserved for those patients who develop G-CSF receptor mutations. Those patients refractory to G-CSF would be transplanted using the best available donor.

**Hematopoietic Stem Cell Transplantation: Donor Evaluation.** Potential HLA-matched sibling donors should be evaluated for neutropenia and, when feasible, neutrophil elastase gene mutations.

## Shwachman Diamond Syndrome

**Pathophysiology and Clinical Features.** Shwachman Diamond syndrome (SDS), first described in 1964, is a rare autosomal recessive disorder characterized by neutropenia, exocrine pancreatic insufficiency, and metaphyseal dysostosis.[122,123] Most of the patients present in infancy or early childhood with failure to thrive and diarrhea. Classic diagnostic criteria require the documentation of pancreatic insufficiency determined by either decreased levels of pancreatic enzymes upon pancreatic stimulation or steatorrhea evidenced by an abnormal 72-hour fecal fat study in a patient with persistent, intermittent or cyclic neutropenia.[16] More recently, low serum levels of trypsinogen and isoamylase (when these tests are available) in a neutropenic patient have been used to confirm the diagnosis. The serum isoamylase remains low throughout life, unlike serum trypsinogen, which tends to increase with age.[124] An imaging study, using computed tomography, ultrasound, or magnetic resonance imaging, that demonstrates pancreatic lipomatosis, is highly suggestive of the diagnosis of SDS (reviewed[125]).

A recent comprehensive review describes the variety of laboratory and clinical findings in patients with SDS.[125] Neutropenia, found in 88% to 100% of patients, is the hematologic hallmark of SDS. The neutropenia is exacerbated in some patients due to a defect in neutrophil chemotaxis and/or immune deficiency.[126] Anemia and reticulocytopenia is present in approximately 80% of patients. The anemia is usually mild; however, some patients do develop a significant macrocytic anemia. A platelet count <150,000/mm$^3$ is common and sometimes severe. Pancytopenia occurs in 10% to 65% of cases and may precede progressive bone marrow dysfunction characterized by SAA, MDS or acute leukemia, usually of myeloid origin.[16,124]

Metaphyseal dysostosis and rib and/or thoracic cage abnormalities are found in 44% to 77% and 32% to 52% of patients, respectively. Poor weight gain, short stature, delayed bone maturation, delayed puberty, developmental delay and learning disabilities, hepatomegaly, elevated liver transaminases, icthyosis, frequent infections, dental caries and dysplastic teeth are consistent features in patients with SDS.[125,127] The differential diagnoses of cystic fibrosis, Pearson syndrome, cartilage hair hypoplasia and celiac disease are relatively easily excluded.

The pathophysiology of SDS is still unclear. However, diminished stem and progenitor cell numbers, manifest by reduced in vitro bone marrow progenitor cell proliferation,[128,129,130] and a decreased CD 34+ count accompanied by defective marrow stroma[131] are features of SDS. As mentioned previously, the underlying pathophysiology of the hematopoietic defect in SDS, in common with the other inherited bone marrow failure syndromes, seems to be a progenitor cell predisposition to undergo apoptosis.[8] Of interest, the mean telomere length in leukocytes of SDS patients is significantly shorter than that found in normal leukocytes. The degree of telomere shortening, however, does not appear to affect the clinical severity of the disease and the significance of this observation is being investigated.[132]

The pancreatic insufficiency seen in SDS patients has been noted to improve with age, and in many cases, SDS patients are able to discontinue supplemental pancreatic enzymes as they get older. However, hematologic dysfunction may progress with age.[124] Patients with SDS should have regular hematologic monitoring. Dror and Freedman recommend a complete blood count every four months.[125] For patients who are hematologically stable, a yearly bone marrow aspirate and biopsy for morphology and cytogenetics is suggested. Although the putative benefits are in debate, the goal of surveillance is to detect progressive aplasia, MDS, or leukemia at the earliest possible time. Chronic transfusion support with iron chelation may be required for patients with clinically significant anemia and/or thrombocytopenia. Erythropoietin has proven ineffective for mitigating anemia.[133] As in Kostmann syndrome, G-CSF has been used, with a decrement in the number and severity of infections and improved quality of life for patients with critical neutropenia.[116] G-CSF appears to be effective also when used during documented infections in SDS patients with less severe neutropenia.[125] Acceptable acute side effects are observed with the use of G-CSF.[116] However, the incremental risk, if any, of MDS/AML for patients with SDS receiving the cytokine is not known. Conventional medical management other than appropriate supportive care is ineffective in the treatment of the severe aplastic anemia and myelodysplasia associated with SDS. Furthermore, the clinical picture is clouded by uncertainty regarding the natural history of hematologic progression. The time from peripheral blood count changes to myelodysplasia is unknown, as is the time from myelodysplasia to overt leukemia. The predictive value of bone marrow cytogenetic abnormalities is also unknown and controversial. Even the ability to define MDS in SDS is questionable, although Dror and Freedman make a strong case that SDS "... is a myelodysplastic disorder from its inception."[125] The true incidence of hematologic malignancy and myelodysplasia is unknown although MDS and/or clonal cytogenetics and leukemia have been described in from 10% to 44% and 5% to 24%, respectively, in patients described in retrospective reviews.[134-137] The most common cytogenetic abnormalities are isochromosome 7 (i7q), monosomy 7 (-7), deletions involving the long arm of 7 (-7q), -5q and other complex abnormalities involving chromosomes 7 or 5. Sometimes chromosomal abnormalities are seen only intermittently. The significance of these abnormalities is at present unclear as not all of the patients undergo leukemic transformation.[138] In a longitudinal prospective study 29% of patients were initially observed to have clonal marrow cytogenetic abnormalities.[139] These abnormalities include i7q, -20q, and a combination of the two. At the time of the report, no patient had progressed into MDS or AML, and one of the patients had no detectable clone at two years of follow-up. Unfortunately, once AML develops, the response to conventional chemotherapy is poor. In addition, intolerance to chemotherapy with untoward side effects has been observed in SDS patients. Thus, HSCT is considered the only curative option for patients with critical neutropenia unresponsive to G-CSF, SAA or "true" MDS and leukemia.

**Genetics.** Shwachman Diamond syndrome is inherited as an autosomal recessive disorder. Recently, Goobie and colleagues defined the SDS locus as a 2.7 cM interval spanning the centromere of chromosome 7. Analysis of multiplex SDS families revealed linkage to this single locus.[140] The same group has refined the SDS locus to a 1.9 cM interval at 7q11 and ultimately identified the previously uncharacterized gene, SBDS.[141]

**Hematopoietic Stem Cell Transplantation: Indications, Outcomes and the Approach to the Patient.** The first transplant for SDS was reported in 1989[142] in a ten-year-old boy with pancytopenia. He was diagnosed with SDS at age eight years but had been anemic, requiring blood transfusions and had infections throughout his life. He underwent HSCT from an HLA-identical sibling after receiving myeloablative conditioning with busulfan, cyclophosphamide and ATG. He developed skin and gut GVHD. On day +12 he was found to have congestive heart failure. The patient engrafted on day +21 but died on day +23 of cardiac failure secondary to cardiomyopathy. Successful engraftment confirmed SDS as a transplantable disease.

▼ Table 17.3 describes the 21 HSCT for SDS that are reported in the literature to date; ten from HLA-identical siblings, one from a mismatched mother, and ten from unrelated donors. The indications for transplantation in these cases were pancytopenia/aplastic anemia and progression to myelofibrosis, MDS or AML.[41,135,142–156] Chromosome 7 abnormalities were found prior to transplant in over 50% of the cases of MDS/AML. Eighteen patients reported engraftment; two patient had primary graft failure. Graft-versus-host disease complicated over half of both HLA-matched sibling and unrelated HSCT. Eleven patients are alive: 5 of 10 sibling HSCT, 0 of 1 maternal HSCT, and 6 of 10 unrelated HSCT. Three patients developed significant liver dysfunction, one requiring a liver transplant for veno-occlusive disease.[147] One SDS patient received an HSCT using an unrelated cord blood donor.[156] Two of the patients noted earlier received a PBSCT, one from a matched sibling and one from a mother.[149,150] Both patients died of severe GVHD.

A mostly unpublished experience of 5 HSCT performed in 4 patients with SDS from a single institution utilized three sibling and two unrelated donors[142] (A Vlachos and JM Lipton; personal communication). All four patients died. The causes of death were cyclophosphamide-associated cardiomyopathy leading to cardiac failure (reported[142]), late graft failure at ten months, secondary leukemia after a second HSCT and veno-occlusive disease/GVHD of the liver with acute respiratory distress syndrome, respectively. Unpublished data from the Shwachman Diamond Syndrome International Registry report nine patients who have undergone an HSCT (personal communication). One matched-sibling HSCT is alive; of two related nonsibling HSCT, one is alive with GVHD and one died of liver failure. Six patients received unrelated HSCT. Of these, four were conditioned with a myeloablative regimen; one is alive with gut GVHD, two died of acute GVHD of the liver, and for one the status is unknown. The remaining two unrelated HSCT were conditioned with a nonmyeloablative regimen consisting of TBI 200 cGy with mycophenolate mofetil/Cyclosporine A posttransplant; one adult died eight months posttransplant of an infection, and one child with nonengraftment died after a second HSCT. Overall crude survival for the reported and unpublished HSCT for SDS is 43%; 7 of 14 for HLA-matched sibling HSCT, 1 of 3 for related nonsibling HSCT and 6 of 16 for unrelated HSCT with one unknown.

HSCT for patients with SDS is fraught with many difficulties. As with all autosomal recessive genetic disorders the probability of finding an HLA-matched sibling donor is only 3 in 16. Hepatic and cardiac toxicity, nutritional deficiencies and preexisting infection as

**TABLE 17.3** Summary of Published/Unpublished Stem Cell Transplants for Shwachman Diamond Syndrome

| Reference | Age/Sex | HLA Match | Conditioning Regimen | Outcome |
|---|---|---|---|---|
| Tsai et al.[142] | 10/M | Sibling | Bu/Cy/ATG | Died (23 days) Cy-induced Pancarditis |
| Barrios et al.[143] | 17/F | Sibling | TLI/ Cy | Alive |
| Seymour and Escudier[144] | 38/M | URD | Bu/Cy | Alive Hepatic dysfunction |
| Smith et al.[145] | 5/M | URD | TBI/ Cy | Died (1 year) BM failure |
| Smith et al.[135] | 14/F | Sibling | Bu/Cy/ Campath | Alive Mild VOD |
| Arseniev et al.[146] | 24/M | Sibling | Bu/Cy | Died (9 mo) Leukemic relapse |
| Bunin et al.[147] | ?/F | URD | TBI/ Cy/Ara-C/ T cell depletion | Alive Liver transplantation for severe VOD |
| Davies et al.[148] | 13/M | URD | TBI/Cy | Alive |
| Davies et al.[148] | 7/M | URD | TBI/Cy | Nonengraftment Died (58 days) Infection |
| Davies et al.[148] | 8/F | URD | TBI/ Cy | Died (2 mo) ARDS |
| Dokal et al.[149] | 25/M | Sibling | TBI/ Cy/ Campath | Gut GVHD Died (6 mo) Fungal pneumonia |
| Okcu et al.[150] | 8/M | URD | TBI/ Cy/ Thiotepa/ T cell depletion | Died (93 days) Grade IV GVHD Pulmonary Hemorrhage |
| Okcu et al.[150] | 9/? | Mother | TBI/ Cy/ Thiotepa/ T cell depletion | Died (32 days) Grade IV GVHD Pulmonary hemorrhage |
| Miano et al.[42] | ?/? | URD | Bu/Cy/Thiotepa | Alive |
| Faber et al.[151] | 5/M | Sibling | Bu/Cy | Alive |
| Cesaro et al.[152] | 5/M | URD | Bu/Cy/Thiotepa/ rabbit ALG | Alive |

*Continued*

**TABLE 17.3** Summary of Published/Unpublished Stem Cell Transplants for Shwachman Diamond Syndrome—cont'd

| Reference | Age/Sex | HLA Match | Conditioning Regimen | Outcome |
|---|---|---|---|---|
| Ritchie et al.[153] | 35/F | Sibling | TBI/Cy | Died (135 days) Liver failure |
| Hsu et al.[154] | 30/M | Sibling | Bu/Cy/ T cell depletion | Died (6 mo) Graft failure Recurrent MDS |
| Park et al.[155] | 21/F | Sibling | TBI/Cy | Alive |
| Fleitz et al.[156] | 3/F | Sibling | Melphalan/Etoposide/ATG | Alive |
| Fleitz et al.[156] | 22 M/F | Unrelated UCB | Melphalan/TLI/ Etoposide/ATG | Alive |
| Unpublished | 7/F | Sibling | BMT #1 Bu/Cy BMT #2 TBI/Cy | Graft failure (9 mo) Died (3 mo) AML |
| Unpublished | 14/M | URD | TBI/Cy | Died (3 mo) VOD/GVHD liver |
| Unpublished | 22 M/F | URD | TBI/Cy | Died (3 mo) Pulmonary infection/ARDS |
| Unpublished | 19/F | ? | ? | Died |
| Unpublished | ?/M | Father | ? | Alive |
| Unpublished | ?/F | Sibling | ? | Died Hemorrhage |
| Unpublished | ?/M | Sibling | ? | Alive |
| Unpublished | 6/F | URD | Cy/fludarabine ATG | Died (330 days) Infection |
| Unpublished | 3/M | URD | Fludarabine/low dose TBI/ CsA/ MMF | Died Graft failure |
| Unpublished | ?/F | Unrelated UCB | ? | Alive |
| Unpublished | 23/M | ? | TBI/Cy/ATG | Died (10 days) Fungal infection |
| Unpublished | 34/M | URD | Fludarabine/low dose TBI/ CsA/ MMF | Died (7 mo) Graft failure Sepsis |
| Unpublished | 10/M | Sibling | Fludarabine/ low dose TBI/ CsA/MMF | Alive Grade IV GVHD Extensive cGVHD |

Abbreviations: CY = cyclophosphamide; Bu = busulfan; GVHD = graft-versus-host disease; TBI = total body irradiation; TLI = total lymphoid irradiation; VOD = venoocclusive disease; ATG = antithymocyte globulin; CsA = cyclosporine; MMF = mycophenylate mofetil; URD = unrelated donor transplant; ARDS = adult respiratory distress syndrome; AML = acute myeloid leukemia.

well as refractory clonal hematologic disease, in particular, severely limit the efficacy of HSCT. Dror and Freedman[125] propose that the poor outcome is a consequence of a marrow stromal defect not corrected and perhaps exacerbated by conditioning regimens as well as critical organ apoptosis induced by radiation and/or chemotherapy. Furthermore, many transplants reported were done as a last resort for patients with advanced disease.

Medical management with G-CSF and appropriate supportive care combined with surveillance for clonal hematologic disease and severe aplastic anemia is the preferred approach for the majority of less severely affected patients. HSCT should be considered only in SDS for patients with clinically significant aplastic anemia or myelodysplasia who fail medical management and for patients with leukemia. The best chance of a successful transplant is with an HLA-matched sibling donor or an unrelated SCT from a molecularly matched donor. A thorough work-up sufficient to rule out SDS should be done for any potential HLA-matched sibling donors.

The patient also must undergo a complete pretransplant evaluation specific for SDS. The assessment should include a cardiac evaluation with electrocardiogram and echocardiogram. Given the myocardial defect in SDS,[16,138] a cardiac biopsy also should be considered. A pulmonary evaluation also is essential with pulmonary function testing, diffusing lung capacity for carbon monoxide (DLCO), and chest radiograph. A CT of the chest should be considered for children who cannot cooperate for pulmonary function testing or for those whose work-up reveals pulmonary pathology. An evaluation of the liver is vital and should include chemistries and possible liver biopsy.[127] Documentation of underlying organ pathology necessitates individualization of the conditioning and anti-GVHD regimens. Thus, clinical trials with less toxic nonmyeloablative preparatory regimens and tailor-made GVHD prophylaxis are indicated with specific attention given to cardiac, hepatic and pulmonary abnormalities found in these patients.

**Hematopoietic Stem Cell Transplantation: Donor Evaluation.** Potential HLA-matched sibling donors should be evaluated for neutropenia and pancreatic insufficiency, and, when indicated, SBDS gene mutation analysis.

## Congenital Amegakaryocytic Thrombocytopenia

**Pathophysiology and Clinical Features.** Congenital amegakaryocytic thrombocytopenia is the rarest of the inherited bone marrow failure syndromes discussed in this chapter. The disorder is characterized by severe hypo-or amegakaryocytic thrombocytopenia presenting during early childhood. Young and Alter described only 37 cases reported in the literature. In addition, they reported  physical anomalies in 16 patients, some consistent with FA or DC. Appropriately it is noted that those disorders could not be ruled out on the basis of a retrospective literature review. Already a number of cases can be reassigned as Hoyeraal-Hreidarsson syndrome, a variant of dyskeratosis congenital.[12] Thus, the number of reported cases is likely overestimated. In comparison there were, at the time of the compilation approximately 170 reported cases of TAR, 850 FA, 200 DC, 450 DBA, 200 SDS, and 150 KS. A more recent update reveals 44 patients with presumed CAT.[157] Of these, 18 had physical anomalies. Although many of the patients had abnormalities inconsistent with other known syndromes, it is most safe to restrict the discussion to those lacking anomalies. Furthermore, although one patient with cerebellar vermis hypoplasia has been described,[158] the majority of cases of CAT confirmed by mutation analysis lack congenital anomalies. Thus, patients with amegakaryocytic thrombocytopenia and congenital anomalies must be carefully evaluated to rule out other inherited bone marrow failure syndromes. In particular, it is critical that the Hoyeraal-Hreidarsson variant of DC (characterized by cerebellar agenesis) as well as FA be ruled out in order to avoid life-threatening transplant conditioning regimen-related toxicity. Thrombocytopenia absent radii syndrome can be excluded on the basis of the defining congenital anomalies. Patients with TAR will improve, usually by one year of age, and can be managed with platelet transfusions[159] except under extreme circumstances.[160]

The 26 patients without anomalies presented with the signs and symptoms of thrombocytopenia at a median age of seven days. Eleven developed aplastic anemia at a median of three years. One developed AML and died and one developed MDS.[157] The median survival was only six years. Of the other 15 deaths, eight died from bleeding or sepsis as a consequence of pancytopenia and seven died with thrombocytopenia from bleeding and/or infection. The hematologic phenotype of CAT is variable. There appears to be two forms, one characterized by both early onset thrombocytopenia and rapid evolution to pancytopenia the other with a later presentation of both thrombocytopenia and pancytopenia.[161] Of the 26 patients reported by Alter and Young, 21 developed thrombocytopenia in the first year of life with the onset in 15 during the first week of life. The other five cases were characterized by a later presentation with thrombocytopenia developing between two and nine years of age. Particular mutations, described in the next section, appear to correlate with severity.

**Genetics.** Recently, in a typical case, CAT was found to be associated with compound heterozygous mutations in exon 10 of the c-mpl gene, each contributed by one parent. Further evaluation showed that these mutations disrupt the function of the thrombopoietin receptor.[158] Additional studies show CAT to be an autosomal recessive disorder in which virtually all cases are due to either homozygous or compound heterozygous mutations of c-mpl.[161–163] Mutation analysis appears to indicate that those patients with complete loss of c-mpl function have more severe thrombocytopenia and more rapid progression to pancytopenia, in contrast to less severely affected patients who maintain some c-mpl activity.[161]

**Hematopoietic Stem Cell Transplantation: Indications, Outcomes and the Approach to the Patient.** The prognosis for patients with CAT is very poor. Alter and Young's recent review of the literature reports approximately 80% of bona fide patients succumbing to complications of thrombocytopenia or pancytopenia by ten years of age.[157] Corticosteroids, androgens, cytokines, and cyclosporine have been tried with, at best, temporary responses.[157,164–167] The only curative treatment has been hematopoietic stem cell transplantation, and as such, it is the treatment of choice. Two patients with CAT developed AML/MDS at 16 and 19 years, respectively. Transplants should be done early enough to avoid blood product sensitization as well as the development of pancytopenia or clonal disease. In contrast to FA, DC, SDS, and perhaps DBA, CAT resembles KS in that c-mpl (like ELA2) expression appears limited (megakaryocyte progenitors, brain, and fetal liver),[168] resulting in no incremental risk of HSCT as a consequence of any nonhematopoietic manifestations of the disorder. This appears to be borne out by the clinical experience. We were able to find 17 reasonably well documented HSCT reported in the literature. Six unrelated and three HLA matched-related HSCT are reported as case reports.[166,169–172] A variety of conditioning regimens and stem cell sources were utilized. Four of six unrelated and three of three matched related donor transplants were alive and well at the time of the reports. Five matched related, one haploidentical parent and two unrelated HSCT are reported from a single center (▼ Table 17.4).[173] All patients were severely thrombocytopenic and two had aplastic anemia at ages 22 months and 6 years 2 months, respectively. The median age at HSCT was 2 years 8 months (range 12 months to 6 years 6 months). The conditioning regimens included busulfan and cyclophosphamide in all cases. All but two received ATG with one receiving thiotepa. GVHD prophylaxis was short-course methotrexate and cyclosporine in all but the peripheral blood stem cell transplants that had been T cell depleted only. The outcome has been excellent. Five of five patients from the single institution and all eight who received an HSCT from an HLA-matched relative are alive and well with full engraftment, minimal acute GVHD and no chronic GVHD at the time of their report. The median follow-up for the single institution patients (including one patient transplanted with a haploidentical mother) was 17 months (range, 3 to 27 months). Of the nine alternative donor HSCT, five are alive; of those five, three for whom such data were available were alive at 7, 16, 31 months.

---

**TABLE 17.4**   **Summary of Stem Cell Transplants for Congenital Amegakaryocytic Thrombocytopenia**

| Age | HLA Match | Conditioning Regimen | Stem Cell Source | Outcome |
|---|---|---|---|---|
| 22 mos | URD | Bu 20 mg/kg<br>Cy 100 mg/kg<br>ATG | BM | Died<br>Bronchiolitis obliterans |
| 24 mos | Mother | Bu 20 mg/kg<br>Cy 200 mg/kg<br>ATG | BM | Alive fully engrafted |
| 4 yrs, 1 mos | Sibling | Bu 16 mg/kg<br>Cy 200 mg/kg | UCB | Alive fully engrafted |
| 2 yrs, 4 mos | Mother | Bu 16 mg/kg<br>Cy 200 mg/kg<br>ATG | T cell depleted<br>PBSC | Alive fully engrafted |
| 12 mos | URD | Bu 20 mg/kg<br>Cy 120 mg/kg<br>ATG | BM | Died<br>Infection |
| 3 yrs, 6 mos | Sibling | Bu 16 mg/kg<br>Cy 200 mg/kg<br>ATG | BM | Alive fully engrafted |
| 6 yrs, 6 mos | Sibling | Bu 16 mg/kg<br>Cy 200 mg/kg<br>ATG | BM | Alive fully engrafted |
| 4 yrs, 4 mos | Haploidentical<br>mother | Bu 16 mg/kg<br>Cy 200 mg/kg<br>Thiotepa | T cell depleted<br>PBSC | Alive fully engrafted |

Table is adapted from Lackner et al.[175] Abbreviations: mos = months; yrs = years; Cy = cyclophosphamide; Bu = busulfan; ATG = antithymocyte globulin; BM = bone marrow; UCB = umbilical cord blood; PBSC = peripheral blood stem cells; URD = unrelated donor transplant.

In conclusion, patients with congenital amegakaryocytic thrombocytopenia should be transplanted as soon as an acceptable donor is found prior to the development of platelet allosensitization, bleeding, or neutropenia-associated infection.

**Hematopoietic Stem Cell Transplantation: Donor Evaluation.** HLA-matched allogeneic donor selection should not present a problem, as it is unlikely those mild phenotypes exist within a family or that heterozygotes are in any way impaired. However, when UCB or a young bone marrow donor are contemplated, c-mpl gene mutation analysis is warranted.

# FUTURE PROSPECTIVES

Over the last decade the "cure" of inherited bone marrow failure syndromes utilizing HSCT has been accomplished, in large part, by the considerable reduction in morbidity and mortality associated with matched-related transplants. In addition, the availability of a variety of well-matched nonrelated stem cell sources has made alternative donor transplantation a viable option under certain circumstances. Furthermore, a comprehensive understanding of the biology and clinical manifestations of the inherited bone marrow failure syndromes has led to necessary improvements in donor selection and conditioning regimens. The outcome for HSCT undoubtedly will continue to improve. Modern molecular genetics and advances in reproductive biology present another opportunity. We anticipate the cloning of virtually all the genes responsible for the inherited bone marrow failure syndromes. Mutation analysis should allow for genotype-phenotype correlations that will better define prognosis and perhaps lead to effective non-HSCT treatment strategies. When mutation analysis is available for a particular syndrome it should be considered as part of the routine patient and donor evaluation.

The young age at diagnosis of the majority of cases of inherited bone marrow failure also permits reproductive strategies. Random genetic screening of couples for the majority of these disorders is currently impractical. This will no doubt change in the future. However, for young families who already have a child diagnosed, the opportunity to have a subsequent unaffected sibling is increasing as specific mutations for many of the inherited bone marrow failure syndromes are described. Preimplantation genetic diagnosis combined with in vitro fertilization provides the chance to have not only an unaffected child, but also one who is genetically selected to be an HLA-matched umbilical cord blood donor. At the time of this writing one case of a successful HSCT using umbilical cord blood stem cells from an HLA-matched, non-FA sibling conceived in this manner had been reported.[174] The ethical arguments surrounding preimplantation genetics[175] and a risk to benefit analysis of in vitro fertilization are complex and beyond the scope of this discussion. However, more and more, as transplanters, we will be asked to weigh in as parents inquire about this approach. Knowledge of pathophysiology, natural history, nontransplant treatment options, and outcomes as well as the epidemiology and genetics of this group of complex disorders is essential in order to guide affected families through the maze of available options.

Statements regarding nonmyeloablative hematopoietic stem cell transplantation must be issued with a caveat. That is, this approach is still considered experimental and rapidly evolving when applied in the context of the inherited bone marrow failure syndromes. The technique has been useful in the elderly and impaired who would not otherwise be transplant candidates. As mentioned earlier, Fanconi anemia, dyskeratosis congenita, and Shwachman Diamond syndrome demand modified conditioning regimens due to disorder-associated intolerance to traditional myeloablative approaches. It remains to be seen whether such a strategy will be advantageous in other bone marrow failure syndromes for which there is no incremental intolerance to myeloablative therapy. This is of special concern in Diamond Blackfan anemia, Kostmann syndrome, and amegakaryocytic thrombocytopenia where the establishment of mixed hematopoietic chimerism may not prevent or may even exacerbate the evolution to clonal hematopoietic disease.

Finally, for each of the inherited bone marrow failure syndromes discussed in this chapter there is a spectrum of hematologic as well as nonhematologic manifestations. This may be the consequence of nonallelic genes within a "family" being mutated as well as different allelic mutations. In addition, the clear demonstration of variable expressivity of these disorders within a particular genotype supports a role for interacting genes and environmental factors. It is likely that there are a number of patients diagnosed with acquired cytopenias for whom a genetic diagnosis would have been made if appropriately investigated. In some instances these cases could represent those with unexpected toxicity (recipient effect) or graft failure (donor effect). These possibilities must be investigated, as technology permits, in presumed cases of acquired bone marrow failure. The choice of nontransplant treatment options, conditioning regimens and donor selection may be influenced considerably. As well, allelic differences or even non-allelic polymorphisms may predict a predisposition to certain HSCT-related toxicities and, in the future, permit patient (genotype)-specific conditioning regimens.

# REFERENCES

1. Akashi K, Traver D, Miyamoto T, Weissman IL. A clonogenic common myeloid progenitor that gives rise to all myeloid lineages. Nature 2000;404:193–197.
2. Williams DA. Ex vivo expansion of hematopoietic stem and progenitor cells: robbing Peter to pay Paul. Blood 1993;81:3169–3172.
3. Orkin SO. Hematopoietic stem cells: Molecular diversification and developmental interrelations. In: Marshak DR, Gardner RL, Gottlieb D (eds). Stem Cell Biology. Cold Spring Harbor NY: Cold Spring Harbor Laboratory Press, 2001:289–306.
4. Lipton JM. The hematopoietic garden: How does it grow? J Pediatr 1998;132: 565–567.
5. Lipton JM, Nathan DG. Aplastic and hypoplastic anemia. Pediatr Clin North Am 1980;27:217–235.
6. Perdahl EB, Naprstek BL, Wallace WC, Lipton JM: Erythroid failure in Diamond-Blackfan anemia is characterized by apoptosis. Blood 1994;83:645–650.
7. Aprikyan AG, Liles WC, Person RE et al. Accelerated apoptosis of bone marrow progenitor cells in severe congenital neutropenia. Blood 1999;94:482a.
8. Dror Y, Freedman MH. Shwachman-Diamond syndrome marrow cells show abnormally increased apoptosis mediated through the Fas pathway. Blood 2001;97: 3011–3016.
9. Pang Q, Christianson TA, Keeble W et al. The anti-apoptotic function of Hsp70 in the interferon-inducible double-stranded RNA-dependent protein kinase-mediated death signaling pathway requires the Fanconi anemia protein, FANCC. J Biol Chem 2002;277:49638–49643.
10. Gluckman E, Devergie A, Dutreix J. Radiosensitivity in Fanconi anemia: Application to the conditioning regimen for bone marrow transplantation. Br J Haematol 1983;54:431–440.
11. Tsai PH, Sahdev I, Herry A, Lipton JM. Fatal cyclophosphamide induced congestive heart failure in a ten year-old boy with Shwachman Diamond syndrome and severe bone marrow failure treated with allogeneic bone marrow transplantation. Am J Pediatr Hematol Oncol 1990;12:472–476.
12. Dokal I. Dyskeratosis congenita in all its forms (Review). Br J Haematol 2000;110:768–779.
13. Botnick LE, Hannon EC, Hellman S. A long lasting proliferative defect in the hematopoietic stem cell compartment following cytotoxic agents. Int J Radiat Oncol Biol Phys 1979;5:1621–1625.
14. Deeg HJ, Storb R, Thomas ED et al. Fanconi's anemia treated by allogeneic marrow transplantation. Blood 1983;61:954–959.
15. Orfali KA, Wynn RF, Stevens RF et al. Failure of red cell production following allogenic BMT for Diamond Blackfan anemia (DBA) illustrates functional significance of high erythrocyte adenosine deaminase (eADA) activity in the donor. Blood 1999;94:414a.
16. Young NS, Alter BP. Aplastic Anemia Acquired and Inherited. Philadelphia: WB Saunders Co., 1994.
17. Fanconi G. Familiare infantile perniziosaartige anämie (perniziöses Blutbild und Konstitution). Jahrbuch Kinderheil 1927;117:257–280.
18. Giampietro PF, Adler-Brecher B, Verlander PC et al. The need for more accurate and timely diagnosis in Fanconi anemia: a report from the International Fanconi Anemia Registry. Pediatrics 1993;91:1116–1120.
19. Butturini A, Gale RP, Verlander PC et al. Hematologic abnormalities in Fanconi anemia: an International Fanconi Anemia Registry study. Blood 1994;84:1650–1655.
20. Kutler DI, Singh B, Satagopan J et al. A 20 year prospective of the International Fanconi Anemia Registry (IFAR). Blood 2003;101:1249–1256.
21. Rosenberg PS, Greene MH, Alter BP. Cancer incidence in persons with Fanconi anemia. Blood 2003;101:822–826.
22. Auerbach AD, Rogatko A, Schroeder-Kurth TM. International Fanconi Anemia Registry: Relation of clinical symptoms to diepoxybutane sensitivity. Blood 1989;73:391–396.
23. Arkin S, Brodtman D, Alter BP, Lipton JM. A screening test for Fanconi Anemia using flow cytometry. Blood 1993;82:10(Suppl 1):688.
24. Cassinat B, Guardiola P, Chevret S et al. Constitutive elevation of serum alpha-fetoprotein in Fanconi anemia. Blood 2000;96:859–863.
25. Alter B, Lipton J. Anemia, Fanconi. eMedicine Journal [serial online]. 2002. Available at: http://www.emedicine.com/ped/topic3022.htm.
26. Grompe M, D'Andrea A. Fanconi anemia and DNA repair. Hum Mol Genet 2001;10:2253–2259.
27. Joenje H, Patel KJ. The emerging genetic and molecular basis of Fanconi anaemia. Nat Rev Genet 2001;2:446–457.
28. Taniguchi T, D'Andrea AD. The Fanconi anemia protein, FANCE, promotes the nuclear accumulation of FANCC. Blood 2002;100:2457–2462.
29. Howlett NG, Taniguchi T, Olson S et al. Biallelic inactivation of BRCA2 in Fanconi anemia. Science 2002;297:606–609.
30. Grompe M. FANCD2: a branch-point in DNA damage response? Nat Med 2002;8:555–556.
31. Futaki M, Yamashita T, Yagasaki H et al. The IVS4 + 4 A to T mutation of the Fanconi anemia gene FANCC is not associated with a severe phenotype in Japanese patients. Blood 2000;95:1493–1498.

32. Faivre L, Guardiola P, Lewis C et al. Association of complementation group and mutation type with clinical outcome in Fanconi anemia. European Fanconi Anemia Research Group. Blood 2000;96:4064–4070.

33. Fanconi anemia. In: Standards for Clinical Care, Owen, J (ed). Eugene, OR: Fanconi Research Fund, Inc., 1999.

34. Gluckman E, Berger R, Dutreix J. Bone marrow transplantation for Fanconi anemia. Semin Hematol 1984;21:20–26.

35. Guardiola P, Socie G, Pasquini R et al. Allogeneic stem cell transplantation for Fanconi anaemia. Severe Aplastic Anaemia Working Party of the EBMT and EUFAR. European Group for Blood and Marrow Transplantation. Bone Marrow Transplant 1998;21(Suppl 2):S24–S27.

36. Kohli-Kumar M, Morris C, DeLaat C et al. Bone marrow transplantation in Fanconi anemia using matched sibling donors. Blood 1994;84:2050–2054.

37. Harris RE. Bone marrow transplantation for Fanconi Anemia. FA Family Newsletter Scientific 1994;(Suppl 17):2.

38. Davies SM, Khan S, Wagner JE et al. Unrelated donor bone marrow transplantation for Fanconi anemia. Bone Marrow Transplant 1996;17:43–47.

39. Guardiola PH, Pasquini R, Dokal I et al. Outcome of 69 allogeneic stem cell transplantation for Fanconi anemia using HLA-matched unrelated donors: a study on behalf of the European Group for Blood and Marrow Transplant. Blood 2000;95:422–429.

40. Kapelushnik J, Or R, Slavin S, Nagler A. A fludarabine-based protocol for bone marrow transplantation in Fanconi's anemia. Bone Marrow Transplant 1997;20:1109–1110.

41. Gluckman E, Auerbach AD, Horowitz MM et al. Bone marrow transplantation for Fanconi anemia. Blood 1995;86:2856–2862.

42. Miano M, Porta F, Locatelli F et al. Unrelated donor marrow transplantation for inborn errors. Bone Marrow Transplant 1998;21(Suppl 2):S37–S41.

43. Wagner JE, MacMillan M. Hematopoietic stem cell transplantation for the treatment of FA. 2002;Science Letter #32:5.

44. Marciniak, R Guarente L. Testing telomerase. Nature 2001;413:370–373.

45. Connor JM, Gatherer D, Gray FC. Assignment of the gene for dyskeratosis congenita to Xq28. Hum Genet 1986;72:348–351.

46. Heiss NS, Knight SW, Vulliamy TJ et al. X-linked dyskeratosis congenita is caused by mutations in a highly conserved gene with putative nucleolar function. Nat Genet 1998;19:32–38.

47. Vulliamy T, Marrone A, Goldman F et al. The RNA component of telomerase is mutated in autosomal dominant dyskeratosis congenita. Nature 2001;413:432–435.

48. Drachtman RA, Alter BP. Dyskeratosis congenita: clinical and genetic heterogeneity. Report of a new case and review of the literature. Am J Pediatr Hematol Oncol 1992;14:297–304.

49. Berthou C, Devergie A, D'Agay MF et al. Late vascular complications after bone marrow transplantation for dyskeratosis congenita. Br J Haematol 1991;79:335–336.

50. Mahmoud HK, Schaefer UW, Schmidt CG et al. Marrow transplantation for pancytopenia in dyskeratosis congenita. Blut 1985;51:57–60.

51. Conter V, Johnson FL, Paolucci P et al. Bone marrow transplantation for aplastic anemia associated with dyskeratosis congenita. Am J Pediatr Hematol Oncol 1988;10:99–102.

52. Rocha V, Devergie A, Socie G et al. Unusual complications after bone marrow transplantation for dyskeratosis congenita. Br J Haematol 1998;103:243–248.

53. Dokal I, Bungey J, Williamson P et al. Dyskeratosis congenita fibroblasts are abnormal and have unbalanced chromosomal rearrangements. Blood 1992;80:3090–3096.

54. Phillips B, Judge M, Webb D, Harper JI. Dyskeratosis congenita: delay in diagnosis and successful treatment of pancytopenia by bone marrow transplantation. Br J Dermatol 1992;127:278–280.

55. Chessells JM, Harper J. Bone marrow transplantation for dyskeratosis congenita. Br J Haematol 1992;81:314.

56. Langston AA, Sanders JE, Deeg HJ et al. Allogeneic marrow transplantation for aplastic anaemia associated with dyskeratosis congenita. Br J Haematol 1996;92:758–765.

57. Ling NS, Fenske NA, Julius RL et al. Dyskeratosis congenita in a girl simulating chronic graft-vs-host disease. Arch Dermatol 1985;121:1424–1428.

58. Storb R, Sanders JE, Pepe M et al. Graft-versus-host disease prophylaxis with methotrexate/cyclosporine in children with severe aplastic anemia treated with cyclophosphamide and HLA-identical marrow grafts. Blood 1991;78:1144–1145.

59. Yabe M, Yabe H, Hattori K et al. Fatal interstitial pulmonary disease in a patient with dyskeratosis congenita after allogeneic bone marrow transplantation. Bone Marrow Transplant 1997;19:389–392.

60. Ghavamzadeh A, Alimoghadam K, Nasseri P et al. Correction of bone marrow failure in dyskeratosis congenita by bone marrow transplantation. Bone Marrow Transplant 1999;23:299–301.

61. Bonfim CMS, Dokal I, de Medeiros CR et al. Allogeneic bone marrow transplantation (allo-BMT) for patients (pts) with dyskeratosis congenita (DC). Blood 2001;98:411a.

62. Lipton JM, Alter BP. Diamond Blackfan anemia. In: Clinical Disorders and Experimental Models of Erythropoietic Failure, Feig SA, Freedman MH (eds), Boca Raton: CRC Press Inc., 1993:39–67.
63. Lipton JM, Kudisch M, Gross R, Nathan DG. Defective erythroid progenitor differentiation system in congenital hypoplastic (Diamond-Blackfan) anemia. Blood 1986;67:963–968.
64. Tsai P, Arkin S, Lipton JM. An intrinsic progenitor defect in Diamond-Blackfan anaemia. Br J Haematol 1989;73:112–120.
65. Josephs HW. Anaemia of infancy and early childhood. Medicine 1936;15:307–402.
66. Diamond LK, Blackfan KD. Hypoplastic anemia. Am J Dis Child 1938;56:464–467.
67. Lipton JM, de Alarcon PA. Louis K. Diamond: an incomparable legacy. J Pediatr Hematol Oncol 2001; 23:371–372.
68. Alter BP. Modern review of congenital hypoplastic anemia. J Pediatr Hematol Oncol 2001;23:383–384.
69. Vlachos A, Alter B, Buchanan G et al. The Diamond Blackfan Anemia Registry (DBAR): preliminary data. Blood 1993;82:88a.
70. Vlachos A, Klein GW, Lipton JM. The Diamond Blackfan Anemia Registry: tool for investigating the epidemiology and biology of Diamond Blackfan anemia. J Pediatr Hematol Oncol 2001;23:377–382.
71. Lipton JM, Federman N, Khabbaze, Y et al. Osteogenic sarcoma associated with Diamond Blackfan anemia: a report from the Diamond Blackfan Anemia Registry. J Pediatr Hematol Oncol 2001;23:39–44.
72. Vlachos A, Federman N, Reyes-Haley C et al. Hematopoietic stem cell transplantation for Diamond Blackfan anemia: a report from the Diamond Blackfan Anemia Registry. Bone Marrow Transplant 2001;27:381–386.
73. Gustavsson P, Willig TN, van Haeringen A et al. Diamond-Blackfan anemia: genetic homogeneity for a gene on chromosome 19q13 restricted to 1.8 Mb. Nat Genet 1997;16:368–371.
74. Draptchinskaia N, Gustavsson P, Andersson B et al. The gene encoding ribosomal protein S19 is mutated in Diamond-Blackfan anemia. Nat Genet 1999;21:169–175.
75. Gazda H, Lipton JM, Willig TN et al. Evidence for linkage of familial Diamond-Blackfan anemia to chromosome 8p23.2-23.1 and non-19q non-8p familial disease. Blood 2001;97:2145–2150.
76. Gasser C. Aplastische anämie (chronische erythroblastophthise) und cortison. Schweiz Med Wochenschr 1951;81:1241–1242.
77. August CS, King E, Githens JH et al. Establishment of erythropoiesis following bone marrow transplantation in a patient with congenital hypoplastic anemia (Diamond-Blackfan syndrome). Blood 1976;48:491–498.
78. Iriondo A, Garijo J, Baro J et al. Complete recovery of hemopoiesis following bone marrow transplant in a patient with unresponsive congenital hypoplastic anemia (Blackfan-Diamond syndrome). Blood 1984;64:348–351.
79. Ash RC, Montgomery T, Moreno H et al. Cure of steroid-refractory congenital hypoplastic anemia. Clin Res 1985;33:334a.
80. Wiktor-Jedrzejczak W, Szczylik C, Pojda Z et al. Success of bone marrow transplantation in congenital Diamond-Blackfan anaemia: a case report. Eur J Haematol 1987;38:204–206.
81. Lenarsky C, Weinberg K, Guinan E et al. Bone marrow transplantation for constitutional pure red cell aplasia. Blood 1988;71:226–229.
82. Gluckman E, Esperou H, Devergie A et al. Pediatric bone marrow transplantation for leukemia and aplastic anemia. Nouv Rev Fr Hematol 1989;31:111–114.
83. Skimada M, Mushigama H, Hara M. Complete recovery of hemopoiesis following bone marrow transplantation in a patient with unresponsive congenital pure red cell anemia. Jpn J Pediatr Hematol 1989;3:276–382.
84. Zintl F, Hermann J, Fuchs D et al. Korrektur lethal verlaufender genetischer erkrankungen mit hilfe der knochenmarktransplantation. Kinderarztl Prax 1991;59:10–15.
85. Mori PG, Haupt R, Fugazza G et al. Pentasomy 21 in leukemia complicating Diamond-Blackfan anemia. Cancer Genet Cytogenet 1992;63:70–72.
86. Saunders EF, Olivieri N, Freedman MH. Unexpected complications after bone marrow transplantation in transfusion-dependent children. Bone Marrow Transplant 1993;12:88–90.
87. Greinix HT, Storb R, Sanders JE et al. Long-term survival and cure after marrow transplantation for congenital hypoplastic anaemia (Diamond-Blackfan syndrome). Br J Haematol 1993;84:515–520.
88. Seip M. Malignant tumors in two patients with Diamond-Blackfan anemia treated with corticosteroids and androgens. Pediatr Hematol Oncol 1994;11:423–426.
89. Lee AC, Ha SY, Yuen KY, Lau YL. Listeria septicemia complicating bone marrow transplantation for Diamond-Blackfan syndrome. Pediatr Hematol Oncol 1995;12:295–299.
90. Mugishima H, Gale RP, Rowlings PA et al. Bone marrow transplantation for Diamond-Blackfan anemia. Bone Marrow Transplant 1995;15:55–58.
91. Van Dijken PJ, Verwijs W. Diamond-Blackfan anemia and malignancy. Cancer 1995;76:517–520.
92. Wagner JE, Rosenthal J, Sweetman R et al. Successful transplantation of HLA-mismatched umbilical cord blood from unrelated donors: analysis of engraftment and acute graft-versus-host disease. Blood 1996;88:795–802.

93. Bonno M, Azuma E, Nakano T et al. Successful hematopoietic reconstitution by transplantation of umbilical cord blood cells in a transfusion-dependent child with Diamond-Blackfan anemia. Bone Marrow Transplant 1997;19:83–85.

94. Vettenranta K, Saarinen UM. Cord blood stem cell transplantation for Diamond Blackfan anemia. Bone Marrow Transplant 1997;19:507–508.

95. Willig T-N, Niemeyer C, Leblanc T et al. Identification of new prognosis factors from the clinical and epidemiologic analysis of a registry of 229 Diamond-Blackfan anemia patients. Pediatr Res 1999;46:553–561.

96. Alter BP. Bone marrow transplant in Diamond-Blackfan anemia (letter). Bone Marrow Transplant 1998;21:965.

97. Dianzani I, Garelli E, Ramenghi U. Diamond Blackfan anemia: a congenital defect in erythropoiesis. Haematologica 1996;81:560–572.

98. Taylor CM, Sharma S, Calderwood S, Olivieri NF. Development of neutropenia, thrombocytopenia, and severe aplastic anemia in patients with Diamond-Blackfan anemia (DBA). Blood 1998;92(Suppl 1):156a.

99. Willig TN, Pérignon JL, Gustavsson P et al. High adenosine deaminase level among healthy probands of Diamond-Blackfan anemia (DBA) cosegregates with the DBA gene region on chromosome 19q13. Blood 1998;92:4422–4427.

100. Deeg HJ, Socie G, Schoch R et al. Malignancies after marrow transplantation for aplastic anemia and Fanconi anemia: a joint Seattle and Paris analysis of results in 700 patients. Blood 1996;87:386–392.

101. Niemeyer CM, Baumgarten E, Holldack J et al. Treatment trial with recombinant human erythropoietin in children with congenital hypoplastic anemia. In: Erythropoietin in Renal and Non-Renal Anemias, Gurland HJ, Moran J, Samtleben W, Scigalla P, Wieczorek L (eds). Basel: Karger 1991;88:276–280.

102. Sumimoto S-I, Kawai M, Kasajima Y, Hamamoto T. Intravenous γ-globulin therapy in Diamond-Blackfan anemia. Acta Paediatr Jpn 1992;34:179–180.

103. Bernini JC, Carillo JM, Buchanan GR. High-dose methylprednisone therapy for patients with Diamond-Blackfan anemia refractory to conventional doses of prednisone. J Pediatr 1995;127:654–659.

104. Alessandri AJ, Rogers PC, Wadsworth LD, Davis JH. Diamond-Blackfan anemia and cyclosporine therapy revisited. J Pediatr Hematol Oncol 2000;22:176–179.

105. Gillio AP, Faulkner LB, Alter BP et al. Treatment of Diamond-Blackfan Anemia with recombinant human interleukin-3. Blood 1993;82:744–751.

106. Abkowitz JL, Schaison G, Boulad F et al. Response of Diamond-Blackfan anemia to metoclopramide: evidence for a role for prolactin in erythropoiesis. Blood 2002;100:2687–2691.

107. Freedman MH, Bonilla MA, Fier C et al. Myelodysplastic syndrome and acute myeloid leukemia in patients with congenital neutropenia receiving G-CSF therapy. Blood 2000;96:429–436.

108. Dale DC. Introduction: severe chronic neutropenia. Semin Hematol 2002;39:73–74.

109. Dale DC, Person RE, Bolyard AA et al. Mutations in the gene encoding neutrophil elastase in congenital and cyclic neutropenia. Blood 2000;96:2317–2322.

110. Berliner N. Molecular biology of neutrophil differentiation. Curr Opin Hematol 1998;5:49–53.

111. Zeidler C, Welte K. Kostmann syndrome and severe congenital neutropenia. Semin Hematol 2002;39:82–88.

112. Kostmann R. Infantile genetic agranulocytosis. Acta Pediatr Scand 1956;45:1–78.

113. Horwitz M, Benson K, Person R et al. Mutations in ELA2 encoding neutrophil elastase, define a 21 day biological clock in cyclic haematopoiesis. Nat Genet 1999;23:433–436.

114. Dale DC, Bonilla MA, Davis MW et al. A randomized controlled phase III trial of recombinant human granulocyte colony-stimulating factor (filgrastim) for treatment of severe chronic neutropenia. Blood 1993; 81:2496–2502.

115. Zeidler C, Boxer L, Dale DC et al. Management of Kostmann syndrome in the G-CSF era. Br J Haematol 2000;109:490–495.

116. Cottle TE, Fier CJ, Donadieu J, Kinsey SE. Risk and benefit of treatment of severe chronic neutropenia with granulocyte colony-stimulating factor. Semin Hematol 2002;39:134–140.

117. Freedman MH, Alter BP. Risk of myelodysplastic syndrome and acute myeloid leukemia in congenital neutropenia. Semin Hematol 2002;39:128–133.

118. Rappeport JM, Parkman R, Newburger P et al. Correction of infantile agranulocytosis (Kostmann's syndrome) by allogeneic bone marrow transplantation. Am J Med 1980;68:605–609.

119. Zeidler C, Welte K, Barak Y et al. Stem cell transplantation in patients with severe congenital neutropenia without evidence of leukemic transformation. Blood 2000;95:1195–1198.

120. Dong F, Brynes RK, Tidow N et al. Mutations in the gene for granulocyte colony-stimulating-factor receptor in patients with acute myeloid leukemia preceded by severe congenital neutropenia. N Engl J Med 1995; 333:487–493.

121. Tschan CA, Pilz C, Zeidler C et al. Time course of increasing numbers of mutations in the granulocyte colony-stimulating factor receptor gene in a patient with congenital neutropenia who developed leukemia. Blood 2001;97:1882–1884.

122. Shwachman H, Diamond LK, Oski FA, Khaw K-T. The syndrome of pancreatic insufficiency and bone marrow dysfunction. J Pediatr 1964;65:645–663.

123. Bodian M, Sheldon W, Lightwood R. Congenital hypoplasia of the exocrine pancreas. Acta Paediatr 1964;53:282–293.
124. Ip WF, Dupuis A, Ellis L et al. Serum pancreatic enzymes define the pancreatic phenotype in patients with Shwachman-Diamond syndrome. J Pediatr 2002;141:259–265.
125. Dror Y, Freedman MH. Shwachman-Diamond syndrome. Br J Haematol 2002;118:701–713.
126. Dror Y, Ginzberg H, Dalal I et al. Immune function in patients with Shwachman-Diamond syndrome. Br J Haematol 2001;114:712–717.
127. Rothbaum R, Perrault J, Vlachos A et al. Diamond syndrome: report from an international conference. J Pediatr 2002;141:266–270.
128. Saunders EF, Gall G, Freedman H. Granulopoiesis in Shwachman's syndrome (pancreatic insufficiency and bone marrow dysfunction). Pediatrics 1979;64:515–519.
129. Woods WG, Krivit W, Lubin BH, Ramsay NKC. Aplastic anemia associated with Shwachman syndrome. In vivo and in vitro observations. Am J Pediatr Hematol Oncol 1981;3:347–351.
130. Suda T, Mizoguchi H, Miura Y et al. Hemopoietic colony-forming cells in Shwachman's syndrome. Am J Pediatr Hematol Oncol 1982;4:129–133.
131. Dror Y, Freedman MH. Shwachman-Diamond syndrome: an inherited preleukemic bone marrow failure disorder with aberrant hematopoietic progenitors and faulty microenvironment. Blood 1999;94:3048–3054.
132. Thornley I, Dror Y, Sung L et al. Telomere shortening in leukocytes of children with Shwachman-Diamond syndrome. Br J Haematol 2002;117:189–192.
133. Seymour JF, Escudier SM. Acute leukemia complicating bone marrow hypoplasia in an adult with Shwachman's syndrome. Leuk Lymphoma 1993;12:131–135.
134. Aggett PJ, Cavanagh NPC, Matthew DJ et al. Shwachman's syndrome. A review of 21 cases. Arch Dis Child 1980;55:331–347.
135. Smith OP, Hann IM, Chessells JM et al. Haematological abnormalities in Shwachman-Diamond syndrome. Br J Haematol 1996;94:279–284.
136. Mack DR, Forstner GG, Wilschanski M et al. Shwachman syndrome: exocrine pancreatic dysfunction and variable phenotypic expression. Gastroenterology 1996;111:1593–1602.
137. Ginzberg H, Shin J, Ellis L et al. Shwachman syndrome: phenotypic manifestations of sibling sets and isolated cases in a large patient cohort are similar. J Pediatr 1999;135:81–88.
138. Smith A, Shaw PJ, Webster B et al. Intermittent 20q- and consistent i(7q) in a patient with Shwachman-Diamond syndrome. Pediatr Hematol Oncol 2002;19:525–528.
139. Dror Y, Durie P, Ginzberg H et al. Clonal evolution in marrows of patients with Shwachman-Diamond syndrome: a prospective 5-year follow-up study. Exp Hematol 2002;30:659–666.
140. Goobie S, Popovic M, Morrison J et al. Shwachman-Diamond syndrome with exocrine pancreatic dysfunction and bone marrow failure maps to the centromeric region of chromosome 7. Am J Hum Genet 2001;68:1048–1054.
141. Boocock GR, Morrison JA, Popovic M et al. Mutations in SBDS are associated with Shwachman-Diamond syndrome. Nat Genet 2003;33:97–101.
142. Tsai PH, Sahdev I, Herry A, Lipton JM. Fatal cyclophosphamide induced congestive heart failure in a ten year-old boy with Shwachman Diamond syndrome and severe bone marrow failure treated with allogeneic bone marrow transplantation. Am J Pediatr Hematol Oncol 1990;12:472–476.
143. Barrios N, Kirkpatrick D, Regueira O et al. Bone marrow transplant in Shwachman Diamond syndrome. Br J Haematol 1991;79:337–338.
144. Seymour JF, Escudier SM. Acute leukemia complicating bone marrow hypoplasia in an adult with Shwachman's syndrome. Leuk Lymphoma 1993;12:131–135.
145. Smith OP, Chan MY, Evans J, Veys P. Shwachman-Diamond syndrome and matched unrelated donor BMT. Bone Marrow Transplant 1995;16:717–718.
146. Arseniev L, Diedrich H, Link H. Allogeneic bone marrow transplantation in a patient with Shwachman-Diamond syndrome. Ann Hematol 1996;72:83–84.
147. Bunin N, Leahey A, Dunn S. Related donor liver transplant for veno-occlusive disease following T-depleted unrelated donor bone marrow transplantation. Transplantation 1996;61:664–666.
148. Davies SM, Wagner JE, Defor T et al. Unrelated donor bone marrow transplantation for children and adolescents with aplastic anaemia or myelodysplasia. Br J Haematol 1997;96:749–756.
149. Dokal I, Rule S, Chen F et al. Adult onset of acute myeloid leukaemia (M6) in patients with Shwachman-Diamond syndrome. Br J Haematol 1997;99:171–173.
150. Okcu F, Roberts WM, Chan KW. Bone marrow transplantation in Shwachman-Diamond syndrome: report of two cases and review of the literature. Bone Marrow Transplant 1998;21:849–851.
151. Faber J, Lauener R, Wick F et al. Shwachman-Diamond syndrome: early bone marrow transplantation in a high risk patient and new clues to pathogenesis. Eur J Pediatr 1999;158:995–1000.
152. Cesaro S, Guariso G, Calore E et al. Successful unrelated bone marrow transplantation for Shwachman-Diamond syndrome. Bone Marrow Transplant 2001;27:97–99.

153. Ritchie DS, Angus PW, Bhathal PS, Grigg AP. Liver failure complicating non-alcoholic steatohepatitis following allogeneic bone marrow transplantation for Shwachman-Diamond syndrome. Bone Marrow Transplant 2002;29:931–933.
154. Hsu JW, Vogelsang G, Jones RJ et al. Bone marrow transplantation in Shwachman-Diamond syndrome. Bone Marrow Transplant 2002;30:255–258.
155. Park SY, Chae MB, Kwack YG et al. Allogeneic bone marrow transplantation in Shwachman-Diamond syndrome with malignant myeloid transformation. A case report. Korean J Intern Med 2002;17:204–206.
156. Fleitz J, Rumelhart S, Goldman F et al. Successful allogeneic hematopoietic stem cell transplantation (HSCT) for Shwachman-Diamond syndrome. Bone Marrow Transplant 2002;29:75–79.
157. Alter BP, Young NS. The bone marrow failure syndromes. Nathan and Oski's Hematology of Infancy and Childhood. In: Nathan DG, Orkin SH (eds). Philadelphia PA: WB Saunders, 1998:281–282.
158. Ihara K, Ishii E, Eguchi M et al. Identification of mutations in the c-mpl gene in congenital amegakaryocytic thrombocytopenia. Proc Natl Acad Sci U S A 1999;96:3132–3136.
159. Hedberg VA, Lipton JM. Thrombocytopenia with absent radii: a review of 100 cases. Am J Pediatr Hematol Oncol 1988;10:51–64.
160. Brochstein JA, Shank B, Kernan NA et al. Marrow transplantation for thrombocytopenia-absent radii syndrome. J Pediatr 1992;121:587–589.
161. Ballmaier M, Germeshausen M, Schulze H et al. c-mpl mutations as the cause of congenital amegakaryocytic thrombocytopenia. Blood 2001;97:139–146.
162. Van den Oudenrijn S, Bruin M, Folman CC et al. Mutations in the thrombopoietin receptor gene (c-mpl) in patients with congenital amegakaryocytic thrombocytopenia. Br J Haematol 2000;110:441–448.
163. Tonelli R, Scardovi AL, Pession A et al. Compound heterozygosity for two different amino-acid substitution mutations in the thrombopoietin receptor (c-mpl gene) in congenital amegakaryocytic thrombocytopenia (CAMT). Hum Genet 2000;107:225–233.
164. Guinan EC, Lee YS, Lopez KD et al. Effects of interleukin-3 and granulocyte-macrophage colony-stimulating factor on thrombopoiesis in congenital amegakaryocytic thrombocytopenia. Blood 1993;81:1691–1698.
165. Gillio AP, Gabrilove JL. Cytokine treatment of inherited bone marrow failure syndromes. Blood 1993;81:1669–1674.
166. Henter JI, Winiarski J, Ljungman P et al. Bone marrow transplantation in two children with congenital amegakaryocytic thrombocytopenia. Bone Marrow Transplant 1995;15:799–801.
167. Hill W. Successful treatment of amegakaryocytic thrombocytopenic purpura with cyclosporine. N Engl J Med 1985;312:1060–1061.
168. Columbyova L, Loda M, Scadden DT. Thrombopoietin receptor expression in human cancer cell lines and primary tissues. Cancer Res 1995;55:3509–3512.
169. MacMillan ML, Davies SM, Wagner JE, Ramsay NK. Engraftment of unrelated donor stem cells in children with familial amegakaryocytic thrombocytopenia. Bone Marrow Transplant 1998;21:735–737.
170. deVries DS, Bruin MC, Bierings M, Revesz T. Congenital amegakaryocytic thrombocytopenia: indication for allogenic stem cell transplantation. Ned Tijdschr Geneeskd 2000;144:1596–1598.
171. Yesilipek MA, Hazar V, Kupesiz A, Yegin O. Peripheral stem cell transplantation in a child with amegakaryocytic thrombocytopenia. Bone Marrow Transplant 2000;26:571–572.
172. Kudo K, Kato K, Matsuyama T, Kojina S. Successful engraftment of unrelated donor stem cells in two children with congenital amegakaryocytic thrombocytopenia. J Pediatr Hematol Oncol 2002;24:79–80.
173. Lackner A, Basu O, Bierings M et al. Haematopoietic stem cell transplantation for amegakaryocytic thrombocytopenia. Br J Haematol 2000;109:773–775.
174. Verlinsky Y, Rechitsky S, Schoolcraft W et al. Preimplantation diagnosis for Fanconi anemia combined with HLA matching. JAMA 2001;285:3130–3133.
175. Joffe S. The expanding indications for preimplantation genetic diagnosis. Oncol Spectrums 2001;2:696–687.

# PART *IV*

# SPECIAL PROCEDURES

# CHAPTER XVIII

# Immune Ablative (Mini) Transplants in Pediatrics

MORRIS KLETZEL

How can a procedure be defined that has multiple names that include "mini" transplant, transplant "lite," "immune" ablative transplant, reduced intensity transplant, nonmyeloablative transplant, and others. To start, there is nothing mini about this approach to transplantation; one may argue that the toxicity of this type of transplant is reduced up front, but there are delayed toxicities that may be as hard to manage as the traditional complications such as vasooclusive disease (VOD), infection, etc. A good way to define this transplant technology is to establish a balance between donor factors and recipient factors in order to achieve a chimerical engraftment (▼ Figure 18.1). On one hand, this means suppressing the immune system of the recipient and, on the other, giving enough immune competent cells from the donor to achieve engraftment. This will represent a zero balance. Since there are no accepted parameters to achieve a zero balance, either the ablation has to be modified (reduce intensity) or the graft modified (selective T cell-depletion; ▼ Figure 18.2). The main purposes of this approach are to decrease acute toxicity, achieve engraftment, minimize the risk of acute and chronic graft-versus-host disease (GVHD), and produce a biological effect of graft-versus-tumor. In this chapter, this approach to transplantation will be referred to as immune ablative.

The combination of high dose chemotherapy and total body irradiation (TBI) followed by bone marrow infusion from a compatible donor has been in use for the past 40 years for the treatment of hematopoietic diseases.[1-5] Recently, studies evaluating the use of combination chemotherapy without TBI report similar results.[6] Engraftment post-marrow infusion occurs in three to four weeks and leads to hematological normalization in three to four months. Bone marrow transplantation has proven to be an effective treatment for some patients with acute or chronic leukemia and nonmalignant diseases. The International Bone Marrow Transplant Registry (IBMTR) results in patients with leukemia show leukemia-free survival as follows: acute lymphoblastic leukemia (ALL) first complete remission (CR) 48 ± 7%; ALL complete second remission (CR2) 43 ± 4%; leukemia in relapse approximately 15%; acute nonlymphoblastic leukemia (ANLL) in relapse 15 + 7%; chronic myelogenous leukemia (CML) in chronic phase approximately 80%. The IBMTR also has reported that bone marrow transplantation (BMT) is a successful modality for the treatment of aplastic anemia with best results in the younger age group.[7] Santos and Tutschka[6] have successfully explored high dose chemotherapy without TBI as a conditioning regimen for allogeneic

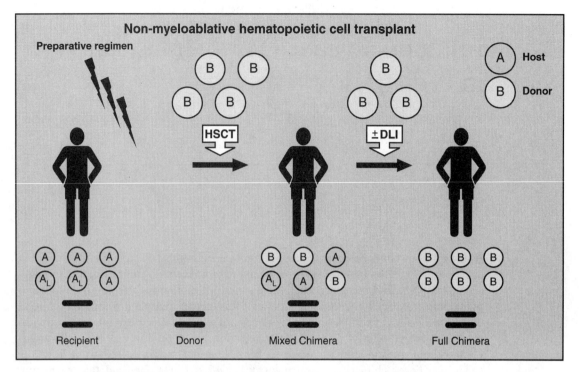

**FIGURE 18.1** Schematic view of how an immune ablative transplant is done, where A represents the host cell and B is the donor cell.

Abbreviations: HSCT = hematopoietic stem cell transplantation; DLI = donor lymphocyte infusion. At the bottom, the molecular transition with variable number tandem repeats (VNTR) can be seen.

BMT. They investigated the combination of busulfan/cytoxan in patients with acute and chronic leukemia who achieved full hematopoietic engraftment and complete remissions. They initially observed significant toxicity that was minimized by reduction of the cytoxan dose, as previously evaluated by Yeager et al.[8] at Johns Hopkins in allogeneic recipients. Since the distribution and serum levels of busulfan in children are lower than in adults, the tolerated dose in children may be higher than in adults and should be calculated on the basis of surface area.[9] In these studies there was a high incidence of relapse posttransplant. This may be due, in part, to suboptimal levels of busulfan. One of the main concerns with these approaches is the peritransplant morbidity and mortality that in some situations may be as high as 40%. The use of immune-ablative regimens may be an alternative to the high morbidity and mortality.

Allogeneic BMT has curative potential in several hematologic malignancies. However, the toxicity of standard BMT techniques limits the approach to younger patients in otherwise good health. Thus, older patients and younger patients with comorbid illnesses or organ dysfunction are not offered potentially curative therapy. It is important to emphasize that even in otherwise healthy young patients, the treatment-related mortality of allogeneic BMT is high.

## Engraftment

| Graft | Host |
|---|---|
| • Stem cell dose | • Immunosuppression |
| • T-cell dose (CD8) | • Preparative regimen |
| • Graft-facilitating cells | • Posttransplant Rx |
| • Stromal stem cells? | • Disease effects |
| | • Sensitization |

## Histocompatibility

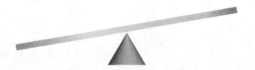

**FIGURE 18.2** Balance that must be achieved for the optimal immune ablative transplant. With reduced immunosuppression in current (NST) regimens, we rely on graft cells (stem T cells and accessory cells) to overcome rejection.

Many observations suggest that much of the curative potential of allogeneic BMT for malignant disease derives from an anti-tumor effect of donor immune cells. It may be possible to purposefully harness this effect by discontinuing immunosuppression after donor cell engraftment has occurred, or by infusing additional immune cells without the cover of immunosuppression.

Allogeneic peripheral blood stem cells may lessen the toxicity of allogeneic transplantation by leading to faster engraftment. In addition, the greater number of stem cells in a peripheral blood stem cell transplant may increase the likelihood of engraftment.

Based on these observations, several groups have begun to investigate new preparative regimens that are much less toxic than traditional transplant regimens, but are nevertheless immunosuppressive enough to allow donor cell engraftment;[10] allogeneic peripheral blood stem cells are given to increase the likelihood of engraftment. Engrafted donor immune cells may eliminate residual tumor cells; if tumor persists, then graft-versus-tumor activity may be enhanced by stopping immunosuppression or by giving additional donor immune cells. The differences between a traditional and an immune ablative transplant are shown in ▼ Table 18.1.

Many of these new preparative regimens are based on nucleoside analogs (especially fludarabine), which have pronounced toxicity for T cells.[10] Other particularly immunosuppressive agents include TBI, cyclophosphamide, and anti-T cell antibodies.

## ANIMAL EXPERIENCE

A major question is whether it will be possible to achieve engraftment following sublethal preparatory regimens in patients whose treatment does not require exposure to supralethal doses of chemotherapy or radiation. This was investigated by Reisner and Martinelli[11] in

| TABLE 18.1 | Differences Between Immune Ablative and Traditional Transplants |
|---|---|
| **Traditional** | **Immune ablative** |
| High doses of chemotherapy and TBI | Lower doses of chemotherapy and TBI |
| Standard cell doses | High doses of cells |
| Intense GVHD prophylaxis | Minimal GVHD prophylaxis |
| Inpatient hospital care | Outpatient care |
| High transplant-related toxicity | Minimal transplant-related toxicity |
| Increased risk of GVHD | Decreased risk of GVHD |
| Rapid engraftment pattern | Slower engraftment |
| Engraftment evaluation by return of counts | Engraftment evaluation of assessment of chimerism |

Abbreviations: TBI = total body irradiation; GVHD = graft-verses-host disease.

the mouse model, where different groups of C3H/HeJ mice were conditioned by a single dose of TBI in the range of 5.5–8.5 Gy and then transplanted with increasing doses of T cell-depleted bone marrow from C57BL/6 donors. The donor type chimerism was determined one month posttransplant. As expected, the results of this study revealed that engraftment was most effective in mice that were conditioned with 8.5 Gy and required a cell dose of $10 \times 10^6$ cells. Donor cell chimerism also could be generated with the lower doses of TBI as long as the cell dose was increased by two- to fourfold or 20-fold.[11]

Storb and Yu[12,13] have developed a nonmyeloablative regimen consisting of a single fraction of TBI 2 Gy delivered at 7 cGy/min in a dog model of dog leukocyte antigen (DLA)-identical transplantation. These investigators found that a nonmyeloablative dose of TBI of 2 Gy was capable of allowing engraftment of donor marrow, provided the recipient received an immunosuppressive regimen of cyclosporine and mycophenolate mofetil (MMF), a combination other studies had shown to have immunosuppressive properties superior to the standard regimen of cyclosporine and methotrexate. The combination of cyclosporine and MMF was intended not only to prevent GVHD, but also to suppress host lymphocytes capable of mediating rejection, which had survived TBI. This combination of low dose TBI and posttransplant cyclosporine/MMF led to stable engraftment-mixed chimeras in 10 of 11 dogs.

# HUMAN EXPERIENCE

## Adults

Giralt et al.[10] reported a nonmyeloablative transplant regimen in fifteen patients [13 with acute myeloid leukemia and 2 with myelodisplastic syndrome (MDS)] who were not candidates for conventional myeloablative therapy because of older age or organ dysfunction.[10] All patients had a human lymphocyte antigen (HLA)-identical or one-antigen mismatched related donor. The median age was 59 years (range 27–71 years). Twelve patients were either refractory to therapy or beyond first relapse. Eight patients received fludarabine at 30 mg/m$^2$/d for four days with idarubicin at 12 mg/m$^2$/d for three days and ara-C at 2 g/m$^2$/d for four days ($N = 7$) or melphalan at 140 mg/m$^2$/d ($N = 1$). Seven patients received 2-chloro-deoxyadenosine at 12 mg/m$^2$/d for five days and ara-C at 1 g/m$^2$/d for five days. Thirteen patients received allogeneic peripheral blood stem cells and 1 received bone marrow after chemotherapy. GVHD prophylaxis consisted of cyclosporine and methylprednisolone. Treatment was generally well tolerated, with only one death from multiorgan failure before receiving stem cells. Thirteen patients achieved a neutrophil count of greater than 0.5 × 10$^9$/L, a median of ten days postinfusion (range 8–17 days). Ten patients achieved platelet counts of 20 × 10$^9$/L a median of 13 days after progenitor cell infusion (range 7–78 days). Eight patients achieved complete remissions (bone marrow blasts were <5% with neutrophil recovery and platelet transfusion independence) that lasted a median of 60 days posttransplantation (range, 34 to 170+ days). Acute GVHD grade ≥2 occurred in three patients. Chimerism analysis of bone marrow cells in six of eight patients achieving remission showed >90% donor cells between 14 and 30 days postinfusion, and three of four patients remaining in remission between 60 and 90 days continued to have >80% donor cells. The conclusion of this study was that this nonmyeloablative transplant approach was well tolerated and resulted in a high incidence of donor cell engraftment. However, overall survival was poor in this very high risk group of patients, the majority of whom had either advanced and refractory leukemia or active infection at the time of transplant; further studies were deemed warranted in a better risk group of patients.

Khouri et al.[14] reported 15 non-Hodgkin's lymphoma (NHL) and chronic lymphocytic leukemia (CLL) patients treated with fludarabine-based preparative regimens. Six patients were in advanced refractory relapse and induction therapy had failed in two patients. Patients with CLL or low-grade lymphoma received fludarabine 90 to 150 mg/m$^2$ and cyclophosphamide 900–2,000 mg/m$^2$. Patients with intermediate high-grade lymphoma or Richter's transformation received cisplatin 25 mg/m$^2$ daily for four days, fludarabine 30 mg/m$^2$, and cytarabine 500 mg/m$^2$ daily for two days. Chemotherapy was followed by allogeneic stem cell infusion from HLA-identical siblings. Patients with residual malignant cells or mixed chimeras could receive a donor lymphocyte infusion of 0.5 to 2 × 10$^8$ mononuclear cells/kg two to three months posttransplantation if graft-versus-host disease was not present.

Eleven patients had engraftment of donor cells, and the remaining four patients promptly recovered autologous hematopoiesis. Eight of 11 patients achieved a complete response. Five of six patients (83.3%) with chemosensitive disease continue to be alive compared with two of nine patients (22.2%) who had refractory or untested disease at the time of study entry ($P = .04$). Additional dose-finding studies by this group have led to the adoption of a regimen that employs fludarabine at 30 mg/m$^2$ daily for three doses and cyclophosphamide at 750 mg/m$^2$ daily for three doses.

Slavin et al.[15] reported 26 patients with acute leukemia ($N = 10$), chronic leukemia ($N = 8$), NHL ($N = 2$), MDS ($N = 1$), multiple myeloma ($N = 1$), and genetic disease ($N = 4$) who were treated with allogeneic peripheral blood stem cell (PBSC) transplantation following a preparative regimen consisting of fludarabine, antithymocyte globulin

(ATG), and low dose busulfan. Patients received cyclosporine alone as GVHD prophylaxis. The regimen was well tolerated with no severe regimen-related toxicity. Donor cells engrafted, resulting in stable partial ($N = 9$) or complete ($N = 17$) chimeras. In nine patients the absolute neutrophil count (ANC) did not decrease to below $0.1 \times 10^9/L$, whereas two patients never experienced ANC $< 0.5 \times 10^9/L$. ANC of $0.5 \times 10^9/L$ was accomplished within 10 to 32 (median, 15) days. Platelet counts did not decrease to below $20 \times 10^9/L$ with four patients requiring no platelet support at all; overall platelet counts $> 20 \times 10^9/L$ were achieved within 0 to 35 (median, 12) days. Fourteen patients experienced no GVHD at all; severe GVHD (grades 3 and 4) was the single major complication and the cause of death in four patients, occurring after early discontinuation of cyclosporine A. Relapse was reversed by infusion of donor lymphocytes in two of three cases. With a median follow-up of eight months, 22 of 26 patients (85%) were alive and 21(81%) were disease free. The actuarial probability of survival at 14 months was 77.5% (95% confidence interval 53%–90%).

Childs et al.[16] reported 11 patients with malignant diseases treated with cyclophosphamide (120 mg/kg) and fludarabine (125 mg/m$^2$) followed by allogeneic PBSC transplantation. Cyclosporine was given for GVHD prophylaxis and tapered beginning at day 30 to produce a graft-versus-malignancy effect. All patients had evidence of donor engraftment at the time of neutrophil recovery, but one patient had late rejection with autologous hematopoietic recovery. Four patients developed grade II–III acute GVHD, while none developed chronic GVHD. Of five patients with hematologic malignancies, three had complete remission and one had a partial remission. One of two renal cell carcinoma patients had complete remission and one of four melanoma patients had evidence of tumor regression.

Storb[13] then tested the approach in a series of patients with genetic diseases and hematologic malignancies. Eight patients were recently reported. Diseases included patients with CLL,[2] MDS,[2] AML,[2] and myeloma.[2] Patients received 2 Gy of TBI with cyclosporine given orally from day $-1$ to day 35, and MMF given orally from day 0 to day 27. Granulocyte colony-stimulating factor (G-CSF) mobilized PBSCs from HLA-identical donors were infused on day 0. Of the first five patients with adequate follow-up, four were treated in the outpatient setting. Posttransplant myelosuppression was generally very mild. All patients had engraftment of donor T cells, with the percent chimeras ranging from 15% to 100% at day 28 and 5% to 100% at day 56. Four patients with persistent malignancy received donor lymphocyte infusion (DLI) at a cell dose of 10$^7$ CD3 positive cells per kilogram, followed by grade II acute GVHD in two. DLI was followed by a complete disease response in two patients. Stable hematopoietic cell engraftment occurred in two patients; however, two patients rejected the graft and the underlying malignancy in two patients relapsed. Additional patients have been treated by Storb et al.:[13] 6 of 43 patients have rejected their grafts including two of six myeloma patients and two of five CML patients.

Thus, several nonmyeloablative preparative regimens have been developed that allow engraftment of donor cells in a significant percentage of patients. Achievement of mixed chimeras can then serve as the platform for additional immunologic maneuvers aimed at eradicating residual tumor cells. Each of the preparative regimens reported has its relative pros and cons. The regimens of Giralt, Kouri, and Slavin are moderately intensive and associated with several days of posttransplant cytopenias; additional significant toxicities have been observed, including venoocclusive disease of the liver. The appeal of the regimen of

Storb et al. is its minimal toxicity; however, rejections were observed in several patients, suggesting that additional immunosuppressive agents may need to be added to the single dose of TBI. An ideal drug might be fludarabine, which in standard doses is associated with only modest myelotoxicity, but has pronounced immunosuppressive activity.

## Pediatrics

There are no specific publications with this technique in pediatric patients. Some pediatric patients are reported in the large adult series in ▼ Table 18.2. Our experience at the Children's Memorial has been published.[15–17]

# MEGADOSE CD34+ CELLS

Megadose CD34 cells may be given to promote engraftment. Recently, several lines of evidence have suggested that CD34+ cells when given in a megadose may decrease graft rejection.[1,18,19] In major histocompatibility complex (MHC) mismatched mouse models, transplantation of megadose CD34 cells (doses 5-fold higher than normal) results in donor chimeras even in sublethally irradiated (650 cGy) recipients. This suggests that there are two major mechanisms of graft rejection: immune rejection and stem cell competition. Theoretically, large doses of CD34 cells may compete with surviving host progenitor cells for hematopoietic space. In one patient clinical trial, T cell-depleted (TCD) grafts with doses of CD34 cells seven- to tenfold greater than usual resulted in rapid engraftment for 16 out of 17 haploidentical recipients. The same pretransplant conditioning regimen failed to promote engraftment in any of five patients receiving conventional CD34 dose TCD haploidentical grafts. Megadose CD34 cells also may decrease GVHD.[1,18,19] Addition of CD34+ cells to primary mixed lymphocyte cultures causes a decrease in cytotoxic T lymphocytes (CTL) precursors against irradiated human lymphocyte antigen (HLA)-mismatched peripheral blood stimulation. Surface membranes of CD34 cells are positive for HLA-DR but negative for B7 co-stimulatory molecules. They may, therefore, induce tolerance by antigen presentation without co-stimulation. Of supporting interest, in one study of TCD haploidentical hematopoietic stem cell transplantation that used megadose CD34 grafts (and no posttransplantation immunosuppression) only one patient developed GVHD more than grade II.[1,18,19]

# HISTOCOMPATIBILITY

The HLA region spans approximately 4000 Kb on the short arm of chromosome 6. The HLA genes can be divided into two major classes: Class I including HLA A, B, and C; and class II including HLA DR, DQ, and DP. Class I molecules are expressed on all nucleated cells, whereas the class II molecules are found on B-lymphocytes, monocytes, and occasionally on activated T lymphocytes. There are over 100 different antigens expressed within the B, C, DR, DQ, and DP loci that have been identified by traditional serological typing. A simple calculation of the number of possible HLA phenotypes has been estimated to be approximately $4 \times 10^{18}$. However, in specific populations, some HLA phenotypes occur with a much higher frequency than others, which affects the opportunity of finding

## TABLE 18.2  Pediatric Experience with Immune Ablative Transplants

| Age | Donor type | Dx | Flu/BU/ATG | Chimerism | Acute GVHD | Chronic GVHD | CsA | Toxicity | Outcome/Days post-TX | Ref. |
|---|---|---|---|---|---|---|---|---|---|---|
| 16 | MRD | Thal | Yes | Yes | Yes | No | Yes | None | A&W | 15 |
| 1 | MRD | ANLL | Yes | Yes | Yes/3 | No | Yes | None | A&W | 15 |
| 2 | MRD | JCML | yes | Yes | Yes/4 | No | Yes | None | A&W | 15 |
| 12 | MRD | ALL CR2 | Yes | N/a | No | Yes | Yes | None | Relapse | 15 |
| 10 | MRD | Fanconi | Yes | Mixed | No | No | Yes | None | A&W | 15 |
| 3 | MRD | Gaucher | Yes | No | No | No | Yes | None | A&W | 15 |
| 15 | MRD | CML | Yes | Yes | No | No | Yes | None | A&W/60 | 16 |
| 13 | MUD | ALL CR3 | Yes | Yes | Yes/1 | No | Yes | None | A&W/75 | 16 |
| 5 | MRD | HIGM | Yes | Yes | No | No | Yes | None | A&W/609 | 16 |
| 7 | MUD | ALL CR3 | Yes | No | No | No | Yes | PTLD | Relapse | 16 |
|  |  |  |  |  |  |  |  |  | Died/27 | 16 |
| 9 | MUD | HIGM | Yes | Mixed | No | No | Yes | None | A&W/553 | 16 |
| 7 | NRD | Thal | Yes | Yes | No | No | Yes | Loss graft | A&W*560 | 16 |
| 3 | MUD | ANLL CR2 | Yes | Yes | Yes/2 | No | Yes | F&N | Relapse | 16 |
|  |  |  |  |  |  |  |  |  | Died/126 | 16 |
| 11 | MRD | ALL CR3 | Yes | Yes | Yes/2 | Yes | Yes | Fungal infection | Died/87 | 16 |
| 17 | MRD | NHL CR3 | Yes | Yes | Yes/1 | No | Yes | None | A&W/420 | 16 |
| 4 | MUD | SCA | Yes | No | No | No | Yes | None | A&W | 16 |
|  |  |  |  |  |  |  |  |  | Auto**/379 | 16 |
| 0.5 | MMRD | Sandhof | Yes | Yes | No | No | Yes | None | A&W/371 | 16 |
| 15 | MUD | SCA | Yes | No | No | No | Yes | None | A&W | 16 |
|  |  |  |  |  |  |  |  |  | Auto**302 | 16 |
| 12 | MRD | NHL Cr3 | Yes | No | No | No | Yes | Pneumonia | A&W/365 | 16 |

Abbreviations: Dx = diagnosis; Flu = fludarabine; BU = busulfan; ATG = antithymocyte globulin; GVHD = graft-versus-host disease; TX = transplantation; MRD = matched related donor; MUD = matched unrelated donor; MMRD= mismatched related donor; NHL= non-Hodgkin's lymphoma; SCA= sickle cell anemia; HIGM= hyper-IGM syndrome; CR2/3 = complete remission 2/3; A&W= alive and well; Auto** = autologous recovery; PTLD =posttransplant lymphoproliferative disease; Thal = Thalasemia; JCML = juvenile chronic myelogenous leukemia; N/a = not applicable; F&N = fever and neutropenia.

a matched unrelated donor in a national or international pool.[11,18] Historically, HLA typing has been accomplished utilizing standard serological techniques. However, new emerging technologies, including isoelectric focusing (IEF), specific sequence oligoprobing (SSOP), restriction fragment length polymorphism (RFLP), and polymerase chain reaction (PCR), have provided a more sensitive approach to identifying genetic disparity between donors and recipients. In addition, these techniques can be accomplished in a more timely and efficient manner.

## PERIPHERAL BLOOD STEM CELLS

Stem cells are present in the peripheral blood, and in some clinical situations PBSCs are used in place of marrow for transplantation.[20–22] Most of the experience with PBSCs has involved autologous transplants but syngeneic PBSC transplants,[23] and at least 25 allogeneic transplants have been performed with PBSCs.[24] There are some advantages of using PBSCs instead of marrow cells in transplantation. These include:

1. The collection of PBSCs does not require the donor to undergo a surgical procedure in an operating room, thus eliminating anesthesia risk.
2. Recovery from marrow donation takes several days and sometimes significant complications may occur.[25,26] Recovery from PBSC collection is immediate.
3. One PBSC product can be collected on an outpatient basis using a blood cell separator in three to four hours.[27]
4. The apheresis procedure to collect PBSCs is very similar to that used to collect platelets from normal donors. In the past, it was projected that to obtain adequate numbers of PBSCs for successful transplants, five to six apheresis collections would have to be performed. However, if the donor is treated with the growth factor filgrastim, the number of circulating stem cells is drastically increased and only one or two apheresis collection procedures are required.[27]

## CHIMERISM

In all HSCT is important to determine the percent chimerism. This term refers to the presence of lymphohematopoietic cells of non-host origin. These cells could be derived incidentally from a fetal-maternal transfusion or a blood transfusion, or, more common today, purposely done after HSCT. Full or complete chimerism refers to complete replacement of host cells by donor lymphohematopoiesis. While mixed chimerism indicates the presence of both donor and recipient cells within a given cellular compartment, in some situations there may be split chimerism, which refers to lineage-specific studies in cases where the myeloid compartment may be 100% donor while the lymphocytes have a mixed chimera. When studies of chimerism are performed, one should refer specifically to the cell type used in the particular study. Another term commonly utilized is the microchimerism that indicates the presence of donor origin cells, but can only be detected with very sophisticated and sensitive techniques.[28,29]

There are multiple techniques to assess chimerism. Early studies rely on techniques such as red cell immunophenotyping, cytogenetics, and immunoglobulin isotypes analysis.[30–34] The problems with these techniques are their lack of sensitivity and difficulty in quantification.

Another very useful technique when there is a sex mismatch is the use of fluorescent in situ hybridization (FISH) (► Figure 18.3); this technique is sensitive and quantitative, but only for sex mismatched transplants.[35]

The most applicable techniques are those dependent on DNA extraction using either restriction length polymorphisms (RFLPs), variable number tandem repeats (VNTRs), and small tandem repeats (STRs). These techniques are very sensitive, allow an accurate quantification, are reproducible in different laboratories, and are inexpensive but labor intensive (► Figure 18.4).[36-39] With these techniques even the different components of the peripheral blood can be separated to determine more specific chimerism (myeloid, T lymphs, B lymphs and even platelets), leaving only red cell determination to be done by immunophenotyping. Together, these techniques provide a full assessment of chimerism.

## Chimerism After Immune Ablative Transplants for Malignant Diseases

A determination of chimerism that is specific to the leukemia cell line of origin becomes very important in this type of transplant because the persistence of detectable recipient hematopoiesis even at extremely low levels is at considerable high risk for relapse. This may represent a surrogate test for minimal residual disease. In the immune ablative transplant, the graft must be pushed to be 100% of donor origin, which can be achieved with multiple infusions either of DLIs or stem cells (▼ Table 18.3).[40]

A recent report from the American Society of Blood and Marrow Transplantation,[41] at the request of the National Marrow Program and the International Bone Marrow Transplant Registry, established guidelines for chimerism analysis. The recommendations are:

1. Chimerism analysis should be undertaken using sensitive (<1%) informative techniques. At present STR/VNTR analysis is the approach most likely to give reproducible informative data. Other techniques are less sensitive and can be utilized when the STR/VNTR are not available. Analysis used for clinical decision making should be performed in Clinical Laboratory Improvement Amendment (CLIA) certified laboratories.

2. Peripheral blood cells are generally more useful than marrow for chimerism studies. Lineage-specific chimerism studies should be considered the assay of choice in the setting of immune ablative or reduced intensity transplants.

3. In immune ablative or reduced intensity transplants, the early pattern of chimerism may be predictive for either GVHD (increase T cell donor chimerism) or graft failure (decline in T cell chimerism to <20% donor cells). Therefore, if therapeutic interventions are based on these patterns of chimerism, the following recommendations apply to protocols in which achieving mixed chimerism as an immunological platform for DLI is a primary goal:

    a. Frequent (every 2–4 weeks) peripheral blood analysis of chimerism by VNTRs or STR analysis until DLI is administered. DLIs are then considered for chimerism.

    b. For patients who develop GVHD, are not DLI candidates, or who have achieved full donor chimerism, infrequent donor chimerism is recommended (3–6 months).

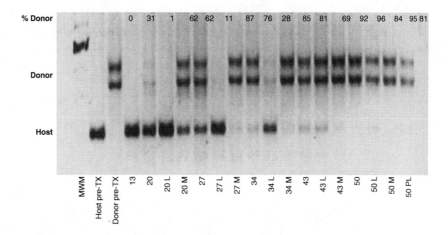

**FIGURE 18.3** Chimerism after an immune ablative transplant.

Abbreviations: MWM = molecular weight marker; TX = transplant; L = lymphoid (T cells); M = myeloid; PL = platelets. (Gel courtesy of Ms. Marie Olszewski, Stem Cell Laboratory, Northwestern University, Chicago, IL.)

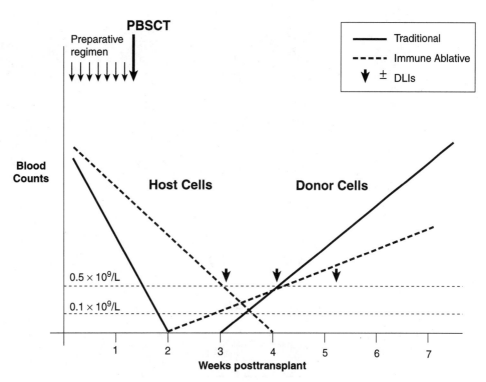

**FIGURE 18.4** Schematic of the pattern of engraftment in a traditional (**solid line**) and immune ablative (**dashed line**) transplant. Arrows denote DLIs.

## TABLE 18.3    Evaluation of Chimerism of Patients with Leukemia

| Case | Days post-BMT | Informative primer pair(s) | Total # of specimens collected | PCR results (%) of donor's DNA | Blast (%) |
|------|---------------|----------------------------|--------------------------------|--------------------------------|-----------|
| 1 | 335 | D17S30 | 4 | 100 | 0 |
| 2 | 61 | D1S80 | 1 | 100 | 0 |
|   | 109 | D1S80 | 1 | 88 | 11.8 |
|   | 131 | D1S80 | 1 | 92 | 15.7 |
|   | 145 | D1S80 | 1 | 92 | 8.5 |
|   | 152 | D1S80 | 1 | 87 | 5 |
| 3 | 1,095 | D17S30 | 1 | 22 | 100 |
| 4 | 1,057 | SRY/ZP3 | 1 | 100 | 0 |
| 5 | 20 | ZP3/SRY | 1 | 98 | 0 |
|   | 37 | ZP3/SRY | 1 | 25 | 11.7 |
|   | 44 | ZP3/SRY | 1 | 90 | 8.6 |
|   | 55 | ZP3/SRY | 1 | 100 | 0 |
|   | 83 | ZP3/SRY | 1 | 100 | 0 |
|   | 104 | ZP3/SRY | 1 | 100 | 0 |
|   | 114 | ZP3/SRY | 1 | 100 | 0 |
|   | 225 | ZP3/SRY | 1 | 100 | 0 |
|   | 272 | ZP3/SRY | 1 | 5 | 88.3 |
| 6 | 474 | D1S80 | 3 | 100 | 0 |
| 7 | 91 | APO-B | 1 | 100 | 0 |
| 8 | 364 | SRY/ZP3 | 1 | 100 | 0 |
| 9 | 350 | D17S30 | 1 | 100 | 0 |
| 10 | 73 | D17S30 | 2 | 100 | 0 |
| 11 | 351 | D17S30 | 1 | 100 | 0 |
| 12 | 267 | SRY/ZP3 | 2 | 100 | 0 |
| 13 | 24 | ZP3/SRY | 1 | 70 | 0 |
|   | 30 | ZP3/SRY | 1 | 95 | 0 |

| TABLE 18.3 | Evaluation of Chimerism of Patients with Leukemia—cont'd |

| Case | Days post-BMT | Informative primer pair(s) | Total # of specimens collected | PCR results (%) of donor's DNA | Blast (%) |
|---|---|---|---|---|---|
| | 198 | ZP3/SRY | 1 | 88 | 10.5 |
| | 219 | ZP3/SRY | 1 | 50 | 27.8 |
| | 236 | ZP3/SRY | 1 | 34 | 73 |
| 14 | 484 | D17S30, APO-B2 | 1 | 100 | 0 |
| 15 | 33 | ZP3/SRY | 1 | 100 | 0 |
| | 61 | ZP3/SRY | 1 | 100 | 0 |
| | 97 | ZP3/SRY | 1 | 26.6 | 2 |
| | 97 BM | ZP3/SRY | 1 | 71.8 | |
| | 112 | ZP3/SRY | 1 | 69.4 | 0 |
| | 124 | ZP3/SRY | 1 | 62 | |
| | 124 BM | ZP3/SRY | 1 | 41 | 10.8 |
| | 151 | ZP3/SRY | 1 | 75 | 1 |
| | 153 | ZP3/SRY | 1 | 50 | 6 |
| | 171 | ZP3/SRY | 1 | 75 | |
| | 171 BM | ZP3/SRY | 1 | 0 | 5.7 |
| | 192 | ZP3/SRY | 1 | 65 | 5 |
| | 241 | ZP3/SRY | 1 | 0 | 34.6 |
| 16 | 225 | SRY/ZP3 | 1 | 100 | 0 |
| 17 | 42 | D17S30 | 1 | 100 | 0 |
| | 140 | D17S30 | 1 | 100 | 0 |
| | 365 | D17S30 | 1 | 100 | 97.5 |
| 18 | 113 | D17S30 | 3 | 100 | 0 |
| 19 | 239 | D17S30 | 1 | 100 | 0 |
| 20 | 126 | D17S30 | 1 | 100 | 0 |
| 21 | 434 | D1S80 | 4 | 100 | 0 |

BM = Samples tested from the bone marrow; otherwise, peripheral blood samples.

c. Multiple chimerism evaluation initially every 2–4 weeks, and then every 3–6 months are recommended following prophylactic DLI both to evaluate the effect of chimerism of the DLI and to discern whether additional DLIs are necessary.

4. For nonmalignant disorders other than aplastic anemia, chimerism analysis should be done 1, 2, and 3 months posttransplantation.[41]

## PATTERNS OF ENGRAFTMENT

In this type of transplant the pattern of engraftment is quite different when compared to the traditional transplant. In the first place, the counts don't usually drop to $< 0.5 \times 10^9$/L, and if only looking at the counts the recovery may not be noticeable. For that reason it is very important to assess quantitatively the chimeras beginning in week 2 posttransplant; in our case we have been doing them weekly to determine if there is a need for DLIs, but the recommendation is q2 weeks. The recovery is quite slow but usually by week 8 patients will have a full chimera. If on the other hand the pattern is slower or there is a decrease in the percent of donor cells at a given point, one may consider giving the patient a boost of stem cells or DLIs in order to push the graft to a full chimera (see Figure 18.4). We show the pattern of engraftment of a patient with sickle cell disease that clearly demonstrates the slow pattern of engraftment (▼ Figure 18.5).

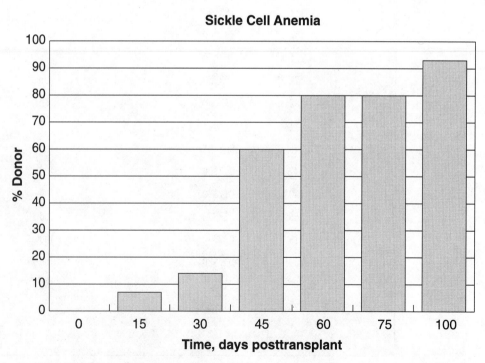

**FIGURE 18.5** Pattern and speed of engraftment in a patient with sickle cell anemia who underwent an immune ablative transplant.

## ISSUES TO BE RESOLVED AND FUTURE DIRECTIONS

There is no doubt in my mind that this technology is here to stay and that in the future we have the obligation to reduce toxicity from the traditional way of doing transplants. The problem is that there are many unresolved issues that need to be addressed scientifically, including randomized clinical trials. These issues include:

- What is the optimal preparative regimen?
- What is the optimal cell dose to be infused?
- What is the optimal GVHD prophylaxis?
- How can acute and chronic GVHD be prevented?
- For what diseases would this approach most likely be beneficial?
- Can this technology be expanded to all age groups?
- Can sources other than bone marrow or peripheral blood stem cells be used (i.e., umbilical cord blood)?

In summary, these are some of the questions to be resolved. In the meantime, we should consider this approach for pediatric patients with comorbid illnesses or for those with benign disorders.

# REFERENCES

1. Thomas ED, Fefer A, Buckner CD et al. Current status of bone marrow transplantation of aplastic anemia and acute leukemia. Blood 1977;49:671–681.
2. Champlin R, Gale RP. Bone marrow transplantation for acute leukemia; recent advances and comparison with alternative therapies. Semin Hematol 1987;24:55–67.
3. Hurd DD. Allogeneic and autologous bone marrow transplantation for acute non-lymphoblastic leukemia. Semin Hematol 1987;14:407–416.
4. Blume KG, Beutler LE, Bross KG et al. Bone marrow ablation and allogeneic marrow transplantation in acute leukemia. N Engl J Med 1950;3012:1041–1046.
5. Gale RP, Kay Hem, Rimm HEM et al. Bone marrow transplantation for acute leukemia in first remission. Lancet 1952;2;1006–1009.
6. Santos GW, Tutschka PJ, Brookmeyer R et al. Marrow transplantation for acute nonlymphocytic leukemia after treatment with busulfan and cyclophosphamide. N Engl J Med 1983;309:1347–1353.
7. Registry report: Report from the International Bone Marrow Transplant Registry: Advisory Committee of the International Bone Marrow Registry. Bone Marrow Transplant 1989;4:221–228.
8. Yeager AM, Kaizer H, Santos GW et al. Autologous bone marrow transplantation in patients with acute non-lymphocytic leukemia using ex vivo marrow treatment with -hydroperoxycyclophosphamide. N Engl J Med 1986;315:141–147.
9. Grochow LB, Krivit W, Whitley CB et al. Busulfan disposition in children. Blood 1990;75:1723–1727.
10. Giralt S, Estey E, Albitar M et al. Engraftment of allogeneic hematopoietic progenitor cells with purine analog-containing chemotherapy: harnessing graft-versus-leukemia without myeloablative therapy. Blood 1997;89:4531–4536.
11. Reisner Y, Martinelli MF. Stem cell escalation enables HLA disparate haematopoietic transplants in leukemia patients. Immunol Today 1999;20:343–347.
12. Storb R, Yu C, Sandmaier B. Mixed hematopoietic chimerism after hematopoietic stem cell allografts. Transplant Proc 1999;31:677–678.
13. Storb R. Non-myeloablative preparative regimens: experimental data and clinical practice. In: Perry MC, ed. American Society of Clinical Oncology Educational Book, Alexandria, VA: American Society of Clinical Oncology, 1999:241.
14. Khouri IF, Keating M, Korblihg M et al. Transplant-lite: induction of graft-versus-malignancy using fludarabine based non-ablative chemotherapy and allogeneic blood progenitor-cell transplantation as treatment for lymphoid malignancies. J Clin Oncol 1998;16:2817–2824.
15. Slavin S, Nagler A, Naparstek E et al. Non-myeloablative stem cell transplantation and cell therapy as an alternative to conventional bone marrow transplantation with lethal cytoreduction for the treatment of malignant and nonmalignant hematologic diseases. Blood 1998;91:756–763.
16. Childs R, Bahceci E, Clave E et al. Non-myeloablative allogeneic peripheral blood stem cell transplants (PBSCT) for malignant diseases reduces transplant-related mortality (TRM) (Abstr). Blood 1998;92(Suppl I, Part 1 of 2):37a.
17. Duerst RE, Haut PR, Venkaterwaran L et al. Hematopoietic chimerism following immunoablative therapy for non-malignant disorders. Outpatient stem cell transplantation (SCT) (Abstr #5171). Blood 2000;96:329b.
18. Bachar-Lustig E, Rachanim N, Li HW et al. Megadose of T cell-depleted marrow overcomes MHC barriers in sublethally irradiated mice. Nat Med 1995;1:1268–1273.
19. Gratwohl A, Baldomero H, John L et al. Pressure cells transplants across a major histocompatibility barrier in rabbits: positive effects of a higher number of precursor cells? Acta Haematol 1996;95:176–180.
20. Kessinger A, Armitage JO, Landmark JD et al. Reconstitution of human hematopoietic function with autologous cryopreserved circulating stem cells. Exp Hematol 1987;14:192–196.
21. Reiffers B, Bernard I, David B. Successful autologous transplantation with peripheral blood hematopoietic cells in patients with leukemia. Exp Hematol 1986;14:312–325.
22. Schmitz N, Linch DC, Goldstone AH et al. Randomized trial of Filgrastim-mobilized peripheral blood progenitor cell transplantation versus autologous bone-marrow transplantation in lymphoma patients. Lancet 1996;347:353–357.
23. Weaver CH, Buckner CD, Longin K. Syngeneic transplantation with peripheral blood mononuclear cells collected after the administration of recombinant human granulocyte colony-stimulating factor. Blood 1993; 82:1981–1984.
24. Bensinger W. Oral communication. Crystal City, VA: American Red Cross Conference on the Use of Peripheral Blood Stem Cell Transplants, June 24, 1994.
25. Buckner CD, Clift RA, Sanders JE et al. Marrow harvesting from normal donors. Blood 1984;64:630–634.
26. Bortin MM, Buckner CD. Major complications of marrow harvesting for transplantation. Exp Hematol 1983;11:916–921.

27. Comenzo RL, Malachowski ME, Miller KB et al. Engraftment with peripheral blood stem cells collected by large-volume leukapheresis for patients with lymphoma. Transfusion 1992;32:729–731.
28. Evans PC, Lambert N, Maloney S et al. Long-term fetal micro-chimerism in peripheral blood mononuclear cell subsets in healthy women and women with scleroderma. Blood 1999;93:2033–2037.
29. Maloney S, Smith A, Fuerst DE et al. Micro-chimerism of maternal origin persist into adult life. J Clin Invest 1999;104:41–47.
30. Walker H, Singer CR, Patterson J. The significance of host hematopoietic cells, detected by cytogenetic analysis of bone marrow from recipients of bone marrow transplants. Br J Haematol 1986;62:385–391.
31. Roy DC, Tantravahi R, Murray C et al. Natural history of mixed chimerism after bone marrow transplantation with CD6-depleted allogeneic marrow: a stable equilibrium. Blood 1990;75:296–304.
32. Lawler SD, Harris H, Miller J et al. Cytogenetic follow up studies of recipients of T cell depleted allogeneic bone marrow. Br J Haematol 1987;65:143–150.
33. Sparkes MC, Crist ML, Sparkes RS et al. Gene markers in human bone marrow transplantation. Vox Sang 1977;33:202–205.
34. Witherspoon RP, Schanfield MC, Storb R et al. Immunoglobulin production of donor origin after marrow transplantation for acute leukemia and aplastic anemia. Transplantation 1978;26:407–408.
35. Dewald G, Staller R, Al Saadi A et al. Multicenter investigation with interphase fluorescence in situ hybridization using X- and Y-chromosome probes. Am J Med Genet 1998;76:318–326.
36. Luhn R, Bellissimo D, Uzqiris A et al. Quantitative evaluation of post bone marrow transplant engraftment status using fluorescent-labeled variable number of tandem repeats. Mol Diagn 2000;5:129–138.
37. Thiede C, Florek M, Bornhauser M et al. Rapid quantification of mixed chimerism using multiplex amplification of short tandem repeat markers and fluorescence detection. Bone Marrow Transplant 1999; 10:1055–1060.
38. Badr P, Holle W, Klingbiel T et al. Quantitative assessment of mixed hematopoietic chimerism by polymerase chain reaction after allogeneic BMT. Anticancer Res 1996;16:1759–1763.
39. Scharf SJ, Smith AG, Hansen JA et al. Quantitative determination of bone marrow transplant engraftment using fluorescence polymerase chain reaction primer for human identity markers. Blood 1995;85:1954–1963.
40. Wang LJ, Chou P, Gonzalez-Ryan L et al. Evaluation of mixed chimerism in pediatric patients with leukemia after allogeneic stem cell transplantation by PCR quantitative analysis of variable number tandem repeats and testis determination gene. Bone Marrow Transplant 2002;29:51–56.
41. Antin JH, Childs R, Filipovich AH et al. Establishment of complete and mixed chimerism after allogeneic lymphohematopoietic transplantation: recommendations from a workshop at the 2001 tandem meeting of the International Bone Marrow Transplant Registry and the American Society of Blood and Marrow Transplantation. Biol Blood Marrow Transplant 2001;7:473–485. Review.

# CHAPTER XIX

# Umbilical Cord Blood Transplantation

DONNA WALL

In the past decade umbilical cord blood (UCB) has developed into an important alternative source of hematopoietic progenitors for transplantation in pediatrics. The field of cord blood transplantation began with the observation that the blood retained in the placenta after separation of the infant was rich in hematopoietic progenitors.[1,2] There soon followed an appreciation that there were sufficient hematopoietic precursors in the blood that could be collected from a single placenta to support allogeneic hematopoietic reconstitution, an alternative source of hematopoietic precursors for transplantations.[3] After initial success with sibling allogeneic transplants,[4,5] efforts to develop inventories of cord blood units for future unrelated donor allogeneic cord blood transplants were initiated in several countries. To date it is estimated that over 3,000 cord blood transplants have been performed, and retrospective and prospective studies are beginning to define the role of this new hematopoietic stem cell source in clinical transplantation.

Conceptually there are several potential benefits to cord blood when compared to other sources of hematopoietic stem cells used in allogeneic transplantation (▼ Table 19.1). Since cord blood is banked and fully characterized prior to initiation of a donor search, it is available for transplantation at the time that is optimal for the patient, without the constraints of donor availability, often within days if necessary.[6] Secondly, the maternal-fetal barrier results in a low rate of viral contamination in cord blood, cytomegalovirus (CMV) and Epstein-Barr virus (EBV) being the most clinically important transplant-related viruses. Equally important has been the observation of less graft-versus-host disease (GVHD) following cord blood transplant, which has allowed the use of less perfectly immunologically matched cord blood units for transplantation, and resulting in an unrelated donor option for a majority of patients with rare immune types.[7] This is of importance since less than 50% of unrelated donor marrow searches identify a suitable immunologically matched donor who is available for donation of hematopoietic stem cells, and this percentage is lower for those not of Northern European descent.[8]

These benefits are balanced by real concerns. The number of hematopoietic precursors contained within a given cord blood unit is limited and is less than conventionally used in allogeneic bone marrow or peripheral blood stem cell transplants. Although there may be relatively higher numbers of the very immature progenitors, the limited intermediate precursor cell number translates into prolonged time to engraftment, which carries with it

> ### TABLE 19.1    Pros and Cons of Cord Blood as an Alternative Donor Hematopoietic Progenitor Cell Source
>
> **Pros**
> - Rapidly available
> - Lower risk of acute and chronic GVHD
> - Lower viral contamination and transfer risk
> - Partially HLA-antigen matching is acceptable for unrelated donor transplantation
>
> **Cons**
> - Prolonged time to hematopoietic recovery
> - Prolonged time to immune recovery
> - Transplant is usually dependent on a single frozen bag of cord blood
> - Inability to obtain more donor hematopoietic progenitor cells if nonengraftment occurs or donor leukocyte infusions needed

increased transplant-related risks. Since there is only one donation at time of birth there is no option for future booster grafts or donor leukocyte infusions.

## CELLULAR COMPOSITION OF CORD BLOOD

Cord blood is the residual blood that had been circulating in the fetus, transporting nutrients from the placenta to the fetus. Its content includes all cellular elements found in blood: platelets, red blood cells, leukocytes. It is not clear why hematopoietic precursors are circulating during fetal development, although there appears to be varying expression of adhesion molecules important in cell trafficking through gestation.[9]

### Hematopoietic Precursors

Based on observations in the mouse, Knudtzon studied the ability of umbilical cord blood to form hematopoietic colonies when cultured on agar with a feeder layer of peripheral blood cells.[1] The numbers and quality of the colonies were similar to those found in bone marrow, and he postulated that cord blood might be used as a source of hematopoietic stem cells for restoration of bone marrow function. There followed work by Boyse, Bard, and Broxmeyer demonstrating that umbilical cord blood contained reconstituting hematopoietic cells (reviewed by Wagner and Kurtzberg[10]) and that there were sufficient numbers of hematopoietic precursors to recover hematopoietic function in patients undergoing allogeneic transplantation.[11] Several groups have noted an increase in very primitive hematopoietic precursors with production of larger colonies and a higher replating capacity[2,12–18] as well as a greater number of severe combined immunodeficiency disease mouse-repopulating cells.[19] These findings suggest that, although fewer cells are available in a given cord blood unit, it is enriched in primitive hematopoietic precursors that are critical for long-term engraftment. Cord blood obtained from the premature infant at the time of delivery contains more hematopoietic precursors.[20] However, since there is less placental blood volume to be collected, there is no increase in the total number of hematopoietic cells in cord blood units from premature infants.[21-23]

## Fewer Intermediate Platelet Precursors in Cord Blood Units

There are fewer megakaryocytic colony-forming units found in cord blood, which likely contributes to the prolonged time to platelet recovery noted after cord blood transplantation (CBT).[24] Bornstein and colleagues compared cord blood and peripheral blood megakaryocytes cultured in the presence of thrombopoietin. While the cord blood proliferated twice as much as peripheral blood, the megakaryocytes remained diploid rather than undergoing endomitosis, suggesting relative immaturity of cord blood megakaryocytic precursors.[25]

## Nucleated Red Blood Cells in Cord Blood Units

On average nucleated red blood cells contribute 8% of CB nucleated cells, with a wide range noted after normal term delivery (range 0% to 42%).[26] With conventional red cell depletion techniques used in cord blood banking (e.g., hetastarch sedimentation), a large proportion of nucleated red blood cells (NRBCs) remain with in the cord blood product and thus contribute to the final total nucleated cells (TNC) (range 0% to 36%). There was concern that high NRBC content in the TNC would have a misleadingly high estimation of hematopoietic potential of a cord blood unit. However, NRBC content correlates with CD34+ cells and, in fact, there is a positive correlation between higher NRBC content and engraftment.[27]

## Defining Hematopoietic Content in Cord Blood Units

For the purposes of cord blood banking the cord blood unit is characterized by the total nucleated cell count, which includes neutrophils and nucleated red blood cells. Clinical decisions and trials have utilized the total nucleated cell count in calculating expected cell dose pretransplant; this is the only hematologic parameter that has been consistent between the various cord blood bank laboratories and hence comparable. The majority of cells counted in the TNC do not have hematopoietic potential, but there is a good correlation between TNC and CD34+ cells and CFU content allowing for the TNC to be used in clinical decision making.[26,28] As banking becomes more standardized it is likely that pre-freeze CD34 quantitation will become more important in clinical decision making.[29]

## IMMUNOLOGIC FEATURES OF CORD BLOOD

The immune cells contained within cord blood have been extensively studied in attempt to explain the clinical observation of lower GVHD. The cord blood T cells have been circulating between the infant and placenta until delivery and thus are exposed to the local immunologic effects of the maternal-placental interface, which by definition must allow the immunologically distinct yet immunocompetent fetus to be tolerated by the mother. From the 14th week of gestation, the fetus is immunocompetent and able to reject grafts.[30]

It has been postulated that the immunoregulatory effect of the placental environment facilitates tolerance of the immunocompetent T cells when transplanted; however, mechanisms have not been elucidated as yet.

As a generalization, there are relatively fewer T cells contained within the UCB graft (due to the limited numbers of cells in a cord blood unit) with a high proportion of those T cells having a naïve phenotype (CD45RA positive).[31–37] The afferent arm of the immune system, including monocytes, antigen presenting B cells are immature and are only partially functional.[38–42] Dendritic cells are immature and are partially or fully functional.[38,43–45]

T cell function of UCB, as measured by the mixed lymphocyte reaction and mitogen proliferation assays, is normal.[46–48] Stimulated CB cells release fewer cytokines compared to adult peripheral blood lymphocytes.[49–54] However, when T cells are separated into CD45RA and RO subsets, the cytokine release by the subsets of mature and immature T cells is similar to marrow cells—suggesting the deficiency is due to immaturity.[55] Garderet and colleagues demonstrated that cord blood T cells, although naïve, have a normal T cell repertoire based on analysis of the T cell receptor β-chain diversity and response to stimulation with staphylococcal superantigens.[56,57] They noted that the cord blood repertoire was more polyclonal compared to adult peripheral blood due to lack of stimulation and expansion of specific clones, postulating possible linkage with the lower risk of GVHD. Wang and colleagues found fewer alloreactive cytotoxic T lymphocyte (CTL) precursors in cord blood, which correlated with less destruction in a skin explant model[58] (▶ Figure 19.1). Similarly, Barbey and colleagues found that the CB CD8 cells had a higher threshold for stimulation and that once stimulated they released less cytokines.[59] Deacock and colleagues noted higher alloreactive T cells compared to adult peripheral blood cells.[60]

It also has been postulated that CB T cells contain more T helper (TH) or T-cytotoxic functional phenotypes which inhibit GVHD.[59,62,63] Cord blood lymphocytes, especially CD4 positive cells, are more likely to undergo apoptosis in response to tumor necrosis factor (TNF) and interleukin-2 (IL-2).[64–66] All these observations support the concept that the UCB T cells are functional but that their responses tend to be blunted, with favorable effects on GVHD but prolonged immunoincompetence after transplant.

The thymus plays an important role in immune recovery post-UCB transplant. A murine model of cord blood transplant across major histocompatibility barriers has been developed by Chen and colleagues.[67] In this model, full term fetal blood was compared to adult peripheral blood and adult T cell-depleted bone marrow as the allogeneic hematopoietic source (C57BL/6 [H-2b] into BALB/c [H-2d]). Fetal blood transplants were associated with decreased numbers of splenic immunocompetent cells, explained in part by lower numbers of thymic output with fewer TREC positive cells. However, the T cells present had similar proliferation and cytokine production when compared to cells after T cell-depleted grafts. This relative immunoincompetence was confirmed by prolonged survival of unrelated heart transplants in the recipients of mismatched CB transplants.

The natural killer (NK) cells in cord blood are functionally active, the NK number and function recover early after transplant.[33,49,55,68–71] El Marsafy and colleagues noted increased natural suppressor activity in cord blood relative to adult blood.[72] Increased suppressor cell function and phenotype was noted also by Han and colleagues.[31]

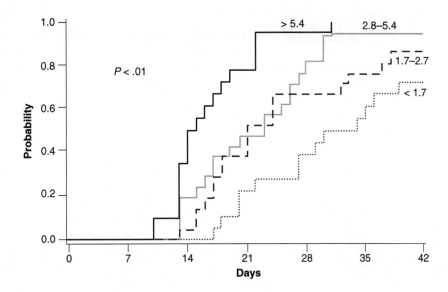

**FIGURE 19.1** Cumulative incidence of neutrophil engraftment after unrelated donor UCB transplantation (n = 102): effect of CD34 cell dose (x $10^5$/kilogram recipient body weight). Wagner, 2002.[102]

## STEM CELL LABORATORY ISSUES

The clinical laboratory has to make adjustments for cord blood. For laboratory personnel experienced with peripheral blood stem cell (PBSC) or marrow products there needs to be appreciation that the full product for transplantation is contained in the single product, often 20 mL or less. There is limited material for restriction fragment length polymorphism (RFLP) and samples for quality control, with the emphasis needing to be on making sure that as much of the product as possible is available for transplantation. Material from the post thaw wash discard may be a useful source of DNA for future testing. There also must be close coordination with the transplant unit as there is not an opportunity to obtain more product from the donor. Utilization of a controlled thaw in the laboratory with the addition of dextran and albumin immediately after rapid thaw has resulted in improved engraftment and has become part of clinical practice.[73]

## CORD BLOOD TRANSPLANTATION RESULTS

### Engraftment Is Dependent on Cell Dose

All CB transplant series that involve myeloablative preparative regimens and unmanipulated CB infusions have demonstrated a relationship between cell dose and engraftment following UCB transplant (▼ Table 19.2). Graft failure rate and time to neutrophil recovery both increase with lower cell doses as defined either by total nucleated cells/kg or CD34

| TABLE 19.2 | Rate and Timing of Engraftment Following Cord Blood Transplant and Factors Associated with Improved Engraftment | | | | |
|---|---|---|---|---|---|
| Reference (number studied) | Age (median) | %ANC >500 | Median time to ANC >500 | Platelet (range) | Factors associated with more rapid engraftment |
| Rubinstein[74] New York Placental Blood Program (562) | 82% <17 y | 81% by d+42 91% by d+60 | 28 d | >50K 90 d (16–250) | • Increased cell dose<br>• Lower recipient weight<br>• Absence of HLA mismatch |
| Gluckman[98] Eurocord (143) | 0.3–45 y | 87% by d+60 | | | • Increased cell dose<br>• No HLA mismatch |
| Wagner[102] Minnesota (102) | 0.2–57 y (7.4 y) | 88% by d+42 | 23 | >50K 86d (29–276) | • Increased CD34 dose<br>• Platelets: also age and lack of severe GVHD<br>• No association with HLA matching |
| Laughlin[135] Multicenter adult experience (68) | 18–58 (31.4 y) | 90% by d+42 | 27 | >20 K 58 d (35–142) for 30 evaluable | • Number of nucleated cells in graft prefreeze |

positive cells/kg. A threshold of a minimum of $1.5 \times 10^7$ nucleated cells/kg is needed to reliably achieve engraftment by day 42 following transplantation. Higher cell doses are associated with more reliable timely neutrophil recovery (▶ Figure 19.2). Cell doses below $1 \times 10^7$ total nucleated cells/kg are associated with unacceptable graft failure and delayed count recovery. However, even with minimal doses there have been reports of durable trilineage durable engraftment. At limiting cell doses, the degree of HLA matching influences engraftment, with more rapid engraftment and lower graft failure following more immunologically matched transplants.[74]

## Prolonged Time to Platelet Recovery

Compared to bone marrow, and especially mobilized peripheral blood allogeneic transplants, CBT is associated with slower platelet recovery. It is unusual to see platelet transfusion independence prior to 35 days posttransplant. This is attributed to fewer intermediate

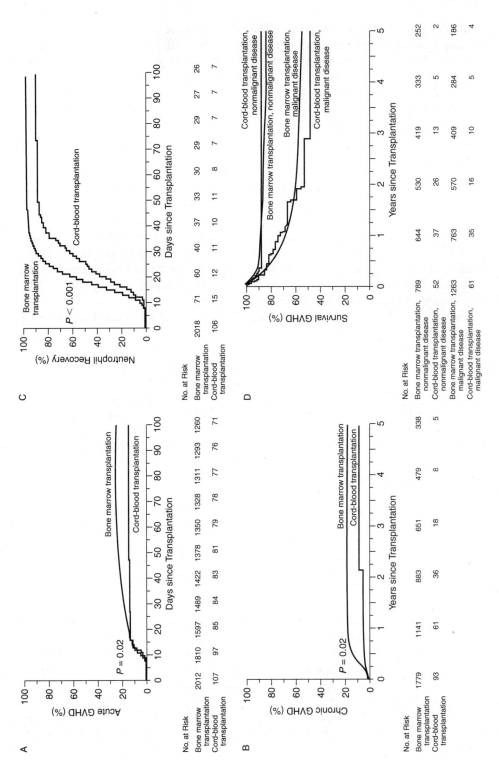

**FIGURE 19.2** Outcomes among Recipients of a Cord-Blood Transplant from an HLA-Identical Sibling and Recipients of a Bone Marrow Transplant from an HLA-Identical Sibling.

The curves indicate censored data. Panel A shows the cumulative incidence of grade II, III, and IV acute graft-versus-host disease (GVHD). Panel B shows the cumulative incidence of chronic GVHD. Panel C shows the cumulative incidence of neutrophil recovery to more than 500 cells per cubic millimeter. Panel D shows the Kaplan-Meier estimate of survival according to the underlying disease. Figures have been reproduced with permission from Rocha et al. 2000.[97]

committed platelet progenitors in graft.[75] The rate of and time to platelet recovery does not correlate with the cell dose in the graft. However, when platelet recovery was compared to that seen in unrelated donor marrow transplant there was no difference seen in a case comparison study by Barker et al.[76] The reasons for delayed platelet recovery are likely related to different causes, and there is slower recovery but less GVHD with the CBT. Unlike neutrophil recovery, platelet recovery has been less sensitive to cell dose, reflecting multiple clinical factors, such as infection, GVHD, drug toxicities, and cell dose.[74]

## Infections

Infections are currently the major cause of transplant-related mortality in cord blood transplantations.[74,77] There are high rates of serious bacterial, fungal, and viral infections that necessitate close monitoring and prevention strategies after treatment.

There is a delayed recovery of T cell number, function, and repertoire in adults compared to children receiving UCBT.[78] The finding of less thymic activity as measured by the number of TREC positive cells suggests a critical role for the thymus in immune recovery following UCBT. Preliminary results suggest that avoiding thymic damage by use of a submyeolablative regimen may result in more rapid immune recovery.[79,80]

Since there is a low rate of transfer of maternal CMV or EBV across the placental barrier, cord blood has a very low rate of CMV or EBV contamination.[81] This is a major benefit in transplanting infants and young children who tend to be viral naïve. However, CMV reactivation from recipient cells posttransplant in a setting where the donor cells have not previously been exposed to CMV can result in posttransplant EBV-related lymphoproliferative disease or lymphoproliferative disorder (LPD).[82–86] Marshall and colleagues failed to find EBV-specific T cells, even in the presence of Epstein-Barr viremia following cord blood or T cell-depleted marrow transplants, in contrast to findings of early recovery in unmanipulated PBSCT.[87] Late viral infections remain problematic post UCB transplant.

## Immunologic Recovery

Recovery of immune function posttransplant is important for control of infections and graft-versus-leukemia (GVL) effect. T cell recovery is a combination of expansion of mature, previously antigen-stimulated T cells from the graft and the later thymus dependent generation of T cells. GVHD impairs the recovery of T cell function. Given that a majority of T cells in the UCB graft are of the immature phenotype, there was concern that immune recovery would be delayed.[88–92]

Neutrophil function, as measured by superoxide generation, bacterial killing, and chemotaxis, recovers with the quantitative recovery of neutrophils.[92,93] B cell recovery starts by three months posttransplant.[91,92] Specific antibody production requires T cell help and in general postvaccination responses can be seen by one year posttransplant.[94] Natural killer cell number and function returns early posttransplant.[91,92] The percentage of NK cells in the lymphocyte populations is high in the first six months posttransplant but absolute numbers are normal.[92]

Recovery of T cell subsets tends to occur between three and nine months posttransplant. A consistent observation has been the recovery of T cell subsets with a high CD4/CD8 ratio.[88,89,91-94] This is the inverse of what is seen after unmanipulated or T cell-depleted bone marrow transplants.[95,96]

Quality of T cell reconstitution has been studied using combined approaches of phenotyping, analysis of T cell receptor diversity, and assessment of ex vivo thymic function by measuring TCR rearrangement excision circles (TRECs).[90] Talvensaari and colleagues found that during the first year after transplantation, TCR repertoires were highly abnormal and TREC values low in both CB and bone marrow (BM) recipients. However, from two years after transplantation onward TREC values as well as TCR diversity were higher in CB recipients than in recipients of bone marrow transplants, supporting both thymic regeneration of the T cell progenitors and complete immune recovery following CB transplant. Klein and colleagues found a similar pattern of TREC and TCR receptor diversity post-CB transplant and postulated that early T cell recovery after UCBT occurs primarily through peripheral expansion of adoptively transferred donor T cells, while later recovery, marked by the reappearance of TREC-containing cells, was associated with increasing numbers of phenotypically naïve T cells, improved mitogen and recall antigen responses, and diversification of the T cell repertoire. They noted a delay in central T cell recovery in adults relative to children that may be due to differences in thymic function resulting from age-related atrophy, GVHD, or the pharmacologic effects of prophylaxis and treatment of GVHD.[78]

## Graft-Versus-Host Disease

The severity of both acute and chronic GVHD is low with cord blood as the donor source (▼ Table 19.3). This has been demonstrated in a retrospective collaboration by Eurocord and the International Bone Marrow Transplantation Registry (IBMTR).[97] In this review, 113 recipients of HLA-identical cord blood transplants were compared to 2,052 bone marrow transplant recipients. Multivariant Cox regression analysis adjusted for factors that could influence GVHD demonstrated that the incidence of grade II–IV GVHD was 14% for CB compared to 24% for bone marrow as shown in Figure 19.2. Similarly, chronic GVHD was lower in CB recipients compared to bone marrow recipients (5% compared to 14%). There was no difference in survival.

Most CB transplants are being performed with one, two, or even three major disparities at HLA A, B or DR. Despite these HLA discrepancies, the incidence of severe GVHD has been less or similar to HLA matched unrelated marrow transplants.[74,76,91,97-103] Most series have failed to find an association with severity of acute/chronic GVHD and the degree of HLA matching. It remains controversial as to whether major class I or class II mismatches are better tolerated.

## Noninherited Maternal Haplotype-Disparate Transplants

Cord blood transplantation presents an interesting situation in the family transplant setting. van Rood suggested that haplotype mismatched cord blood in the infant who was exposed in utero to the mismatched organ should result in tolerance.[104,105] In fact, in a series of haplotype-mismatched sibling UCB transplants, no serious GVHD occured if the mismatched antigen was one to which the fetus had been exposed compared to 80% serious GVHD if the fetus had not been exposed to the mis-matched antigen.

| | | | | Factors associated with |
|---|---|---|---|---|
| **Reference** | **N** | **% acute GVHD** | **Chronic GVHD** | **a GVHD risk** |
| Rubinstein[74] | 381 | 0–I—56%<br>II—22%<br>III—11%<br>IV—11% | 25% mostly limited | • Increased risk for age >12y or peritrans-plant infection<br>• Lower if 6/6 match but otherwise no difference between 1, 2, or 3 antigen mismatches |
| Gluckman[98] | 65 | II—12%<br>III–IV—20% | 14% | • No association with number of HLA mismatches<br>• Lower risk of CMV seronegative |
| Wagner[102] | 102 | II—12%<br>III–IV—20% | 9% all extensive | • No association with HLA matching or CD3 cell dose |
| Laughlin[135] | 55 | II—40%<br>III–IV—20% | 12 of 33 evaluable; 11/12 limited | • No correlation with degree of HLA matching or CMV status |

**TABLE 19.3 Acute and Chronic GVHD Risk After Unrelated Donor Cord Blood Transplantations with Factors Affecting GVHD**

## Graft-Versus-Leukemia

Graft-versus-host disease has been associated with the graft-versus-leukemia (GVL) effect.[106,107] Since there was a lower rate of both acute and chronic GVHD with cord blood as the donor source, there was concern that the GVL effect associated with UCBT also would be diminished. This has been studied as best as possible in the laboratory. Joshi and colleagues demonstrated strong tumor cell killing by cord blood NK cells that was enhanced by the addition of IL-2.[68] Harris and colleagues demonstrated an antileukemic effect of CB in both in vitro and animal models.[108] Clinically, several anecdotal reports have described leukemia regression following withdrawal of immunosuppression post-CB transplantation.[109]

Since there are as yet no prospective comparisons of cord blood to other HSCT sources, it is difficult to address the GVL effect. Since CB transplants can be arranged within days, there has been a greater representation of patients with resistant disease in the CB series. However disease control appears to be similar to other unrelated donor sources—perhaps related to the fact that major HLA mismatches are routinely accepted for CB transplantation. In a retrospective review comparing matched sibling cord blood transplant to bone marrow transplant in children, Rocha and colleagues reported similar survivals with persistent or recurrent disease accounting for 48% of deaths in the CB group and 49% in the bone marrow group.[97] In a review of their experience at the University of Minnesota, Wagner et al. reported a 37% cumulative incidence of relapse at 2 years posttransplant. Age at transplant and high risk malignancy were associated with higher relapse risks.[102] Similar relapse rates between unrelated donor CB and BM transplants in the Eurocord sponsored retrospective analysis comparing outcomes at a variety of programs.[77] In that series the relapse rate at 2 years was 38% for CB and 39% for BM recipients. The main differences in adjusted outcomes between the three transplant groups appeared in the first 100 days after transplant. After day 100, CB, bone marrow, and T cell-depleted bone marrow transplant (T-UBMT) achieved similar results in terms of relapse, but chronic GVHD occurred more frequently after unmanipulated BMT and death after T cell-depleted BMT.

There are several possible explanations for the GVL/GVHD disparity when cord blood is utilized as the stem cell source. While the donor inoculum has fewer T lymphocytes and a greater number of naïve lymphocytes (RA+ cells), lymphocytic function is normal in vitro. The fact that there tends to be a greater HLA mismatch accepted between donor and recipient in cord blood transplant increases the antigenic differences that could potentially act as targets for a GVL effect.

## SURVIVAL FOLLOWING CORD BLOOD TRANSPLANTS

Survival following unrelated donor CBT ranges between 35 to 60%.[74,91,102] Several case control trials have demonstrated similar transplant outcomes for patients with acute leukemia receiving CB and BM transplants. Interpretation of these studies is complicated by the different patients who are receiving CB transplants due to the ability to undergo transplant quickly.

Several series have analyzed factors that affect survival following CB transplantation and have all demonstrated that increase cell dose (TNC/kg or CD34+ cells/kg) is the major influence on survival.[29,74,76,77,91,98,99,101,102,110,135] It is interesting that degree of HLA matching has not correlated strongly with survival in a majority of reports. Two larger reviews have demonstrated a significant improvement in survival with greater degrees of HLA matching, but the magnitude of the differences in survival has not been great.[74,102] Improved definition of HLA matching between donor and recipient at the high resolution DNA level is needed and is a major focus of the NHLBI-sponsored COBLT trial.[126]

## CLINICAL SITUATIONS AMENABLE TO CORD BLOOD TRANSPLANTATION

### Infants

The indications for allogeneic transplantation are varied and include high risk leukemia, immunodeficiency syndromes, and metabolic disorders. In general there is an urgency to proceed to transplant quickly. The cell doses achievable with CB result in reliably rapid recovery of hematopoiesis (personal observation). Many infants are naïve for CMV and EBV, as is the CB unit, decreasing the risk of viral transfer.

## Immunodeficiency Syndromes

The immunodeficiency syndromes, especially severe combined immunodeficiency syndromes, are well suited to be treated with CB as the unrelated, and if possible, related donor source. The lack of viral contamination, high cell dose, low GVHD risk, and rapid availability are all well suited to the clinical needs of this patient population. Knutsen and colleagues have reported excellent outcomes in this disease setting.[94,111]

## Urgent Clinical Situations

In settings of primary nonengraftment following allogeneic transplant or severe marrow aplasia following therapy, CB offers the possibility of a rapidly available stem cell source.

## Rare HLA Antigens

Since CB transplant can be safely performed across HLA mismatches, individuals with uncommon HLA antigens for whom a marrow donor is extremely unlikely to be identified can be approached with CB as an alternative stem cell source.

# ISSUES UNIQUE TO CORD BLOOD TRANSPLANTATION

## Undetected Hematologic/Metabolic Disorders

A serious concern with cord blood as an alternative stem cell source is that the inheritable medical problems of the donor are not yet known. Current CB banking procedures include careful family histories, screening of CB for hemoglobinopathies, assessment of hematologic potential by CFU and CD34 cell count, and often lymphocyte count. Donor families are encouraged to self-report serious medical problems of the infants or may be actively interviewed later in infancy. Despite these efforts there are some disorders that are likely not to be identified at the time of birth that could cause serious posttransplant complications, primary immunodeficiency syndromes being the most critical. While a large number of these disorders will be detected by family history and lymphocyte count, most can not be detected so early in life.

In general, an undetected metabolic disorder is not likely to cause serious harm, given the ubiquitous nonhematopoietic expression of many enzymes. However, in the setting of transplantation for metabolic disorders where the metabolic correction of the patient depends on the CB unit, identification of carrier or affected state in the CB unit is important. deGasperi and colleagues have demonstrated feasibility of testing CB companion samples for specific defects prior to transplant.[112]

## One Time Donation

The CB banking process relies on the anonymity of the donor and family. Thus, there is not an opportunity to return to that donor for further cells in the event of nonengraftment or for donor leukocyte infusions.[113,114] All CB transplants should be entered into with a plan for rescue donor source in case of nonengraftment. There are strategies being developed to retain some CB cells for in vitro expansion and subsequent adoptive immunotherapy.[115]

# GUIDANCE ON SELECTION OF CORD BLOOD UNIT

## Cell Dose Is as Important as HLA Match

All reports thus far have demonstrated improved outcomes with higher cell doses. The cell dose of $1.5 \times 10^7$/kg should be considered as a minimum cell dose and cell doses in the $3.5 \times 10^7$/kg range result in more rapid engraftment and improved survival.[102,116] Cell dose is more important than immunologic match.

## Chosing HLA Mismatches

There has been little effect on CB transplant outcomes with partially HLA matched CB. At least one antigen at HLA A, B, and DR foci should match. Further understanding of the immunogenicity of HLA types is needed before a rational approach to CB can be standardized.

# CORD BLOOD BANKING

## Unrelated Donor Banks

Pablo Rubinstein and the New York Blood Center founded the first unrelated donor cord blood bank in the United States.[101,117,118] Currently there are dozens of active public banks and several private facilities worldwide, capturing multiple ethnicities.[119]

Generally, cord blood units are collected from volunteer donor families after the delivery of a healthy infant, either in utero (before placental separation) or after the placenta is delivered. Extensive screenings of donor mothers predelivery and of the cord blood unit itself are performed before a unit considered for transplantation (▼ Table 19.4). In general, the parents of the infant donating the cord blood relinquish all rights to the collected unit and the unit is stored anonymously for use by transplant centers worldwide. The units are defined by information from the parents as well as by the cord blood itself; and units may be stored for 10 or more years. Cord blood banks are developing processes that will ensure the hematopoietic viability and product identity for years to come. Organizations such as NETCORD, the National Marrow Donor Program (NMDP), Foundation for Accreditation of Cellular Hematopoietic Therapies (FACHT) and the American Association of Blood Banks (AABB) are developing standards for banking procedures, quality control, and ways to coordinate the exchange of cord blood units between the banks and transplant programs.[120,121] National regulatory bodies such as the Food and Drug Administration are developing regulations to ensure product safety.[122–124] Central to the development of the field of cord blood transplantation have been the research organizations Eurocord, IBMTR, and COBLT, which are critically analyzing the outcomes of cord blood transplantation, especially as they pertain to the qualities of the cord blood unit.[77,98,125,126]

---

**TABLE 19.4**    Key Elements in Cord Blood Unit Screening and Testing

*Maternal*
- Infectious disease risk factor screening
- Labor and delivery risk factors for infection
- Testing maternal blood for syphilis, HIV 1 and 2, HIV p24, hepatitis B and C, CMV

*Family*
- Genetic screening with focus on inherited hematologic and immunologic disorders and cancer risk

*Cord Blood*
- Total nucleated cell count with differential including mononuclear cell count and nucleated RBC quantitation
- Testing for syphilis, HIV 1 and 2, HIV p24, HTLV, hepatitis B and C, CMV
- Culture for bacterial and fungal contamination
- Hematopoietic potential: CD34 and/or CFU content
- Hemoglobinopathy screening for sickle cell and thalassemia
- HLA testing

---

## Autologous and Related Donor Collections and Banks

Several groups have established public banking programs for autologous and related cord blood units.[127,128] These programs bank cord blood for a sibling with hematologic malignancies or for autologous use. An NHLBI-sponsored comprehensive program for sibling cord blood collection and banking has been developed by Reed and Lubin, the Sibling Cord Blood Program in Oakland (see Chapter VIII). This national resource coordinates collection, banking, storage, and release of cord blood units for use in transplantation of siblings with hematologic or malignant disorders utilizing cord blood collected from healthy siblings.[128,129]

More controversial are the private, for-profit storage companies that will, for a fee, collect and store cord blood for a family. In this setting, cord blood from healthy infants is stored for the potential future use in case aplastic anemia, leukemia, or genetic defects are deteced anytime later in life. This area has been a focus of intense debate and at present has limited utility.[130–134]

### Aging CB Inventory

Many CB banks are aging. Duration of CB viability is not known and older units are at risk of accidental thaws. Banks are developing strategies to address these issues.

## FUTURE DIRECTIONS FOR CORD BLOOD TRANSPLANTATION

The major limitations of CB transplantation is the low cell number, which are insufficient for transplantation of the older child or the adult.[135] Two approaches have been explored thus far: infusion of multiple cord blood units at time of transplant and in vitro expansion of committed progenitors.

Transplanting multiple cord blood units allows early hematopoiesis with one unit ultimately becoming dominant. Early experience supports hypothesis. Murine[136] and human studies support the feasibility of multiple unit infusions.[137–140] Several human trials involving multiple cord transplants are currently taking place, however, clinical conclusions cannot yet be drawn.

It may be possible to expand CB precursor populations. McNiece and colleagues demonstrated the capacity to expand large numbers of committed progenitors with a cytokine cocktail, but no expansion of the immature progenitors.[141] When tested in clinical trial, durable engraftment was observed with very limited cell doses.[142] There are other promising expansion possibilities using antibody-based cell selections and combinations of new growth factors.[143]

Cord blood has been studied as a target for gene therapy, because of the relative ease in transferring genes into cord blood cells.[144–147] The first successful application of gene therapy involved insertion of the adenosine deaminase gene into autologous CB cells of infants affected by that form of severe combined immunodeficiency. Kohn and colleagues were able to demonstrate durable engraftment and long-term enzyme production in their patients.[148–150]

## CONCLUSION: ROLE OF CORD BLOOD

Umbilical cord blood is an alternative source of hematopoietic stem cells for related and unrelated donor allogeneic hematopoietic stem cell transplantation. At this point, its role is greatest in pediatrics. The impact of CB in adult transplantation will depend on the ability to expand cells. The choice of unrelated cord blood depends on patient age, weight, size, cord blood availability, urgency of transplant, impact of GVHD on outcome (malignant vs. nonmalignant disease), and experience of the transplant center. Importantly, cord blood currently provides a viable transplant option for those without HLA-matched adult donor options.

# REFERENCES

1. Knudtzon S. In vitro growth of granulocytic colonies from circulating cells in human cord blood. Blood 1974;43:357–361.
2. Nakahata T, Ogawa M. Hemopoietic colony-forming cells in umbilical cord blood with extensive capability to generate mono- and multipotential hemopoietic progenitors. J Clin Invest 1982;70:1324–1328.
3. Broxmeyer HE, Douglas GW, Hangoc G et al. Human umbilical cord blood as a potential source of transplantable hematopoietic stem/progenitor cells. Proc Natl Acad Sci USA 1989;86:3828–3832.
4. Gluckman E, Broxmeyer HA, Auerbach AD et al. Hematopoietic reconstitution in a patient with Fanconi's anemia by means of umbilical-cord blood from an HLA-identical sibling. N Engl J Med 1989;321:1174–1178.
5. Wagner JE, Broxmeyer HE, Byrd RL et al. Transplantation of umbilical cord blood after myeloablative therapy: analysis of engraftment. Blood 1992;79:1874–1881.
6. Barker JN, Krepski TP, DeFor TE et al. Searching for unrelated donor hematopoietic stem cells: availability and speed of umbilical cord blood versus bone marrow. Biol Blood Marrow Transplant 2002;8:257–260.
7. Beatty PG, Boucher KM, Mori M, Milford EL. Probability of finding HLA-mismatched related or unrelated marrow or cord blood donors. Hum Immunol 2000;61:834–840.
8. Confer DL. Unrelated marrow donor registries. Curr Opin Hematol 1997;4:408–412.
9. Surbek DV, Steinmann C, Burk M et al. Developmental changes in adhesion molecule expressions in umbilical cord blood CD34 hematopoietic progenitor and stem cells. Am J Obstet Gynecol 2000;183:1152–1157.
10. Wagner JE, Kurtzberg J. Allogeneic umbilical cord blood transplantation. In: Cellular Characteristics of Cord Blood and Cord Blood Transplantation, Broxmeyer HE (ed), Bethesda, MD: AABB Press, 1998:113–145.
11. Broxmeyer HE, Hangoc G, Cooper S et al. Growth characteristics and expansion of human umbilical cord blood and estimation of its potential for transplantation in adults. Proc Natl Acad Sci USA 1992;89:4109–4113.
12. Leary AG, Ogawa M. Blast cell colony assay for umbilical cord blood and adult bone marrow progenitors. Blood 1987;69:953–956.
13. Almici C, Carlo-Stella C, Wagner JE et al. Clonogenic capacity and ex vivo expansion potential of umbilical cord blood progenitor cells are not impaired by cryopreservation. Bone Marrow Transplant 1997;19:1079–1084.
14. Almici C, Carlo-Stella C, Wagner JE et al. Biologic and phenotypic analysis of early hematopoietic progenitor cells in umbilical cord blood. Leukemia 1997;11:2143–2149.
15. Traycoff CM, Abboud MR, Laver J et al. Evaluation of the in vitro behavior of phenotypically defined populations of umbilical cord blood hematopoietic progenitor cells. Exp Hematol 1994;22:215–222.
16. Payne TA, Traycoff CM, Laver J et al. Phenotypic analysis of early hematopoietic progenitors in cord blood and determination of their correlation with clonogenic progenitors: relevance to cord blood stem cell transplantation. Bone Marrow Transplant 1995;15:187–192.
17. De Bruyn C, Delforge A, Bron D et al. Comparison of the coexpression of CD38, CD33 and HLA-DR antigens on CD34+ purified cells from human cord blood and bone marrow. Stem Cells 1995;13:281–288.
18. Bender JG, Unverzagt K, Walker DE et al. Phenotypic analysis and characterization of CD34+ cells from normal human bone marrow, cord blood, peripheral blood, and mobilized peripheral blood from patients undergoing autologous stem cell transplantation. Clin Immunol Immunopathol 1994;70:10–18.
19. Wang JC, Doedens M, Dick JE. Primitive human hematopoietic cells are enriched in cord blood compared with adult bone marrow or mobilized peripheral blood as measured by the quantitative in vivo SCID-repopulating cell assay. Blood 1997;89:3919–3924.
20. Surbek DV, Holzgreve W, Jansen W et al. Quantitative immunophenotypic characterization, cryopreservation, and enrichment of second- and third-trimester human fetal cord blood hematopoietic stem cells (progenitor cells). Am J Obstet Gynecol 1998;179:1228–1233.
21. Wyrsch A, dalle Carbonare V, Jansen W et al. Umbilical cord blood from preterm human fetuses is rich in committed and primitive hematopoietic progenitors with high proliferative and self-renewal capacity. Exp Hematol 1999;27:1338–1345.
22. Haneline LS, Marshall KP, Clapp DW. The highest concentration of primitive hematopoietic progenitor cells in cord blood is found in extremely premature infants. Pediatr Res 1996;39:820–825.
23. Campagnoli C, Fisk N, Overton T et al. Circulating hematopoietic progenitor cells in first trimester fetal blood. Blood 2000;95:1967–1972.
24. Drygalski A, Xu G, Constantinescu D et al. The frequency and proliferative potential of megakaryocytic colony-forming cells (Meg-CFC) in cord blood, cytokine-mobilized peripheral blood and bone marrow, and their correlation with total CFC numbers: implications for the quantitation of Meg-CFC to predict platelet engraftment following cord blood transplantation. Bone Marrow Transplant 2000;25:1029–1034.
25. Bornstein R, Garcia-Vela J, Gilsanz F et al. Cord blood megakaryocytes do not complete maturation, as indicated by impaired establishment of endomitosis and low expression of G1/S cyclins upon thrombopoietin-induced differentiation. Br J Haematol 2001;114:458–465.

26. Alonso JM 3rd, Regan DM, Johnson CE et al. A simple and reliable procedure for cord blood banking, processing, and freezing: St Louis and Ohio Cord Blood Bank experiences. Cytotherapy 2001;3:429–433.

27. Stevens CE, Gladstone J, Taylor PE et al. Placental/umbilical cord blood for unrelated-donor bone marrow reconstitution: relevance of nucleated red blood cells. Blood 2002;100:2662–2664.

28. Armitage S, Fehily D, Dickinson A et al. Cord blood banking: volume reduction of cord blood units using a semi-automated closed system. Bone Marrow Transplant 1999;23:505–509.

29. Migliaccio AR, Adamson JW, Stevens CE et al. Cell dose and speed of engraftment in placental/umbilical cord blood transplantation: graft progenitor cell content is a better predictor than nucleated cell quantity. Blood 2000;96:2717-2722.

30. Zanjani ED, Almeida-Porada G, Ascensao JL et al. Transplantation of hematopoietic stem cells in utero. Stem Cells 1997;15:79–92; discussion 93.

31. Han P, Hodge G, Story C, Xu X. Phenotypic analysis of functional T-lymphocyte subtypes and natural killer cells in human cord blood: relevance to umbilical cord blood transplantation. Br J Haematol 1995;89:733–740.

32. Mills KC, Gross TG, Varney ML et al. Immunologic phenotype and function in human bone marrow, blood stem cells and umbilical cord blood. Bone Marrow Transplant 1996;18:53–61.

33. Theilgaard-Monch K, Raaschou-Jensen K, Palm H et al. Flow cytometric assessment of lymphocyte subsets, lymphoid progenitors, and hematopoietic stem cells in allogeneic stem cell grafts. Bone Marrow Transplant 2001;28:1073–1082.

34. Paloczi K. Immunophenotypic and functional characterization of human umbilical cord blood mononuclear cells. Leukemia 1999;13(Suppl 1):S87–S89.

35. D'Arena G, Musto P, Cascavilla N et al. Flow cytometric characterization of human umbilical cord blood lymphocytes: immunophenotypic features. Haematologica 1998;83:197–203.

36. Beck R, Lam-Po-Tang PR. Comparison of cord blood and adult blood lymphocyte normal ranges: a possible explanation for decreased severity of graft versus host disease after cord blood transplantation. Immunol Cell Biol 1994;72:440–444.

37. Keever CA. Characterization of cord blood lymphocyte subpopulations. J Hematother 1993;2:203–206.

38. Liu E, Tu W, Law HK, Lau YL. Decreased yield, phenotypic expression and function of immature monocyte-derived dendritic cells in cord blood. Br J Haematol 2001;113:240–246.

39. Paloczi K, Batai A, Gopcsa L et al. Immunophenotypic characterisation of cord blood B-lymphocytes. Bone Marrow Transplant 1998;22(Suppl 4):S89–S91.

40. Garban F, Ericson M, Roucard C et al. Detection of empty HLA class II molecules on cord blood B cells. Blood 1996;87:3970–3976.

41. Schroeder HW Jr, Zhang L, Philips JB 3rd. Slow, programmed maturation of the immunoglobulin HCDR3 repertoire during the third trimester of fetal life. Blood 2001;98:2745–2751.

42. Varis I, Deneys V, Mazzon A et al. Expression of HLA-DR, CAM and co-stimulatory molecules on cord blood monocytes. Eur J Haematol 2001;66:107–114.

43. Sorg RV, Kogler G, Wernet P. Identification of cord blood dendritic cells as an immature CD11c- population. Blood 1999;93:2302–2307.

44. Sorg RV, Kogler G, Wernet P. Functional competence of dendritic cells in human umbilical cord blood. Bone Marrow Transplant 1998;22(Suppl 1):S52–S54.

45. Sato K, Nagayama H, Takahashi TA. Generation of dendritic cells from fresh and frozen cord blood CD34+ cells. Cryobiology 1998;37:362–371.

46. Umemoto M, Azuma E, Hirayama M et al. Cytokine-enhanced mixed lymphocyte reaction (MLR) in cord blood. Clin Exp Immunol 1998;112:459–463.

47. D'Arena G, Cascavilla N, Carotenuto M. Blastogenic response of activated human umbilical cord blood T-lymphocytes. Haematologica 1998;83:1048–1050.

48. Risdon G, Gaddy J, Broxmeyer HE. Allogeneic responses of human umbilical cord blood. Blood Cells 1994;20:566–570.

49. Krampera M, Tavecchia L, Benedetti F et al. Intracellular cytokine profile of cord blood T- and NK-cells and monocytes. Haematologica 2000;85:675–679.

50. Garcia Vela JA, Delgado I, Bornstein R et al. Comparative intracellular cytokine production by in vitro stimulated T lymphocytes from human umbilical cord blood (HUCB) and adult peripheral blood (APB). Anal Cell Pathol 2000;20:93–98.

51. D'Arena G, Musto P, Cascavilla N et al. Inability of activated cord blood T lymphocytes to perform Th1-like and Th2-like responses: implications for transplantation. J Hematother Stem Cell Res 1999;8:381–385.

52. Cohen SB, Perez-Cruz I, Fallen P et al. Analysis of the cytokine production by cord and adult blood. Hum Immunol 1999;60:331–336.

53. Chalmers IM, Janossy G, Contreras M, Navarrete C. Intracellular cytokine profile of cord and adult blood lymphocytes. Blood 1998;92:11–18.

54. Qian JX, Lee SM, Suen Y et al. Decreased interleukin-15 from activated cord versus adult peripheral blood mononuclear cells and the effect of interleukin-15 in upregulating antitumor immune activity and cytokine production in cord blood. Blood 1997;90:3106–3117.

55. Nomura A, Takada H, Jin CH et al. Functional analyses of cord blood natural killer cells and T cells: a distinctive interleukin-18 response. Exp Hematol 2001;29:1169–1176.

56. Garderet L, Dulphy N, Douay C et al. The umbilical cord blood alph-abeta T-cell repertoire: characteristics of a polyclonal and naive but completely formed repertoire. Blood 1998;91:340–346.

57. Toubert A, Douay C, Chalumeau N et al. Effects of superantigenic stimulation on the cord blood alpha-beta T cell repertoire. Bone Marrow Transplant 1998;22(Suppl 1):S36–S38.

58. Wang XN, Sviland L, Ademokun AJ et al. Cellular alloreactivity of human cord blood cells detected by T-cell frequency analysis and a human skin explant model. Transplantation 1998;66:903–909.

59. Barbey C, Irion O, Helg C et al. Characterisation of the cytotoxic alloresponse of cord blood. Bone Marrow Transplant 1998;22(Suppl 1):S26–S30.

60. Deacock SJ, Schwarer AP, Bridge J et al. Evidence that umbilical cord blood contains a higher frequency of HLA class II-specific alloreactive T cells than adult peripheral blood. A limiting dilution analysis. Transplantation 1992;53:1128–1134.

61. Marcus H, Dekel B, Arditti FD et al. T cells from newborn humans are fully capable of developing into cytotoxic T lymphocyte effector cells in adoptive hosts. Transplantation 2002;73:803–810.

62. Han P, Hodge G. Intracellular cytokine production and cytokine receptor interaction of cord mononuclear cells: relevance to cord blood transplantation. Br J Haematol 1999;107:450–457.

63. Chipeta J, Komada Y, Zhang XL et al. Neonatal (cord blood) T cells can competently raise type 1 and 2 immune responses upon polyclonal activation. Cell Immunol 2000;205:110–119.

64. Yang YC, Hsu TY, Chen JY et al. Tumour necrosis factor-alpha-induced apoptosis in cord blood T lymphocytes: involvement of both tumour necrosis factor receptor types 1 and 2. Br J Haematol 2001;115:435–441.

65. Lin SJ, Wang LY, Huang YJ, Kuo ML. Effect of interleukin (IL)-12 and IL-15 on apoptosis and proliferation of umbilical cord blood mononuclear cells. Bone Marrow Transplant 2001;28:439–445.

66. Lin SJ, Chao HC, Yan DC. Phenotypic changes of T-lymphocyte subsets induced by interleukin-12 and interleukin-15 in umbilical cord vs. adult peripheral blood mononuclear cells. Pediatr Allergy Immunol 2001;12:21–26.

67. Chen BJ, Cui X, Sempowski GD et al. A comparison of murine T-cell-depleted adult bone marrow and full-term fetal blood cells in hematopoietic engraftment and immune reconstitution. Blood 2002;99:364–371.

68. Joshi SS, Tarantolo SR, Kuszynski CA, Kessinger A. Antitumor therapeutic potential of activated human umbilical cord blood cells against leukemia and breast cancer. Clin Cancer Res 2000;6:4351–4358.

69. Brahmi Z, Hommel-Berrey G, Smith F, Thomson B. NK cells recover early and mediate cytotoxicity via perforin/granzyme and Fas/FasL pathways in umbilical cord blood recipients. Hum Immunol 2001;62:782–790.

70. Umemoto M, Azuma E, Hirayama M et al. Two cytotoxic pathways of natural killer cells in human cord blood: implications in cord blood transplantation. Br J Haematol 1997;98:1037–1040.

71. Chargui J, Masao H, Yoshimura R et al. NK/cytotoxic T cells: major effector cells in GVHD after umbilical cord blood allotransplantation. Transplant Proc 2000;32:2454–2455.

72. El Marsafy S, Dosquet C, Coudert MC et al. Study of cord blood natural killer cell suppressor activity. Eur J Haematol 2001;66:215–220.

73. Rubinstein P, Dobrila L, Rosenfield RE et al. Processing and cryopreservation of placental/umbilical cord blood for unrelated bone marrow reconstitution. Proc Natl Acad Sci USA 1995;92:10119–10122.

74. Rubinstein P, Carrier C, Scaradavou A et al. Outcomes among 562 recipients of placental-blood transplants from unrelated donors. N Engl J Med 1998;339:1565–1577.

75. Kanamaru S, Kawano Y, Watanabe T et al. Low numbers of megakaryocyte progenitors in grafts of cord blood cells may result in delayed platelet recovery after cord blood cell transplant. Stem Cells 2000;18:190–195.

76. Barker JN, Davies SM, DeFor T et al. Survival after transplantation of unrelated donor umbilical cord blood is comparable to that of human leukocyte antigen-matched unrelated donor bone marrow: results of a matched-pair analysis. Blood 2001;97:2957–2961.

77. Rocha V, Cornish J, Sievers EL et al. Comparison of outcomes of unrelated bone marrow and umbilical cord blood transplants in children with acute leukemia. Blood 2001;97:2962–2971.

78. Klein AK, Patel DD, Gooding ME et al. T-cell recovery in adults and children following umbilical cord blood transplantation. Biol Blood Marrow Transplant 2001;7:454–466.

79. Rizzieri DA, Long GD, Vredenburgh JJ et al. Successful allogeneic engraftment of mismatched unrelated cord blood following a nonmyeloablative preparative regimen. Blood 2001;98:3486–3488.

80. Chao NJ, Liu CX, Rooney B et al. Nonmyeloablative regimen preserves "niches" allowing for peripheral expansion of donor T-cells. Biol Blood Marrow Transplant 2002;8:249–256.

81. Wall DA, Noffsinger JM, Mueckl KA et al. Feasibility of an obstetrician-based cord blood collection network for unrelated donor umbilical cord blood banking. J Matern Fetal Med 1997;6:320–323.

82. Haut PR, Kovarik P, Shaw PH et al. Detection of EBV DNA in the cord blood donor for a patient developing Epstein-Barr virus-associated lymphoproliferative disorder following mismatched unrelated umbilical cord blood transplantation. Bone Marrow Transplant 2001;27:761–765.

83. Sirvent N, Reviron D, de Lamballerie X, Michel G. First report of Epstein-Barr virus lymphoproliferative disease after cord blood transplantation. Bone Marrow Transplant 2000;25:120–121.

84. Ohga S, Kanaya Y, Maki H et al. Epstein-Barr virus-associated lymphoproliferative disease after a cord blood transplant for Diamond-Blackfan anemia. Bone Marrow Transplant 2000;25:209–212.

85. Barker JN, Martin PL, Coad JE et al. Low incidence of Epstein-Barr virus-associated posttransplantation lymphoproliferative disorders in 272 unrelated-donor umbilical cord blood transplant recipients. Biol Blood Marrow Transplant 2001;7:395–399.

86. Curtis RE, Travis LB, Rowlings PA et al. Risk of lymphoproliferative disorders after bone marrow transplantation: a multi-institutional study. Blood 1999;94:2208–2216.

87. Marshall NA, Howe JG, Formica R et al. Rapid reconstitution of Epstein-Barr virus-specific T lymphocytes following allogeneic stem cell transplantation. Blood 2000;96:2814–2821.

88. Moretta A, Maccario R, Fagioli F et al. Analysis of immune reconstitution in children undergoing cord blood transplantation. Exp Hematol 2001;29:371–379.

89. Locatelli F, Maccario R, Comoli P et al. Hematopoietic and immune recovery after transplantation of cord blood progenitor cells in children. Bone Marrow Transplant 1996;18:1095–1101.

90. Talvensaari K, Clave E, Douay C et al. A broad T-cell repertoire diversity and an efficient thymic function indicate a favorable long-term immune reconstitution after cord blood stem cell transplantation. Blood 2002;99:1458–1464.

91. Thomson BG, Robertson KA, Gowan D et al. Analysis of engraftment, graft-versus-host disease, and immune recovery following unrelated donor cord blood transplantation. Blood 2000;96:2703–2711.

92. Giraud P, Thuret I, Reviron D et al. Immune reconstitution and outcome after unrelated cord blood transplantation: a single paediatric institution experience. Bone Marrow Transplant 2000;25:53–57.

93. Abu-Ghosh A, Goldman S, Slone V et al. Immunological reconstitution and correlation of circulating serum inflammatory mediators/cytokines with the incidence of acute graft-versus-host disease during the first 100 days following unrelated umbilical cord blood transplantation. Bone Marrow Transplant 1999;24:535–544.

94. Knutsen AP, Wall DA. Umbilical cord blood transplantation in severe T-cell immunodeficiency disorders: two-year experience. J Clin Immunol 2000;20:466–476.

95. Kook H, Goldman F, Padley D et al. Reconstruction of the immune system after unrelated or partially matched T-cell-depleted bone marrow transplantation in children: immunophenotypic analysis and factors affecting the speed of recovery. Blood 1996;88:1089–1097.

96. Small TN, Papadopoulos EB, Boulad F et al. Comparison of immune reconstitution after unrelated and related T-cell-depleted bone marrow transplantation: effect of patient age and donor leukocyte infusions. Blood 1999;93:467–480.

97. Rocha V, Wagner JE Jr, Sobocinski KA et al. Graft-versus-host disease in children who have received a cord-blood or bone marrow transplant from an HLA-identical sibling. Eurocord and International Bone Marrow Transplant Registry Working Committee on Alternative Donor and Stem Cell Sources. N Engl J Med 2000;342:1846–1854.

98. Gluckman E, Rocha V, Boyer-Chammard A et al. Outcome of cord-blood transplantation from related and unrelated donors. Eurocord Transplant Group and the European Blood and Marrow Transplantation Group. N Engl J Med 1997;337:373–381.

99. Gluckman E, Rocha V, Chevret S. Results of unrelated umbilical cord blood hematopoietic stem cell transplantation. Rev Clin Exp Hematol 2001;5:87–99.

100. Ooi J, Iseki T, Takahashi S et al. A clinical comparison of unrelated cord blood transplantation and unrelated bone marrow transplantation for adult patients with acute leukaemia in complete remission. Br J Haematol 2002;118:140–143.

101. Rubinstein P, Adamson JW, Stevens C. The Placental/Umbilical Cord Blood Program of the New York Blood Center. A progress report. Ann N Y Acad Sci 1999;872:328–334; discussion 334–335.

102. Wagner JE, Barker JN, DeFor TE et al. Transplantation of unrelated donor umbilical cord blood in 102 patients with malignant and nonmalignant diseases: influence of CD34 cell dose and HLA disparity on treatment-related mortality and survival. Blood 2002;100:1611–1618.

103. Yu LC, Wall DA, Sandler E et al. Unrelated cord blood transplant experience by the pediatric blood and marrow transplant consortium. Pediatr Hematol Oncol 2001;18:235–245.

104. van Rood JJ, Claas F. Noninherited maternal HLA antigens: a proposal to elucidate their role in the immune response. Hum Immunol 2000;61:1390–1394.

105. van Rood JJ, Loberiza FR Jr, Zhang MJ et al. Effect of tolerance to noninherited maternal antigens on the occurrence of graft-versus-host disease after bone marrow transplantation from a parent or an HLA-haploidentical sibling. Blood 2002;99:1572–1577.

106. Weiden PL, Flournoy N, Sanders JE et al. Antileukemic effect of graft-versus-host disease contributes to improved survival after allogeneic marrow transplantation. Transplant Proc 1981;13:248–251.
107. Horowitz MM, Gale RP, Sondel PM, et al. Graft-versus-leukemia reactions after bone marrow transplantation. Blood 1990;75:555–562.
108. Harris DT. In vitro and in vivo assessment of the graft-versus-leukemia activity of cord blood. Bone Marrow Transplant 1995;15:17–23.
109. Howrey RP, Martin PL, Driscoll T et al. Graft-versus-leukemia-induced complete remission following unrelated umbilical cord blood transplantation for acute leukemia. Bone Marrow Transplant 2000;26:1251–1254.
110. Wagner JE, Kurtzberg J. Cord blood stem cells. Curr Opin Hematol 1997;4:413–418.
111. Knutsen AP, Wall DA. Kinetics of T-cell development of umbilical cord blood transplantation in severe T-cell immunodeficiency disorders. J Allergy Clin Immunol 1999;103:823–832.
112. deGasperi R, Raghavan SS, Sosa MG et al. Measurements from normal umbilical cord blood of four lysosomal enzymatic activities: alpha-L-iduronidase (Hurler), galactocerebrosidase (globoid cell leukodystrophy), arylsulfatase A (metachromatic leukodystrophy), arylsulfatase B (Maroteaux-Lamy). Bone Marrow Transplant 2000;25:541–544.
113. Collins RH Jr, Goldstein S, Giralt S et al. Donor leukocyte infusions in acute lymphocytic leukemia. Bone Marrow Transplant 2000;26:511–516.
114. Porter DL, Collins RH Jr, Hardy C, et al. Treatment of relapsed leukemia after unrelated donor marrow transplantation with unrelated donor leukocyte infusions. Blood 2000;95:1214–1221.
115. Robinson KL, Ayello J, Hughes R et al. Ex vivo expansion, maturation, and activation of umbilical cord blood-derived T lymphocytes with IL-2, IL-12, anti-CD3, and IL-7. Potential for adoptive cellular immunotherapy post-umbilical cord blood transplantation. Exp Hematol 2002;30:245–251.
116. Gluckman E. Hematopoietic stem-cell transplants using umbilical-cord blood. N Engl J Med 2001;344:1860–1861.
117. Rubinstein P, Stevens CE. The New York Blood Center's Placental/Umbilical Cord Blood Program. Experience with a 'new' source of hematopoietic stem cells for transplantation. Ernst Schering Res Found Workshop 2001;33:47–70.
118. Rubinstein P, Stevens CE. Placental blood for bone marrow replacement: the New York Blood Center's program and clinical results. Baillieres Best Pract Res Clin Haematol 2000;13:565–584.
119. Ballen K, Broxmeyer HE, McCullough J et al. Current status of cord blood banking and transplantation in the United States and Europe. Biol Blood Marrow Transplant 2001;7:635–645.
120. Menitove JE, Chambers LA, Gjertson DW et al. AABB Standards for Cord Blood Services (1st ed). Bethesda, MD: American Association of Blood Banks, 2001.
121. FACT: Standards for hematopoietic progenitor cell collection, processing, and transplantation (2nd ed). In: Founation for the Accreditation of Cellular Therapy, 2002.
122. Proposed rule: Current good tissue practices for manufacturers of human cellular and tissue-based products: inspection and enforcement (21 CFR Part 1271). Fed Regist 2001;66:1508–1559.
123. Proposed rule: Suitability determination for donors of human cellular and tissue-based products (21 CRF Parts 210, 211, 820, and 1271). Fed Regist 1999;52:696–723.
124. Harvath L. Food and Drug Administration's proposed approach to regulation of hematopoietic stem/progenitor cell products for therapeutic use. Transfus Med Rev 2000;14:104–111.
125. Gluckman E, Rocha V, Chastang CL. Umbilical cord blood hematopoietic stem cell transplantation. Eurocord-Cord Blood Transplant Group. Cancer Treat Res 1999;101:79–96.
126. Wagner JE, Kurtzberg J. Banking and transplantation of unrelated donor umbilical cord blood: status of the National Heart, Lung, and Blood Institute-sponsored trial. Transfusion 1998;38:807–809.
127. Kato S, Nishihira H, Sako M et al. Cord blood transplantation from sibling donors in Japan. Report of the national survey. Int J Hematol 1998;67:389–396.
128. Reed W, Walters M, Lubin BH. Collection of sibling donor cord blood for children with thalassemia. J Pediatr Hematol Oncol 2000;22:602–604.
129. Reed W, Smith R, Dekovic F et al. Comprehensive banking of sibling donor cord blood for children with malignant and nonmalignant disease. Blood 2003;101:351–357.
130. Harris DT. Experience in autologous and allogeneic cord blood banking. J Hematother 1996;5:123–128.
131. Sugarman J, Kaalund V, Kodish E et al. Ethical issues in umbilical cord blood banking. Working Group on Ethical Issues in Umbilical Cord Blood Banking. JAMA 1997;278:938–943.
132. Fernandez MN. Eurocord position on ethical and legal issues involved in cord blood transplantation. Bone Marrow Transplant 1998;22(Suppl 1):S84–S85.
133. Cord blood banking for potential future transplantation: subject review. American Academy of Pediatrics. Work Group on Cord Blood Banking. Pediatrics 1999;104:116–118.
134. Fisher CA, McGrath MB, Cannon ME. Related and autologous cord blood banking. In: Cellular Characteristics of Cord Blood and Cord Blood Transplantation, Broxmeyer HA (ed). Bethesda, MD: AABB Press, 1998:199–216.

135. Laughlin MJ, Barker J, Bambach B et al. Hematopoietic engraftment and survival in adult recipients of umbilical-cord blood from unrelated donors. N Engl J Med 2001;344:1815–1822.
136. Chen BJ, Cui X, Chao NJ. Addition of a second, different allogeneic graft accelerates white cell and platelet engraftment after T-cell-depleted bone marrow transplantation. Blood 2002;99:2235–2240.
137. Fernandez MN, Regidor C, Cabrera R et al. Cord blood transplants: early recovery of neutrophils from co-transplanted sibling haploidentical progenitor cells and lack of engraftment of cultured cord blood cells, as ascertained by analysis of DNA polymorphisms. Bone Marrow Transplant 2001;28:355–363.
138. Barker JN, Weisdorf DJ, Wagner JE. Creation of a double chimera after the transplantation of umbilical-cord blood from two partially matched unrelated donors. N Engl J Med 2001;344:1870–1871.
139. Kogler G, Nurnberger W, Fischer J et al. Simultaneous cord blood transplantation of ex vivo expanded together with non-expanded cells for high risk leukemia. Bone Marrow Transplant 1999;24:397–403.
140. Shen BJ, Hou HS, Zhang HQ, Sui XW. Unrelated, HLA-mismatched multiple human umbilical cord blood transfusion in four cases with advanced solid tumors: initial studies. Blood Cells 1994;20:285–292.
141. McNiece IK, Almeida-Porada G, Shpall EJ, Zanjani E. Ex vivo expanded cord blood cells provide rapid engraftment in fetal sheep but lack long-term engrafting potential. Exp Hematol 2002;30:612–616.
142. Shpall EJ, Quinones R, Giller R et al. Transplantation of ex vivo expanded cord blood. Biol Blood Marrow Transplant 2002;8:368–376.
143. Liu J, Li K, Yuen PM et al. Ex vivo expansion of enriched CD34+ cells from neonatal blood in the presence of thrombopoietin, a comparison with cord blood and bone marrow. Bone Marrow Transplant 1999;24:247–252.
144. Oki M, Ando K, Hagihara M et al. Efficient lentiviral transduction of human cord blood CD34(+) cells followed by their expansion and differentiation into dendritic cells. Exp Hematol 2001;29:1210–1217.
145. Wu MH, Smith SL, Dolan ME. High efficiency electroporation of human umbilical cord blood CD34+ hematopoietic precursor cells. Stem Cells 2001;19:492–499.
146. Woods NB, Mikkola H, Nilsson E et al. Lentiviral-mediated gene transfer into haematopoietic stem cells. J Intern Med 2001;249:339–343.
147. Sonderbye L, Feng S, Yacoubian S et al. In vivo and in vitro modulation of immune stimulatory capacity of primary dendritic cells by adenovirus-mediated gene transduction. Exp Clin Immunogenet 1998;15:100–111.
148. Kohn DB. Adenosine deaminase gene therapy protocol revisited. Mol Ther 2002;5:96–97.
149. Kohn DB, Hershfield MS, Carbonaro D et al. T lymphocytes with a normal ADA gene accumulate after transplantation of transduced autologous umbilical cord blood CD34+ cells in ADA-deficient SCID neonates. Nat Med 1998;4:775–780.
150. Kohn DB, Weinberg KI, Nolta JA et al. Engraftment of gene-modified umbilical cord blood cells in neonates with adenosine deaminase deficiency. Nat Med 1995;1:1017–1023.

# CHAPTER XX

# Ex Vivo Expansion of Hematopoietic Stem Cells

PETER H. SHAW AND SETH J. COREY

Delayed and failed engraftment remain important causes of morbidity and mortality in pediatric stem cell transplantation. However, overall engraftment rates have been improved with the infusion of larger doses of mononuclear cells (MNC) and CD34+ stem cells per kilogram of body weight.[1-3] In smaller pediatric patients and when bone marrow (BM) or granulocyte-colony stimulating factor (G-CSF)-mobilized peripheral blood (PB) is the cell source, sufficient cell dose is rarely a cause of engraftment failure.

Over the last ten years, with the increase in the use of umbilical cord blood (UCB) in pediatric and adult stem cell transplantation as an alternative stem cell source, engraftment delay and failure is more prevalent. UCB is now being used more frequently as a hematopoietic stem cell source for a variety of malignant and nonmalignant conditions with success.[4-6] It is a good stem cell option for several reasons: it is more rapidly available than unrelated bone marrow and there is a lower incidence of acute, chronic, and severe graft-versus-host disease (GVHD)[4-6] even with less than a 6 of 6 HLA (Human Leukocyte Antigen) match. Its major drawback is that even with a cell dose sufficient to engraft, patients have delayed platelet and neutrophil engraftment when compared to BM and PB recipients.[4-6] In the largest published unrelated cord blood transplant series the median time to neutrophil engraftment, as defined by an absolute neutrophil count of $500/\mu l$ for three consecutive days, occurred at day 28 for the 81% of UCB recipients who engrafted by 42 days. Platelet engraftment, as defined by a count of $50,000/\mu l$ on seven successive days, was more markedly delayed, with a median time of approximately 90 days for UCB recipients at a rate of 85% at 180 days.[4]

In transplanting larger children (>40 kg) and adolescents, the stem cell dose of an UCB unit can be inadequate. Ex vivo expansion can allow wider use of UCB in patients where cell dose was previously a limiting factor. Several other strategies have been pursued to address this cell dose inadequacy, but this chapter will primarily focus on the expansion of stem cells and discuss other novel approaches in the last section. Not limited to UCB stem cells, ex vivo expansion has been found to increase the MNC and CD34+ cell dose in peripheral blood, and consequently quickens engraftment while not decreasing its overall success rate.[7,8] Enrichment of specific cell populations in addition to stem cells, such as megakaryocyte (MK) precursors, T cell progenitors, and B cell progenitors, is now possible and may be able to specifically accelerate platelet engraftment[9,10] and immune reconstitution, respectively.

Since hematopoiesis occurs in an intricate microenvironment of stem cells, fibroblasts, lymphocytes, and blood vessels with growth factors and stromal factors, ex vivo manipulation of stem cells requires considerable technological development. As in any biological system, it is impossible to perfectly mimic the milieu in which blood stem cells proliferate and differentiate. Temperature, pH, blood flow, intercellular interactions, known and unknown cytokines in specific concentrations, the extracellular matrix of glycosaminoglycans, and stromal cells all play important roles in guiding pluripotent stem cells into mature hematopoietic elements. Furthermore, the regenerative and expansive qualities of the cultured hematopoietic progenitor cell are variable and will change during the course of ex vivo manipulation. Many researchers have performed ex vivo expansion experiments with UCB, BM, and PB with a variety of cytokines in a variety of conditions, all with varying results.

## MOUSE MODELS

Basic research on murine hematopoiesis has revealed features of hematopoietic stem cells that have paved the way for expansion trials in humans. As a precursor to human trials, the use of ex vivo expanded hematopoietic human stem cells in mouse transplant models has proven its safety and efficacy. Serial transplants have established the self-renewal capacity of blood stem cells in mice.[11] Ratajczak and colleagues found that marrow cells primed with thrombopoietin (TPO), interleukin-3 (IL-3), stem cell factor (SCF), and IL-1α formed colonies in vitro faster than unprimed cells. Mice transplanted with marrow, 1/10th of which had been treated with the same cytokines prior to cryopreservation, had platelet and neutrophil recovery three to five days earlier than those that received unmanipulated marrow.[12] Schipper et al. transplanted nonobese diabetic severe combined immune deficiency (NOD-SCID) mice with human UCB incubated with TPO and unmanipulated human UCB. Mice that received the incubated cells had first signs of platelet recovery at three days and a plateau at 19 days versus 10 and 40 days for mice that received unmanipulated UCB.[13] Drygalski et al. compared the ex vivo expansion and mouse engraftment potential of the human cells incubated with TPO, Flt3 ligand (Flt3L), IL-3, and SCF versus IL-11, Flt3L, IL-3, and SCF. Their group found that the former combination had significantly better colony-forming cell (CFC) expansion than the latter, which correlated to faster platelet engraftment.[14] Lastly, Piacibello's group demonstrated one of the most essential aspects of ex vivo expanded cord blood in murine transplant recipients: its repopulating and self-renewal capacity, even after six weeks in culture.[11]

Fibbe et al. took a novel and promising approach by priming donor stem cells in vivo. Donor mice were treated with TPO intraperitoneally for five days prior to BM harvesting. These mice had an impressive thrombocytosis and more CFCs in their marrow than controls when harvested. This marrow was transplanted into lethally irradiated mice, and when compared to controls, the recipients had significantly faster platelet recovery and higher platelet nadirs. There was comparable enhancement in erythrocyte engraftment.[15] This work led to a comprehensive review of the subject, which concluded that such a strategy, as well as, ex vivo expansion, were both effective at enhancing engraftment in mice.[16]

# EX VIVO EXPANSION EXPERIMENTS
# ON HUMAN HEMATOPOIETIC STEM CELLS

The critical components of any ex vivo expansion approach include: the hematopoietic stem cell, growth medium and cytokines, stroma or scaffolding properties, length of time in culture, and biophysical variables such as oxygen tension and pH. The composition of the starting cell population is an important aspect of such expansion experiments, whether the source is UCB, PB, or BM. Ideally cells should be fresh, but in the case of PB and UCB, they are usually frozen then thawed at the time of expansion. Fortunately frozen hematopoietic stem cells retain their proliferative and differentiating capacity after freezing and thawing. A population enriched for CD34+ cells demonstrates more proliferative potential than an unselected cell population.[17] CD34+ cells can be positively selected and purified on small and large scales using immunomagnetic beads[18-20] for both experimental and clinical expansion, respectively.

Clinical ex vivo expansion may be either allogeneic or autologous. For autologous transplantation, the recipient may have poor bone marrow capacity due to poor stem cell regeneration and/or stromal injury, resulting in poor mobilization and a consequent inadequate stem cell harvest. Autologous transplantation also may be complicated by the presence of tumor cells, which can be expanded ex vivo with growth factor support. A theoretical, but clinically unproven advantage of CD34+ selection in the autologous setting is the purging of these tumor cells. The major drawback of such selection is the loss of total nucleated and CD34+ cells. Accordingly, several researchers have performed successful small and large-scale ex vivo expansion on unselected hematopoietic stem cells.[7,21,22] Currently, CD34-selected cells are used more frequently because of their excellent proliferative capacity.

Whether selected or unselected cells are used, cell seeding density is an important component of the culture system. If the seeding density is too high, the cells will deplete all of the nutrients and cytokines in the media and start to die. Waste products accumulate and the environment becomes more acidic. In addition, too much intercellular contact can lead to contact inhibition and growth arrest. To dilute a culture may compromise the intercellular interactions that need to occur in cell growth and differentiation. When cell density was greater than $1 \times 10^6$ CD34+ cells/ml of media cell death increased considerably.[23] Most researchers therefore start with approximately 1 to $2 \times 10^4$ CD34+ UCB cells/ml,[10,11,24] $5 \times 10^4$ CD34+ BM cells/ml,[11,23,25] and 2 to $5 \times 10^4$ CD34+ PB cells/ml.[26] Unselected hematopoietic cells have been cultured at a density of 1 to $3 \times 10^6$ MNC/ml by Paquette et al.[7] and Naparstek et al.[22] in their clinical trials.

The next essential component in mimicking the marrow environment in guiding expansion is the growth medium. From extensive work in both the liquid and semi-solid phases, it appears that a serum-free medium leads to greater cell proliferation.[24,27] This probably is due to the fact that serum contains inhibitory factors in serum that hinder rapid cell division (i.e., TGF-$\beta$, Interferons, etc.). Concerns about regulatory rules have eliminated the use of animal serum and have favored the development of defined medium. In addition, cultures in the liquid phase, whether in wells, culture dish, culture flask, or in a gas-permeable closed bag, have greater potential for overall expansion than collagen-based and other semi-solid media.[24]

Ex vivo expansion experiments have been performed in stromal cell-containing cultures as well with some success,[28–31] but there is evidence that stroma maintains hematopoietic cells in an undifferentiated state by direct inhibition.[32] Stromal cells therefore seem to maintain stem cells' long-term repopulating ability but hinder large-scale expansion, although the topic is controversial. The use of stromal cells in cell expansion is more physiological and may enhance intercellular interactions, which play a partially-understood role in the growth and production of blood cells. However, this is not essential because ex vivo expansion can produce cell clusters and colonies, both on the floor of the vessel and free-floating in the media of matrix-free liquid culture. In human pre-clinical expansion experiments, liquid culture in serum-free media continues to be the preferred method, although the use of stromal cells in large-scale cultures may yet prove to be more effective. The contribution of mesenchymal cells in facilitating engraftment is being tested in multiple transplant centers.

The next important variable of ex vivo expansion is establishing how many days in culture are required to achieve a peak in cell proliferation. Many laboratories have cultured cells in a static system for 7 to 14 days, with most agreeing that the maximum expansion of progenitors occurs at days 10 to 12.[10,11,33,34] After that, there is a decrease in proliferative capacity and increased senescence.[10,27,35] Static systems are the most easily maintained. In experiments where re-feeding of cytokines and refreshing of media occurs, cell cultures can be maintained for weeks without significant cell death occurring,[23] including many long-term culture-initiating cells (LT-CICs), but it is unclear if the there is a clinical advantage to this approach.

The incubator temperature and gaseous environment for ex vivo expansion have been typically set at 37°C with 21% $O_2$, 5% $CO_2$ and >95% humidity. However, oxygen tension has a profound effect on maturation and proliferation of hematopoietic stem cells. Mostafa and colleagues examined its specific effects on megakaryocytopoiesis. They selected PB and BM cells for CD34 expression and grew them in recombinant human cytokines at two different $O_2$ concentrations: 5% and 20%. By day 15, the cells grown in 20% oxygen had significantly more CD41(gpIIbIIIa)+ cell expansion and higher ploidy, indicative of more maturation. Cells grown in 5% $O_2$ had a greater number of megakaryocyte colony-forming units (CFU-Mks). Changing the $O_2$ from 20% to 5% at days 5 and 7 led to similar delayed megakaryocyte maturation.[36] This may be explained physiologically in that oxygen tension is lower in the marrow, the primary site of early megakaryocytic development, than the peripheral circulation (most notably the pulmonary vessels). Likewise other researchers have found that more physiologic oxygen tensions enhance colony-forming units of other cell lines as well.[37,38] LaIuppa et al. also found that $O_2$ concentration has a profound effect on cytokine-mediated proliferation and differentiation in culture.[39] To date, no researcher has studied the effects of physiological $O_2$ tension on clinical-scale expansion, but such environmental alteration will probably have comparable effects.

The choice of exogenous cytokines to be used is most crucial for ex vivo expansion experiments. While no ideal cytokine or cytokine combination has been established for expanding all hematopoietic cell lines, a significant amount of research has been performed to define the best combination to drive the proliferation and differentiation of stem cells and specific cell lines. In expanding stem and early progenitor cells, it is most logical and effective to use established early-acting cytokines including SCF,[40–43] IL-3,[40–42] and Flt3L.[40–44] These cytokines prove to be synergistic with each other and other later-acting cytokines.

Some controversy exists regarding IL-3's influence on the ability of ex vivo manipulated cells to form LTC-ICs in vitro and home to the marrow space in vivo,[45] although most published data show no negative effects.[46–48] IL-6 and IL-11 have been used extensively as well in different combinations, but they tend to result in more terminal differentiation of cell lines, which is not desirable in the transplant setting.[49–51]

If a more lineage-specific expansion for transplantation is required, other cytokine combinations have been tested. For example, B cell precursors have been grown from CD34+ UCB cells in IL-10, IL-4, Flt3L, and IL-2. These cells developed normal function and had normal marrow reconstituting ability.[52] To enrich a stem cell product for myeloid progenitors, G-CSF and granulocyte-macrophage-colony stimulating factor (GM-CSF) have been used in various combinations of cytokines.[26,33,34,53,54] Such a strategy would be effective if neutrophil engraftment was the investigator's goal. Expansion of megakaryocytic precursors is being widely investigated to address the issue of delayed platelet engraftment. TPO and megakaryocyte growth and development factor (MGDF), a slightly modified form of TPO, are potent and platelet-specific[55] and in various combinations with SCF, IL-3, and Flt3L result in excellent expansion of megakaryocyte precursors,[24,36,56,57] which have been correlated with platelet engraftment in the clinical setting.[9,10,58] Erythropoietin (Epo) in combination with early-acting cytokines is a potent stimulant for erythroid progenitor expansion. It can override the influence of other lineage-specific cytokines, even at small concentrations,[24] but erythroid engraftment is the least troublesome of the three cell lines examined in the transplant setting. Therefore, its use in clinical ex vivo expansion is unclear. Prior to instituting any combination in a clinical trial, it is important to document all cell lines expanded, as the inadvertent proliferation of T cell subsets may increase the severity of GVHD in cell recipients.

In summary, the cytokine combination can be tailored to the clinical requirement, but whether it is specific cell lines or stem cells, SCF, Flt3L, and IL-3 should be included in the "cocktail." The cells ideally should be CD34-selected while maximizing the yield. The cell expansion should be performed in a closed system (thus far, static systems have shown superior results to refeeding systems) in a serum-free liquid medium and infused after 10 to 12 days in culture. Prior to infusion into a patient, the cells should be washed to remove remnants of cytokines and the medium for both medical and regulatory purposes.

# HUMAN CLINICAL TRIALS — CHILDREN AND ADULTS

Ex vivo hematopoietic cell expansion would be of little use to stem cell transplantation physicians if it could not be used consistently to enhance short- and long-term engraftment in their patients. Bertolini and colleagues were one of the first groups to report the safety and efficacy of this strategy in human subjects. They incubated autologous PBSCs of 10 adult solid tumor patients for one week with SCF, TPO, IL-3, IL-6, IL-11, Flt3L, and macrophage inflammatory protein-alpha (MIFP-α) prior to infusion after high-dose chemotherapy for various solid tumors. Patients required less platelet transfusions than historical controls and two did not require any platelet support.[59]

Some researchers have used closed automated systems (referred to as "bioreactors" or "perfusion cultures") that replenish the growth media and cytokines periodically. While devices such as Aastrom's Replicell™ System have proved safe for transplant recipients, thus far their expansion capabilities have been unimpressive in their ability to improve engraftment kinetics.[60-62] On the other hand, closed, static systems involving gas-permeable Teflon™-coated bags have resulted in good clinical expansion of stem cells that have shown promising early results in the UCB setting. In 37 UCB transplant recipients (12 children and 25 adults), Shpall and colleagues infused an unexpanded aliquot of UCB at day 0 and then gave a boost at day 10 with the remaining cells, which were CD34-selected and cultured in a static system containing recombinant human (rh)SCF, rhG-CSF, and rhMGDF. They documented a median 111-fold expansion of total nucleated cells and a four-fold expansion of CD34+ cells. Clinically, this resulted in a median time to an absolute neutrophil count (ANC) greater than 500/$\mu$lof 28 days (range 15 to 49) days (35 days for adult and 25 days for pediatric patients; $P = .0774$) and a median time to platelets > 20,000/$\mu$l of 113 days (range 38 to 345; 261 days for adult and 58 days for pediatric patients; $P = .0008$).[63] In this small series, the pediatric population had statistically faster engraftment, possibly due to their smaller stem cell requirement.

Using a similar static closed-bag system as Shpall, several other researchers reported encouraging results as well. McNiece et al., who work closely with Shpall, likewise documented the safety of expanding CD34-selected PBSCs for 10 days in SCF, G-CSF, and MGDF in a closed-bag static serum-free system, washing them in phosphate-buffered saline (PBS) and reinfusing them into breast cancer patients at day 0 of transplant. They then infused unexpanded cells on day +1 of transplant. Patients who received expanded cells had neutrophil engraftment at a median of 6 (range 4 to 14 days) versus 9 (range 7 to 24 days) days in historical controls.[26] No effect on platelet engraftment was seen. However, Naparstek et al. noted a hastened platelet recovery in 20 adult leukemic bone marrow transplant recipients who received an aliquot of unmanipulated marrow on day 0 and the rest after short-term (3-day) incubation with IL-3 and GM-CSF. Patients receiving the incubated cells had significantly faster platelet recovery and shorter hospital stays when compared with the control subjects. The platelet count reached greater than 25,000/$\mu$l at a median of day 17.[22] Paquette et al. infused ex vivo expanded (SCF, MGDF, and G-CSF) PBSCs into 24 adult breast cancer patients after high-dose chemotherapy and reported that they had statistically faster neutrophil and platelet engraftment than 48 historical controls. There was no increased incidence of posttransplantation complications seen in these patients.[7] ► Table 20.1 summarizes the results of pediatric and adult clinical trials using ex vivo expansion in stem cell transplantation compared to internal and historical controls, and illustrates that this technique can lead to faster engraftment of platelets and neutrophils, especially in smaller patients.

With an overall smaller body mass and therefore smaller cell dose needed overall, pediatric stem cell transplant patients would seem to benefit most from efficient ex vivo expansion strategies. This concept is supported by the preliminary data presented by Shpall's group.[64] The ideal approach seems to be the expansion of an aliquot of selected cells and the simultaneous infusion of these with unselected cells at day 0 of the transplant. This had been difficult previously with UCB frozen in a single bag, but will be feasible with the relatively recent introduction of compartmentalized bags. In the future there needs to be multi-institutional ex vivo expansion trials in both children and adults for an increased patient accrual to allow for more statistical power in assessing whether there is a true difference in both short- and long-term neutrophil and platelet engraftment. Expansion techniques need to be improved for consistent, successful applicability to the adult patient population.

| | | | | Median Time to ANC > 500/μL | Median Time to Platelets > 20,000/μL |
|---|---|---|---|---|---|
| Series | Patient Population | Number of Patients | Stem Cell Source | (days) | (days) |
| Rubinstein et al.[4] | Pediatric and Adult | 562 | UCB | 42 | 95 |
| Wagner et al.[70] | Pediatric and Adult | 92 | UCB | 24 | 86# |
| Shpall et al.[63] | Pediatric | 12 | Ex vivo UCB | 25 | 58 |
| | Adult | 25 | Ex vivo UCB | 35 | 261 |
| | Pediatric and Adult (total) | 37 | Ex vivo UCB | 28 | 93 |
| Paquette et al.[7] | Adult | 48 | PB | 9 | 10 |
| | Adult | 24 | Ex vivo PB | 7& | 9& |
| McNiece et al.[26] | Adult | 175 | PB | 9 | N.R. |
| | Adult | 12 | Ex vivo PB | 6 | N.R. |
| Naparstek et al.[22] | Adult | 40 | Allo-BM | N.R.* | 23 |
| | Adult | 20 | Ex vivo Allo-BM | N.R.* | 17 |
| Engelhardt et al.[60] | Adult | 10 | Ex vivo Auto-BM | 17 | 28 |

**TABLE 20.1 Ex Vivo Expansion Clinical Trials and Historical Controls**

Abbreviations: UCB = umbilical cord blood; Allo-BM = allogeneic bone marrow; Auto-BM = autologous bone marrow; PB = autologous peripheral blood stem cells; N.R. = not reported. Symbols: * = no statistically significant difference between expanded and unexpanded sources; # = platelet engraftment documented at 50,000/μL; & = differences between expanded and unexpanded sources statistically significant.

## NEW DIRECTIONS

The future use of ex vivo expansion will be based on three indications: expansion of UCB as an alternative source of allogeneic stem cells, expansion of genetically corrected autologous stem cells, and expansion of a stem cells and selective cell types in allogeneic or autologous transplants. Because of medical urgency to transplant a patient with recurrent leukemia, a lower risk of viral transmission, and decreased incidence of graft-versus-host disease, UCB provides an attractive source. Greater banking of UCB is clearly needed, as only 30,000 units have been collected worldwide. A larger network of cord blood banks will permit greater ease in finding a donor that closely approximates a complicated HLA match. Until UCB can be safely, quickly, and effectively expanded, its use in adult stem cell transplantation will remain limited. As described here, using custom cytokine combinations and environmental manipulations, specific cell types such as cytotoxic lymphocytes, dendritic cells, or megakaryocytes probably will serve as the most common targets for cell line-specific expansion.

Because the manipulation of cytokine combinations, stromal components, and culture facilities has met with limited success thus far, newer strategies to expand ex vivo stem cells are being developed. Basic research into the biology and transcriptional profile of the hematopoietic stem cell (HSC) may translate into their being genetically engineered to achieve better expansion. The finding of telomerase shortening has suggested mechanisms for stem cell senescence, which must be prevented to achieve a better stem cell product.

Identification of Notch as a signaling pathway in hematopoietic stem cells that inhibits differentiation has been used to expand stem cells.[65]

There are presently several alternate approaches to ex vivo expansion being investigated to aid speed and rate of engraftment. Fibbe et al., in work discussed earlier, demonstrated the effectiveness in a murine model of in vivo expansion of platelet precursors in the donor prior to harvesting.[15] The donor mice were pretreated with TPO in their experiment, which was not FDA approved in 2002. If this cytokine was approved, it would be worthwhile to test this hypothesis in allogeneic human transplantation. In addition, TPO also conceivably could hasten platelet engraftment when given to the recipient after transplant with other cytokines, such as G- and GM-CSF. Unfortunately, the development of TPO and other cytokines for clinical use has not been progressing rapidly since the approval of these latter two recombinant human cytokines.

There also has been work in murine models where UCB transplant recipients were given all-*trans* retinoic acid from day −2 to day +2 and were found to have both up-regulation of intercellular adhesion molecule-1 (ICAM-1) expression and increased engraftment rates versus controls.[66] This oral medication is well tolerated in humans and its use merits further investigation in the transplant setting. One newer strategy does not expand UCB stem cells per se, but rather attempts to overcome the problem of cell dose by transplanting patients with multiple cord blood units simultaneously. This has been used in a mouse model[67] and several case reports and small adult series with some evidence of early mixed chimerism, but no evidence of improved clinical outcome.[68-70]

Several of the new strategies described in this last section seem promising in the pursuit to decrease the morbidity and mortality in the stem cell transplant setting, but there is still unrealized potential in the use of ex vivo expanded hematopoietic stem cells that will only be fully realized through rigorous preclinical and clinical investigations.

## ACKNOWLEDGMENTS

This work is supported by grants from Children's Oncology Group (P.S.), Children's Hospital of Pittsburgh (P.S., S.C.), Pittsburgh Foundation (S.C.), Pittsburgh Tissue Engineering Initiative (S.C.), and the National Institutes of Health (S.C).

# REFERENCES

1. Shpall EJ, Camplin R, Glaspy JA. Effect of CD34+ peripheral blood progenitor cell dose on hematopoietic recovery. Biol Blood Marrow Transplant 1998;4:84–92.
2. Pecora AL. Progress in clinical application of use of progenitor cells expanded with hematopoietic growth factors. Curr Opin Hematol 2001;8:142–148.
3. Kletzel M, Haut PR, Olszewski M, Figuerres E. Analysis of parameters affecting engraftment in children undergoing allogeneic BM transplants. Cytotherapy 1999;1:417–422.
4. Rubinstein P, Carrier C, Scaradavou A et al. Outcomes among 562 recipients of placental blood transplants from unrelated donors. N Engl J Med 1998;339:1565–1577.
5. Kurtzberg J, Laughlin M, Graham ML et al. Placental blood as a source of hematopoietic stem cells for transplantation into unrelated recipients. N Engl J Med 1996;335:157–166.
6. Gluckman E, Rocha V, Boyer-Chammard A et al. Outcome of cord-blood transplantation from related and unrelated donors. Eurocord Transplant Group and the European Blood and Marrow Transplantation Group. N Engl J Med 1997;337:373–381.
7. Paquette RL, Dergham ST, Karpff E et al. Ex vivo expanded unselected peripheral blood: progenitor cells reduce posttransplant neutropenia, thrombocytopenia, and anemia in patients with breast cancer. Blood 2000;96:2385–2390.
8. Bertolini F, Battaglia M, Pedrazzoli P et al. Megakaryocytic progenitors can be generated ex vivo and safely administered to autologous peripheral blood progenitor cell transplant recipients. Blood 1997;89:2679–2688.
9. Feng R, Shimazaki C, Inaba T et al. CD34+/CD41a+ cells best predict platelet recovery after autologous peripheral blood stem cell transplantation. Bone Marrow Transplant 1998;21:1217–1222.
10. Dercksen MW, Rodenhuis S, Dirkson MK et al. Subsets of CD34+ cells and rapid hematopoietic recovery after peripheral-blood stem-cell transplantation. J Clin Oncol 1995;13:1922–1932.
11. Piacibello W, Sanavio F, Severino A et al. Engraftment in nonobese diabetic severe combined immune deficiency mice of human CD34+ cord blood cells after ex vivo expansion: evidence for amplification and self-renewal of repopulating stem cells. Blood 1999;93:3736–3749.
12. Ratajczak MZ, Ratajczak J, Machalinski B et al. In vitro and in vivo evidence that ex vivo cytokine priming of donor marrow cells may ameliorate posttransplant thrombocytopenia. Blood 1998;91:353–359.
13. Schipper LF, Reniers NCM, Brand A, Fibbe WE. In-vivo thrombopoietic capacity of ex-vivo expanded human megakaryocytes from cord blood in NOD-SCID mice (Abstr #2548). Blood 1999;94(10 part 1):571a.
14. Drygalski A, Savatski LL, Eastwood D et al. The rate of platelet (PLT) and leukocyte (WBC) recovery and percent donor engraftment in mice transplanted with ex vivo-expanded marrow cells are differentially affected by the cytokine combination used (Abstr #3296). Blood 2000;96(11 part 1):762a.
15. Fibbe WE, Heemskerk DPM, Laterveer L et al. Accelerated reconstitution of platelets and erythrocytes after syngeneic transplantation of bone marrow cells derived from thrombopoietin pretreated mice. Blood 1995;86:3308–3313.
16. Fibbe WE, Noort WA, Schipper F, Willemze R. Ex vivo expansion and engraftment potential of cord blood-derived CD34+ cells in NOD/SCID mice. Ann N Y Acad Sci 2001;938:9–17.
17. Briddell RA, Kern BP, Zilm KL et al. Purification of CD34+ cells is essential for optimal ex vivo expansion of umbilical cord blood cells. J Hematother 1997;6:145–150.
18. Miltenyi S, Muller W, Weichel W, Radbruch A. High-gradient magnetic cell separation with MACS. Cytometry 1990;11:231–238.
19. Hildebrandt M, Serke S, Meyer O et al. Immunomagnetic selection of CD34+ cells: factors influencing component purity and yield. Transfusion 2000;40:507–512.
20. Martin-Henao GA, Picon M, Amill B et al. Isolation of CD34+ progenitor cells from peripheral blood by use of an automated immunomagnetic selection system: factors affecting the results. Transfusion 2000;40:35–43.
21. McNiece IK, Harrington JA, James RI et al. Ex vivo expansion of CB cells without CD34+ selection using co-culture on MSC (Abstr #3537). Blood 2001;98(11 part 1):851a.
22. Naparstek E, Hardan Y, Ben-Shahar M et al. Enhanced marrow recovery by short preincubation of marrow allografts with human recombinant interleukin-3 and granulocyte-macrophage colony-stimulating factor. Blood 1992;80:1673–1678.
23. Douay L. Experimental culture conditions are critical for ex vivo expansion of hematopoietic stem cells. J Hematother Stem Cell Res 2001;10:341–346.
24. Shaw PH, Olszewski M, Kletzel M. Expansion of megakaryocyte precursors and stem cells from umbilical cord blood CD34+ cells in collagen and liquid culture media. J Hematother Stem Cell Res 2001;10:391–403.
25. Ladd AC, Pyatt R, Gothot A et al. Orderly process of sequential cytokine stimulation is required for activation and maximal proliferation of primitive human bone marrow CD34+ hematopoietic progenitor cells residing in G0. Blood 1997;90:658–668.
26. McNiece I, Jones R, Cagnoni P et al. Ex-vivo expansion of hematopoietic progenitor cells: preliminary results in breast cancer. Hematol Cell Ther 1999;41:82–86.

27. Poloni A, Giarratana MC, Kobari L et al. The ex vivo expansion capacity of normal human bone marrow cells is dependent on experimental conditions: role of the cell concentration, serum and CD34+ cell selection in stroma-free cultures. Hematol Cell Ther 1997;39:49–58.

28. Kanai M, Hirayama F, Yamaguchi M et al. Stroma cell-dependent ex vivo expansion of human cord blood progenitors and augmentation of transplantable cell activity. Bone Marrow Transplant 2000;26:837–844.

29. Liesveld JL, Martin BA, Harbol AW et al. Effect of stromal cell coculture on progenitor cell expansion and myeloid effector function in vitro. J Hematother 1998;7:127–139.

30. Tsuji T, Nishimura-Morita Y, Watanabe Y et al. A murine stromal cell line promotes the expansion of CD34high+-primitive progenitor cells isolated from human umbilical cord blood in combination with human cytokines. Growth Factors 1999;16:225–240.

31. Breems DA, Blocklande AW, Cybell KE et al. Stromal contact prevents loss of hematopoietic stem cell quality during ex vivo expansion of CD34+ mobilized peripheral blood stem cells. Blood 1998;91:111–117.

32. Goldfarb AN, Delehanty LL, Wang D et al. Stromal inhibition of megakaryocytic differentiation correlates with blockade of signaling by protein kinase C-ε and ER/MAPK. J Biol Chem 2001;276:29526–29530.

33. Kobari L, Giarratana MC, Poloni A et al. Flt3 ligand, MGDF, Epo and G-CSF enhance ex-vivo expansion of hematopoietic cell compartments in the presence of SCF, IL-3 and IL-6. Bone Marrow Transplant 1998;21:759–767.

34. Haylock DN, To LB, Dowse TL et al. Ex vivo expansion and maturation of peripheral blood CD34+ cells into myeloid lineage. Blood 1992;80:1405–1412.

35. Bregni M, Magni M, Siena S et al. Human peripheral blood hematopoietic progenitors are optimal targets of retroviral-mediated gene transfer. Blood 1992;80:1418–1422.

36. Mostafa SS, Miller WM, Papoutsakis ET. Oxygen tension influences the differentiation, maturation and apoptosis of human megakaryocytes. Br J Haematol 2000;111:879–889.

37. Ishikawa Y, Ito T. Kinetics of hemopoietic stem cells in a hypoxic culture. Eur J Haematol 1988;40:126–129.

38. Maeda H, Hotta T, Yamada H. Enhanced colony formation of human hemopoietic stem cells in reduced oxygen tension. Exp Hematol 1986;14:930–934.

39. LaIuppa JA, Papoutsakis ET, Miller WM. Oxygen tension alters the effects of cytokines on the megakaryocyte, erythrocyte, and granulocyte lineages. Exp Hematol 1998;26:835–843.

40. Warren MK, Rose WL, Beall LD, Cone J. CD34+ cell expansion and expression of lineage markers during liquid culture of human progenitor cells. Stem Cells 1995;13:167–174.

41. Kogler G, Callejas J, Sorg RV et al. The effect of different thawing methods, growth factor combinations and media on the ex vivo expansion of umbilical cord blood primitive and committed progenitors. Bone Marrow Transplant 1998;21:233–241.

42. Ohmizono Y, Skabe H, Kimura T et al. Thrombopoietin augments ex vivo expansion of human cord blood-derived hematopoietic progenitors in combination with stem cell factor and flt3 ligand. Leukemia 1997;11:524–530.

43. De Felice L, Di Pucchio T, Breccia M et al. Flt3L enhances the early stem cell compartment after ex vivo amplification of umbilical cord blood CD34+ cells. Bone Marrow Transplant 1998;22(Suppl 1):S66–S67.

44. Rusten LS, Lyman SD, Veiby OP, Jacobsen SEW. The FLT3 ligand is a direct and potent stimulator of the growth of primitive and committed human CD34+ bone marrow progenitor cells in vitro. Blood 1996;87:1317–1325.

45. Piacibello W, Snavio F, Garetto L et al. Differential growth factor requirement of primitive cord blood hematopoietic stem cell for self-renewal and amplification vs proliferation and differentiation. Leukemia 1998;12:718–727.

46. Bryder D, Jacobsen SE. Interleukin-3 supports expansion of long-term multilineage repopulating activity after multiple stem cell divisions in vitro. Blood 2000;96:1748–1755.

47. Rossmanith T, Schroder B, Bug G et al. Interleukin 3 improves the ex vivo expansion of primitive human cord blood progenitor cells and maintains the engraftment potential of SCID repopulating cells. Stem Cells 2001;19:313–320.

48. Ratajczak MZ, Ratajczak J, Machalinski B et al. In vitro and in vivo evidence that ex vivo cytokine priming of donor marrow cells may ameliorate posttransplant thrombocytopenia. Blood 1998;91:353–359.

49. Tanaka R, Koike K, Imai T et al. Stem cell factor enhances proliferation, but not maturation, of murine megakaryocytic progenitors in serum-free culture. Blood 1992;80:1743–1749.

50. Perez LE, Rinder HM, Wang C et al. Xenotransplantation of immunodeficient mice with mobilized human blood CD34+ cells provides an in vivo model for human megakaryocytopoiesis and platelet production. Blood 2001;97:1635–1643.

51. Cardier JE, Murphy MJ, Erickson-Miller CL. IL-6 interferes with stimulation of HPP-CFC and large CFU-Mk in conjunction with cytokine combinations from primitive murine marrow cells. Stem Cells 1997;15:437–442.

52. Fluckiger AC, Sanz E, Garcia-Lloret M et al. In vitro reconstitution of human B-cell ontogeny: from CD34(+) multipotent progenitors to Ig-secreting cells. Blood 1998;92:4509–4520.

53. Denning-Kendall PA, Nicol A, Horsley H et al. Is in vitro expansion of human cord blood cells clinically relevant? Bone Marrow Transplant 1998;21:225–232.
54. Kobari L, Pflumio F, Giarratana MC et al. In vitro and in vivo evidence for the long-term multilineage (myeloid, B, NK and T) reconstitution capacity of ex vivo expanded human CD34+ cord blood cells. Exp Hematol 2000;28:1470–1474.
55. Kaushansky K, Broudy VC, Lin N et al. Thrombopoietin, the Mpl ligand, is essential for full megakaryocyte development. Proc Natl Acad Sci USA 1995;92:3234–3248.
56. Pick M, Nagler A, Grisaru D et al. Expansion of megakaryocyte progenitors from human umbilical cord blood using a new two-step separation procedure. Br J Haem 1998;103:639-650.
57. Hoffman R. Regulation of megakaryocytopoiesis. Blood 1989;74:1196–1212.
58. Meldgaard KL, Jensen L, Jarlbaek L et al. Subsets of CD34+ hematopoietic progenitors and platelet recovery after high dose chemotherapy and peripheral blood stem cell transplantation. Haemotologica 1999;84: 517–524.
59. Bertolini F, Battaglia M, Pedrazzoli P et al. Megakaryocytic progenitors can be generated ex vivo and safely administered to autologous peripheral blood progenitor cell transplant recipients. Blood 1997;89:2679–2688.
60. Engelhardt M, Douville J, Behringer D et al. Hematopoietic recovery of ex vivo perfusion culture expanded bone marrow and unexpanded peripheral blood progenitors after myeloablative chemotherapy. Bone Marrow Transplant 2001;27:249–259.
61. Kurtzberg J, Jaroscak J, Martin PL et al. Augmentation of umbilical cord blood (UCB) transplantation with ex vivo expanded cells, a phase I trial using the Replicell system (Abstr #2574). Blood 1999;94(10 part 1): 571a.
62. Bachier CR, Gokmen E, Teale J et al. Ex-vivo expansion of bone marrow progenitor cells for hematopoietic reconstitution following high-dose chemotherapy for breast cancer. Exp Hematol 1999;27:615–623.
63. Shpall EJ, Quinones R, Giller et al. Transplantation of adult and pediatric cancer patients with cord blood progenitors expanded ex vivo (Abstr #882). Blood 2000;96(11 part 1):207a.
64. Milner LA, Bigas A. Notch as a mediator of cell fate determination in hematopoiesis: evidence and speculation. Blood 1999;93:2431–2448.
65. Huang S-L, Mai H-R, Fang J-P et al. All-trans retinoic acid up-regulates ICAM-1 expression and enhances engraftment of hematopoietic stem cells in murine model for unrelated umbilical cord blood transplantation (Abstr #727). Blood 2001;98(11 part 1):173a.
66. Jaroscak JJ, Laughlin MJ, Gerson SL. Engraftment competition between umbilical cord blood (UCB) units in NOD/SCID mice (Abstr #2704). Blood 2001;98(11 part 1):645a.
67. Barker JN, Weisdorf DJ, DeFor TE et al. Impact of multiple unit unrelated donor umbilical cord blood transplantation in adults: preliminary analysis of safety and efficacy (Abstr #2791). Blood 2001;98(11 part 1):666a.
68. Gryn J, Harris DT, Shadduck RK et al. Multiple unmatched cord units (MUCs) for adult allogeneic transplantation (Abstr #2792). Blood 2001;98(11 part 1):666a.
69. De Lima M, Komanduri K, St. John L et al. Using two mismatched unrelated donor cord blood units for transplantation: analysis of chimerism and immune reconstitution (Abstr #5308). Blood 2001;98(11 part 2): 382b.
70. Wagner JE, Davies SM, DeFor TE et al. Unrelated donor umbilical cord blood transplantation (UD-UCBT) in 92 patients at the University of Minnesota: analysis of risk factors (Abstr #2788). Blood 2001;98(11 part 1): 665a.

# PART V

# COMPLICATIONS

# CHAPTER XXI

# Immunotherapy Options for Relapse After Bone Marrow Transplantation

DENNIS P. M. HUGHES AND JOHN E. LEVINE

Since the advent of bone marrow transplantation (BMT), many diseases that previously seemed hopeless now can be treated with considerable fractions of patients achieving durable remissions and long periods of disease-free survival. Initially the main therapeutic effect of BMT was thought to result from the direct cytotoxic effects of intensive chemotherapy and/or irradiation, but we have come to understand the importance that the immune responses of donor cells have in controlling disease. By manipulating this graft-versus-leukemia (GVL) effect[1,2] and attempting to separate it from graft-versus-host disease (GVHD),[3] outcomes have improved further. Still, by the very nature of the diseases that merit BMT, many patients do suffer relapse after transplant.

When disease recurs in a bone marrow transplant patient, the clinician must consider multiple factors in recommending further treatment options. No single solution or response will be appropriate for all patients. Rather, one must know the latest data about several modalities and consider these data in the context of the particular patient and disease presented. Therapies that are highly effective for patients with low tumor burden or very slow-growing tumors might be inappropriate for someone with a marrow replaced by leukemia blasts. Likewise, intense, myeloablative or sub-myeloablative approaches that may yield a good expectation of long-term remission for a patient whose relapse occurs years after BMT might be too toxic for a patient with the same disease but recurring after just a few months. New agents also may become available, such as imitanib mesylate (Gleevec),[4,5] arsenic trioxide,[6-8] or all-*trans* retinoic acic (ATRA),[9-13] whose efficacy against particular malignancies can abruptly change the standard of care for that disease.

In addition to the patient-related factors of age, diagnosis, tumor burden, performance, and prior treatment, one must know the mechanisms of action behind the various treatment modalities and the data regarding their efficacy, both alone and in combination, for the disease in question. Unfortunately for the pediatric transplant physician, there are few large, well-designed studies of children who relapse after BMT. Most of the data available come from adult patients or from reports that combine outcomes from adults and children into a single manuscript. One should exercise caution in making these extrapolations, particularly since children may respond differently than adults given similar therapy. This paucity of data also should spur creation of more large-group protocols specific for children. While preference should be given for enrolling patients in multicenter research trials or in single-institution studies, the decision process for each patient must be made on an individual basis. This chapter discusses several of the factors that must be considered in recommending therapy for the child who relapses after BMT.

## PATIENT CHARACTERISTICS

### Age

Young age appears beneficial for patients relapsing after BMT.[14,15] The bulk of these data comes from reports mixing outcomes of adults and children, where neither treatment nor pathology was uniform among the study patients. In addition, there have been no reports comparing outcomes of younger children to teenagers. These caveats noted, there seems to be a trend in the literature that the younger the patient, the better the outcome. This effect is most clear when considering a second BMT; the Société Française de Greffe de Moelle (SFGM),[15] in a study of 150 patients, showed that children younger than 16 had better overall survival and better disease-free survival at two years. Further, adults aged 16 to 30 years fared better than those over 30. This improved outcome was due almost entirely to a large increase in treatment-related mortality (TRM) as patients aged (20% of patients under 16 vs. 56% of patients over 30). These findings are supported by the report by Dazzi and colleagues[14] that patients older than 35 receiving donor leukocyte infusions (DLI) were much more likely to get GVHD than those under 35, regardless of cell dose. An earlier report by Mrsic and colleagues[16] of patients receiving a second transplant found that patients under 26 years of age had a slightly better two-year event-free survival compared to those over 26. In this study a large difference in TRM (25% vs. 56%) was partially offset by an increase in relapse among the younger patients (70% vs. 57%). One possible explanation for this finding is that older patients who would have relapsed following transplant instead died earlier from the second BMT itself. However, selection bias as to who was offered a second transplant also may have played a critical role. Mrsic et al. did not provide information on differences between those who underwent second transplant compared to patients who relapsed who were not considered for the procedure. In contrast, Kolb et al. reported no difference in outcome between patients less than 36 years of age and those older, who received DLI.[17] Most other studies and reports were either too small to make the analysis or contained too few children to see any effect. Taking these data together, treatment-related toxicities for pediatric patients appear to be no higher than those reported in adult studies of the same treatment, and may be lower. Unfortunately, evidence to support the premise that a decrease in TRM contributes to increases in event-free and overall survival has not been demonstrated convincingly.

### Disease

Different diseases have vastly different outcomes and responses to treatment of relapse after BMT that reflect aspects of their underlying biology. In general, myeloid malignancies respond better to treatments in which immunologic reactions are thought to be important, such as second BMT,[18] DLI,[17] antibody therapy,[19] and cytokine treatment[20–23] than lymphoid malignancies. No biologic explanation for this clinical observation has been rigorously tested, but one might be that the increased expression of Class I human lymphocyte antigen (HLA) molecules by myeloid cells allows for easier recognition by cytotoxic T lymphocytes.[24] Another explanation may be the finding that acute lymphoblastic leukemia (ALL) is resistant to natural killer (NK) cell-mediated killing.[25] Alternatively, rapid rates of progression for some conditions, such as ALL, can preclude using interventions like DLI where the mean time to response[26–28] is longer than the mean time to death in the untreated patient.[27,29] Of course, treatments can be used in combination, and groups are now reporting studies in which DLI is used to consolidate remissions secured with conventional chemotherapy.[30,31]

## Tumor Burden

The total tumor burden for a patient, not surprisingly, has a significant impact upon outcome, with patients who have only a cytogenetic relapse doing better than those with overt hematologic relapse.[18,21,23,32,33] The magnitude of disease burden probably affects several aspects of the patient's response to treatment. More treatment will be required to achieve remission in those who bear more disease. In addition, many treatments rely on antitumor immune responses by T cells and NK cells from the donor. It is well known from experimental models that the presence of overwhelming antigen can lead to T cell anergy rather than activation.[34–39] In these cases, T cells that would otherwise have good antitumor responses might be rendered specifically nonresponsive by the sheer excess of antigenic signaling. For those patients with a large tumor burden after BMT, durable remissions may be achieved only if patients are effectively cytoreduced prior to initiating any form of cellular immunotherapy.

## Prior Treatment

While prior therapy is intricately tied to the disease, tumor burden at relapse and performance status, consideration of this variable will still play an important role in choosing current therapy options. It is generally assumed that recurrent disease will have greater resistance to those chemotherapeutic agents previously used in its treatment, so different drugs or classes of drugs are often chosen. Likewise, each body tissue has a maximum tolerated radiation dose, so the x-ray therapy (XRT) approaches used both during the initial treatment and the first BMT may make radiation therapy unavailable for relapse after BMT. Prior anthracycline dose may preclude the further use of these drugs. A good first step in approaching the relapsed BMT patient would be to assemble a complete record of all prior treatments given, including agents used and total lifetime doses, radiation doses, and fields used, into an easily read chart form. This information will make it easier to know which options will be available for the individual patient.

# TREATMENT OPTIONS

Multiple options for therapy are available for the relapsed BMT patient, each with important advantages and disadvantages. Knowing these, the physician can combine the patient-specific information discussed above with an awareness of the most recent outcomes data for each therapy for a given disease to generate an intelligent set of choices for the child whose cancer returns after BMT.

## Chemotherapy Alone

There have been two studies focused on children whose relapse after BMT was treated with chemotherapy alone, both now more than 12 years old. In 1987, Bostrom et al. reported a series of 65 ALL patients who had relapsed after BMT.[29] Of these, 61 were less than 18 years of age, and most were transplanted in their second or third relapse. Of these patients, 12 elected to receive no additional therapy and had a median survival of 36 days. Not including one patient who received palliative steroids, the remaining patients received induction regimens consisting mostly of vincristine, prednisone, L-asparaginase ± daunomycin. Twenty-nine of 52 patients (56%) achieved a complete remission, 4% had partial remissions, 17% died due to complications, and 23% succumbed to progressive disease without achieving a response. Patients then received various maintenance therapies that usually failed to control the disease, and the overall survival (OS) at 2.5 years postrelapse was 8%. Of the four long-term survivors, one had an isolated testicular relapse and the others had received cytarabine during induction or maintenance. One of these had a prolonged period of marrow suppression after induction, necessitating a repeat infusion of donor bone marrow, which may have significantly altered the disease course (see DLI below). All survivors had been in complete remission (CR) of at least 100 days after the first BMT.

Mortimer et al. found a duration of remission of 100 days or more posttransplant to be important to the success of subsequent therapy.[40] In their series, 95 of 455 acute myeloid leukemia (AML) patients transplanted in Seattle relapsed after BMT, and 62 of those 95 received salvage therapy. Of the 14 patients who relapsed within 100 days of transplant, there were six toxic deaths and only one remission achieved, with no long-term survivors. Of the 23 whose posttransplant remission lasted at least a year, 15 (65%) achieved remission, and this group had a median disease-free survival of six months with several long-term survivors. Reinduction therapies consisting of cytarabine and daunomycin were most successful. They also included data on the 130 of 366 (36%) of ALL patients who relapsed after BMT, of whom 94 received further therapy; 55% of these achieved a remission, with success being much more common among patients whose posttransplant remission lasted at least one year (65%) than in those whose relapse occurred within 100 days of transplant (7%).

Mehta et al. reported a series of acute leukemia patients treated at the Royal Marsden Hospital in Surrey, United Kingdom, for relapse after BMT.[41] This mixed group of children and adults demonstrated the overall poor outcome for all patients and highlighted the difficulties with chemotherapy use in this population. In their study, 127 of 195 relapse patients received reinduction chemotherapy, and only 45% of these (57 of 127) achieved a complete remission. Of 78 patients who received only chemotherapy (standard dose or palliative), OS was 6.7% and 1.3% at one and three years following relapse, respectively. There were no long-term survivors in the chemotherapy-alone group. Keil et al., from Vienna, reported a series of 47 adult patients with acute leukemia who experienced a recurrence following BMT.[27] Of these, ten (6 AML and 4 ALL) elected to receive no further treatment and had a mean time to death of one month. Fourteen patients were treated with reinduction chemotherapy. Only two patients achieved a complete remission, both of short duration.

The mean time to death for this group was two months, and the disease-free survival (DFS) and OS at one year was zero.

Though the data are incomplete, one might expect that about 55% of ALL patients who relapse after BMT will be able to achieve remission with a standard three or four drug reinduction.[27,29,40] Outcomes are better for patients with longer durations of remission after BMT.[29,40] The findings are similar for relapsed AML patients treated with cytarabine and anthracyclines.[15,18,27] The addition of maintenance chemotherapy prolonged the survival of ALL patients who achieve remission, though remissions were rarely durable.[29] The site of disease also affects outcome, though there are so few patients who experience an isolated testicular relapse following transplant that it is difficult to make definitive statements about expected outcomes. In all, the statement of Mortimer and colleagues still stands after 13 years, "reinduction should be attempted for all patients relapsing greater than one year from marrow transplantation. The decision for treatment of patients relapsing earlier than one year should be made on an individual basis."[40] Depending upon the severity of relapse, the type of disease, and the response to therapy, additional kinds of therapy might be considered.

## Immunomodulation

With greater experience in BMT from allogeneic donors, it has become clear that much of the success of this approach in many diseases is due not only to the cytotoxic effects of conditioning, but also to the immunologic recognition of malignant cells by the infused lymphocytes. Even when donor and recipient are molecularly matched for all HLA antigens, the myriad allelic differences in thousands of non-HLA encoded genes provide the peptides that are minor histocompatibility antigens. Host T cells would have been selected to not recognize these antigens during thymic education, while donor T cells would have been educated to those antigens unique to the donor. It is believed that the recognition by donor T cells of these peptides in the context of host HLA precipitates the reactions that culminate in GVHD.[24] Since malignant cells also will express some of these same peptide antigens or leukemia specific antigens, they also are susceptible to immune-mediated cytotoxicity from donor cells: the GVL effect. While a great deal of research has attempted to separate the GVL effect from those responses that cause GVHD,[42–46] there is still no reliable method in the clinic to achieve one without the other. Several studies have noted that the risk of relapse is lower in patients who experienced acute and/or chronic GVHD compared to those who experienced no GVHD,[47,48] supporting the idea that immune reactions of donor T cells help to control disease. To exploit this activity, many clinicians remove immunosuppression as the first step when a relapse is detected, especially if the tumor burden is relatively low or if the GVHD response was low or delayed.

Further steps can be taken to enhance the recognition of leukemic cells by donor lymphocytes. Interferon-α2b can increase the reactions of infused T cells and is known to worsen GVHD.[20,49] It also has been shown in some studies to improve outcomes for relapsed leukemias after transplant,[20,41] while others show little or no benefit.[50,51] Granulocyte-macrophage colony-stimulating factor (GM-CSF) can improve the antigen-presentation abilities of myeloid blasts, and in one study the addition of GM-CSF was thought to give a slight improvement in overall outcomes when combined with DLI.[52] Interleukin-2 (IL-2) is known to promote T cell proliferation and survival, and has been used successfully in the treatment of melanoma and other solid tumors.[53] In the studies of both Slavin et al.[21] and Singhal et al.,[50] the addition of IL-2 to DLI therapy led to improved DFS and OS. However, given the heterogeneity of the patients treated in these studies and the low numbers of patients overall, no firm conclusions can be made yet about the role of exogenous cytokines in treating the patient who relapses after BMT. As further laboratory research identifies ways to separate the GVH and GVL responses, we may see an increased role for the manipulation of the immunologic milieu with growth factors and cytokines as well as more exotic treatments like tumor vaccines. These approaches await large, controlled trials to demonstrate their efficacy. In the meantime, more direct approaches for inducing a GVL response may be undertaken.

## Donor Leukocyte Infusion

If allogeneic transplantation owes much of its success to the immunologic recognition of tumor cells by donor T cells, then a relapse after allo-BMT can be viewed as a failure of these T cells to achieve effective immune surveillance. There are multiple ways in which this immune control might fail, both for the T cells and for the tumor cells. Tumors can escape immune detection by down-regulation of immune recognition molecules like HLA or of death-related genes such as *Fas*.[54] They also may begin to express inhibitory cytokines or other molecules that directly kill responding lymphocytes.[55-57] T cells may become specifically nonresponsive to particular antigens, especially if the antigens are present in overwhelming abundance.[34-39] Once these T cells cease to respond to their antigenic target, it is difficult if not impossible to overcome their anergy.

It is likely that multiple cell types beyond classical, HLA-restricted, $\alpha\beta$ T cells contribute to both the GVL effect and the GVH effect. NK cells are lymphocytes that can mediate cytotoxic reactions against a variety of cellular targets, including leukemic cells.[58] These cells utilize class I HLA molecules for their recognition but, in contrast to classical $\alpha\beta$ T cells, it is the absence of HLA molecules on the surface of target cells that renders them susceptible to NK-mediated cytolysis.[59] Thus, those leukemic clones that down-regulate HLA expression and evade T cell surveillance may become targets for NK-mediated killing. NK cell recognition also may be restricted to self-HLA, and these cells may be potent mediators of GVHD and GVL. Ruggeri et al.[25] have shown that alloreactive NK cell clones could kill 100% of acute and chronic myeloid leukemia clones they tested. ALL lines have been more resistant to NK-mediated killing. ALL clones may be targets of $\alpha\beta$ T cells in patients with good response to allo-BMT.[60] While neither NK cells nor $\alpha\beta$ T cells are subject to anergy in the way that classical $\alpha\beta$ T cells are, both of these cell types are subject to T cell regulatory influences. Thus, when donor $\alpha\beta$ T cells cease to respond to the host's cancer, multiple mechanisms of response may fail.

For the allo-BMT patient who relapses, however, a fresh infusion of donor lymphocytes may be useful. Kolb et al. reported the first large series of patients with relapse after BMT who were treated with DLI in 1995.[17] In their series, chronic myelogenous leukemia (CML) patients in cytogenetic relapse or hematologic relapse had outstanding response rates to DLI alone (82% and 78%, respectively), with a probability of survival at five years of 67%. However, only one patient of 14 with transformed phase CML achieved a CR with DLI. Outcomes for other diseases were less promising, however, perhaps due to the rapid growth rates of these diseases and higher tumor burden at the time of DLI. Patients with relapsed AML and myelodysplastic syndrome (MDS) showed some response to DLI (CR rates of

29% and 25%, respectively). These patients still had a median survival of less than one year, however. There was little benefit shown for ALL patients in this study, with no patients achieving remission from DLI alone, a median survival of less than six months after DLI, and a 100% probability of relapse at 15 months following treatment. A follow-up report from the same group three years later confirmed these findings. Since the bulk of Kolb's patients were adults, some caution should be exercised about extrapolating these results to acute leukemias in children.

Subsequent studies have revealed some of the mechanisms behind BMT failures and DLI efficacy. Baurmann et al. have shown that CML patients can relapse despite persistent donor-derived T cells,[26] presumably because these T cells were either not host-reactive or were anergic. Serial analyses of these patients demonstrated complete conversion from recipient hematopoiesis to donor hematopoiesis between 9 and 13 weeks. Smit et al. demonstrated that outcomes for relapsed CML patients treated with DLI correlated with the frequency of T cell progenitors specific for CD34+ CML precursors.[24] Several groups have noted patients with severe or fatal aplasia after DLI,[17,33,61–63] and Keil et al. found that a lack of donor hematopoiesis at the time of DLI was predictive of aplasia. This finding suggested that outcomes could be improved with simultaneous infusion of T cells and G-CSF-mobilized CD34+ hematopoietic progenitors at the time of DLI64.

The first large North American study of DLI was reported by Collins and colleagues in 1997.[33] In their group of 140 children and adults, CML patients were again shown to have excellent responses to DLI: 60% CR rate overall at two years, with much better responses for those with cytogeneic (100% CR) or hematologic relapse (73.5% CR) compared to those with accelerated phase (33.3% CR) or blast phase (16.7% CR). Similar to Kolb's findings, patients with AML or ALL treated with DLI after relapse had much lower response rates: 15.4% and 18.2%, respectively. The major complications included acute and chronic GVHD (60% each) and pancytopenia (18.6%). These symptoms were manageable in most patients, as only 28 of 125 patients experienced grade III or grade IV GVHD. Both acute and chronic GVHD were correlated with better disease responses.

The outcomes from DLI may be better if patients receive their infusion at a state of minimal residual disease, as suggested by the CML outcomes.[23] For patients with more advanced malignancies, their outcome can be improved if chemotherapy is used for cytoreduction prior to DLI.[23] Levine et al. reported a prospective trial of chemotherapy and DLI for patients with relapse of advanced myeloid disease.[30] This treatment was similar to undergoing a second BMT, except that the chemotherapy was sub-myeloablative and no immunosuppression was given after cells are infused. The median T cell dose was $1 \times 10^8$ CD3+ cells per kg. Overall survival at two years for the entire cohort was 19%, with a median follow-up of 871 days. Of 57 evaluable patients, 27 achieved a CR with the planned therapy (47%). Patients with a complete response were more likely to survive, with one- and two-year survival rates of 51% and 41%, respectively, compared to a one-year survival for nonresponders of only 5%. The only pretreatment factor that correlated favorably with survival was the duration of the post-BMT remission. Patients who remained in remission for at least six months following BMT were more likely to become survivors than patients with shorter remissions (▼ Figure 21.1). This finding suggests that duration of posttransplant remission should be a factor for consideration when planning strategies for posttransplant relapse.

Donor leukocyte infusion, whether given in conjunction with chemotherapy or alone, is potentially highly toxic. Treatment-related mortality ranges from 23%[30] to 15%.[65] Graft-versus-host disease occurs in 56%[30] to 42%.[31,65,66] Therefore, the toxicity of DLI should be

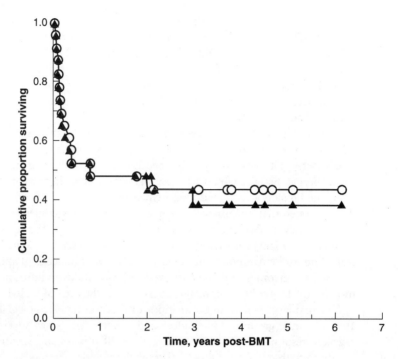

**FIGURE 21.1** Disease-free survival (▲) and survival (○) rate for 23 patients receiving a second bone marrow transplant for hematological relapse.

carefully balanced against the potential benefit when considering its use in the management of post-BMT relapse. One strategy to minimize the risk of GVHD has been to give initial low cell doses and escalate to effect. Mackinnon and colleagues at Memorial Sloan Kettering Cancer Center treated relapsed CML patients with escalating-dose DLI, starting as low as $1 \times 10^5$ T cells per kilogram.[62] If no response was observed, higher cell doses were administered. Of 22 patients treated on this protocol, 19 achieved a CR, some with a cell dose of as low as $1 \times 10^7$. Only one of 19 patients developed acute GVHD (1 of 19 patients), but 9 of 19 patients did develop chronic GVHD. Subsequently, Dazzi and colleagues in the United Kingdom reported similar results with escalating dose DLI for relapsed CML,[66] where they had identical response rates but the incidence of chronic GVHD was much lower for escalating dose treatment (10%) than for bulk-dose (44%). The rates of grades II, III, and IV acute GVHD also were higher in bulk-dose DLI. An escalating cell dose strategy has not been well studied for acute leukemia relapse.

## Second Bone Marrow Transplant

For the patient who relapses following BMT, a second transplant can reproduce all the anticipated benefits of an initial transplant. Chemotherapy, with or without irradiation, may either achieve or consolidate a remission. Allogeneic stem cells, together with donor T cells, should both regenerate the hematopoietic compartment and further reduce or eliminate leukemic clones. The GVL effect should provide both additional cytoreduction and long-term disease control.

Unfortunately, a second BMT is capable also of reproducing all the toxicities and hazards of the first transplant, and these are often more severe in patients who have been previously transplanted. The shorter the remission following the first transplant, the more severe the toxicities of BMT are likely to be, and the more resistant the disease will be to additional therapy. Furthermore, certain treatments, such as radiation and anthracyclines, have total lifetime doses that should not be exceeded, and this can limit therapeutic choices in the preparative regimen.

Reports of patients receiving a second BMT were made as early as 1976, and both the high incidence of toxicities and the high incidence of further relapse were evident from the start. Wright et al. described a series of 15 patients with acute leukemia (along with 10 patients with aplastic anemia) who received a second transplant.[67] While their series reported two patients who survived longer than a year, these were both patients who received a second bone marrow infusion due to primary graft failure. All patients in their series treated with second BMT for relapsed disease died within a year, either from infection or recurrent disease. Ten years later an Australian group reported another small series of eight leukemia patients given second transplants for relapse, including three long-term survivors: the only patient with CML, one of five patients with AML, and one of two patients with ALL.[68] One presumes that they chose the patients who received therapy very carefully. It is noted also that, while the two survivors with myeloid disease had good performance scores, the ALL patient had a Karnofsky score of 60 three years after her second transplant. Other reports from this period showed either very few or no survivors of acute leukemia one year after second transplant.[69] However, none of these protocols included reinduction prior to second BMT, and the only long-term survivors from any of these studies were those who had a low tumor burden at the time of transplant and who were at least 100 days from their first transplant at the time of relapse.

In 1989, Mortimer and colleagues from Seattle made an updated report on their results with second transplants, and the importance of GVHD in the efficacy of allo-BMT became clearer.[40] In this study 18 patients were given a second transplant, seven of which were autologous. The two patients who achieved durable, long-term remissions were AML patients conditioned with cyclophosphamide-based therapies who experienced grade III or IV GVHD. Another patient had no GVHD and had a three-year remission from the second transplant before dying from recurrent disease. None of the other patients had significant GVHD reported, and all died within a year.

Several reports in the next few years further demonstrated the importance of GVHD and identified additional factors contributing to outcome for patients receiving a second BMT.[16,18,70] While GVHD seemed important as a measure of the GVL effect, chronic GVHD seemed more predictive than acute GVHD, and neither of these was helpful if the relapsed patients had experienced GVH symptoms with the first transplant. Outcomes were much worse for patients relapsing within six months of the first transplant, and over time such patients came to be excluded from subsequent studies. This exclusion is appropriate, since the toxic death rate for these patients is 50% or more in some studies, and the median survival with transplant may be shorter than with palliation or no treatment for patients with very early relapse. However, these restrictions have led to the progressive increase in the proportion of CML patients in case series being reported. Again, for the pediatric transplanter, these data must be interpreted with caution.

One important benefit that arose from understanding the role of GVH and GVL in patients with relapsed disease is the improved management of children who relapse after

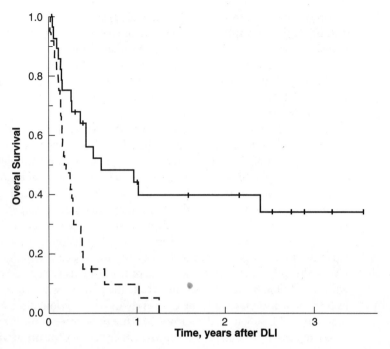

**FIGURE 21.2** Overall survival rate over time after donor leukocyte infusion in (dashed line) patients and (solid line) patients.

autologous BMT. With autologous transplants the sole mechanism of action is intensive therapy with subsequent rescue from myeloablation. Recurrent disease in this case might still be controlled by the immune responses of infused allogeneic T cells. Mehta et al. studied the outcomes of 117 acute leukemia patients treated with autologous transplant at the Royal Marsden Hospital in the United Kingdom who subsequently relapsed.[41] Of this large group, four ALL patients received allografts as a second transplant and two of four became long-term survivors. By comparison, four patients had a second transplant with autologous or syngeneic (identical twin) BMT. All four relapsed, three within a year. Only 5% of patients receiving standard treatment survived. Patients with AML given an autologous first BMT and an allogeneic BMT for their second transplant had even better outcomes. Other groups also have reported using allogeneic BMT for patients who relapse after autologous transplant, with similar outcomes. These outcomes are depicted in ▲ Figure 21.2.[71,72]

It also became clear that, similar to the findings in DLI, outcomes are superior for patients who receive their second BMT in a CR or minimal residual disease state. Mrsic and colleagues examined data from the International Bone Marrow Transplant Registry and identified 114 patients who received a second BMT for relapsed leukemia.[16] They showed that receiving a second transplant in a CR state, as opposed to transplants with overt disease, led to improved outcomes in two ways: patients had a lower incidence of treatment-related mortality (26% vs. 55%) and, for those surviving transplant, had a lower rate of relapse (54% vs. 95%). In Mrsic et al.'s study, these factors combined to give a very large difference in two-year EFS: 34% for acute leukemia patients transplanted in CR versus 2% EFS for those not in a CR at the time of transplant. Other groups found similar results in smaller series.[18,71]

An additional prognostic factor confirmed by Mrsic's report was the time interval between the first BMT and subsequent relapse.[16] The numbers are quite stark: for any leukemia patient retransplanted within six months, the two-year EFS was zero. As with the findings about tumor burden above, both toxicity and relapse rate contribute to the failures of those who relapse early. Patients retransplanted within six months face a 90% treatment-related mortality, and survivors face an 88% chance of relapse. These findings, along with others confirming them, have led most researchers to avoid second BMT for patients whose recurrence appears within six months.

While early reports of second BMT did not examine age as a prognostic factor, the larger studies of the late 1980s and the 1990s showed that younger people tended to do better with second transplants because of lower treatment-related mortality.[15,16,70] For most of these reports, the vast majority of deaths following a second BMT occurred within one year of the treatment.

A newer development that exploits this information to improve outcomes is the use of reduced-intensity conditioning prior to second transplant for selected patients. These reduced intensity transplants utilize lower dosages and less myeloablative agents to reduce the disease burden and consolidate remissions. Patients then receive stem cells together with allogeneic T cells for their second transplant. Recovery of hematopoiesis is rapid with myeloid recovery on average at 13.5 days and platelet recovery averaging 21 days.[73] In the report from Pawson and colleagues, where fludarabine, cytarabine, and anthracyclines were used for conditioning, there were no toxic deaths from this approach.[73] Other reports have tried similar low-intensity conditioning regimens, and the early results are encouraging.[74–76] This therapy blurs the distinction between a second transplant and DLI, revealing a spectrum of therapeutic options that balance the respective contributions of cytotoxic and immunologic controls for recurrent disease.

## SUMMARY

Relapse after BMT in children represents a difficult challenge requiring consideration of multiple factors before the best approach may be chosen. Particular aspects of the child's health and performance will affect the response to various therapies. Tumor burden, localization of disease, and duration of remission will all affect how likely a given patient is to respond to treatment, and how much therapy will be needed for those patients who might yet have a good outcome. Localized relapse, such as isolated testicular disease or a single chloroma, might benefit from specific local treatment with less need for intensive systemic measures. Newer, disease-specific agents like gemtuzumab ozogamacin (Mylotarg) for AML,[77–80] rituximab for NHL,[81,82] and imitanib mesylate (Gleevec) for CML[4,5,83] can be tried, as malignant clones may not have developed resistance to such agents and the toxicities might be better tolerated than those of intensive therapy. For patients with a very low tumor burden, such as those with only cytogenetic relapse, remissions may be achieved with a reduction of immunosuppression alone in some cases.

The higher the tumor burden, the more intensive the treatments will need to be, and most patients may benefit from exploiting both cytotoxic and immunotherapeutic mechanisms. Patients with good performance status whose posttransplant remission lasted at least six months to a year deserve a trial of chemotherapy to attempt cytoreduction. For those who respond, additional therapy may be chosen to consolidate the remission, taking into account all of the information discussed in this chapter. For those with the most aggressive disease but with good performance, choices will likely lie somewhere in the spectrum from DLI to fully myeloablative BMT. As always, consideration should be given to enrolling patients on larger, multicentered clinical trials or single institution studies where appropriate. Patients should understand the risks and benefits, however. No studies to date have therapies for overt relapse from acute leukemias that give even a 50% two-year event-free survival.

As was true more than a century ago,[84] the physician's role sometimes is to break the bad news to the patient and family and to console them afterwards. For patients whose disease recurs within perhaps six months of transplant, and certainly for those who relapse within 100 days, this may be our biggest job. Given the poor outcomes for this group, we would do patients and their families a kindness by conveying accurate information about further treatment, and help families to plan realistic goals for themselves.

# REFERENCES

1. Russell L, Jacobsen N, Heilmann C et al. Treatment of relapse after allogeneic BMT with donor leukocyte infusions in 16 patients. Bone Marrow Transplant 1996;18:411–414.
2. Tringali S, Vasta S, Scime R et al. Testicular relapse of AML during chronic graft-versus-host disease induced by donor leukocyte infusion. Haematologica 1996;81:339–342.
3. Mehta J, Powles R, Kulkarni S et al. Induction of graft-versus-host disease as immunotherapy of leukemia relapsing after allogeneic transplantation: single-center experience of 32 adult patients. Bone Marrow Transplant 1997;20:129–135.
4. Buchdunger E, Cioffi CL, Law N et al. Abl protein-tyrosine kinase inhibitor STI571 inhibits in vitro signal transduction mediated by c-kit and platelet-derived growth factor receptors. J Pharmacol Exp Ther 2000; 295:139–145.
5. Thiesing JT, Ohno-Jones S, Kolibaba KS et al. Efficacy of STI571, an Abl tyrosine kinase inhibitor, in conjunction with other antileukemic agents against Bcr-Abl-positive cells. Blood 2000;96:3195–3199.
6. Chen G, Zhu J, Shi X et al. In vitro studies on cellular and molecular mechanisms of arsenic trioxide (As2O3) in the treatment of acute promyelocytic leukemia: As2O3 induces NB4 cell apoptosis with down regulation of Bcl-2 expression and modulation of PML-RAR alpha/PML proteins. Blood 1996;88:1052–1061.
7. Chen G-Q, Shi X-G, Tang W et al. Use of arsenic trioxide (As2O3) in the treatment of acute promyelocytic leukemia (APL): I. As2O3 exerts dose-dependent dual effects on APL cells. Blood 1997;89:3345–3353.
8. Shen Z-X, Chen G-Q, Ni J-H et al. Use of arsenic trioxide (As2O3) in the treatment of acute promyelocytic leukemia (APL): II. Clinical efficacy and pharmacokinetics in relapsed patients. Blood 1997;89:3354–3360.
9. Chen Z, Tao R, Xia X. The present status in all-trans retinoic acid (ATRA) treatment for acute promyelocytic leukemia patients: further understanding and comprehensive strategy are required in the future. Leuk Lymphoma 1992;8:247–252.
10. Degos L. All-trans retinoic acid (ATRA) therapeutical effect in acute promyelocytic leukemia. Biomed Pharmacother 1992;46:201–209.
11. Degos L. All-trans-retinoic acid treatment and retinoic acid receptor alpha gene rearrangement in acute promyelocytic leukemia: a model for differentiation therapy. Int J Cell Cloning 1992;10:63–69.
12. Dombret H, Sutton L, Duarte M et al. Combined therapy with all-trans-retinoic acid and high-dose chemotherapy in patients with hyperleukocytic acute promyelocytic leukemia and severe visceral hemorrhage. Leukemia 1992;6:1237–1242.
13. Hofmann S. Retinoids "differentiation agents" for cancer treatment and prevention. Am J Med Sci 1992; 304:202–213.
14. Dazzi F, Cwynarski K, Craddock C et al. Factors influencing acute GVHD after donor lymphocyte infusion (Abstr). Blood 1999;94:668a.
15. Michallet M, Tanguy M, Socie G et al. Second allogeneic haematopoietic stem cell transplantation in relapsed acute and chronic leukaemias for patients who underwent a first allogeneic bone marrow transplantation: a survey of the Societe Francaise de Greffe de moelle (SFGM). Br J Haematol 2000;108:400–407.
16. Mrsic M, Horowitz M, Atkinson K et al. Second HLA-identical sibling transplants for leukemia recurrence. Bone Marrow Transplant 1992;9:269–275.
17. Kolb H, Schattenberg A, Goldman J et al. Graft-versus-leukemia effect of donor lymphocyte transfusions in marrow grafted patients. European Group for Blood and Marrow Transplantation Working Party Chronic Leukemia. Blood 1995;86:2041–2050.
18. Wagner J, Vogelsang G, Zehnbauer B et al. Relapse of leukemia after bone marrow transplantation: effect of second myeloablative therapy. Bone Marrow Transplant 1992;9:205–209.
19. de Vetten M, Jansen J, van der Reijden B et al. Molecular remission of Philadelphia/bcr-abl-positive acute myeloid leukaemia after treatment with anti-CD33 calicheamicin conjugate (gemtuzumab ozogamicin, CMA-676). Br J Haematol 2000;111:277–279.
20. Grigg A, Kannan K, Schwarer A et al. Chemotherapy and granulocyte colony stimulating factor-mobilized blood cell infusion followed by interferon-alpha for relapsed malignancy after allogeneic bone marrow transplantation. Intern Med J 2001;31:15–22.
21. Slavin S, Naparstek E, Nagler A et al. Allogeneic cell therapy with donor peripheral blood cells and recombinant human interleukin-2 to treat leukemia relapse after allogeneic bone marrow transplantation. Blood 1996;87:2195–2204.
22. Slavin S, Nagler A. Cytokine-mediated immunotherapy following autologous bone marrow transplantation in lymphoma and evidence of interleukin-2-induced immunomodulation in allogeneic transplants. Cancer J Sci Am 1997;3(Suppl 1):S59–S67.
23. Kolb HJ. Donor leukocyte transfusions for treatment of leukemic relapse after bone marrow transplantation. EBMT Immunology and Chronic Leukemia Working Parties. Vox Sang 1998;74(Suppl 2):321–329.
24. Smit WM, Rijnbeek M, van Bergen CAM et al. T cells recognizing leukemic CD34+ progenitor cells mediate the antileukemic effect of donor lymphocyte infusions for relapsed chronic myeloid leukemia after allogeneic stem cell transplantation. Proc Natl Acad Sci U S A 1998;95:10152–10157.

25. Ruggeri L, Capanni M, Casucci M et al. Role of natural killer cell alloreactivity in HLA-mismatched hematopoietic stem cell transplantation. Blood 1999;94:333–339.
26. Baurmann H, Nagel S, Binder T et al. Kinetics of the graft-versus-leukemia response after donor leukocyte infusions for relapsed chronic myeloid leukemia after allogeneic bone marrow transplantation. Blood 1998; 92:3582–3590.
27. Keil F, Prinz E, Kalhs P et al. Treatment of leukemic relapse after allogeneic stem cell transplantation with cytotoreductive chemotherapy and/or immunotherapy or second transplants. Leukemia 2001;15:355–361.
28. Frassoni F, Barrett A, Granena A et al. Relapse after allogeneic bone marrow transplantation for acute leukemia: a survey by the E.B.M.T. of 117 cases. Br J Haematol 1988;70:317–320.
29. Bostrom B, Woods W, Nesbit M et al. Successful reinduction of patients with acute lymphoblastic leukemia who relapse following bone marrow transplantation. J Clin Oncol 1987;5:376–381.
30. Levine JE, Braun T, Penza SL et al. Prospective trial of chemotherapy and donor leukocyte infusions for relapse of advanced myeloid malignancies after allogeneic stem-cell transplantation. J Clin Oncol. 2002;20: 405–412.
31. Collins R, Goldstein S, Giralt S et al. Donor leukocyte infusions in acute lymphocytic leukemia. Bone Marrow Transplant 2000;26:511–516.
32. Verdonck L, Petersen E, Lokhorst H et al. Donor leukocyte infusions for recurrent hematologic malignancies after allogeneic bone marrow transplantation: impact of infused and residual donor T cells. Bone Marrow Transplant 1998;22:1057–1063.
33. Collins RH Jr, Shpilberg O, Drobyski WR et al. Donor leukocyte infusions in 140 patients with relapsed malignancy after allogeneic bone marrow transplantation. J Clin Oncol 1997;15:433–444.
34. Falb D, Briner T, Sunshine G et al. Peripheral tolerance in T cell receptor-transgenic mice: evidence for T cell anergy. Eur J Immunol 1996;26:130–135.
35. Cardoso A, Schultze J, Boussiotis V et al. Pre-B acute lymphoblastic leukemia cells may induce T cell anergy to alloantigen. Blood 1996;88:41–48.
36. Staveley-O'Carroll K, Sotomayor E, Montgomery J et al. Induction of antigen-specific T cell anergy: An early event in the course of tumor progression. Proc Natl Acad Sci U S A 1998;95:1178–1183.
37. Switzer S, Wallner B, Briner T et al. Bolus injection of aqueous antigen leads to a high density of T cell-receptor lig and in the spleen, transient T-cell activation and anergy induction. Immunology 1998;94:513–522.
38. LaSalle J, Hafler D. T cell anergy. FASEB J. 1994;8:601–608.
39. Gimmi C, Freeman G, Gribben J et al. Human T cell clonal anergy is induced by antigen presentation in the absence of B7 costimulation. Proc Natl Acad Sci U S A 1993;90:6586–6590.
40. Mortimer J, Blinder M, Schulman S et al. Relapse of acute leukemia after marrow transplantation: natural history and results of subsequent therapy. J Clin Oncol 1989;7:50–57.
41. Mehta J, Powles R, Treleaven J et al. Outcome of acute leukemia relapsing after bone marrow transplantation: utility of second transplants and adoptive immunotherapy. Bone Marrow Transplant 1997;19:709–719.
42. Hill GR, Teshima T, Gerbitz A et al. Differential roles of IL-1 and TNF-{alpha} on graft-versus-host disease and graft-versus-leukemia. J Clin Invest 1999;104:459–467.
43. Teshima T, Hill GR, Pan L et al. IL-11 separates graft-versus-leukemia effects from graft-versus-host disease after bone marrow transplantation. J Clin Invest 1999;104:317–325.
44. Boyer MW, Vallera DA, Taylor PA et al. The role of B7 costimulation by murine acute myeloid leukemia in the generation and function of a CD8+ T cell line with potent in vivo graft-versus-leukemia properties. Blood 1997;89:3477–3485.
45. Billiau AD, Fevery S, Rutgeerts O et al. Crucial role of timing of donor lymphocyte infusion in generating dissociated graft-versus-host and graft-versus-leukemia responses in mice receiving allogeneic bone marrow transplants. Blood 2002;100:1894–1902.
46. Sefrioui H, Billiau A, Waer M. Graft-versus-leukemia effect in minor antigen mismatched chimeras given delayed donor leukocyte infusion: immunoregulatory aspects and role of donor T and ASGM1-positive cells. Transplantation 2000;70:348–353.
47. Carlens S, Ringden O, Remberger M et al. Factors affecting risk of relapse and leukemia-free survival in HLA-identical sibling marrow transplant recipients with leukemia. Transplant Proc 1997;29:3147–3149.
48. Horowitz M, Gale R, Sondel P et al. Graft-versus-leukemia reactions after bone marrow transplantation. Blood 1990;75:555–562.
49. Slavin S, Naparstek E, Nagler A et al. Allogeneic cell therapy for relapsed leukemia after bone marrow transplantation with donor peripheral blood lymphocytes. Exp Hematol 1995;23:1553–1562.
50. Singhal S, Powles R, Kulkarni S et al. Long-term follow-up of relapsed acute leukemia treated with immunotherapy after allogeneic transplantation: the inseparability of graft-versus-host disease and graft-versus-leukemia, and the problem of extramedullary relapse. Leuk Lymphoma 1999;32:505–512.
51. Aviles A, Talavera A, Diaz N et al. Interferon as maintenance therapy in refractory malignant lymphoma. J Hematother. 1999;8:263–267.

52. Kolb HJ, Schmid C, Muth A et al. Donor cell transfusion for the treatment of recurrence – Adoptive immunotherapy using donor cells and GM-CSF for recurrent acute leukemia and acute phase CML after allogeneic marrow transplantation (Abstr). Blood 1998;92:344b.
53. Rosenberg SA, Yang JC, White DE, Steinberg SM. Durability of complete responses in patients with metastatic cancer treated with high-dose interleukin-2: identification of the antigens mediating response. Ann Surg 1998;228:307–319.
54. Kourilsky P, Jaulin C, Ley V. The structure and function of MHC molecules. Possible implications for the control of tumor growth by MHC-restricted T cells. Semin Cancer Biol 1991;2:275–282.
55. Bennett MW, O'Connell J, O'Sullivan GC et al. The Fas counterattack in vivo: apoptotic depletion of tumor-infiltrating lymphocytes associated with Fas ligand expression by human esophageal carcinoma. J Immunol 1998;160:5669–5675.
56. Buzyn A, Petit F, Ostankovitch M et al. Membrane-bound Fas (Apo-1/CD95) ligand on leukemic cells: A mechanism of tumor immune escape in leukemia patients. Blood 1999;94:3135–3140.
57. Cardi G, Heaney JA, Schned AR, Ernstoff MS. Expression of Fas(APO-1/CD95) in tumor-infiltrating and peripheral blood lymphocytes in patients with renal cell carcinoma. Cancer Res 1998;58:2078–2080.
58. Ruggeri L, Capanni M, Martelli M, Velardi A. Cellular therapy: exploiting NK cell alloreactivity in transplantation. Curr Opin Hematol 2001;8:355–359.
59. Lowdell M, Lamb L, Hoyle C et al. Non-MHC-restricted cytotoxic cells: their roles in the control and treatment of leukaemias. Br J Haematol 2001;114:11–24.
60. Lamb L, Musk P, Ye Z et al. Human gammadelta(+) T lymphocytes have in vitro graft vs leukemia activity in the absence of an allogeneic response. Bone Marrow Transplant 2001;27:601–606.
61. Garicochea B, van Rhee F, Spencer A et al. Aplasia after donor lymphocyte infusion (DLI) for CML in relapse after sex-mismatched BMT: recovery of donor-type haemopoiesis predicted by non-isotopic in situ hybridization (ISH). Br J Haematol 1994;88:400–402.
62. Mackinnon S, Papadopoulos E, Carabasi M et al. Adoptive immunotherapy evaluating escalating doses of donor leukocytes for relapse of chronic myeloid leukemia after bone marrow transplantation: separation of graft-versus-leukemia responses from graft-versus-host disease. Blood 1995;86:1261–1268.
63. Keil F, Haas OA, Fritsch G et al. Donor leukocyte infusion for leukemic relapse after allogeneic marrow transplantation: lack of residual donor hematopoiesis predicts aplasia. Blood 1997;89:3113–3117.
64. Mandanas R, Saez R, Selby G, Confer D. G-CSF-mobilized donor leukocyte infusions as immunotherapy in acute leukemia relapsing after allogeneic marrow transplantation. J Hematother 1998;7:449–456.
65. Porter DL, Collins RH Jr, Shpilberg O et al. Long-term follow-up of patients who achieved complete remission after donor leukocyte infusions. Biol Blood Marrow Transplant 1999;5:253–261.
66. Dazzi F, Szydlo RM, Craddock C et al. Comparison of single-dose and escalating-dose regimens of donor lymphocyte infusion for relapse after allografting for chronic myeloid leukemia. Blood 2000;95:67–71.
67. Wright S, Thomas E, Buckner C et al. Experience with second marrow transplants. Exp Hematol 1976;4:221–226.
68. Atkinson K, Biggs J, Concannon A et al. Second marrow transplants for recurrence of haematological malignancy. Bone Marrow Transplant 1986;1:159–166.
69. Blume K, Forman S. High dose busulfan/etoposide as a preparatory regimen for second bone marrow transplants in hematologic malignancies. Blut 1987;55:49–53.
70. Barrett A, Locatelli F, Treleaven J et al. Second transplants for leukaemic relapse after bone marrow transplantation: high early mortality but favourable effect of chronic GVHD on continued remission. A report by the EBMT Leukaemia Working Party. Br J Haematol 1991;79:567–574.
71. Blau I, Basara N, Bischoff M et al. Second allogeneic hematopoietic stem cell transplantation as treatment for leukemia relapsing following a first transplant. Bone Marrow Transplant 2000;25:41–45.
72. Chiang K, Weisdorf D, Davies S et al. Outcome of second bone marrow transplantation following a uniform conditioning regimen as therapy for malignant relapse. Bone Marrow Transplant 1996;17:39–42.
73. Pawson R, Potter M, Theocharous P et al. Treatment of relapse after allogeneic bone marrow transplantation with reduced intensity conditioning (FLAG ± Ida) and second allogeneic stem cell transplant. Br J Haematol 2001;115:622–629.
74. Nagler A, Ackerstein A, Kapelushnik J et al. Donor lymphocyte infusion post-non-myeloablative allogeneic peripheral blood stem cell transplantation for chronic granulomatous disease. Bone Marrow Transplant 1999;24:339–342.
75. Slavin S, Nagler A, Shapira M et al. Non-myeloablative allogeneic stem cell transplantation focusing on immunotherapy of life-threatening malignant and non-malignant diseases. Crit Rev Oncol Hematol 2001;39:25–29.
76. Michallet M, Bilger K, Garban F et al. Allogeneic hematopoietic stem-cell transplantation after nonmyeloablative preparative regimens: Impact of pretransplantation and posttransplantation factors on outcome. J Clin Oncol 2001;19:3340–3349.

77. Sievers EL, Appelbaum FR, Spielberger RT et al. Selective ablation of acute myeloid leukemia using antibody-targeted chemotherapy: A phase I study of an anti-CD33 calicheamicin immunoconjugate. Blood 1999;93: 3678–3684.

78. van der Velden VHJ, te Marvelde JG, Hoogeveen PG et al. Targeting of the CD33-calicheamicin immunoconjugate Mylotarg (CMA-676) in acute myeloid leukemia: in vivo and in vitro saturation and internalization by leukemic and normal myeloid cells. Blood 2001;97:3197–3204.

79. Sievers EL, Larson RA, Stadtmauer EA et al. Efficacy and safety of gemtuzumab ozogamicin in patients with CD33-positive acute myeloid leukemia in first relapse. J Clin Oncol 2001;19:3244–3254.

80. Hogge DE, Willman CL, Kreitman RJ et al. Malignant progenitors from patients with acute myelogenous leukemia are sensitive to a diphtheria toxin-granulocyte-macrophage colony-stimulating factor fusion protein. Blood 1998;92:589–595.

81. Maloney DG. Preclinical and phase I and II trials of rituximab. Semin Oncol 1999;26:74–78.

82. Kunkel L, Wong A, Maneatis T et al. Optimizing the use of rituximab for treatment of B-cell non-Hodgkin's lymphoma: a benefit-risk update. Semin Oncol 2000;27:53–61.

83. Countouriotis A, Moore TB, Sakamoto KM. Cell surface antigen and molecular targeting in the treatment of hematologic malignancies. Stem Cells 2002;20:215–229.

84. McGregor-Robertson J. Cancer. In: McGregor-Robertson J (ed). The Household Physician (2nd ed.) London: The Gresham Publishing Company 1899:433–435.

# CHAPTER XXII

# Infectious Complications After Hematopoietic Cell Transplantation

JOHN R. WINGARD AND ELIAS ANAISSIE

Infectious complications pose important challenges to the transplant clinician. They cause severe morbidity and are an important cause of death following hematopoietic cell transplantation (HCT). Despite this challenge, one could argue that advances in supportive care, especially progress in antimicrobial therapy, have been responsible for much of the improvements in HCT outcomes over the last two decades. The introduction of new antimicrobial agents, gains in knowledge of the epidemiology of infectious complications, and the testing of strategies of how to use antimicrobial agents to minimize infectious morbidity all have played important roles in this progress. Notwithstanding, shifts in the types of infectious complications and their timing after transplant have occurred and continue to pose new and changing challenges for clinicians. The emergence of antimicrobial resistance, the increasing use of mismatched or volunteer donors as sources of graft cells, new sources of stem cells including cord blood and peripheral blood, the introduction of hematopoietic growth factors, the use of technologies that remove T lymphocytes, or other immune constituents of the graft and changing immunoprophylaxis strategies all impact infectious complications in different ways. These changes in transplant practices necessitate vigilance for transplant clinicians to meet shifting infectious complications. This chapter reviews the dynamic changes in host defenses at various times after transplant, the types of infectious complications encountered during these periods, the strategies one can use to minimize the adverse sequelae of infection during each phase, and the shifts in infectious syndromes that have occurred during the past two decades and are continuing to occur.

## DEFICITS IN HOST DEFENSES AFTER HCT

There are several constituents of HCT, including conditioning regimen, stem cell graft, and immunoprophylaxis. Each of these, plus certain HCT complications, affect host defenses in different ways (▼ Table 22.1).

Conditioning regimens for HCT are designed to reduce tumor burden to a minimum (for those for which neoplastic disease is the reason for HCT) and to suppress host/recipient immunity to prevent graft rejection in the case of allogeneic HCT. Conventional

| TABLE 22.1 | Host Defenses Impacted by Hematopoietic Cell Transplantation Practices | |
|---|---|---|
| *Stem Cell Procedures* | *Host Defense Affected* | *Factors Influencing Severity of Immunosuppression* |
| Conditioning regimen | Granulocytes, monocytes, mucosal injury | Intensity of cytoreductive therapy Use of certain agents (e.g., etoposide, TBI) |
| Stem cell graft | Hematopoiesis, cell-mediated and humoral immunity | Number of hematopoietic precursors In vivo or ex vivo manipulations that remove T lymphocytes or other immune cells |
| Post-transplant graft-versus-host disease immunoprophylaxis | Cell-mediated immunity | Degree of histocompatibility between donor and recipient |
| *Transplant complications* | | |
| Graft-versus-host disease | Cell-mediated and humoral immunity Reticulo-endothelial function | Severity of GVHD Duration and dose of corticosteroid use Duration of immunosuppressive therapy |
| Viral infections | Cell-mediated immunity | CMV, HSV and EBV |

Abbreviations: TBI = total body irradiation; CMV = cytomegalovirus; HSV = herpes simplex virus; EBV = Epstein-Barr virus.

conditioning regimens typically incorporate cytoreductive agents, including alkylating agents, podophyllotoxins, antimetabolites, and total body irradiation (TBI), which cause ablation of hematopoiesis and immunity of the recipient in preparation for replacement by the donor graft. Tissues with rapidly dividing cell populations are incidentally injured, particularly the mucosal stem cells, resulting in loss of mucosal integrity. The intensity of cytoreductive therapy influences the degree of myelosuppression and mucosal injury. In addition, certain agents, such as etoposide, melphalan, and TBI, have greater impact on the mucosa than other agents given at similar dose intensity.

In recent years, reduced intensity conditioning regimens (so-called nonablative or "mini" transplants) contain new purine analogs with profound immunosuppressive properties, anti-T cell antibodies and/or low dose TBI in the conditioning regimen of allogeneic HCT in place of intensive cytotoxic agents. Such conditioning regimens have much less myelosuppression and little mucosal injury. Therefore, such individuals are less susceptible for the infectious sequelae early after HCT related to the conditioning regimen. However, later infectious complications appear comparable, according to scattered reports to date.

The makeup of the stem cell product influences the rapidity of hematopoietic recovery and immune reconstitution. Hematopoietic progenitors are routinely enumerated today as the number of CD34+ cells per kilogram of recipient body weight and numerous studies show a correlation with the rapidity of neutrophil recovery. Increasingly, transplant clinicians strive to optimize the stem cell content to facilitate rapid engraftment. Engineering of the graft to remove T cells or by selection of hematopoietic precursors only (by CD34 selection procedures) profoundly affects immune reconstitution. Even though such manipulations are associated with a lower risk for graft-versus-host disease (GVHD) in the allogeneic setting, immune reconstitution is retarded and infectious complications are increased. The degree of histocompatibility between donor and recipient also profoundly affects the rapidity of immune reconstitution. Individuals with major or minor histocompatibility differences have very prolonged immunodeficient states and the duration is influenced by greater disparity.

The immunoprophylaxis regimen for prevention of GVHD also impedes immune reconstitution. Multiple immunosuppressive agents, inclusion of corticosteroids, and posttransplant administration of antibodies against T cells in the prophylactic regimen all increase the severity and duration of immunodeficiency.

Several transplant complications increase susceptibility for infectious complications. Chief among these is the occurrence of acute or chronic GVHD. In patients with chronic GVHD, impaired reticulo-endothelial function, immunoglobulin deficiency, and poor opsonization persist for many months, even years. Certain viral infections, particularly herpes virus infections, suppress cell-mediated immunity. Patients with cytomegalovirus (CMV) infections are particularly susceptible to bacterial and fungal superinfections.

# INFECTIOUS COMPLICATIONS AT DIFFERENT TIMES AFTER TRANSPLANT

Three distinct risk periods have been characterized (▼ Figure 22-1). Each is marked by a different set of deficits in host defenses and different types of infectious syndromes. The first risk period is the preengraftment phase extending from the stem cell infusion to time of engraftment interval, typically two to four weeks in duration. The second phase is the early postengraftment period extending from engraftment to approximately three months after transplant. The third phase is the late postengraftment period extending onward from three months.

## First Phase

In the pre-engraftment phase, neutropenia and mucosal injury are the predominant host defenses compromised. The patient frequently has an indwelling central venous catheter and this foreign body presents an additional risk for nosocomial infection. Bacterial infections predominate during this first phase. Historically, gram-negative organisms were both most frequent and most deadly. Over the past decade, most centers have seen a gradual decline in the proportion of bacteremias caused by gram-negative organisms with an emergence of gram-positive organisms as the most frequent causes of infection during this first phase. The reasons for this shift are not entirely clear, but explanations proposed include the increasing use of indwelling venous catheters and the more prevalent practice of prophylactic antibiotics that selectively suppress gram-negative bacteria, allowing a competitive advantage for gram-positive organisms. Many of the gram-positive bacterial

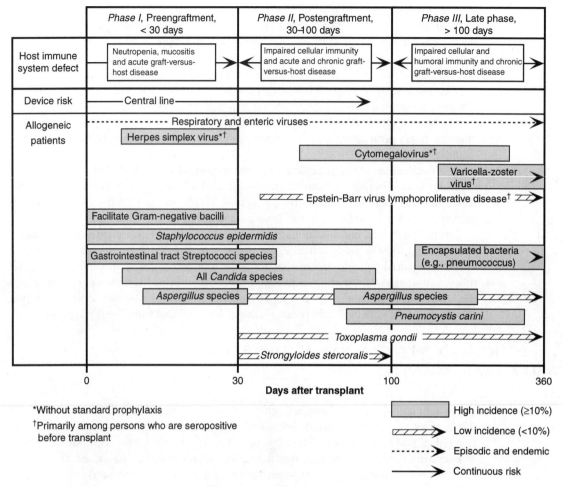

**FIGURE 22.1**   Phases of opportunistic infections among allogenic hematopoietic stem cell transplant recipients.

pathogens have a more indolent course than the gram-negative pathogens, but several, including *Staphylococcus aureus* and *Streptococcus viridans,* may have fulminant, life-threatening manifestations if not treated promptly.[1,2] Over time, emergence of antibiotic resistance will continue to influence the type and susceptibility of organisms contributing to these infectious complications.

The chief manifestation of infection during this first phase is fever. The manifestations of infection are attenuated because of the inability to mount an inflammatory response.[3] Evaluation should include a targeted history for infection with special attention to cutaneous, oral, gastrointestinal, respiratory, sinus, and genitourinary symptomology. A physical examination should be performed with particular attention to oral cavity, lungs, and skin. Examination of the exit site and tunnel of any indwelling catheter should be performed carefully. Blood cultures should be obtained. A chest radiograph or computed tomography (CT) scan is indicated in patients with respiratory symptoms and a urinalysis and urine culture for those with urinary symptoms. Even in the absence of any symptoms or signs suggestive of infection, studies in chemotherapy-induced myelosuppression many years ago demonstrated that the majority of episodes of neutropenic fever were caused by infections and the longer one waits before antimicrobial intervention, the greater morbidity and mortality from such infections. Accordingly, both the evaluation and initiation of antimicrobial therapy should be prompt.[4]

Fungal pathogens are infrequent causes of the first fever during neutropenia. However, with increasing duration of neutropenia the risk for fungal infection increases. The vast majority of fungal pathogens are *Candida* species. Their manifestation is primarily persistent or recurrent fever; occasionally cutaneous papules or macronodular nodules, new onset azotemia, and polymyalgias or polyarthralgias can occur and should alert the clinician to the possibility of candidemia. Evaluation should include fungal blood cultures and culture or biopsy of any suspected lesions. Occasionally, *Aspergillus* species or other mold fungal pathogens can occur, but the risk is quite small during the first two to three weeks of neutropenia, unless the patient has been heavily pretreated for his underlying disease or had invasive aspergillosis during prior chemotherapy. If engraftment is delayed, however, this risk grows with increasing duration of neutropenia. The usual portal of entry is the nasal passages and respiratory tract, and less frequently the skin and the gastrointestinal tract. The most common site of infection is the lungs, but skin, the sinuses, and nasal passages also can be affected. Clinical manifestations can include fever, skin lesions, epistaxis, nasal pain, nasal eschar, hemoptysis, cough, pleuritic pain, pleural friction rub, and localized wheezes or signs of consolidation. Radiographs of chest and/or sinuses are important. CT scans have been shown to be much more sensitive indicators of early disease than plain radiographs and are strongly urged.[5-7] Several studies show that early initiation of therapy is associated with improved outcomes.[5,8-13] In recent years, other fungal pathogens are increasingly emerging causes of infection both in the first and second phases of transplant.[14,15]

Herpes simplex virus (HSV) is the only viral pathogen that predictably causes symptomatic infection during the pre-engraftment period. HSV seropositive patients develop active infection an average of one week after transplant in two-thirds of instances,[16] manifest as ulcerative stomatitis, indistinguishable from oral ulcerations produced by cytotoxic agents.

## Second Phase

In the second phase, the early postengraftment period, the predominant deficit in host defenses is cell-mediated immunity. Residual host cell-mediated immune responses are on the decline and insufficient time has lapsed for the donor immune system to produce robust protective immune responses. Viral infections, especially by herpes viruses, are historically the most important and serious infections during this period.[17-21] CMV infection is common in CMV seropositive patients or in seronegative patients who receive grafts from seropositive donors.[22] The most common clinical manifestation is pneumonitis presenting with nonproductive cough, low-grade fever, and dyspnea. Other less common presentations include enterocolitis (increasing in recent years), rarely chorioretinitis, hepatitis, fever, leukopenia, leptomeningitis, or encephalitis. Weekly surveillance blood specimens assayed by the CMV antigen test or a polymerase chain reaction (PCR) assay for CMV should be performed from engraftment until day 100, since viremia often precedes clinical illness and allows early therapy to prevent morbidity and mortality.[23,24]

Invasive fungal infections are quite common also during this period, particularly in patients receiving corticosteroids or experiencing GVHD.[17,20,21,25–27] In addition, recipients of T cell-depleted stem cell grafts, those who receive anti-T lymphocyte antibody post-transplant and those who receive grafts from mismatched donors are especially vulnerable. Patients receiving steroids for several weeks in duration are especially susceptible. Bacteremias from any source (including those associated with the venous catheter) may occasionally occur. *Pneumocystis carinii* can cause interstitial pneumonitis during this phase if prophylaxis is not used. BK virus, a polyoma virus that replicates in genitourinary epithelial cells, occasionally can cause hemorrhagic cystitis, especially in patients with acute GVHD.

## Third Phase

The late postengraftment period (beyond 100 days), is characterized by gradual reconstitution of cellular and humoral immune responses with tapering and discontinuation of immunoprophylaxis at six months for most patients. Immune recovery is largely complete by one year. There are several situations in which prolonged immunodeficiency persists. Patients with chronic GVHD, recipients of T cell-depleted grafts, and recipients of alternate donor grafts, all have persisting immune defects with continuing susceptibility for opportunistic infections. Varicella zoster virus (VZV) infections typically occur at a median of five months after transplant and are more likely in patients who experience chronic GVHD. Late-onset CMV has become increasingly frequent in patients who receive ganciclovir early. Risk factors for late-onset CMV infection are GVHD and early CMV viremia. Susceptibility to *Pneumocystis carinii* persists for as long as the patient remains on active immunosuppressant therapy. Patients with chronic GVHD have poor opsonization and impaired reticuloendothelial function and are particularly vulnerable for severe infection by encapsulated bacteria, including *Streptococcus pneumoniae, Haemophilus influenzae,* and *Neisseria meningitides.*

Although there is a temporal sequence of infectious complications that characterizes most of the major infections, not all occur at predictable times after transplant. Certain infections occur seasonally. This is particularly true for the respiratory viruses where infection patterns mirror those in the community. Respiratory syncitial virus (RSV) infections and influenza infections occur typically during the winter months. Parainfluenza infections, in contrast, occur throughout the year. Enteric viruses typically occur in bone marrow transplant (BMT) patients when an outbreak is happening in the community as well. For both the respiratory and gastrointestinal viral pathogens, awareness of what infections are present in the community (as well as the staff in the BMT unit) is important in narrowing the differential diagnostic possibilities.

## TREATMENT STRATEGIES

The most important strategies for prophylaxis and treatment are described in ▸ Table 22.2. The Center for Disease Control, along with the American Society of Blood and Marrow Transplantation and the Infectious Disease Society of America jointly formulated guidelines

| TABLE 22.2 | Antimicrobial Treatment and Prophylactic Strategies |  |
|---|---|---|

| Viruses | Situation | Strategy |
|---|---|---|
| HSV | Seropositive recipient | Acyclovir, valacyclovir or famciclovir prophylaxis in Phase I |
| CMV | Seropositive recipient | Weekly serum testing for CMV antigen<br>Ganciclovir prophylaxis or preemptive therapy |
|  | Seronegative recipient given graft from seronegative donor | Blood transfusions from only seronegative donors (or use of leukocyte filtration) |
|  | CMV pneumonia | Ganciclovir plus IVIG or CMV immuneglobulin |
| VZV | VZV seronegative recipient exposed to actively infected person | VZIG (within 96 hours of exposure)<br>Postexposure acyclovir |
| Bacteria | Neutropenic fever | Empiric antibiotics according to IDSA Guidelines[27] |
|  | Chronic GVHD | Prophylaxis using agent active against encapsulated bacteria |
| Fungi | Allogeneic and high-risk autologous HCT recipients | Fluconazole prophylaxis in Phase I |
|  | Candidemia | Amphotericin B (or lipid formulation) or fluconazole in susceptible species |
|  | Aspergillosis | Amphotericin B (or lipid formulation) or voriconazole |
| Pneumocystis carinii | All HCT recipients | Prophylaxis with trimethoprim-sulfamethoxazole for 6 months, and beyond if active chronic GVHD or steroids continue to be used |

Abbreviations: HSV = herpes simplex virus; CMV = cytomegalovirus; IVIG = intravenous immunoglobulin; GVHD = graft-versus-host disease; HCT = hematopoietic stem cell transplantation.

for infection control for HCT patients.[28] These guidelines were based on the strength of evidence from studies published in peer-reviewed literature supplemented by expert opinion in situations where evidence was scant, but there was evidence in other patient populations or standards of care were sufficiently developed to provide strong inferences.

## Viral infections

Acyclovir prophylaxis is recommended for patients who are HSV seropositive. This should be started just prior to the transplant and continue until engraftment.

For CMV, ganciclovir is the chief therapeutic option, given either prophylactically or preemptively. Prophylaxis involves institution of ganciclovir in at-risk patients (seropositive recipients or recipients of seropositive grafts) at the time of engraftment and continuing during the chief risk period up to 100 days. Alternatively, patients can be tested weekly for asymptomatic CMV antigenemia, and for those with antigenemia, ganciclovir can be started preemptively to avert the subsequent occurrence of CMV disease. Once started preemptively, ganciclovir should be continued either through day 100 or for at least several weeks until clearance of viremia and then reinstitution of weekly monitoring. Both strategies have been validated in controlled trials.[23] The prophylaxis strategy has generally been associated with fewer breakthrough viremias, but has been associated with greater toxicity (more frequent myelosuppression) and some series suggest a greater likelihood of late-onset CMV infection and disease (beyond 100 days). Surveys of various BMT centers show that the preemptive strategy is more commonly used. Some centers use the prophylaxis approach in very high risk patients (seropositive recipients of unrelated donor transplants or T cell-depleted transplants) where the risk for CMV disease is extremely high and employ the preemptive approach for those at somewhat lesser risk. An increase in late-onset CMV infection has led many to recommend that surveillance beyond day 100 also be performed at least twice monthly for as long as chronic GVHD, steroid use, or very low CD4 counts persist. Controlled trials are underway to evaluate strategies in this third phase. For patients who are seronegative and whose donor is also seronegative, provision of CMV negative blood products is recommended to avoid acquisition of CMV from blood transfusions. If a CMV negative blood product is not available, then use of a leukocyte filter is a suitable substitute since removal of leukocytes reduces the risk, as CMV is a cell associated virus.[29]

Although CMV infection is frequent in seropositive autologous patients, the risk for CMV disease is substantially lower than after allogeneic HCT.[22] Accordingly, in the past, no routine precautions were exercised by most centers in this low risk group. However, recent studies suggest that recipients of CD34 selected stem cell grafts are at substantial risk for CMV disease (and other opportunistic infections) and this situation warrants vigilance by the transplant clinician. In addition, the prior use of immunosuppressive purine analogs (such as fludarabine or cladribine) and the increasing use of anti-B or T cell antibodies in the therapy of lymphohematopoietic malignancies is associated with profound and prolonged immunodeficiency, and sporadic reports of increasing CMV and other opportunistic infections associated with T cell deficiency are occurring. Thus, such individuals are at risk and vigilance is warranted. For CMV pneumonia, ganciclovir plus immune globulin is the preferred therapy. Both conventional lots of intravenous immunoglobulin (IVIG) and CMV immune globulin have been used with success but no head to head comparison has been conducted. Ganciclovir resistance is infrequent in HCT recipients but foscarnet is an alternative for ganciclovir resistant isolates or for patients unable to tolerate ganciclovir.[30]

Acyclovir prophylaxis for six months has shown a beneficial reduction in VZV infection during prophylaxis. However, after discontinuation recurrences resumed at the same rate as would be expected without prophylaxis, with no substantial net benefit. Thus, it is not routinely recommended. Very prolonged administration (one year) is being evaluated. For children who are VZV-naïve and are exposed to individuals with active VZV infection, VZIG (given within 96 hours of exposure) or preferably acyclovir should be given as postexposure prophylaxis.

Epstein-Barr virus (EBV)-associated posttransplant lymphoma (PTL) is uncommon after HCT, but recipients of T cell-depleted grafts, recipients of mismatched transplants, and those who receive posttransplant anti-T cell antibodies are at risk, especially if they were seronegative prior to transplant and received grafts from seropositive donors.[31] Transfusions of donor lymphocytes or enriched anti-EBV cytotoxic T cells have been shown in small series to be effective treatment for PTL and as preemptive therapy in patients with high viral burden to reduce the subsequent occurrence of EBV-PTL. The mainstay therapy of EBV-associated PTL is a reduction in immunosuppression if possible. In some cases cytotoxic chemotherapy regimens is required as well. Rituximab also has been found to be an effective therapy.

## Bacterial Infections

Awareness of antibiotic resistance patterns is crucial for optimal antibiotic selection. Studies of antibiotic prophylaxis during the first phase of transplant have shown delays in fever onset and reduced bacteremia rates, but no overall reduction in mortality. Practices vary from center to center as to the routine use of antibiotic prophylaxis. If antibiotic prophylaxis is used, selection of an agent should be made with knowledge of the spectrum of organisms that will be covered and vigilance for the emergence of antibiotic resistance as well as impact on the spectrum of superinfections over time. Some studies have suggested that flouroquinolone prophylaxis has been associated with increased likelihood of alpha streptococcal bacteremia, especially in children and where conditioning regimens that produce ulcerative mucositis are employed.

Consensus guidelines also have been developed for the routine management of neutropenic fever.[4] The use of a third or fourth generation cephalosporin (such as cefepime or ceftazidime), a carbapenem (such as imipenem or meropenem), or a combination of aminoglycoside plus an antipseudomonal carboxypenicillin or ureidopenicillin offers broad spectrum coverage effective in most situations of first fever during neutropenia. Because of the emergence of vancomycin-resistant enterococci (VRE), the routine use of vancomycin has been discouraged by multiple consensus expert panels. Superinfection by staphylococci is frequent. For *Staphylococcus epidermidis,* in vitro tests for methicillin susceptibility are not reliable and vancomycin should be used. For *Staphylococcus aureus* infections, the clinician can be guided by susceptibility testing instituted by beta lactam or vancomycin. For patients in septic shock, broad spectrum antibiotics, including vancomycin and agents to cover antibiotic-resistant gram-negative bacteria, may be quite justified until the etiologic agent is identified. Once the pathogen is identified, then antibiotic coverage should be narrowed to retain only those antimicrobial agents needed for the specific pathogen so as to avoid the emergence of antibiotic resistance.

Responses to the empiric antibiotic regimen as well as results of the cultures guide further actions as to continuation of the initial antibiotic regimen or modification. For persistent or recurrent fever, guidelines have been developed to guide management and have recently been updated.[4] The specifics are beyond the scope of this chapter.

## Fungal Infections

Fluconazole prophylaxis provides protection against most *Candida* pathogens and is routinely recommended prior to engraftment for allogeneic recipients and autologous recipients treated for hematologic malignancies, those who have undergone intense conditioning regimens likely to result in mucosal damage, those who have received stem cell grafts subjected to CD34 selection, and those who have received prior fludarabine or cladrabine.[32–36] In one study, continuation of fluconazole to 75 days conferred longer protection that persisted even beyond cessation of the drug.[33,34] Unfortunately, fluconazole has not quelled the increasing problem of mold fungal infections. Today the major invasive fungal pathogen is aspergillosis. To date, there are no proven effective preventive strategies, although one recent report suggested that itraconazole prophylaxis through the first 100 days was able to reduce both yeast and filamentous fungal infections.[37] Further study is needed. For breakthrough *Candida* or *Aspergillus* infections, polyene therapy with either amphotericin B or one of the lipid formulations is indicated. Caspofungin, a member of the new echinocandin family of antifungal agents that acts on biosynthesis of glucan, a major constituent of the fungal cell wall, is quite active for invasive *Candida* infections and has been licensed on the basis of its activity as salvage therapy for invasive *Aspergillus* infections. Voriconazole was licensed for the treatment of aspergillosis after demonstration of superior efficacy, improved survival, and less toxicity to amphotericin as first-line therapy.[38] Other broad spectrum triazoles are in clinical development. Posaconazole, another triazole, appears to have good activity against mucormycosis, a group of organisms against which voriconazole has little activity. Both of these new triazoles may have activity against *Fusarium* spp. and *Scedosporium* spp., pathogens that are notoriously difficult to treat.

## CONCLUSIONS

Although infectious complications continue to pose formidable challenges for the transplant clinician, tremendous strides in prevention and treatment of infectious complications have occurred over the past two decades and this progress has accounted for part of the improved outcomes after HCT. Notwithstanding, changes in transplant practices and the emergence of resistant organisms under selection pressures from changing antimicrobial practices necessitate further inquiry and the development of new drugs and strategies of antimicrobial use to continue progress. The chief obstacle for bacterial infections is emergence of antibiotic resistance. HSV and VZV have been subdued by acyclovir. Early CMV disease has been largely controlled but strategies to prevent the increasing occurrence of late-onset CMV disease are needed. *Pneumocystis carinii* pneumonia can be effectively controlled by trimethoprim-sulfamethoxazole. *Candida* infections have been largely controlled with fluconazole. To date, the most formidable challenge is effective therapies for mold fungal infections. Despite enormous progress over the past two decades, work is yet needed.

# REFERENCES

1. Bochud PY, Calandra T, Francioli P. Bacteremias due to viridans streptococci in neutropenic patients: a review. Am J Med 1994;97:256–264.
2. Pizzo PA, Ladisch S, Robichaud K. Treatment of gram-positive septicemia in cancer patients. Cancer 1980;45:206–207.
3. Sickles EA, Green WH, Wiernick PH. Clinical presentation of infection in granulocytopenic patients. Arch Intern Med 1975;135:715–719.
4. Hughes WT, Armstrong D, Bodey GP et al. 2002 guidelines for the use of antimicrobial agents in neutropenic patients with cancer. Clin Infect Dis 2002;34:730–751.
5. Kuhlman JE, Fishman EK, Burch PA et al. Invasive pulmonary aspergillosis in acute leukemia. The contribution of CT to early diagnosis and aggressive management. Chest 1987;92:95–99.
6. Heussel CP, Kauczor HU, Heussel GE et al. Pneumonia in febrile neutropenic patients and in bone marrow and blood stem cell transplant recipients: use of high resolution computed tomography. J Clin Oncol 1999; 17:796–805.
7. Janzen DL, Padley SPG, Adler BD et al. Acute pulmonary complications in immunocompromised non-AIDS patients: Comparison of diagnostic accuracy of CT and chest radiography. Clin Radiol 1993;47:159–165.
8. Burch PA, Karp JE, Merz WG et al. Favorable outcome of invasive aspergillosis in patients with acute leukemia. J Clin Oncol 1987;5:1985–1993.
9. Goodrich JM, Reed EC, Mori M et al. Clinical features and analysis of risk factors for invasive candidal infection after marrow transplantation. J Infect Dis 1991;164:731–740.
10. Aisner J, Schimpff SC, Wiernick PH. Treatment of invasive aspergillosis: relation of early diagnosis and treatment to response. Ann Intern Med 1977;86:539–543.
11. Fisher BD, Armstrong D, Yu B et al. Invasive aspergillosis: progress in early diagnosis and management. Am J Med 1981;71:571–577.
12. von Eiff M, Roos M, Schulten R et al. Pulmonary aspergillosis: early diagnosis improves survival. Respiration 1995;62:341–347.
13. Caillot D, Mannone I, Cuisenier B et al. Role of early diagnosis and aggressive surgery in the management of invasive pulmonary aspergillosis in neutropenic patients. Clin Microbiol Infect 2001;7(Suppl 2):54–61.
14. Walsh TJ, Goll AH. Emerging fungal pathogens: evolving challenges to immunocompromised patients for the 21st century. Transplant Infect Dis 1999;1:247–261.
15. Anaissie E. Opportunistic mycoses in the immunocompromised host: experience at a cancer center and review. Clin Infect Dis 1992;14(Suppl 1):S43–S53.
16. Saral R, Burns WH, Laskin OL et al. Acyclovir prophylaxis of herpes simplex virus infections. N Engl J Med 1981;305:63–67.
17. Winston DJ, Gale RP, Meyer DV, Young LS. Infectious complications of human bone marrow transplantation. Medicine (Baltimore) 1979;58:1–31.
18. Meyers JD, Flournoy N, Thomas ED. Risk factors for cytomegalovirus infection after human marrow transplantation. J Infect Dis 1986;153:478–488.
19. Wingard JR, Piantadosi S, Burns WH et al. Cytomegalovirus infections in patients treated by intensive cytoreductive therapy with marrow transplant. Rev Infect Dis 1990;12:805–810.
20. Peterson PK, McGlave P, Ramsay NKC et al. A prospective study of infectious diseases following bone marrow transplantation: Emergence of aspergillus and cytomegalovirus as the major causes of mortality. Infect Control 1983;4:81–89.
21. Meyers JD. Infections in marrow recipients. In: Mandell GL, Douglas RG, Bennett JE, eds. Principles and Practice of Infectious Diseases. New York: John Wiley and Sons, 1985;1674–1676.
22. Wingard JR, Chen DY-H, Burns WH et al. Cytomegalovirus infection after autologous bone marrow transplantation: Comparison to infection after allogeneic bone marrow transplantation. Blood 1988;71: 1432–1437.
23. Boeckh M, Gooley TA, Myerson D et al. Cytomegalovirus pp65 antigenemia-guided early treatment with ganciclovir versus ganciclovir at engraftment after allogeneic marrow transplantation: a randomized, double blind study. Blood 1996;88:4063–4071.
24. Einsele H, Ehninger G, Hebart H et al. Polymerase chain reaction monitoring reduces the incidence of cytomegalovirus disease and the duration and side effect of antiviral therapy after bone marrow transplantation. Blood 1995;86:2815–2820.
25. Jantunen E, Ruutu P, Niskanen L et al. Incidence and risk factors for invasive fungal infections in allogeneic BMT recipients. Bone Marrow Transplant 1997;19:801–808.
26. Marr KA, Carter RA, Crippa F et al. Epidemiology and outcome of mould infections in hematopoietic stem cell transplant recipients. Clin Infect Dis 2002;34:909–917.
27. Grow WB, Moreb JS, Roque D et al. Late onset of invasive aspergillus infection in bone marrow transplant patients at a university hospital. Bone Marrow Transplant 2002;28:59–62.

28. Centers for Disease Control and Prevention. Guidelines for preventing opportunistic infections among hematopoietic stem cell transplant recipients: recommendations of CDC, the Infectious Disease Society of America, and the American Society of Blood and Marrow Transplantation. MMWR Morb Mortal Wkly Rep 2000;49(RR-10):1–128.

29. Bowden RA, Slichter SJ, Sayers M et al. Comparison of filtered leukocyte-reduced and cytomegalovirus (CMV) seronegative blood products for the prevention of transfusion-associated CMV infection after marrow transplantation. Blood 1995;86:3598–3603.

30. Moretti S, Zikos P, Can Lint MT et al. Foscarnet vs ganciclovir for cytomegalovirus (CMV) antigenemia after allogeneic hematopoietic stem cell transplantation (HSCT): a randomized study. Bone Marrow Transplant 1998;22:175–180.

31. Curtis RE, Travis LB, Rowlings PA et al. Risk of lymphoproliferative disorders after bone marrow transplantation: A multi-institutional study. Blood 1999;94:2208–2216.

32. Goodman JL, Winston DJ, Greenfield RA. A controlled trial of fluconazole to prevent fungal infections in patients undergoing bone marrow transplantation. N Engl J Med 1992;326:845–851.

33. Slavin MA, Osborne B, Adams R et al. Efficacy and safety of fluconazole prophylaxis for fungal infections after marrow transplantation – a prospective, randomized, double-blind study. J Infect Dis 1995;171: 1545–1552.

34. Marr KA, Seidel K, Slavin MA et al. Prolonged fluconazole prophylaxis is associated with persistent protection against candidiasis-related death in allogeneic marrow transplant recipients: long-term follow-up of a randomized, placebo-controlled trial. Blood 2000;96:2055–2061.

35. Rotstein C, Bow EJ, Laverdiere M et al. Randomized placebo-controlled trial of fluconazole prophylaxis for neutropenic cancer patients: benefit based on purpose and intensity of cytotoxic therapy. Clin Infect Dis 1999;28:331–340.

36. Ellis ME, Clink H, Ernst P et al. Controlled study of fluconazole in the prevention of fungal infections in neutropenic patients with hematological malignancies and bone marrow transplant recipients. Eur J Clin Microbiol Infect Dis 1994;13:3–11.

37. Winston DJ, Maziarz RT, Pranatharthi H et al. Long-term antifungal prophylaxis in allogeneic bone marrow transplant patients: a multicenter, randomized trial of intravenous/oral itraconazole versus intravenous/oral fluconazole (Abstr). Blood 2001;98:479a.

38. Herbrecht R, Denning DW, Patterson TF et al. Open, randomized comparison of voriconazole (VRC) and amphotericin B (AmB) followed by other licensed antifungal therapy (OLAT) for primary therapy of invasive aspergillosis (IA). Abstracts 41st Interscience Conference on Antimicrobial Agents and Chemotherapy 2001;378.

# CHAPTER XXIII

# Graft-Versus-Host Disease After Stem Cell Transplantation in Children

PAULETTE MEHTA

Acute graft-versus-host disease (GVHD) was first described following allogeneic bone marrow transplantation in the 1960s.[1] According to the classical definitions, GVHD occurs in the setting of immunocompetent tissue transferred into an immunoincompetent recipient stimulating the cytokine cascade, which results in epithelial and endothelial cell apoptosis and end organ damage. Since the time of its recognition, there have been many prevention and treatment trials of both acute and of chronic GVHD. Nevertheless, GVHD remains one of the major limiting factors to survival after bone marrow transplantation. The absence of GVHD disease, paradoxically, is also a problem as this is associated with deficient graft-versus-leukemia (GVL) effect.[2] Thus, the goal of prevention and treatment trials is to minimize GVHD while still allowing some GVHD to confer a graft-versus-cancer effect. There is good evidence already that the graft-versus-leukemia effect is present also as a graft-versus-cancer effect in other malignancies including lymphomas, myeloma and solid tumors.

## ACUTE GRAFT-VERSUS-HOST DISEASE

### Definitions

Acute GVHD has been differentiated from chronic GVHD in that the former occurs within 100 days of bone marrow transplantation and the latter after 100 days. In practice, however, the time periods overlap with each other and this is seen especially in doses of donor lymphocytes that are used to boost donor chimerism, displace host lymphocytes, or eradicate minimal residual disease or relapse. The two syndromes are clinically different and the differentiation is predicated more on the presentation of disease rather than the time from bone marrow transplantation (▼ Table 23.1).

### Clinical Findings

Acute GVHD is an inflammatory disease in which the skin, liver, and gastrointestinal tract are usually involved.[3-5] The skin is the most commonly affected tissue and the skin rash is usually maculopapular, can be evanescent and usually involves ears, neck, shoulders, chest,

| TABLE 23.1 | Clinical Grading of Acute Graft-Versus-Host Disease |

| Organ | Grade |
| --- | --- |
| Skin | 1: maculopapular rash occupying <25% of body surface area<br>2: rash occupying 25–50% of body surface area<br>3: generalized (i.e., 50%–100%) rash<br>4: stage 3 with bullous formation and/or desquamation |
| Liver | 1: bilirubin 2–3 mg/dL<br>2: bilirubin 3–6 mg/dL<br>3: bilirubin 6.1–15 mg/dL<br>4: bilirubin >15 mg/dL |
| Gastrointestinal tract | 1: persistent nausea and/or diarrhea >30 mL/kg<br>2: diarrhea >60 mL/kg<br>3: diarrhea >90 mg/kg<br>4: diarrhea >90 kg or >2,000 mL/day or severe abdominal pain and/or ileus |
| Overall grade of acute graft-versus-host disease | I: skin 1–2; liver 0; g-i tract 0<br>II: skin 1–3; liver 1 and/or g-i tract 1<br>III: skin 2–3; liver and/or g-i tract 2–3<br>IV: skin 2–4; liver and/or g-i tract 2–4 |

If there is no skin disease, then the overall grade is the higher single organ grade.

and back, palms and soles.[6] The changes resemble those that occur due to hypersensitivity of drugs and due to engraftment, and can be best differentiated by biopsy showing infiltrating mononuclear cells or dyskeratotic cells in the absence of other confounding situations such as drug rashes or viral infections. Biopsy results, however, are not always conclusive and need to be evaluated in clinical context.

The gastrointestinal tract and the liver are commonly involved, usually in association with skin changes.[7,8] Gastrointestinal GVHD presents as crampy abdominal pain and diarrhea. The diarrhea is often voluminous, watery, can be bloody, and can contain large amounts of mucus. Rectal biopsy can be diagnostic and shows lymphocytic infiltrates at the crypts, with necrosis and dropout of crypt cells. Computed tomography (CT) scan findings include multiple, diffuse, fluid-filled bowel loops with a thin, enhancing layer of bowel wall mucosae.[9] Bowel wall thickening often is absent. Pathologic evaluation of acute GVHD includes histological apoptosis and gland destruction, sparse inflammatory infiltrates, and granular eosinophilic debris in dilated glands.[7] False positive findings, however, occur in cytomegalovirus (CMV) gastritis, human immunodeficiency virus (HIV) infection, primary immunodeficiency, and after renal transplantation.

Liver involvement is usually manifested as increased unconjugated bilirubin; pathology of specimens show lymphocytic infiltrates in the interlobular and marginal bile ducts, characteristic of cholestasis. Other conditions need to be excluded, including drug toxicity, viral disease, and venoocclusive disease. Venoocclusive disease, although clinically resembling GVHD, is associated with endothelial damage and with clinical signs of ascites, hepatomegaly, and hepatic pain.

## Hyperacute Graft-Versus-Host Disease

Hyperacute GVHD is an exaggerated form of acute GVHD and usually occurs within the first 72 hours after bone marrow transplantation.[10–12] Where acute GVHD can be thought of as a cytokine storm, this, in contrast, is a cytokine hurricane. The cytokines produced include interleukin-2 (IL-2), tumor necrosis factor (TNF), and interferon γ (IFN-γ). It occurs usually in the setting of human lymphocyte antigen (HLA) mismatched donor recipients and is an extremely exaggerated form of acute graft-versus-host disease. Patients usually have fever, skin changes, diarrhea, hyperbilirubinemia, and may have sudden lung collapse.

## Involvement of Cytokines

Cytokine secretion, especially IL-2, TNF and INF-γ, accompany the changes due to GVHD and mediate much of the endothelial and organ damage.[1–3,13–16] Mononuclear cells infiltrate into involved tissue; lymphocytes and natural killer (NK) cells mobilize into target tissues. Infiltrating NK cells contribute to tissue damage by releasing cytokines; TNF-α induces expression of adhesion molecules on endothelium (i.e., E-selectin, vascular cell adhesion molecule-1 [VCAM-l]), which stimulate leukocytes, and is a ligand for vascular leukocyte adhesion molecule-4 (VLA-4). Leukocytes attach to the endothelium, and infiltrate into tissue parenchyma. Lymphocytes home into skin following stem cell transplantation and the skin eruptions are due to binding of peripheral blood monocytes to skin.

## Risk Factors

Risk factors for GVHD include older age, immune disparity between host and graft, and female cells into male donors.[4,5,17,18] Cytokine polymorphisms are also potentially risk factors.

Polymorphisms of TNF-α, IL-10, IFN-γ, IL-1 receptor antagonist, and IL-6 genes have been shown to predict for GVHD. In one study, cytokine gene polymorphisms were assessed in 242 sibling matched transplants; IL-10 and IL-6 were the major risk factors for developing chronic GVHD, and none were found in association with acute GVHD.[13,16,18]

## Staging

Standard staging criteria for acute and chronic GVHD are shown in ◄ Table 23.1 and ▼ Table 23.2, respectively.[19] The staging of acute GVHD was discussed at the 1994 consensus conference.[19] At that conference, bone marrow transplant experts agreed to modify the standard GVHD criteria to include persistent nausea with histological evidence of GVHD

**TABLE 23.2**    Clinical Staging of Chronic Graft-Versus-Host Disease

*Limited:* localized skin involvement and/or hepatic dysfunction

*Extensive:* (must have at least one from list A and/or one from list B)

List A: generalized skin involvement, or

limited skin involvement + any item from list B

hepatic involvement + any item from list B

List B: liver histology showing chronic progressive hepatitis, bridging necrosis or cirrhosis

eye involvement (positive Schirmer test)

minor salivary glands involved

oral mucosa involved

any other organ involved

even without diarrhea as stage 1. It was recommended that accurate staging be done, and that actual rates of grades II–IV and III–IV corrected for graft failure and potential interventions for early relapse be reported. Also, the indications for therapy of GVHD and the response needed to be accurate should be recorded. At another conference in 1994, the Working Party Chronic Leukemia of the European Group for Blood and Marrow Transplantation[5] also reconsidered staging for acute GVHD. They analyzed data of 1,294 patients transplanted from an allogeneic donor for chronic myelogenous leukemia (CML) in first chronic phase, and tested the predictive value of acute GVHD grading for day 100 mortality; transplant-related mortality; relapse incidence; leukemia-free survival; and overall survival. The staging corresponded to outcome and confirmed the validity of the five point grading system currently in practice.

## PREVENTION TRIALS

Many attempts have been made to prevent excessive GVHD, including pharmacologic agents, T cell depletion, or manipulation of the donor-host cell environment.

### Pharmacologic Trials

*Methotrexate and Cyclosporine and Steroids*

Methotrexate was the first drug shown to prevent GVHD in dogs and to some extent in humans.[3,20,21] In the 1980s cyclosporine-based preventive regimens were developed and greatly reduced the amount of clinical GVHD.[21] When the combination of cyclosporine and methotrexate were studied in head to head comparisons with methotrexate alone, the combination was more efficacious in preventing GVHD. The combination is most effective in human lymphocyte antigen (HLA)-identical siblings and least effective in HLA-mismatched bone marrow transplantation.

Subsequently a third drug was added to the cyclosporine-methotrexate combination. Steroids plus the combination were found to be better than the prior two-drug regimen alone for hematological malignancies, and is commonly used in HLA nongenotypically identical donor transplants. Another advance in the pharmacologic preventive regimen armamentarium is tacrolimus. We recently evaluated the pharmacokinetics of tacrolimus in children undergoing bone marrow transplantation.

Tacrolimus acts in a similar fashion to cyclosporine, and has less renal toxicity, but more neurotoxicity. It is cleared more quickly in infants and young children, and doses therefore need to be modified. We studied pharmacokinetics of tacrolimus in seven patients (age 8 to 17 years) undergoing allogeneic stem cell transplantation. Four patients received matched unrelated donor (MUD) transplants, two underwent HLA-matched related donor transplants, and one underwent an umbilical cord blood donor transplant. All patients received tacrolimus by continuous infusion at 0.03 to 0.04 mg/kg/day beginning on the day prior to transplant. Tacrolimus whole blood concentrations were monitored by micropar-ticle enzyme immunoassay. Our goal was to maintain a blood tacrolimus level of 10 to 20 µg/mL. Once patients were tolerating oral medications, tacrolimus infusion was converted to oral dosing using a 4:1 conversion. Dose of tacrolimus and resulting tacrolimus concen-trations were recorded and the total body clearance of tacrolimus was calculated retro-spectively. The mean clearance, based on first steady-state tacrolimus concentrations nec-essary for achieving a therapeutic level (10 to 20 µg/mL), was 108.1 mL/h/kg (range 79.7 to 142.0 mL/h/kg), greater than that reported in adult BMT patients (71 ± 34 mL/h/kg). The average dose required to achieve that therapeutic range was 0.0354 mg/kg/day as an intravenous continuous infusion. Over the entire course of intravenous tacrolimus, mean clearance was 97.0 mL/h/kg (range 33.4 to 153.3 mL/h/kg). In six of the seven patients, clearance values dropped after two to four weeks of therapy by an average of 32.5 mL/h/kg. In two patients, sharp drops in clearance were temporally related to changes in liver func-tion tests. Three of the seven patients died of severe acute GVHD; all of these patients had undergone matched unrelated donor transplantation, and two of these three had initial clearance levels over 120 mL/h/kg. Thus, children appear to have more rapid tacrolimus clearance than adults and may need to begin therapy earlier in order to obtain stable and optimal levels.

## TREATMENT OF ACUTE GRAFT-VERSUS-HOST DISEASE

There are several conventional and several experimental methods of treating acute GVHD.[20,22–24] Steroids are the mainstay of treatment for acute GVHD, especially if they were not used initially to prevent GVHD. Patients with cutaneous GVHD have the best responses (up to ~66%) compared to those with gut and/or liver GVHD (response rates of 2–40%). Steroids need to be used until the GVHD has completely resolved, and then needs to be slowly tapered over weeks to months to the smallest amount necessary to prevent sympto-matic GVHD. This is sometimes difficult to do because of the many toxic effects of steroid treatment, such as infection (especially fungal and viral), cataracts, bone decalcification, osteoporosis, diabetes mellitus, and hypertension.

## Daclizumab

Daclizumab, a humanized monoclonal IgG1 directed against the alpha chain of the interleukin-2 receptor (IL-2R), is a competitive inhibitor of IL-2 on activated lymphocytes.[21,22,25,26] To test the hypothesis that specific inhibition of activated lymphocytes in patients with ongoing acute GVHD might ameliorate the process, Przepiorka and colleagues treated 43 patients with advanced or steroid-refractory GVHD with daclizumab.[25] The first cohort of 24 patients was treated with daclizumab 1 mg/kg on days 1, 8, 15, 22, and 29. On day 43, the complete response (CR) rate was 29%. Survival on day 120 was 29%. A second cohort of 19 patients was treated with daclizumab 1 mg/kg on days 1, 4, 8, 15, and 22. For these patients, the CR rate on day 43 was 47% and survival on day 120 was 53%. There were no infusion-related reactions and no serious side effects related to daclizumab. Following treatment, there was a reduction in serum concentrations of soluble IL-2R and peripheral blood CD3(+)25(+) lymphocytes, but these changes were not predictive of response. Daclizumab has substantial activity for the treatment of acute GVHD, and the second regimen evaluated is recommended for a controlled study.[25]

## Other Drugs Being Studied for Efficacy Against Acute Graft-Versus-Host Disease

New agents such as mycophenolate mofetil, tresperimus, rapamycin, and basiliximab are being studied. Improved understanding of tolerance has resulted in new approaches to prevention of GVHD. Anti-CD40L, CTLA-4-Ig, tresperimus, and rapamycin are agents that are being explored in this area and have shown impressive results in animal models. In vivo T cell depletion, Campath-1 or ATG is being used in high risk patients. Data on its efficacy are anecdotal so far. Due to the variation in grading of GVHD between centers, randomized studies are needed to quantify the relative merits of different regimens, and participation in such studies is encouraged.

Several other therapies have been tried but only anecdotal information about their efficacy is known at this time. These therapies include antibody therapy with anti-T cell, anti-TNF, and anti-IL-1 receptor antagonists.

## A New Approach to Reducing Acute Graft-Versus-Host Disease After Bone Marrow Transplantation: Staggering CD34 and CD3+ Cells

Another way of reducing graft-versus-host disease is by infusion small numbers of T cells (i.e., less than 1 to $5 \times 10^{-5}$ T cells/kg). However, depletion of T cells from bone marrow harvests predisposes to more infections and to a greater risk of nonengraftment. Alternatively, depletion of subpopulations of T cells (i.e., CD8 T cells) has been tried, but still results in a higher risk of engraftment failure than with whole T cell populations. An interesting variation of this is early institution of T cell infusions followed by subsequent delayed T cell "addback." This strategy relies on achieving early engraftment, without GVHD, followed by T cell feedback 30 days after engraftment, for the graft-versus-cancer effect. Another model is to achieve partial microchimerism as an end point of treatment, at least for the nonmalignant hematological conditions such as sickle cell disease. Mixed chimerism allows for less thorough eradication of the host myeloid and lymphoid host system, and still increases the amount of hemoglobin from donor cells sufficiently to prevent the signs of symptoms of sickle cell disease.

Patients with hematological malignancy also can be transplanted with the goal of limited donor chimerism initially, later to be followed by measured doses of donor lymphocyte infusions, to increase chimerism to full donor chimerism over time, and thereby eliminate clonal host cells. We recently reported on our series of patients treated with late infusions of CD3+ T-lymphocytes.[27,28] We used G-CSF primed peripheral blood stem cell enriched leukocyte infusions with CD3+ lymphocytes to provide a graft-versus-leukemia effect, and progenitor cells to restore donor hematopoiesis and prevent pancytopenia. We studied the effects in six children and suggested that donor leukocyte infusions should be considered for all children who relapse after bone marrow transplantation, especially in those with myeloid malignancies. Moreover, we suggested that patients who exhibit suboptimal graft function early or late should be considered for additional measured doses of CD3+ lymphocytes from their original donors.

## Suicide Gene Transfer

Another interesting model of treating acute GVHD is through suicide gene transfer.[2,29,30–34] In this model, donor lymphocytes are engineered with the HSV-TK herpes simplex thymidine kinase suicide gene to confer sensitivity to ganciclovir. In cases of severe GVHD, giving ganciclovir can then eliminate the T cells that were infused and caused the GVHD.

# CHRONIC GRAFT-VERSUS-HOST DISEASE

Chronic GVHD also occurs after bone marrow transplantation when an immunocompetent graft is given to an immunoincompetent host and there is disparity between host and donor. Unlike acute GVHD, this starts after the first 100 days (by conventional definition but not always in actual practice). While it has less of an acute presentation and is less immediately life threatening, it can lead to crippling and sometimes fatal disease. It is a systemic multiorgan syndrome that resembles autoimmune vasculitis.[1,35,36] The mechanism of its development is attack by donor T cells causing epithelial cell damage, mononuclear cell inflammation, fibrosis, and in the lymphoid system hypocellularity and atrophy. The major problem is causing life-threatening viral infections, especially CMV.

The most commonly involved organs in GVHD are skin, mouth, eye, sinus, and gastrointestinal tract. After that, lungs, muscles, tendons, serous surfaces, vagina, and bone marrow may become involved. It is not clear as to whether kidney, bladder, and brain can become involved in this process. Chronic GVHD can occur as a consequence of acute GVHD, as de novo disease (no preceding GVHD) or as a subsequent consequence of prior acute GVHD. Unlike acute GVHD, the classification is usually only limited versus widespread, and without specific grading of each organ. Skin involvement is typically hyperpigmentation, hypopigmentation, erythematosis with scaling, and erythematosis that may or may not be covered by lichen planus-like striae. Dermal and subcutaneous fibrosis can cause thickening and hardening of the skin, and it can resemble scleroderma. The fibrosis can result in joint contractors. The mouth is often affected with stray on the mucosal the cheeks, lips or palate, erythematosis of mucous membranes, decreased salivary flow, dryness of mouth. Eyes are often involved with keratoconjunctivitis sicca and can resemble Sjögren's syndrome. Hepatic involvement by chronic GVHD usually presents as bile duct abnormalities and can progress to cirrhosis or hepatic failure. Sinuses can be involved as part of the sicca syndrome and esophagus can be involved with mucosal inflammation and fibrosis and clinically as difficulty in swallowing and retrosternal pain. Although the upper and lower gastrointestinal tract may be involved, it is less common than in acute GVHD. Bronchiolitis obliterans is a very serious complication of chronic GVHD and can occur in up to 26% of bone marrow transplant recipients.

## Pathology

Pathologically there are three main processes that mediate chronic GVHD: epithelial injury, mononuclear cell infiltrate, and fibrosis. Epithelial injury in skin or lip is characterized by basal layer degeneration. In the skin there may be hyperkeratosis and hypertrophy. Fibrosis of epithelial and subepithelial tissues has been described in skin, mouth, esophagus, intestines, lungs, liver, marrow, and other organs.

## Risk Factors for GVHD

The main predisposing factor for development of chronic GVHD after bone marrow transplantation is preceding acute GVHD.[1,18,35-39] Other factors are age of patient, receipt of HLA nonidentical grafts peripheral administration of donor buffy coats in addition to donor marrow cells, and possibly use of a blood stem cell allograft. At this time it appears from most, but not all, reports that granulocyte colony-stimulating factor (G-CSF) mobilized peripheral blood stem cells is associated with a higher incidence of chronic GVHD than historically with the use of bone marrow. The reason for which young children are less at risk for chronic GVHD compared to older children or to adults is unknown. It has been hypothesized that the deteriorating thymic function that occurs with increasing age may be one factor.

# TREATMENT OF CHRONIC GRAFT-VERSUS-HOST DISEASE

## Steroids

Long-term immunosuppressive therapy is usually used in the setting of long-term chronic GVHD.[20,22,40,41] Steroids (daily or every other day) are usually used and can be paired with cyclosporine, thalidomide, mycophenolate or other similar agents. Very slow tapering of cyclosporine after its introduction for GVHD prophylaxis seems to be very helpful in preventing chronic GVHD (or acute flares of acute GVHD). Flares after cyclosporine discontinuation should be treated by reinstitution of full dosage of cyclosporine (i.e., ~12.5 mg/k/day) to which prednisolone can be added. Alternatively, prednisone can be started in full therapeutic doses, to which cyclosporine can be added either on a daily or alternate day basis. Tacrolimus can be used in patients unresponsive to cyclosporine and/or other immune suppressants and shows a response rate of approximately 10%. Daclizumab is proving to be a valuable adjunct in both acute and chronic GVHD and is usually well tolerated.

## Daclizumab

As mentioned in the section on acute GVHD, daclizumab is an inhibitor of Il-2 on activated lymphocytes. It has been used extensively in patients with solid organ transplantation and has been used also for patients with chronic GVHD after bone marrow transplantation. In one published paper, three of four patients with chronic GVHD after bone marrow transplantation had a good response to daclizumab;[44] in another combination of daclizumab with anti-CD20 resulted in complete remission of bullous pemphigoid in a patient with chronic graft-versus-host disease.[45] Patients, including the very young and the elderly, tolerate daclizumab well and some investigators are considering using the drug early in transplant (i.e., prior to steroidresistance and/or as use for prophylaxis).

## Thalidomide

Thalidomide can be used safely in children. We recently reported on our experience with thalidomide therapy in children undergoing bone marrow transplantation.[42] We studied six patients, two with chronic GVHD, two with acute GVHD, and two with chronic progressive GVHD. One patient with chronic GVHD had a complete response, whereas the others had a partial response. Side effects consisted primarily of sedation and constipation. None had neuropathy, which has been reported frequently in adults. One patient had rash, eosinophilia, and early pancreatitis that began shortly after initiation of thalidomide, and persisted and resolved only after discontinuation of thalidomide. In reviewing the literature we found three major studies of thalidomide in GVHD.[42] Overall results showed efficacy in at least 50% of children with chronic GVHD and little or no efficacy in children with exclusively acute GVHD.

The reasons for which thalidomide appears to be effective in chronic as opposed to acute GVHD probably relate to a variety of factors. First, thalidomide is only available as an oral drug and may not be well absorbed when acute GVHD is present because the gastrointestinal tract is not intact. Secondly, antiangiogenesis (the presumed mechanism of thalidomide effect) may be detrimental in the early phase after chemotherapy-induced injury from bone marrow transplant conditioning, and the detrimental effect in preventing healing of the gastrointestinal tract and other organs may obscure any benefit. Conversely, later during the course of bone marrow transplantation recovery when angiogenesis is not as needed for repair of toxicity-related organ damage, the benefit may be much greater than the detriment.

## PUVA Treatment

Ultraviolet irradiation of methoxypsoralen (PUVA) to sensitized patients is helpful for the cutaneous manifestations of chronic GVHD, and extracorporeal photophoresis also can be used.[20,40] Dall'Amico and Messina recently reported on photochemotherapy for their patients with GVHD in children and in adults.[43] They reviewed 31 studies where this was used in the treatment of acute and chronic GVHD. They studied 75 acute GVHD patients: 59 with skin involvement, 47 with liver, and 28 with gastrointestinal manifestations. Treatment duration was from 1 to 24 months. Regression of skin disease occurred in 83% of patients (CR = 67%). A complete remission of liver and gastrointestinal manifestations occurred in 38% and 54%, respectively. Overall patient survival was 53%. Of the 43 patients alive, eight developed chronic GVHD manifestations. A total of 204 chronic GVHD patients treated with extracorporeal phototherapy (ECP) 1 to 11 months from transplantation were considered in 20 series. A regression of skin disease was found in 76% of patients (CR in 38%); an improvement in liver and lung disease was found in 48% and 39%, respectively, and an improvement in oral manifestations was found in 63% of the cases.

## Supportive Care

Chronic GVHD is often incurable either because of resistance to therapy or because of risk of leukemia relapse with complete eradication of chronic GVHD. Supportive care is therefore an important component of care.[20,40,41] Supportive treatment for chronic GVHD involving lungs includes bronchodilators, immune suppressants, infection prophylaxis, immunoglobulin replacement, and sometimes lung transplantation. Physical therapy is important to alleviate the muscle weakness, fasciitis, and contractures that occur. Prophylactic treatment of infections is sometimes needed because of suppression of endogenous immunity to fight infections. Pneumonitis related to CMV and to *Pneumocystis carinii* have both been implicated in the pulmonary syndromes accompanying chronic GVHD.

Patients who have chronic GVHD and who are on immunosuppressive drugs need to have proper supportive care with prevention of infection using trimethoprim/sulfamethoxazole for prevention of *Pneumocystis carinii* pneumonia, and may need oral penicillin or other antibiotics for bacterial infections. Post-bone marrow transplant vaccinations should be deferred in these patients until after the chronic GVHD has abated.

# REFERENCES

1. Klingebiel T, Schlegel PG. GVHD: Overview on pathophysiology, incidence, clinical and biological features. Bone Marrow Transplant 1998;21(Suppl 2):S45–S49.
2. Munker R, Gunther W, Kolb HJ. New concepts about graft-versus-host and graft-versus-leukaemia-reactions. A summary of the 5th International Symposium held in Munich, March 21 and 22, 2002. Bone Marrow Transplant 2002;30:549–556.
3. Bron D. Graft-versus-host disease. Curr Opin Oncol 1994;6:358–364.
4. Crawford SW, Longton G, Storb R. Acute graft-versus-host disease and the risks for idiopathic pneumonia after marrow transplantation for severe aplastic anemia. Bone Marrow Transplant 1993;12:225–231.
5. Gratwohl A, Hermans J, Apperley J et al. Acute graft-versus-host disease: grade and outcome in patients with chronic myelogenous leukemia. Working Party Chronic Leukemia of the European Group for Blood and Marrow Transplantation. Blood 1995;86:813–818.
6. Takatsuka H, Takemoto Y, Yamada S et al. Similarity between eruptions induced by sulfhydryl drugs and acute cutaneous graft-versus-host disease after bone marrow transplantation. Hematology 2002;7:55–57.
7. Washington K, Bentley RC, Green A et al. Gastric graft-versus-host disease: a blinded histologic study. Am J Surg Pathol 1997;21:1037–1046.
8. Mentzel HJ, Kentouche K, Kosmehl H et al. US and MRI of gastrointestinal graft-versus-host disease. Pediatr Radiol 2002;32:195–198.
9. Donnelly LF, Morris CL. Acute graft-versus-host disease in children: abdominal CT findings. Radiology 1996;199:265–268.
10. Tanaka Y, Kami M, Ogawa S et al. Hyperacute graft-versus-host disease and NKT cells. Am J Hematol 2000;63:60–61.
11. Takeda H, Mitsuhashi Y, Kondo S et al. Toxic epidermal necrolysis possibly linked to hyperacute graft-versus-host disease after allogeneic bone marrow transplantation. J Dermatol 1997;24:635–641.
12. Imamura M, Hashino S, Kobayashi S et al. Hyperacute graft-versus-host disease accompanied by increased serum interleukin-6 levels. Int J Hematol 1994;60:85–89.
13. Tambur AR, Yaniv I, Stein J et al. Cytokine gene polymorphism in patients with graft-versus-host disease. Transplant Proc 2001;33:502–503.
14. Hill GR, Krenger W, Ferrara JL. The role of cytokines in acute graft-versus-host disease. Cytokines Cell Mol Ther 1997;3:257–266.
15. Deeg HJ. Cytokines in graft-versus-host disease and the graft-versus-leukemia reaction. Int J Hematol 2001;74:26–32.
16. Akalin E, Murphy B. Gene polymorphisms and transplantation. Curr Opin Immunol 2001;13:572–576.
17. Huang X, Chen Y, Guo N et al. Hyperacute graft versus host disease after allo-stem cell transplantation, analysis of 118 cases (in Chinese). Zhonghua Yi Xue Za Zhi 2002;82:511–514.
18. Dickinson AM, Cavet J, Cullup H et al. GVHD risk assessment in hematopoietic stem cell transplantation: role of cytokine gene polymorphisms and an in vitro human skin explant model. Hum Immunol 2001;62:1266–1276.
19. Przepiorka D, Weisdorf D, Martin P et al. 1994 Consensus Conference on Acute GVHD Grading. Bone Marrow Transplant 1995;15:825–828.
20. Zecca M, Locatelli F. Management of graft-versus-host disease in paediatric bone marrow transplant recipients. Paediatr Drugs 2000;2:29–55.
21. Simpson D. Drug therapy for acute graft-versus-host disease prophylaxis. J Hematother Stem Cell Res 2000;9:317–325.
22. Simpson D. New developments in the prophylaxis and treatment of graft versus host disease. Expert Opin Pharmacother 2001;2:1109–1117.
23. Lazarus HM, Vogelsang GB, Rowe JM. Prevention and treatment of acute graft-versus-host disease: the old and the new. A report from the Eastern Cooperative Oncology Group (ECOG). Bone Marrow Transplant 1997;19:577–600.
24. Arranz R, Conde E, Rodriguez-Salvanes F et al. CsA-based post-graft immunosuppression: the main factor for improving outcome of allografted patients with acquired aplastic anemia. A retrospective survey by the Spanish Group of Hematopoietic Transplantation. Bone Marrow Transplant 2002;29:205–211.
25. Przepiorka D, Kernan NA, Ippoliti C et al. Daclizumab, a humanized anti-interleukin-2 receptor alpha chain antibody, for treatment of acute graft-versus-host disease. Blood 2000;95:83–89.
26. Carswell CI, Plosker GL, Wagstaff AJ. Daclizumab: a review of its use in the management of organ transplantation. BioDrugs 2001;15:745–773.
27. Reddy V, Moreb J, Mehta P. Donor lymphocyte infusions for CML: possible effects of age and mobilization. Blood 2000;95:2994–2995.
28. Mehta PA, Roberts C, Fisk D et al. Donor leukocyte infusions after bone marrow transplantation in children: series from a single institution and review of the literature. Int J Pediatr Hematol Oncol 2001;72:71–79.

29. Tiberghien P, Reynolds CW, Keller J et al. Ganciclovir treatment of herpes simplex thymidine kinase-transduced primary T lymphocytes: an approach for specific in vivo donor T cell depletion after bone marrow transplantation? Blood 1994;84:1333–1341.

30. Tiberghien P. Use of suicide gene-expressing donor T-cells to control alloreactivity after haematopoietic stem cell transplantation. J Intern Med 2001;249:369–377.

31. Tiberghien P. "Suicide" gene for the control of graft-versus-host disease. Curr Opin Hematol 1998;5:478–482.

32. Cohen JL, Boyer O, Thomas-Vaslin V, Klatzmann D. Suicide gene-mediated modulation of graft-versus-host disease. Leuk Lymphoma 1999;34:473–480.

33. Cohen JL, Boyer O, Klatzmann D. Suicide gene therapy of graft-versus-host disease: immune reconstitution with transplanted mature T cells. Blood 2001;98:2071–2076.

34. Bonini C, Ferrari G, Verzeletti S et al. HSV-TK gene transfer into donor lymphocytes for control of allogeneic graft-versus-leukemia. Science 1997;276:1719–1724.

35. Zecca M, Prete A, Rondelli R et al. Chronic graft-versus-host disease in children: incidence, risk factors, and impact on outcome. Blood 2002;100:1192–1200.

36. Penas PF, Jones-Caballero M, Aragues M et al. Sclerodermatous graft-vs-host disease: clinical and pathological study of 17 patients. Arch Dermatol 2002;138:924–934.

37. Patey-Mariaud de Serre N, Reijasse D, Verkarre V et al. Chronic intestinal graft-versus-host disease: clinical, histological and immunohistochemical analysis of 17 children. Bone Marrow Transplant 2002;29:223–230.

38. Jacobsohn DA, Montross S, Anders V, Vogelsang GB. Clinical importance of confirming or excluding the diagnosis of chronic graft-versus-host disease. Bone Marrow Transplant 2001;28:1047–1051.

39. Visentainer JE, Lieber SR, Persoli LB et al. Correlation of mixed lymphocyte culture with chronic graft-versus-host disease following allogeneic stem cell transplantation. Braz J Med Biol Res 2002;35:567–572.

40. Siadak M, Sullivan KM. The management of chronic graft-versus-host disease. Blood Rev 1994;8:154–160.

41. Currie DM, Ludvigsdottir GK, Diaz CA et al. Topical treatment of sclerodermoid chronic graft vs. host disease. Am J Phys Med Rehabil 2002;81:143–149.

42. Mehta P, Kedar A, Graham-Pole J et al. Thalidomide in children undergoing bone marrow transplantation: series at a single institution and review of the literature. Pediatrics 1999;103:e44.

43. Dall'Amico R, Messina C. Extracorporeal photochemotherapy for the treatment of graft-versus-host disease. Ther Apher 2002;6:296–304.

44. Willenbacher W, Basara N, Blau IW et al. Treatment of steroid refractory acute and chronic graft-versus-host disease with daclizumab. Br J Haematol 2001;112:820–823.

45. Szabolcs P, Reese M, Yancey KB et al. Combination treatment of bullous pemphigoid with anti-CD20 and anti-CD25 antibodies in a patient with chronic graft-versus-host disease. Bone Marrow Transplant 2002;30:327–329.

CHAPTER *XXIV*

# Late Effects After Hematopoeitic Cell Transplantation

PAUL A. CARPENTER AND JEAN E. SANDERS

Over the past three decades hematopoietic cell transplantation (HCT) has been administered to children of all ages in an attempt to cure a variety of malignant and nonmalignant disorders. An increasing number of these children have survived into adulthood and have been followed for the development of late complications. The development of chronic graft-versus-host disease (GVHD) and delayed immune reconstitution relates directly to the allogeneic graft, while the underlying disease primarily determines the probability of recurrent disease. Delayed effects that are related to the chemoradiotherapy preparative regimens include neuroendocrine dysfunction and damage to target organs such as the lung, heart, eye, skeletal growth plates and brain. Late effects that more likely have combined etiologies include chronic lung disease, osteoporosis, and secondary malignancies. It is often difficult to ascertain to what extent therapies given prior to HCT contribute to posttransplant late effects. This chapter focuses on the pathophysiology of late effects that have combined etiologies, or which arise predominantly as a result of the preparative regimen. Late events including recurrent disease and chronic GVHD are covered elsewhere (see Chapters 21–23). An understanding of posttransplant delayed effects that relate to the patient's history of chemoradiotherapy is especially relevant to the long-term follow-up of children because of their unique developmental status. Anticipation of problems that may occur is necessary so that prevention or early intervention is possible.

## ENDOCRINE EFFECTS

Endocrine disturbances have been documented in 20% to 80% of survivors of childhood cancer and frequently occur as late effects of therapy. Total body irradiation (TBI) or local external radiation to the whole brain, orbit, face, or nasopharynx frequently disturbs the hypothalamic-pituitary axis.[1–3] The larger the dose-fraction and total cumulative dose, and the longer the duration from therapy, the greater the likelihood for endocrinopathy.

### Growth Hormone Deficiency and Final Adult Height

Growth in children and the attainment of normal adult height is a complex process that requires an appropriate balance of nutritional, genetic, endocrine, and other physical and psychosocial factors. During infancy, growth is highly dependent on nutrition and thyroid hormone. During childhood, growth hormone (GH) predominates, and in puberty the synergistic interplay of GH and sex steroids are critical for attainment of final adult height.[4] During all stages, any prolonged disturbance of physical or psychosocial well-being may adversely impact growth and development.[4-7] For the child who undergoes HCT, such disturbances occur following prior cranial irradiation, TBI, and prolonged glucocorticoid therapy.

Short stature has been defined as height below the third percentile for age, however, linear growth failure also may be present when a child's height growth decreases from their established height channel percentile. For longitudinal studies of growth, the height standard deviation (SD) score, or z-score, is a better expression of the gain or loss in height for individuals, or groups of individuals. The height z-score considers patient sex and age and is a standardized way to express height deviation relative to the mean.

## Growth Hormone Deficiency

Growth impairment has been well documented after exposure to single or fractionated doses of TBI.[8-14] The association of growth failure with GH deficiency appears to be important, but the true incidence of GH deficiency after HCT remains unknown because analyses have been retrospective and GH testing has often been limited to the subset of children who demonstrated poor growth. Therefore, reported incidences of GH deficiency have varied

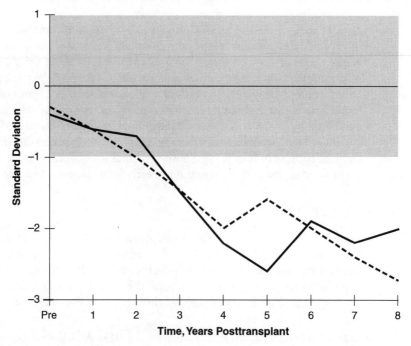

**FIGURE 24.1A** Height standard deviation (SD) scores following pediatric hematopoietic cell transplantation for malignancy. Height SD scores are shown for 101 children who received 1000 cGy total body irradiation (TBI). Fifty-four children received 1800 to 3600 cGy cranial (CNS) irradiation prior to TBI (—) and 47 children received only TBI (--).

from 20% to 85%.[2,15-21] Besides loss of height velocity and final adult height, other clinical problems reported in nontransplanted but GH-deficient individuals include obesity and decreased lean body mass, elevated serum lipids, decreased bone mineral density, and reduced quality of life.[22]

## Preparative Regimen Effects on Growth Hormone Deficiency and Linear Growth

**Irradiation.** Growth hormone deficiency occurs after cranial irradiation in a dose and time dependent manner and is irreversible.[23-27] External beam radiation doses of more than 3000 cGy typically produce GH deficiency within five years of treatment. Doses of 1800 to 2400 cGy administered for the treatment of central nervous system (CNS) leukemia may take longer to result in GH deficiency.[27] Growth in 491 children has been evaluated after single or fractionated dose TBI-containing preparative regimens[15] (updated analysis). One hundred sixty-three of these children who were shorter at the time of transplant had received an additional 1000 to 2400 cGy of cranial irradiation to specifically address CNS leukemia. A 1000 cGy single exposure of TBI was particularly deleterious to growth rates and final adult height in 101 children, and impaired growth manifested between two and eight years posttransplant (◄ Figure 24.1A). Fractionated, total cumulative TBI exposures of 1200 to 1575 cGy also compromised final adult height in 390 children (▼ Figure 24.1B), albeit less significantly than single exposures of 1000 cGy.[13-15] Cranial irradiation further impaired final adult height beyond the effect of TBI alone. Consistent with other reports, the

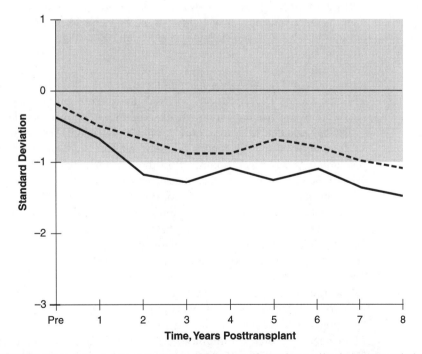

**FIGURE 24.1B** Height standard deviation (SD) scores following pediatric hematopoietic cell transplantation for malignancy. Height SD scores are shown for 390 children given 1200 to 1575 cGy fractionated TBI. One hundred nine children received 1000 to 2400 cGy cranial (CNS) irradiation prior to TBI (—) and 281 children received only TBI (--).

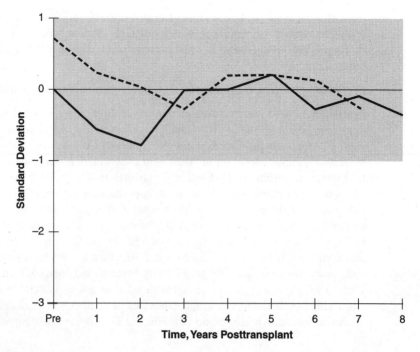

**FIGURE 24.1C** Height standard deviation (SD) scores following pediatric hematopoietic cell transplantation for malignancy. Height SD scores are for 18 boys (—) and 18 girls (--) given busulfan at 16 mg/kg and cyclophosphamide at 200 mg/kg.

impact of cranial radiation was apparent throughout one to eight years following fractionated TBI exposure.[2,12,14,16] In contrast, cranial irradiation did not substantially lower height standard deviation (SD) scores until approximately eight years following single exposure TBI.

**Cyclophosphamide.** Normal growth rates and height SD scores have been observed in 91 children with aplastic anemia whose transplant preparative regimen was cyclophosphamide (CY; 200 mg/kg) alone.[15,28] In these children temporary decrements in growth velocity were observed during periods of active GVHD, but catch-up growth was observed following control of GVHD and discontinuation of glucocorticoid therapy.

**Busulfan.** The reported data pertaining to height growth of children who had Busulfan (BU) added to their CY-containing preparative regimen is limited to small case series. Despite the observation that BU is highly gonadotoxic to the postpubertal ovary, normal growth rates have been observed in both males and females for up to eight years.[12,15,29,30] In one series, 10 children have been reported who have achieved normal final adult height following a BU/CY regimen.[14] We have followed 36 children who underwent marrow transplant for malignant disease at a median age of 10.4 years (range 1.4 to 17.0 years) preceded by a preparative regimen containing 16 mg/kg BU and 200 mg/kg CY (▲ Figure 24.1C; J.E. Sanders, personal communication). The median age of these children is currently 17.3 years (range 7.0 to 28.4 years) and final adult height is evaluable in sixteen. Seven of the girls and nine boys achieved median final adult heights at the 50th (range 5th to 95th) and 25th (range 10th to 50th) percentiles, respectively.

## Diagnosis of Growth Hormone Deficiency

The diagnosis of growth failure is confirmed by documenting a reduction in height velocity. The most accurate and consistent height measurements are obtained with a Harpenden stadiometer. The patient with growth failure will have decreasing height growth and falling height percentile channel. Because the secretion of GH normally follows a diurnal and pulsatile pattern, the diagnosis of biochemical GH deficiency may be confirmed by documenting the absence of normal peaks in GH serum levels as determined from multiple overnight blood samples. More convenient than this labor-intensive sampling procedure are several standardized tests that assess GH secretion in response to provocative stimuli.[31] Because 20% of normally growing children fail to increase GH secretion after one provocative stimulus, and 4% fail after two stimuli, it is standard practice to have two positive GH provocation test results before declaring GH deficiency.[4,32–35] There remains a paucity of normative data about GH response to the entire range of provocative stimuli, but clonidine and arginine are easily administered and have been used extensively in children. The clonidine and arginine stimulation tests may cause mild somnolence or vomiting in 35% and 2% of children, respectively,[35] but are considered safer than the insulin-induced hypoglycemia test, which requires the blood sugar nadir to be less than 50% of baseline levels. The insulin-induced hypoglycemia test must be performed under close supervision and is contraindicated in children with seizure disorders.[4] Insulin Growth Factor-1 blood levels that are controlled for age and gender may be used to confirm GH deficiency and to monitor response to GH therapy but are not sufficiently sensitive or specific to make the diagnosis. The Insulin Growth Factor-1 results are influenced by nutritional status and have generally been unreliable after central nervous system irradiation.[22]

## Treatment of Growth Hormone Deficiency

Even though GH deficiency has been observed in up to 85% of children following HCT, less than half have received GH therapy.[15] No prospective studies have evaluated the impact of early GH replacement therapy on growth and final adult height. Most retrospective studies have indicated that GH therapy may improve growth rates, but most children achieve a final height below their target adult height.[10,14,17,36] In one study, 13 children received a TBI-containing preparative regimen, eight of whom also received prophylactic cranial irradiation for acute leukemia, and were administered GH posttransplant (0.02 to 0.03 mg/kg/day).[17] GH therapy restored normal height velocity but there was no "catch-up" growth and final height SD scores remained impaired. In these children a mean of 3.2 years had elapsed between TBI and initiation of GH therapy, which began at a mean age of 12.2 years (range 5.8 to 18. 2 years). Cohen et al. reported growth in one study of 25 TBI recipients and in another study of 145 TBI recipients, and found that final height SD was significantly lower than both pre-HCT height and corrected mid-parental height.[14,36] These two studies concluded that GH therapy was unnecessary because final height SD was not more than 2 SD below the mean,[36] or because GH treated children did not have significantly improved growth.[14] The poor response to GH therapy has been attributed to factors such as spinal irradiation, early puberty, suboptimal GH dosing schedules and to the older age of most patients when started on GH therapy. Recent data suggest that improvements in growth and final height can be achieved with contemporary dosing regimens that employ daily doses in the range of 0.04 mg/kg, increasing to 0.06 mg/kg at puberty.[16,37–39]

The total height gained from GH therapy has been found to relate inversely to patient age at the start of treatment, and relate positively to the duration of therapy. We have observed that the interval change in height SD score between transplant and diagnosis of GH deficiency was –0.2 and, that an additional –0.2 SD decrement occurred during the median eight month interval between diagnosis and treatment of GH deficiency. Children who received GH therapy subsequently maintained height SD scores, while untreated children experienced a further –0.9 decrement in height SD score by the time they reached final adult height. Factors that were predictive of an improved final height after GH therapy were prior cranial irradiation, age >10 years, or a height SD above –1.5 at the time of transplant. Further loss in height SD was at least prevented in children who were younger than 10 years or whose height SD score was –1.5 or below. The final height SD in GH treated children was ±0.52 SD more compared to untreated children ($P = .003$) in a multiple linear regression model, which adjusted for gender, age at transplant, and height SD score at time of GH deficiency diagnosis. Because growth before puberty is the major determinant of final adult height, treatment during the prepubertal period should be optimized.

Nontransplanted GH deficient individuals have reduced lean body mass, omental obesity, reduced bone mineral density, hyperlipidemia, and a threefold increase in cardiovascular mortality.[22] In addition, GH deficient children have manifested behavioral problems, anxiety, depression, social isolation and academic underachievement, with subsequent difficulties as adults in maintaining gainful employment.[22,40,41] In these patients GH-replacement therapy resulted in increased lean body mass, increased bone mineral density, improved lipid metabolism, and improved overall quality of life.[22,42] Decreased bone mineral density, reduced physical functioning, and low income have emerged also as significant problems after pediatric HCT.[43–45] Longitudinal prospective studies are underway to test the hypothesis that GH replacement therapy has other clinically significant benefits in addition to promoting linear growth.

Concerns that GH therapy may increase the risk for recurrent malignancy have not been validated in large studies of brain tumor survivors.[46,47] Among our 73 children who received more that 268 patient-years of GH therapy, none developed recurrent leukemia and two developed a brain tumor. This incidence of secondary malignancy is less than that observed among children treated for acute lymphoblastic leukemia and is less than that observed at five to ten years after HCT.[48]

## Puberty, Gonadal Function, and Fertility

There is considerable normal variation in the timing and sequence of pubertal events making it difficult to assess a child's pubertal development based only on chronological age-related norms. Pubertal development correlates more reliably with osseous maturation as measured by bone age. An intact hypothalamic-pituitary-gonadal axis is required for initiation and completion of puberty, and maintenance of fertility. Radiation may be toxic to the gonads and hypothalamic-pituitary axis while chemotherapy, particularly alkylating agents, may be gonadotoxic. Therefore, puberty may be disturbed by those chemoradiotherapies administered as the initial treatment for an underlying malignancy, those administered with the transplant preparative regimen, or both. The most common disturbance is pubertal delay secondary to premature gonadal failure. Less commonly, precocious puberty may result from prior cranial irradiation.

## Females

Human oocytes are nonreplaceable and their number is a function of age, peaking at about mid-gestation, and declining from about 2 million at birth to about 2,000 at menopause.[49] The ootoxic effects of radiation and chemotherapy are related to the nonreplaceable population of cells within the ovary. Because most therapies deplete ova rather than ablate them entirely the prepubertal gonad may be more resistant than the postpubertal gonad to damage by alkylating agents and radiation.[50] The half lethal dose (LD50) for the human oocyte is about 400 cGy. Unlike antimetabolites, alkylating agents also affect resting cells and cause dose-dependent oocyte toxicity.[51,52]

**Preparative Regimen Effects on Female Puberty.** Puberty in girls begins with thelarche at a mean age of 11.7 ($\pm$1.2) years and is followed by the development of secondary sexual characteristics. Peak height velocity is achieved at 12.4 ($\pm$1.1) years and results from the synergism between augmented sex hormones and GH production. Ninety percent of girls have had menarche by 12.9 ($\pm$1.05) years, after which there is relatively little gain in height. Attainment of final height occurs by 14.4 ($\pm$1.1) years, or about the time that bony epiphyses fuse.[53] It follows that delayed or absent puberty may significantly impact the development of secondary sex characteristics, growth velocity, and final adult height.

**Irradiation.** Approximately 50% of prepubertal girls given 1200 to 1575 Gy fractionated TBI entered puberty spontaneously and achieved menarche at the normal age.[15] Increased serum follicle-stimulating hormone (FSH) and luteinizing hormone (LH) have been seen in up to two-thirds early posttransplant, but normalization of gonadotropin levels has occurred over time.[54] Almost all of the remaining prepubertal females fail to develop secondary sexual characteristics unless adequate hormone replacement is administered.[15] Delayed puberty is typically associated with blunting of the pubertal growth spurt. The inadequate sex hormone production that results from delayed puberty may lead to a tall and thin body habitus if there is sufficient GH to allow height growth beyond the usual chronological age at which bony epiphyses close.

Precocious puberty is a much less common delayed effect of irradiation than is normal or delayed puberty but has been reported in children, especially girls, who received cranial irradiation between the ages of one to eight years.[54-56] Thirty-six females who received 1800 to 2400 cGy of prophylactic cranial irradiation for acute lymphoblastic leukemia (ALL) at a mean age of 3.9 years manifested precocious puberty at a mean age of 8.6 years. Seven of the 12 tested also had biochemical GH deficiency.[56] These children should be considered to have co-existing GH deficiency that may be obscured by apparently normal growth rates that occur with precocious puberty. Insufficient GH coupled with premature fusion of the epiphyses in these children may severely reduce final adult height.

**Cyclophosphamide.** Nearly all 27 prepubertal girls who were given 200 mg/kg CY and bone marrow transplantation (BMT) for aplastic anemia demonstrated normal pubertal development and all have had normal gonadotropin levels and ovarian function.[15,57,58] However, primary ovarian failure has been reported in prepubertal girls after total cumulative CY doses of above 500 mg/kg.[59]

**Busulfan.** Thirteen of 15 still prepubertal girls who had been transplanted for thalassemia major had hypergonadotropic hypogonadism after preparative regimens containing 14 to 16 mg/kg BU and 200 mg/kg CY.[60] All had low estradiol levels before and after transplant. Interpretation of this data is confounded by the fact that delayed or absent puberty is observed in conventionally treated thalassemia. Combined data from small case series provides limited information for 36 prepubertal girls who were followed after BU-containing preparative regimens for acute myeloid leukemia or solid tumors. Pubertal nonprogression or delay followed in 22 (76%) of the 29 who were evaluable[15,29,30,61,62] (J.E. Sanders, personal communication).

**Diagnosis and Treatment of Delayed Puberty in Girls.** Delayed puberty is defined as the 3% of girls who have not developed the first signs of puberty by 13.2 years.[22] Evaluation of girls at 13 years of age for gonadal failure is advised if there is no evidence of thelarche, or at age 14 if there has been no progression to Tanner Stage 2 or 3, and at age 16 if there has been no evidence of menarche. Constitutional delay in maturation may be present and can be ascertained by inquiry about parental height, weight, onset of maternal menarche, and sex maturational milestones. Hypothyroidism also should be excluded. Hypogonadal individuals often grow normally in childhood, but then fail to undergo the adolescent growth spurt and usually have a weight age greater than their height age. Tanner developmental staging and the color of vaginal mucosae and secretions may be informative. It is important to realize that some androgenic manifestations may reflect adrenarche rather than gonadal function. Useful laboratory investigations include serum FSH, LH, and estradiol levels. A pelvic ultrasonogram can help to define ovarian size and morphology, the presence of cysts and follicles. A wrist radiograph for bone age, and serum for free T4 and thyroid-stimulating hormone (TSH) can help to rule out alternative diagnoses.

Management of abnormal puberty is best done in collaboration with a pediatric endocrinologist. The promotion of sexual maturation in girls with delayed puberty can be achieved by supplementing with daily estrogen. Estrogen is also necessary for the development of peak adult bone mass, which continues to occur into the early twenties. An important additional benefit of estrogen therapy is promotion of the pubertal growth spurt, but doses of estrogen should initially be low, and gradually increased to mimic natural hormone production to prevent premature closure of bony epiphyses and compromised final adult height. In the less common situation of precocious puberty, or normal onset but rapidly progressing puberty, GH deficiency is usually also present. More complicated regimens have integrated gonadotropin-releasing hormone (GnRH) analogs to suppress puberty while GH therapy is concomitantly administered in an attempt to improve final adult height.[56,63,64]

**Preparative Regimen Effects on Ovarian Follicles and Hormonal Function.** Radiation effects on ovarian function are dose and age dependent. The relative contribution of the chemotherapy preparative regimen to ovarian failure is difficult to establish since many patients treated for malignant disease received conventional, alkylating agent chemotherapy before HCT. In general, younger women are less likely to develop premature ovarian failure, although the specific alkylating agent and dose appear to be important.

**Irradiation.** Radiation doses to the ovaries of 250 to 500 cGy will cause temporary amenorrhea in women aged less than 40 years. In women older than 40 years of age artificial menopause usually follows doses of 400 to 700 cGy, but doses of 1000 to 2000 cGy are required to induce ovarian follicle failure in most prepubertal children.[54,65] Therefore, myeloablative TBI doses may produce oligomenorrhea, amenorrhea, and symptoms of premature menopause in all postpubertal females. Ovarian recovery, heralded by spontaneous return of menses, normalization of LH, FSH, and estradiol levels, has been documented in 53 (10%) of 532 women between three and seven years after TBI and was not influenced by the presence or absence of chronic GVHD.[15,57,58,66] Many of the women with ovarian recovery were younger than 26 years of age at the time of TBI administration.

**Cyclophosphamide.** All 103 females aged between 13 and 48 years at the time of receiving CY at 200 mg/kg and HCT for aplastic anemia subsequently developed amenorrhea.[15] Ovarian function recovered in 54% at a median of 9 months (range 3 to 36 months), with a return of normal gonadotropin and estrogen levels and normal spontaneous menstruation. Almost all of the women who recovered ovarian function were less than 26 years of age at the time of transplant.

**Busulfan.** De Sanctis et al. first implicated BU as a cause of ovarian failure in girls transplanted for thalassemia, but interpretation of these data was confounded by the possibility that thalassemia per se may be associated with gonadal failure.[60] Ovarian function was evaluated in 21 girls with solid tumors who were treated with moderate to high cumulative doses of CY or ifosfamide followed by myeloablative autologous HCT.[61] The 10 girls whose preparative regimen contained high-dose BU all had severe and persistent ovarian failure compared to 2 of the 11 who did not receive BU. At least 20 other girls have had ovarian function evaluated after BU/CY preparative regimens and all have demonstrated ovarian failure.[29,30,58,62,67–69] In the largest series reported so far, all but one of 73 women who received BU and CY (200 mg/kg) at a median age of 38 years developed ovarian failure.[66] BU and lower dose CY (120 mg/kg) resulted in a similar outcome when administered to 19 women whose median age was 30 years.[70]

**Evaluation and Treatment of Ovarian Failure.** In the postpubertal female, evaluation of ovarian function should occur by three to six months posttransplant. From postmenarche into the reproductive age, hormonal replacement therapy has been recommended beginning approximately three months after myeloablative doses of TBI or after BU/CY regimens. Hormone replacement therapy may be indicated also after CY-only regimens in those who do not recover normal serum estradiol levels. In women with a uterus, and who are 50 years of age, hormone replacement therapy (HRT) generally comprises daily conjugated equine estrogen with monthly cycles of progestogen because unopposed estrogen increases the risk of endometrial carcinoma. The risk of ovarian or cervical cancer does not appear to be increased with estrogen therapy. All women should be informed about the risks and benefits of receiving hormone replacement therapy. Because 50% of young women recover ovarian follicular function after a regimen of CY alone, it is appropriate to attempt withdrawal of HRT between one to three years posttransplant if serum gonadotropins are not markedly elevated. Potential clinical manifestations that may indicate recovery include premenstrual symptoms and subsequent break-through bleeding while on HRT. Therefore, it follows that successful withdrawal of HRT is indicated by the return of regular menstrual cycles and maintenance of normal serum estrogen and gonadotropin levels. Because ovarian follicle recovery is infrequent and occurs late after myeloablative TBI regimens it is generally not worthwhile to attempt HRT withdrawal before six years posttransplant.

**Preparative Regimen Effects on Female Fertility: Irradiation.** Doses of 500 to 600 cGy produce permanent sterility in 60% of females 15 to 40 years of age and 100% of premenopausal females 40 years and older.[71] Women treated with TBI or with alkylating agents may undergo menopause as early as age 30 and be unable to become pregnant. Among 16 pregnancies and 8 infants born to 13 women who received TBI as children, there was a high risk for spontaneous abortion (8 of 16), preterm labor, and low birth weight but no increase in the frequency of birth defects compared to population norms.[66] Damage to the vasculature and elastic properties of the uterus may impair adequate expansion and lead to positional deformities and early delivery. Cardiovascular and pulmonary late effects may complicate delivery.

**Cyclophosphamide.** Among 56 pregnancies and 44 infants born to 28 women who received high-dose CY alone and BMT as children, the risk of spontaneous abortion was not higher than expected when compared to the general population.[66] Others also have reported pregnancies after chemotherapy alone preparative regimens.[72–74]

**Busulfan.** None of 73 adult women who received BU/CY has become pregnant,[15] and we are not aware of any reported cases of either pregnancy or live births following therapy with myeloablative doses of busulfan. Therefore, currently it seems reasonable to state that busulfan therapy is not compatible with subsequent fertility.

**Evaluation and Treatment of Female Infertility.** The return of spontaneous menses and normalization of FSH, LH, and estradiol levels are indicative of a chance for future pregnancy. However, it is important to note that there is no definitive link between the serum hormonal profile and quality of oocytes. The possibility of becoming pregnant is higher in patients who are younger at the time of transplant.

Despite the reports of pregnancy post-HCT, most women experience ovarian failure and infertility. Frozen embryo storage is currently the best preemptive approach for infertility and has been a standard procedure for in vitro fertilization centers since 1983,[75] but is generally only applicable to women who have a partner to provide sperm. Moreover, the time required for pharmacological stimulation of the ovary before egg retrieval is often contraindicated by the need to initiate chemotherapy for the underlying malignancy. Oocyte banking may offer additional possibilities in the future but is currently experimental and remains limited by poor survival of oocytes and low fertilization rates.[76] An additional area of research is the cryopreservation of ovarian tissue prior to high dose chemotherapy. A landmark case report has documented the transient restoration of ovarian function in one woman following the reimplantation of previously harvested autologous ovarian cortical strips.[77] Further research is required to improve vascular supply to the graft and maintain prolonged activity of the transplanted ovarian tissue.

## Males

Puberty in boys begins with testicular enlargement at a mean age of 13.44 ($\pm$1.04) years. Pubic hair and the first appearance of spermatozoa in early morning urine specimens occur at a mean age of about 13.90 ($\pm$1.04) years. Most dramatic is the rapid linear growth spurt, which peaks in late puberty at 14.36 ($\pm$1.08) and is complete by 15.18 ($\pm$1.07) years.[53]

**Preparative Regimen Effects on Male Puberty: Irradiation.** Sklar et al.[78] noted that 51 of 57 nontransplanted prepubertal boys who received ALL chemotherapy and testicular irradiation exposures ranging from 0-1200 cGy underwent puberty at the normal time. Curiously, constitutional growth delay was responsible for 5 of the 6 cases of delayed puberty. Delayed puberty was also similarly distributed among the patients who received no testicular irradiation (3 of 24 patients), doses of 36 to 360 cGy (2 of 22 patients) and 1200 cGy (1 of 11 patients). However, serum FSH was elevated in 6 of the 53 evaluated, including 4 of 8 (50%) who received 1200 cGy TBI. All 14 evaluable prepubertal boys treated with 1375 to 1500 cGy of hyperfractionated TBI and a 400 cGy radiation boost to the testes entered puberty spontaneously and have manifested normal secondary sexual characteristics, although a third of the survivors had elevated serum LH levels.[54] Sanders et al. observed that 39 (56%) of 70 prepubertal males who were greater than 12 years of age at the time of assessment experienced delayed puberty and blunted height velocity following fractionated TBI doses of 1200 to 1575 cGy without additional testicular irradiation.[15]

Several authors have reported substantially lower rates of delayed puberty following fractionated TBI and have reported that Leydig cell dysfunction did not manifest until total cumulative doses to the testes exceeded 2000 cGy.[79,80] We have observed that fractionated TBI boosted with a 400 cGy testicular exposure did not increase the incidence of delayed puberty above that of TBI alone; however, prior treatment of testicular leukemia with doses of 1800 to 2400 cGy followed by TBI almost always induced testicular failure and pubertal delay.[15]

**Cyclophosphamide.** Standard preparative regimens for aplastic anemia that use 200 mg/kg of CY have not had a measurable affect on male puberty.[58,65] Almost all boys have had normal Leydig cell function with normal serum levels of LH and testosterone.[58] Even cumulative CY doses of 350 mg/kg did not affect progression through puberty.[81]

**Busulfan and Cyclophosphamide.** An initial report analyzed gonadal function in 15 boys transplanted for thalassemia following BU/CY at a time when they were still prepubertal.[60] Unstimulated posttransplant gonadotropin levels were normal as was Leydig cell function. More recently, boys transplanted for acute myeloid leukemia (AML) using BU (16 mg/kg) and CY (120 to 200 mg/kg) have been evaluated. Five of nine evaluable boys had delayed puberty and required sex hormone replacement therapy (J.E. Sanders, personal communication). Others have reported that approximately 50% of boys following BU-containing preparative regimens developed elevated serum gonadotropin levels but have not required sex steroid replacement to promote development of secondary sexual characteristics.[30,82]

**Diagnosis and Treatment of Delayed Puberty in Boys.** Evaluation of boys at 14 years of age for gonadal failure is recommended if there is no evidence of secondary sexual development.[22] Constitutional delay in maturation and hypothyroidism should be excluded. Hypogonadal individuals often grow normally in childhood, but then fail to augment growth at puberty and usually have a weight age greater than their height age. Tanner developmental staging and a history of nocturnal ejaculation and erectile function may be informative. Examination of males should note the absence of acne, comedones, mustache, axillary or pubic hair, penile and testicular development, and change in voice. Useful laboratory investigations include serum FSH, LH and testosterone levels. A wrist radiograph for bone age, and serum for free T4 and TSH can help to rule out other diagnoses.

Management of delayed puberty is best done in collaboration with a pediatric endocrinologist. The promotion of sexual maturation in boys with delayed puberty can be achieved by supplementing with gradually escalated doses of depotestosterone in order to also prevent premature closure of bony epiphyses and compromised final adult height.

**Preparative Regimen Effects on Leydig Cells and Testosterone: Irradiation.** Although more resistant to the damaging effects of irradiation than the germinal epithelium, Leydig cells are susceptible.[71,83] The damage to Leydig cells is directly related to radiation dose and inversely related to age at treatment.[78,84] Doses of 200 to 300 cGy can produce slight increases in LH only, but doses greater than or equal to 2000 cGy produce both increased LH and reduced serum testosterone levels in most patients. The treatment of ALL testicular relapses with 2400 cGy of testicular radiation has caused most prepubertal males to need testosterone replacement therapy. Most, but not all boys who are older and/or in early puberty at the time they are treated with 2400 cGy also will ultimately need therapy with testosterone.[85]

**Cyclophophamide.** Leydig and Sertoli cell function in prepubertal and adolescent boys treated for aplastic anemia has not appreciably been altered by standard preparative regimens using only 200 mg/kg of CY.[86] Subtle forms of Leydig cell dysfunction may be observed following high doses of one of several alkylating agents.[65]

**Busulfan and Cyclophosphamide.** Limited available data indicate that approximately 50% of boys have developed abnormal serum gonadotropin levels following BU containing preparative regimens but have not required sex steroid replacement.[29,30]

**Evaluation and Treatment of Leydig Cell Failure.** Inadequate Leydig cell function triggers negative feedback regulation of the pituitary gland, which raises the serum level of luteinizing hormone (LH), often before there is measurable decrease in the serum level of testosterone. Testosterone replacement therapy is available by either intramuscular injection or by topical skin patch to cause virilization and may increase the sense of well-being in postpubertal hypogonadal males. Over replacement may result in gynecomastia and decreased libido.

**Preparative Regimen Effects on Male Germinal Epithelium and Fertility.** The seminiferous epithelium comprises germinal cells (spermatogonia) and nongerminal, Sertoli (supporting) cells. The process by which germ cell precursors are renewed is poorly understood; however, both intact Leydig cell function and pituitary derived FSH are essential for completion of spermatogenesis. Chemoradiotherapy induced germ cell failure is frequent with 40% to 60% of young adult male survivors having impaired fertility. Alkylating agents such as cyclophosphamide, busulfan, ifosfamide, melphalan, procarbazine, and thiotepa are the major gonadotoxic chemotherapies and both the pre- and postpubertal testes are vulnerable.[87] The commonly used preparative regimens have used CY alone or in combination with either BU or TBI.

**Irradiation.** Germ cell dysfunction is observed in almost all males treated with TBI and most will have elevated serum FSH and reduced testicular volumes.[66] Radiation-induced germ cell damage is dose-dependent but age does not appear to be a risk factor.[88] Doses of 10 to 30 cGy may produce temporary oligospermia, but doses of 200 to 300 cGy may produce testicular shrinkage and azoospermia of several years duration.[66] Permanent azoospermia may occur with doses as low as 1000 cGy and almost always occurs after doses above 2400 cGy.[71] Of note, multiple small fractionated radiation doses appear to inhibit spermatogenesis more than large, single fractions. A few men have fathered children mostly after single dose (1000 cGy) TBI.[66,89] Rarely, late recovery of spermatogenesis has occurred even after pelvic doses as high as 4400 cGy.[90]

**Cyclophosphamide.** The plasma concentrations of FSH became elevated in all postpubertal boys who were treated with 200 mg/kg of CY before the onset of puberty compared to only 50% of boys who were treated after puberty[58]. Despite this observation, irrespective of age at treatment, semen analysis is normal in approximately two-thirds and at least 51 normal infants were fathered by 28 men who had previously been treated with high dose CY[66]. Others have shown that that cumulative CY exposures of more than 20 to 25 g/m$^2$ have a high probability of azoospermia and infertility, whereas a dose of less than 7.5 to 10 g/m$^2$ have improved potential for retaining normal sperm production.[88,91]

**Busulfan and Cyclophosphamide.** Limited data exist, but most males appear to sustain damage to germ cells.[29,30] Of 46 men who were evaluated between one and five years after a BU (16 mg/kg) and CY preparative regimen, the majority had normal LH and testosterone levels, but 75% had elevated FSH and azoospemia. Eight men (17%) recovered testicular function, defined by high-normal serum FSH and low-normal sperm counts, but only two men fathered children.[66]

**Evaluation and Treatment of Male Infertility.** Many males with documented azoospermia fail to have either a decrease in testicular volume or elevation in serum FSH. For patients old enough to produce a semen sample, paternity, or a sperm count of more than 10 × $10^6$/mL or 26 × $10^6$ per ejaculate are the best overall indicators of normal gonadal function. Otherwise, elevated FSH and decreased inhibin serum levels are indicative of damage to germinal epithelium and Sertoli cells, respectively.[83] Such patients may have progressed normally through puberty and have normal erectile and ejaculatory function but are infertile on the basis of nonobstructive oligo- or azoospermia. Serial sperm counts have been shown to increase and fertility may recover five to ten years after therapy.

Sperm banking is possible in males able to provide ejaculate but usually requires five to eight days for the banking of at least three semen samples, each separated by approximately 48 hours of abstinence. Quantitative and qualitative sperm defects may be present at the time of initial diagnosis; however, newer in vitro fertilization techniques make storage of all samples with any live sperm appropriate. Male patients who are azoospermic as a result of hypothalamic or pituitary injury may be treated with recombinant gonadotropins. The offspring of male survivors of childhood and adolescent cancer have similar rates of birth defects as the general population or as sibling controls, but so far there has been no increased risk for perinatal mortality or for low birth weight.[66,92] Following high-dose alkylating therapy, a subgroup of men with nonobstructive azoospermia have had sperm retrieval from testicular biopsies. Sperm obtained by this approach have been used for direct injection into oocytes and led to successful pregnancies in some cases.[93]

# Thyroid Function

Approximately 10% to 40% of children will have measurable abnormalities of thyroid function following the most commonly used HCT preparative regimens.[29,94–97] The most common abnormalities are compensated or overt hypothyroidism, but sick euthyroid syndrome, hyperthyroidism and autoimmune thyroiditis have occasionally been reported.[95,98,99]

## Hypothyroidism

External beam irradiation to the neck or mediastinum has long been known to cause thyroid dysfunction.[100,101] In children who received neuraxis radiation for brain tumors the addition of intensive chemotherapy significantly increased the risk of thyroid dysfunction.[97,102] Of 1791 children treated for Hodgkin's disease, the incidence of hypothyroidism at 15 years was approximately 50% after a thyroid radiation exposure of at least 4500 cGy, 30% after 3500 to 4499 cGy and 17% after less than 3500 cGy. Increasing dose of radiation, older age at diagnosis, and female sex were all independently associated with an increased risk of hypothyroidism.[98] In another large study the actuarial incidence of compensated (increased TSH, normal free T4) and overt hypothyroidism at 20 years was 31% and 21%, respectively, with approximately half of this risk manifesting within five years of therapy.[103,104]

Conventional myeloablative-dose TBI preparative regimens deliver 1.5 to threefold less radiation to the thyroid gland than the total dose associated with the treatment of Hodgkin's disease. Nonetheless, 28% to 37% of children have developed compensated hypothyroidism, and up to 13% have developed overt hypothyroidism after a 700 to 1000 cGy single-exposure of TBI.[96,105–108] Following fractionated TBI exposures of 1200 to 1575 cGy 10% to14% of children have developed compensated and 3% to 7% have developed overt hypothyroidism with up to 49 months follow-up.[19,94,96,106] Hyperfractionated TBI does not appear to further reduce the incidence of hypothyroidism.[94] The cumulative incidence of postradiation hypothyroidism increases with time from exposure. For fractionated TBI schedules the timing of the peak incidence of thyroid dysfunction remains to be established.

Preparative regimens comprising CY alone do not appear to cause thyroid function abnormalities at a frequency greater than expected in the normal population.[28,106,109] Five of 48 (10%) children followed for six to ten years after a BU/CY preparative regimen developed elevated TSH levels but none developed overt hypothyroidism.[29,30,94] At a single institution, eight of 60 adults had elevated TSH between one and five years after BU/CY preparative regimens; in these eight patients the total T4 was normal in three, decreased or increased, one each, and not measured in three.[110]

Annual thyroid screening is recommended by examining for thyroid lumps and by measuring the serum TSH and free T4. Patients who develop overt clinical hypothyroidism, or who have an elevated TSH and low T4 should receive thyroxine replacement therapy. In the few cases where the free T4 is borderline low and the TSH remains normal, it is reasonable to repeat thyroid function studies, including a measure of the free T3, in four to six weeks to help determine the need for thyroid hormone therapy. It is prudent to avoid iatrogenic suppression of the serum TSH because adverse metabolic consequences such as reduced bone mineral density have been reported in some studies.[111,112] The treatment of compensated hypothyroidism has varied. Children who have received prior mediastinal or neuraxis radiation in addition to the transplant preparative regimen may more readily progress to overt hypothyroidism, and treatment with thyroxine is reasonable. In other settings the benefit of thyroid hormone replacement therapy is unclear and elevated TSH levels may be transient.[96]

## Sick Euthyroid Syndrome

Thyroid function has been prospectively monitored during the first posttransplant year in a number of patients.[95,113,114] In two studies, approximately 43% of patients developed a sick euthyroid syndrome (SES) within three to six months posttransplant characterized by low total thyroxine, reduced free T3 or T4 and a normal TSH.[95,114] The SES is a well recognized, possibly adaptive response to severe systemic illness or major surgical procedures, and thyroid function tends to normalize as the illness subsides. Vexiau et al. suggested that SES is significantly less common in children than in adults because SES developed after transplant in only two (8%) of 26 children compared to 31 (60%) of 52 adults.[95] Compared to patients with a normal thyroid function panel patients with SES were receiving significantly higher glucocorticoid doses when thyroid function was tested ($P < .01$). However, since glucocorticoids were used to treat GVHD it was unclear to what extent high-dose glucocorticoid therapy and acute GVHD were interdependent. For reasons that are unclear, survival at 30 months was significantly poorer in patients with thyroid abnormalities compared to patients without ($P < .001$). In the multivariate analysis acute GVHD grade and the presence of thyroid abnormalities remained independently predictive of survival.

## Hyperthyroidism and Autoimmune Thyroiditis

Approximately 5% of children who received at least 3500 cGy radiation to the thyroid developed hyperthyroidism at an average of eight years.[98] Some of these patients were treated with antithyroid medication and 20% underwent thyroidectomy. Permanent hyperthyroidism following HCT is even less common.

Isolated case reports and small case series have documented "autoimmune" hyperthyroidism in two adults[115,116] and hypothyroidism in one child[99] following allogeneic HCT. Adoptive transfer of abnormal donor lymphocyte clones has been suggested as a possible mechanism. Eight of 57 prospectively monitored adults who had normal thyroid function immediately before marrow transplantation developed transient hyperthyroidism at a median of 111 days posttransplant. Seven of the eight survived beyond one year and all became hypothyroid at a median of 12 months posttransplant.[114] Elevated serum thyroglobulin and thyroid autoantibodies in most of these patients suggested that immune mediated thyroid injury ultimately contributed to the hypothyroidism.

## Obesity

Child and adolescent obesity is an increasing problem within the population at large.[117–119] The survivor of HCT is at increased risk for obesity due to prior cranial irradiation,[120] growth hormone deficiency,[121] glucocorticoid therapy,[122] and lower activity levels as a result of physical or other limitations. A metabolic syndrome of obesity combined with hyperinsulinemia, low HDL cholesterol levels, and reduced spontaneous GH secretion was seen in eight of 50 childhood cancer survivors and in none of the cases seen in 50 age- and sex-matched controls; this difference was statistically significantly different.[123] Whether or not GH therapy might reverse this metabolic syndrome remains to be studied. Seven obese prepubertal boys who received six months of GH therapy, without additional dietary or exercise modifications, experienced a 5% increase in lean body mass which lends support to the hypothesis that GH may provide other benefits in addition to promoting height growth.[121]

## GROWTH AND DIRECT TISSUE EFFECTS

### Skeletal Dysplasia

Skeletal dysplasia may result from damage to epiphyseal plates as consequence of TBI and intensive chemotherapy. It contributes at least in part to growth disturbance, and to a disproportionate effect on spinal growth compared with other epiphyses.[124] The ultimate impact on final height depends on the dose of radiation therapy, the volume irradiated, and the age of the child at the time of treatment.

### Orofacial

The combination of chemotherapy and radiation to the head and neck can cause growth impairment of deciduous or permanent teeth.[125–129] Micrognathia and mandibular hypoplasia may occur, especially in those less than seven years of age.[130,131] Radiation may result in diminished secretion of saliva, which contributes to the already increased risk for tooth decay. Impaired dentine and enamel formation may lead to tooth and root shortening and, in some cases, complete lack of tooth development depending on the age of the patient at the time of irradiation. Regular dental examination and attention to oral hygiene and diet are mandatory.

## Alopecia

Temporary alopecia is universal after myeloablative chemotherapeutic or radiation-based preparative regimens, but hair regrowth is usually occurring between four and six months later. Permanent alopecia after marrow transplant was initially recognized in adults as a manifestation of chronic GVHD.[132,133] Incomplete hair regrowth also has been reported in adults following non-TBI, BU-containing preparative regimens, and either autologous or allogeneic BMT, in the absence of chronic GVHD.[134,135] In one pediatric study, Vowels et al.[136] prospectively classified the degree of alopecia with respect to pretransplant status as severe (<50% hair regrowth), moderate (50 to 75%) or mild (>75% but less than pretransplant). Overall 18 (24%) of 74 children developed alopecia after either TBI or BU-containing preparative regimens. Permanent alopecia was not seen in children who were transplanted for non-malignant disease and had not received prior chemoradiotherapy. The 13 (18%) with moderate to severe alopecia had received prior cranial irradiation and/or developed chronic GVHD, whereas the five with mild alopecia had not. The risk factors were chronic GVHD ($P < .001$), older age ($P < .001$), prior cranial irradiation ($P = .03$), and there was a trend toward more frequent alopecia with BU ($P = .15$). Ljungman et al. observed that mean minimal BU concentrations were $656 \pm 222$ ng/mL in patients who developed alopecia compared to $507 \pm 224$ ng/mL in those who did not ($P = .005$).[137] Busulfan clearance declines with age and is consistent with the observation that older age is a risk factor for alopecia. Unfortunately, in the case of HCT for leukemia, it is likely that BU levels, which minimize the risk for alopecia, may be insufficient to also minimize the risk for relapse.[137,138] In summary, these studies allow reasonable speculation that permanent damage to hair follicles is cumulative. During pretransplant counseling it is appropriate to mention the possibility of permanent alopecia, especially for children who previously had cranial irradiation, those who are to be conditioned with BU, and those who are of older age and at increased risk for chronic GVHD.

## PULMONARY EFFECTS

Late onset pulmonary complications develop in at least 15% to 25% of all HCT recipients. Before the use of cotrimoxazole and ganciclovir was routine, *Pneumocystis carinii* and cytomegalovirus (CMV) pneumonias accounted for most of the late onset pulmonary complications and death from pulmonary failure. More recently, "noninfectious" late pulmonary complications have been equally appreciated. Consideration of relationships between histopathology, pulmonary physiology, and associations with regimen-related toxicity, GVHD and infection are helpful in recognizing which patients are likely to have noninfectious late pulmonary complications and with management (▶ Figure 24.2). It follows that the exclusion of infection must be considered in the diagnostic evaluation of all late pulmonary complications.

Noninfectious late pulmonary complications comprise four major disease entities, the most common of which is physiologically-defined restrictive lung disease. The remaining three diagnoses are clinicopathologic syndromes whose exact pathogenesis remains poorly understood: bronchiolitis obliterans (BO), BO with organizing pneumonia (BOOP), and late idiopathic pneumonia syndrome (IPS). Clinically significant noninfectious late pulmonary complications occur in 10 to 15% of adult HCT recipients[139,140] (D. Madtes, personal communication), but it remains unclear if the overall incidence of noninfectious late

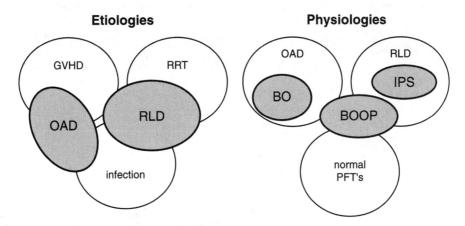

**FIGURE 24.2** Interrelationships between clinicopathological syndromes, pulmonary physiology and etiologies. Abbreviations: GVHD = graft-versus-host disease; RRT = regimen-related toxicity; OAD = obstructive airways disease; RLD = restrictive lung disease; BO = bronchiolitis obliterans; BOOP = bronchiolitis obliterans organizing pneumonia; IPS = idiopathic pneumonia syndrome; PFTs = pulmonary function tests.

pulmonary complications in children is different. One large single institution study reported a 7% aggregate incidence of severe BO, restrictive lung disease, and IPS in pediatric recipients of mainly allogeneic bone marrow.[141] Evaluation of 528 BMT recipients at St Jude Children's Research Hospital in the 1990s indicated that 16% developed posttransplant radiographic pulmonary infiltrates.[142] Approximately 75% of these were further investigated and caused by infection in 30%, BOOP in 26% and IPS in 21%.

A patient may exhibit features of more than one noninfectious late pulmonary complication for which pathognomonic clinical features and histologies are lacking. Clinically, noninfectious late pulmonary complications also may mimic infection, further causing diagnostic dilemmas. Therefore, diagnosis requires consideration of the various known temporal associations, clinical symptoms, and signs, and whether there are recognizable patterns of radiographic and pulmonary function tests (▼ Table 24.1). Bronchoalveolar lavage with the use of fluorescent antibody stains, and shell vial cultures, is usual in the work-up of noninfectious late pulmonary complications other than restrictive lung disease, and permits sensitive and specific detection of viral, bacterial and *Pneumocystis carinii* infections, although negative results neither exclude the presence of fungal infection nor confirm a diagnosis of noninfectious late pulmonary complications.[143,144] Thorascopic lung biopsy is generally required to continue the work-up of a focal pulmonary infiltrate after a negative bronchoalveolar lavage, with the likely diagnoses being BOOP or infection. A lung biopsy is usually not warranted when idiopathic pneumonia syndrome is suspected and an acceptable bronchoalveolar lavage specimen is negative.

## Restrictive Lung Disease

Restrictive lung disease is indicated by a total lung capacity (TLC) of less than 80% predicted. Restrictive lung disease at three months posttransplant or a greater than or equal to 15% loss of TLC in one large study has been associated with a twofold increase in nonrelapse

# TABLE 24.1  Pulmonary Clinicopathological Syndromes

| Feature | IPS | | BOOP | | BO | |
|---|---|---|---|---|---|---|
| **Onset** | Early | Late | | | Early | Late |
| Days from transplant[a] | 21 | 197 | 108 | | 88 | 397 |
| Range days | 1–117 | 106–1639 | 5–2819 | | 54–147 | 165–783 |
| **Incidence (%)** | 6–8 | 4 | ~1 | | 4.0–4.5 | 6.0–6.5 |
| **Symptoms (%)** | | | | | | |
| Dyspnea | | 100 | 45 | | 51 | |
| Fever | | 87 | 61 | | 0 | |
| Cough | | 46 | 59 | | 60 | |
| Wheeze | | 18 | 0 | | 23 | |
| Flu-like | | ND | 0 | | 23 | |
| Asymptomatic | | 0 | 23 | | 20 | |
| **Signs (%)** | | | | | | |
| Crackles | | ND | 48 | | 14 | |
| Tachypnea | | ND | 12 | | ND | |
| Wheeze | | ND | 2 | | 40 | |
| None | | 0 | 50 | | 0 | |
| Reduced SaO$_2$ | | 100 | ND | | ND | |
| Ventilatory support | | 79 | end-stage | | end-stage | |
| **Abnormal radiography (%)** | | 100 | 100 | | 20 | |
| **Pulmonary function tests** | | noncontributory[b] | restrictive | 43% | obstructive | |
| | | | obstructive | 11% | | |
| | | | mixed | 8% | | |
| | | | DLCO ↓ | 64% | | |
| | | | normal | 38% | | |
| **Associations** | | | | | | |
| Infection | | 28%[c] | 13%[d] | | 69%[e] | |
| GVHD | | > 65%[d] | > 80% | | 74% | |
| GE reflux | | ND | ND | | Yes | |
| **Therapy** | | | | | | |
| Immunosupression | | Yes | Yes | | Yes | |
| Directed antibiotics | | No | Unusual | | Consider | |
| Antifungal prophylaxis | | Yes | Unusual | | Unusual | |
| PCP prophylaxis | | Yes* | Yes | | Yes | |
| ECO prophylaxis | | Yes* | Yes | | Yes | |
| Gastric acid inhibitor | | Yes | Unusual | | Consider | |
| **Pulmonary Prognosis (%)** | Early | Late | | | | |
| Improved | 26 | 25 | 78 | | 17 | |
| Stable | 5 | 12.5 | 0 | | 17 | |
| Progessive | 69 | 62.5 | 22 | | 42 | |
| **Survival (%)** | 13[f] | 25[g] | 55[f] | | 35[h] | |

Abbreviations: IPS = idiopathic pneumonia syndrome; BOOP = bronchiolitis obliterans with organizing pneumonia; BO = bronchiolitis obliterans; PCP = *Pneumocystis carinii* pneumonia; ECO = encapsulated organism prophylaxis; ND = no data.

[a]Median for IPS and BOOP, mean for BO.
[b]Usually too ill to perform and BAL results are sufficient.
[c]The 1993 NHLBI definition of IPS excludes infection,[176] but 28% of autopsy specimens were infected, usually with fungus.[177]
[d]Viral infection in 6 of 7 cases.
[e]Sinusitis in 50%.
[f]One-year survival.
[g]Two of 8 patients.
[h]Three-year survival.

mortality related to respiratory failure.[145] Reductions in diffusing capacity also may be observed. One large pediatric study found that 26% of children who were more than six years of age and at least five years after HCT developed restrictive lung disease.[146] The factors most strongly predictive for restrictive lung disease were 1000 cGy of single-dose or 1575 cGy of fractionated TBI, or more than five years from diagnosis to BMT. A smaller study from Denmark documented asymptomatic restrictive lung disease in 10 of 25 (40%) children at a median of eight years after TBI-containing preparative regimens.[147] Kaplan et al. monitored pulmonary function tests for up to seven years in 46 children who had undergone marrow transplant either for aplastic anemia, or for acute leukemia or lymphoma. Only the latter group, who received an 800 cGy dose or eight fractions of 165 cGy TBI, developed restrictive lung disease.[148] Chronic GVHD is not a risk factor for restrictive lung disease (RLD) except in rare instances when restrictive lung disease is due to BOOP or scleroderma involving the chest wall. Likewise, the incidence of restrictive lung disease or diffusing capacity abnormalities has not differed between autologous and allogeneic HCT recipients.[149]

Children do not attain final adult thoracic dimensions nor a full complement of alveoli before eight years of age.[150] Therefore, children younger than eight years of age who are exposed to chemoradiotherapeutic or other lung insults might be more likely to develop severe RLD than adults because of stunted growth and nonrecuperable damage to and loss of pulmonary structures. Surprisingly, age at transplant age was not associated with development of restrictive lung disease.[146] Exertional dyspnea has been observed in patients with more severe RLD consistent with there being reduced pulmonary reserve. Deaths from pulmonary failure have been reported, and at least two patients have received lung allografts for end-stage restrictive lung disease[141,151] (J.E. Sanders, personal communication). Therefore, long-term monitoring of pulmonary function tests, aggressive pulmonary hygiene, and prompt therapy of infection is warranted.

## Obstructive Airways Disease and Bronchiolitis Obliterans

Pulmonary function tests that reveal an actual forced expiratory volume-1/forced vital capacity (FEV1/FVC) ratio of less than 70% and FEV1 of less than 80% predicted are indicative of airways obstruction. Although some patients have airways obstruction pre-transplant, new obstructive airways disease occurs in at least 10% of adult patients with chronic GVHD, and has been seen rarely in recipients of autologous HCT.[152–154] One study of 89 pediatric recipients of allogeneic marrow transplantation reported that 13 of 67 (19%) who survived beyond 90 days developed obstructive airways disease; three of which were transient.[155]

Bronchiolitis obliterans (BO), characterized by fibrinous obliteration of bronchioles, is the histology most commonly found in lungs of patients with obstructive airways disease.[152,153] Patients usually present without fever but with dyspnea and a nonproductive cough, and often with wheeze or "flu-like" symptoms. The chest x-ray is usually normal although pneumothoraces have been noted. High-resolution computerized tomography (CT) has been helpful in evaluating children with suspected BO, particularly when they are unable to perform pulmonary function tests.[155] High-resolution CT scans usually reveal bronchial dilatation, a mosaic pattern of attenuation, and may show evidence of air-trapping during expiration.[156]

Risk factors for obstructive airways disease in adults are chronic GVHD, older age of patient at transplantation and prolonged use methotrexate for GVHD prophylaxis.[152] The striking similarity between histopathologic features of BO after marrow transplant and the BO associated with lung transplant rejection as well as reports of improved lung function after immunosuppressive therapy is compelling.[152,155,157] Although the strong association of chronic GVHD with BO after transplantation is now well accepted,[139,158] the absence of defined target antigens or hallmark epithelial cell apoptosis in lung biopsy specimens has not enabled causality between GVHD and obstructive airways disease/BO to have been ratified.

It is important to establish the rate of progression of airways obstruction in patients with suspected BO. Clark et al. demonstrated that patients whose FEV1 declined by more than 30% predicted for a rapid course and worse outcome during the first year, whereas no patient died of respiratory failure if the decrement in FEV1 was less than 30%.[159] Those with less severe obstructive airways disease usually present beyond day 150; 50% may show stabilization of pulmonary function tests but reversal of obstructive airways disease is uncommon. Palmas et al.[139] likewise found that mild airflow limitation was associated with durable remissions, whereas a reduction in FEV1 to less than 45% predicted was associated with poor response.

In the absence of data from prospective studies evaluating the treatment of BO, a prednisone-containing immunosuppressive regimen suitable for chronic GVHD is applied. Aerosolized bronchodilator treatment for symptomatic patients also may be appropriate. Early and aggressive antibiotic therapy for concomitant sinopulmonary disease should be considered given the high frequency of infection in these patients. A history of gastro-esophageal reflux is often elicitable in patients with GVHD involving the upper intestinal tract. An empiric trial of a proton-pump blocker plus avoidance of a completely horizontal posture may relieve heartburn and reduce covert episodes of pulmonary aspiration.[155,160] Antibiotic prophylaxis for *Pneumocystis carinii* and encapsulated organisms is recommended, as is treatment of hypogammaglobulinemia or IgG subclass deficiencies.[161] The successful application of extracorporeal photopheresis (ECP) to treat refractory BO after lung allografting has been reported in at least 27 patients.[162–164] Three small case series have indicated efficacy for BO after HCT also.[165–167] Finally, lung transplantation has been reported in five patients with pulmonary failure related to BO. Four of these patients had marked improvement in lung function and were alive between 23 months and six years at time of the report.[168–170]

## Bronchiolitis Obliterans Organizing Pneumonia

The syndrome of BOOP was first described as a distinct entity by Epler and co-workers in 1985.[171] Subsequently, a number of case reports have described BOOP in children and adults who have undergone HCT.[172–175] Patients with BOOP present with fever, cough, dyspnea and crackles on auscultation, with disease severity ranging from a mild illness to respiratory failure and death. Histologically, BOOP is defined by plugs of granulation tissue that fill distal airway lumina, extending in to the alveolar ducts and sacs. Alveolar septa may be widened with monocytic infiltrates, and foamy macrophages may accumulate in alveoli. Histological features of BOOP and BO have been observed at different sites of the same lung biopsy specimen, suggesting that these entities represent a spectrum of lung pathology. In the largest series reported to date in the HCT setting, fever, cough, dyspnea, and crackles on physical exam were typical clinical features, and both prior acute and chronic GVHD were strongly associated with development of BOOP, which occurred in about 1% of allogeneic

HCT recipients[140] (D. Madtes, personal communication). Of note, in 22% of patients BOOP arose in the setting of a glucocorticoid taper that had been prescribed for chronic GVHD, and was associated with a viral infection in 13%. Chest radiography or high-resolution CT scans are abnormal; most often showing multifocal patchy opacities or solitary focal pneumonia, and less often, diffuse asymmetric infiltrates[140,156] (D. Madtes, personal communication). The pattern of pulmonary function test results is usually restrictive, although may be normal when BOOP pathology is isolated and focal in distribution. Most small case series indicate that BOOP usually responds to steroids and is associated with a good prognosis.[139] Freudenberger et al. confirmed the findings of others that resolution of BOOP was usual, but could not confirm the conclusions of small case series that found glucocorticoid therapy to be beneficial. In contrast, they found that 22% of BOOP cases progressed despite glucocorticoids. Their case-control analysis was not suitable for evaluation of efficacy, and it is possible that mild cases of focal BOOP did as well without glucocorticoids as more clinically severe cases that received glucocorticoids. Despite the observations that resolution of BOOP is usual, the benefit of glucocorticoids remains unconfirmed. Survival after BOOP appears to fall from 55% at one year down to 33% at five years and possibly relates to the broader sequelae of underlying chronic GVHD.

## Late Onset Idiopathic Pneumonia Syndrome

Idiopathic pneumonia syndrome (IPS) has been defined as a diffuse lung injury for which no infectious etiology is identified[176] and occurs in 6% to 8% of HCT recipients with a median onset during the second to third week,[177] although late onset IPS has been reported 3 to 24 months after HCT.[139,178] The pathogenesis likely involves cytokine-induced and alloreactive T cell-mediated lung injury with a subsequent widespread interstitial inflammatory response and/or alveolar damage associated with the recruitment of other leukocytes. In advanced stages of the IPS, macrophage-induced fibroproliferation contributes to irreversible damage.[176] As mentioned earlier in reference to BO, a definitive casual link between GVHD and the idiopathic pneumonia syndrome is lacking. Recent animal models have demonstrated that IPS developed in irradiated mice transplanted with allogeneic but not syngeneic marrow, and that high concentrations of proinflammatory cytokines were found in BAL fluid of mice with IPS.[179,180] Donor T cell alloreactivity per se, in the absence of systemic GVHD, was sufficient to mediate lung damage after allogeneic BMT.[180] More recently, high levels of tumor necrosis factor-alpha (TNF-α), interleukin-1 (IL-1), IL-2, and IL-6 were identified in the alveolar lung fluid of patients with the idiopathic pneumonia syndrome, but not in patients without idiopathic pneumonia syndrome or normal volunteers.[181] Although grade IV acute GVHD has been strongly associated with IPS, the incidence of IPS is only slightly lower among autologous than allogeneic HCT recipients.[182] TBI-containing preparative regimens in patients who have received prior chest radiotherapy[183] appear to increase the risk of IPS and both increased dose and dose rate of TBI are risk factors.[184,185] In contrast, the idiopathic pneumonia syndrome occurs infrequently in patients receiving non-TBI regimens for aplastic anemia.[186] Overall, the major risk factors for idiopathic pneumonia syndrome include high-dose radiotherapy and multiorgan dysfunction associated with alloreactivity.[177]

The clinical presentation of idiopathic pneumonia syndrome is usually dramatic and marked by dyspnea, fever, and hypoxemia. Chest radiographs are diffusely abnormal, and in cases where the patient was not too ill, pulmonary function tests have indicated a pattern of restriction and impaired diffusing capacity. Approximately 70% of patients require ventilatory support, 50% within two days of presentation. Anecdotal reports have suggested that very high dose methylprednisolone (2 to 10 mg/kg/day) may be beneficial in the therapy of idiopathic pneumonia syndrome, but methylprednisolone at doses of less than 2 mg/kg/day was no more efficacious than no steroids.[177] Concomitant antifungal prophylaxis is usual based on autopsy results indicating that 28% of patients with the idiopathic pneumonia syndrome died with infection that was mostly fungal. Mortality rate approaches 70% for the idiopathic pneumonia syndrome, almost 100% if mechanical ventilation is required.[177]

# CARDIAC EFFECTS

Survivors of childhood malignancy represent one of the largest risk groups for premature cardiovascular disease.[187] Much of the knowledge about late effects of chemotherapy and fractionated mediastinal radiation has come from the study of Hodgkin's disease in childhood. Since the beginnings of HCT in the 1970s late cardiac sequelae have been infrequent. Subclinical abnormalities in the electrocardiograms and myocardial contractility of children have been reported in children evaluated between six months and 16 years posttransplant.[188,189] Treadmill testing appears to be the most sensitive test and detects abnormal cardiac output and oxygen consumption during exercise. In one series of 63 pediatric patients, 40 of whom had previously received anthracyclines, 8 (12.7%) developed late cardiac symptoms, were classifiable as New York Heart Association Class II or III, and had abnormal exercise tests. Because only 20 to 30 years have elapsed since the first decade of HCT in children and young adults, it is conceivable that cardiovascular complications may not yet have presented. Therefore, it is wise for physicians to fully evaluate suspicious cardiovascular symptoms.

## Irradiation Effects on the Heart

Although conventional doses of TBI deliver approximately 25% to 40% less cumulative dose to the mediastinum than traditional doses of mediastinal radiation delivered to the patient with Hodgkin's disease, the delivery of fractionated TBI involves shorter dose intervals, and therefore may still be damaging. Radiation may directly affect all structures of the heart including the pericardium, myocardium, valves, conduction tissues, and coronary blood vessels causing functional abnormalities.[187] Two children who are surviving more than 10 years following TBI-containing preparative regimens have coronary artery disease (J. Sanders, personal communication).

## Chemotherapy Effects on the Heart

Initial preclinical studies in rhesus monkeys conditioned with high-dose cyclophosphamide for BMT indicated the potential for myocardial failure.[190] The risk factors for anthracycline-related cardiac damage after conventional chemotherapy in childhood include age less than four years and female gender.[191] A cumulative anthracycline dose of more that 550 mg/m$^2$ is also a significant risk factor,[192] but the relationship of cardiac toxicity to dose is not linear and reduced cardiac contractility has been reported even after total doses less than 300 mg/m$^2$.[193] In a subcohort of 635 participants drawn from the Childhood Cancer Survivor Study, among those who received anthracyclines, only 30% recalled receiving daunomycin therapy and 52% recalled receiving doxorubicin therapy even after prompting with the drug's names.[194] HCT recipients who previously received anthracyclines for an underlying malignancy may be at greater risk for cardiomyopathy if administered cyclophosphamide and/or irradiation with the HCT preparative regimen.[195] Cardiomyopathies have been reported after cyclophosphamide at 200 mg/kg but usually early during the peritransplant period.[196] At least two children at our institution have died from late cardiomyopathy (J. Sanders, personal communication).

## SKELETAL EFFECTS

Two posttransplant sequelae that involve the skeleton are iatrogenic complications of reduced bone mineral density[44,197,198] and avascular necrosis.[199,200] The incidence of these problems in children is similar and the risk factors for both may include therapies administered before and after the transplant preparative regimen. Prior chemotherapy and TBI may cause skeletal dysplasia as the result of epiphyseal plate damage (Section B). Less commonly, osteochondromata may develop in the long-term survivors of TBI.

In our series of more than 400 children surviving long-term, 14 have reported exostosis and 32 have reported osteochondromata. Lesions developed in long bones, digits, ankles, and scapulae. Radiation osteochondromata are more often multiple than single and are indistinguishable from the more common idiopathic type. Malignant change has not been reported after TBI-induced osteochondromata,[201,202] but in our series one patient developed malignant change in a TBI-induced osteochondroma of the scapula. GH therapy has altered the natural history of osteochondromata.[202]

### Bone Mineral Density

Dual-energy X-ray absorptiometry (DEXA) is a validated semiquantitative method for assessing bone mineral density (BMD). Osteopenia, or reduced BMD, is defined in children by a z-score of −1.0 to 2.4 standard deviations below age-related mean BMD, osteoporosis is defined by a z-score of less than or equal to −2.5. Until recently, normative BMD data have not been available for children and thus, most studies have included only adult patients who demonstrated significant decreases in BMD after HCT. Approximately 40% of 104 adults were reported to be osteopenic at 12 months after HCT.[203] The only study that has reported BMD in children following HCT has indicated that median BMD z-scores were significantly lower, −0.5 (−2 to 1.0) SD, than in adults, 1.0 (−2 to 3; $P < .03$).[44] This is of particular concern because large epidemiological studies have shown that osteopenia and osteoporosis are associated with an increased risk of fracture.[204] The cumulative incidence of non-traumatic fractures in 714 children transplanted over the last three decades and surviving at least two years after HCT is 6% with 74% occurring in the first five years after HCT (J.E. Sanders, personal communication). In descending order of frequency fractures occurred in the radius, humerus, tibia or fibula, vertebrae, femur, ankle, or bones of the feet.

One of the most critical factors in determining involutional osteoporotic fracture risk is the magnitude of peak bone mass that rapidly accumulates during adolescence and early adulthood under the influence of GH and sex steroids. It remains unknown to what extent radiation and chemotherapy contribute to reduced BMD; however, children with decreased BMD carry the increased risk for fractures into adulthood.[205]

The risk factors for reduced BMD in adults are cumulative dose and duration of glucocorticoid therapy,[203,206] and the amount of bone loss is greatest in the first year of glucocorticoid therapy.[207,208] Other risk factors include the duration of cyclosporine and tacrolimus therapy,[203,209] sex hormone insufficiency,[50,197] and a history of prior cranial irradiation.[210] Interestingly, Gilzanz et al. reported that vertebral trabecular BMD was 10% lower in ALL survivors who were 6 to 98 months (mean 42 months) off therapy than in non-leukemic controls who were matched for age, sex, and ethnicity. This decrease could be completely accounted for by those patients who had received cranial radiation.[210] In adults, total body irradiation did not appear to impact BMD.[203] In the analysis by Sanders et al. (personal communication), 19 of the 39 children who developed nontraumatic posttransplant fractures were tested and found to be GH deficient and 18 of the 39 who underwent DEXA scanning had osteoporosis. Of interest, GH-deficient adults treated with GH were found to have a decreased incidence of fractures.[211] Mauseth et al. have reported that the mean hip and lumbar-spine BMD z-scores of 23 GH deficient children who were osteopenic at three years posttransplant improved significantly following treatment with GH.[43]

Dual energy x-ray absorptiometry scans are advised for children at three months and one year posttransplant to enable early detection of reduced BMD. It is reasonable to check a serum calcium, magnesium, and 1, 25-hydroxyvitamin D level in those patients who are shown to have osteoporosis. Supplementation with calcium, vitamin D, and weight-bearing exercise based on guidelines of national organizations[212–214] are recommended, although alone, these measures have not proven effective in preventing osteopenia, osteoporosis, or fractures. Wherever possible, glucocorticoid therapy should be tapered to an alternate day steroid regimen. Sex hormone replacement therapy has increased bone mass in both women and men.[215–217] Prospective studies evaluating the impact of bisphosphonates, sex hormone therapy, and GH replacement on posttransplant BMD and fracture rates are required.

## Avascular Necrosis

Avascular necrosis (AVN) develops in 4% to 10.4% of allogeneic HCT survivors at a median of 12 months (range 2 to 132 months) after transplantation.[199,200,203,218] Nontraumatic AVN is considered to have an ischemic origin but the exact pathogenesis remains poorly understood. Contributing etiologies to bone ischemia have included obliterative arteritis, thrombophilia, hyperlipidemia and fat embolism, repeated microfractures of weight-bearing bone, and increased intramedullary pressure that is possibly secondary to increased intramedullary fat (reviewed[219]). Animal studies have demonstrated that glucocorticoid treatment causes increased intramedullary fat[220,221] and may potentiate the effects of co-existing etiologies because an immunological insult, alone or in combination with glucocorticoids, caused AVN in experimental animals but glucocorticoids or placebo alone did not.[222,223] Glucocorticoid therapy has been associated with approximately 50% of AVN cases in humans[224] and was the factor most associated with increased risk for developing AVN among 1939 adult long-term HCT survivors at the Fred Hutchinson Cancer Research Center. Interestingly, increased duration of steroid use did not provide additional risk.[225] TBI-preparative regimens have also increased the risk for AVN whereas posttransplant use of cyclosporine did not. The largest reported study of posttransplant AVN has involved 4388 patients and in the multivariate analysis three major risks were identified: age older than 16 years, an initial diagnosis of aplastic anemia or acute leukemia, and GVHD.[199] Consistent with these observations Koc et al. have recently reported that patients randomized to alternate-day prednisone for the treatment of chronic GVHD were significantly more likely to develop AVN than those randomized to prednisone and daily cyclosporine (22% vs. 13%, $P = .04$).[226]

In HCT recipients AVN occurs most frequently in weight-bearing bones; the hip in 88%,[199] followed by the humerus. On average approximately two joints, and up to seven joints are affected.[199,227] Compared to idiopathic AVN the joint involvement of glucocorticoid-associated AVN is often bilateral and more severe.[224] AVN is recognized clinically by the presentation of persistent or progressive pain in a typically affected joint, especially in a patient who has received glucocorticoids for GVHD. Plain film radiography lags approximately six months behind pathophysiology and is therefore usually insufficient to detect the early lesions of AVN.[224] Early and accurate diagnosis is best confirmed by MRI imaging of the suspected joints.[218] Attempts at defining early and potentially reversible, or more treatable stages of hip AVN have lead to several classification schema. The early Ficat schema relied on plain film radiography.[228] More recent schema also have utilized information from MRI to distinguish Stage I (abnormal MRI, normal radiograph) and Stage II (abnormal MRI, structurally abnormal radiograph), which occur prior to collapse of the femoral head, from more advanced lesions that are identified by abnormal MRI and radiography showing loss of femoral head contour, and often loss of joint space.[229] In addition to stage, the extent and location of the necrotic portion of bone have been shown to predict outcomes.[230,231]

In the first instance, management of AVN involves provision of pain medications and avoidance of exacerbating factors. A reduction in glucocorticoid therapy should be attempted. Despite the potential benefit of bisphosphonates and statins in the prevention and treatment of early AVN, neither agent has been sufficiently studied for this purpose in adults, nor have they been used extensively in children. Almost half of patients with AVN in the large French study ultimately required joint replacement.[199] In children and young adults it is preferable to avoid early placement of artificial joints that have a finite lifespan. Based on the hypothesis that AVN results from bone ischemia secondary to an intramedullary compartment syndrome, a core decompression procedure has been used to promote revascularization of the femoral head, and to avoid or delay joint replacement.[219,224,231] Core decompression is a well-tolerated, short-stay procedure; complications have occurred in 5% of non-HCT patients and have mainly comprised intertrochanteric fractures and local wound infections.[224] Debate continues about the merits of core decompression, but recent studies, including one meta-analysis that compared 22 studies of core decompression to eight studies of nonoperative treatment, found that core decompression was 84% successful in Stage I disease compared to 61% for nonoperatively treated patients ($P = .0001$).[224] The authors cautioned that nonoperatively treated patients included significantly more cases with steroid-associated and bilateral AVN. Although core decompression provides excellent and immediate pain relief, it does not alter the progression of AVN in Stage II hips and is not appropriate for advanced stage AVN which is best treated by total joint replacement.[224,231] Mont et al. reviewed 42 reports that comprised 1206 hips treated by core decompression and 819 hips treated nonoperatively.[232] They found that satisfactory clinical results were reported in 63.5% of hips in 24 studies of core decompression and in 22.7% of hips in 21 studies of nonoperative management. When looking only at Stage I and II (pre-collapse) hips there were 71% versus 34.5% good results, respectively. If reports from the four centers that do the most core decompression procedures were excluded from the analysis the clinical success rates for core decompression versus nonoperative management were 53% versus 22.7%. Randomized studies comparing core decompression to nonoperative treatment have been limited to two small studies that have yielded conflicting results. The first study of 36 patients confirmed core decompression to be of benefit for early stage AVN[233] and the second study of 33 patients found that core decompression provided prompt relief of pain in symptomatic hips, but was no better that nonoperative treatment in preventing collapse of the femoral head.[234] In summary, until large prospective randomized double-blinded studies are performed, the treatment of early-stage AVN will remain controversial. In the meantime, if core decompression is to be considered then timely referral to an orthopedist experienced in core decompression is recommended before there is extensive irreversible damage to the femoral head or other target epiphysis.

# EYE EFFECTS

The most common late complications of HCT include lens cataracts and the ocular sicca syndrome which are the sequelae of TBI and chronic GVHD. Less commonly occurring infectious sequelae such as ophthalmic herpes zoster and symptomatic CMV retinitis need to be remembered, particularly in high-risk seropositive patients with chronic GVHD.

## Cataracts

The lenses of children who have undergone HCT have frequently been exposed to a variety of physicochemical insults before, during, or after the transplant preparative regimen. Insults that have potential to cause cataracts include prior antineoplastics,[235] cranial, orbital and/or TBI,[236] and glucocorticoids.[237,238] Whether the pediatric lens is more susceptible to these insults remains an open question. Following TBI, posterior subcapsular cataracts are first evident by slit lamp evaluation at approximately one year after BMT[239] and most are visible by three to four years. Following single, 920 to 1000 cGy doses of TBI, 80% of patients developed cataracts at five to six years. Following fractionated TBI cumulative doses of more than 1200 cGy the incidence is lower, approximately 50%, and 30% to 35% for doses of 1200 cGy or below. In a recent very large study from the European Group for Bone Marrow Transplantation (EBMT), the incidence of cataracts after TBI was less than 10% in patients who received either hyperfractionated (more than six fractions) or fractionated and low dose rate schedules (six or less fractions and 0.04 cGy/min).[240] This study confirms earlier observations that fractionation and dose rate are important to cataractogenesis.[241,242] Following chemotherapy preparative regimens and no prior cranial radiation, the incidence is 12% to 20%, almost exclusively related to the use of glucocorticoids.[239,243]

Prevention of cataracts has been limited by reluctance to attempt eye shielding because of the concern for leukemic relapse within the orbit.[244] Young children with monocular and even binocular cataracts are at risk for amblyopia. Close follow-up with an ophthalmologist is especially recommended for children less than two years of age in whom the assessment of vision can be difficult. Older children should continue regular standard checks for visual acuity and cataracts up until age 6 to 7 years, after which neurovisual pathways become fixed. The management of cataracts in the very young child is complex but cataract surgery is generally delayed as long as possible. However, for cataracts that significantly impair vision the treatment of choice usually involves phacoemulsification, removal of the damaged lens and implantation of an artificial intraocular lens.[240] The pediatric eye tends to be far-sighted and is reliant on normal lens flexibility to achieve emmetropia until sufficient growth of the ocular refractive structures makes this no longer necessary.[245] Artificial intraocular lenses are unable to accommodate making the choice of lens strength an issue for the ophthalmologist.[246] Surgical refinements in intraocular lens placement have lessened the problem of posterior capsule opacification that frequently complicated pediatric cataract surgery.[247] Contact lenses are not usually provided because ocular sicca often coexists.

## Ocular Sicca Syndrome

The development of dry eyes associated with insufficient tear production is seen in about one third of patients with, and about 10% of those without, chronic GVHD. Late-onset keratoconjunctivitis sicca in patients without chronic GVHD is usually a sequela of TBI and occurs more frequently in older patients, females, and after single fraction TBI regimens.[248] Untreated, sicca syndrome can be associated with infection, scar formation, and corneal damage. In patients with clinical extensive chronic GVHD, systemic immunosuppression is an essential component in the prevention of progressive sicca. Meticulous ocular hygiene, use of artificial tears, and follow-up with an ophthalmologist are essential. Topical glucocorticoids or immunosuppressive eye drops are infrequently used. Interruption of nasolacrimal drainage to prolong exposure of the cornea to lacrimal fluid should be considered also for patients with significant sicca syndrome and a Schirmer test, which reveals markedly reduced tear production. Nasolacrimal duct puncta can be plugged temporarily, or the canaliculi may be ligated permanently as it often improves symptoms. Nasolacrimal duct occlusion also has been a recognized complication of chronic GVHD.

# NEUROPSYCHOLOGICAL EFFECTS

Late treatment-related neurologic sequelae are well recognized after intensive conventional chemoradiotherapy.[246,249] Children under the age of five years, and especially under the age of three years, are at greater risk for significant neuropsychological deficits after HCT which may result from prior cranial irradiation, intrathecal or systemic chemotherapy, or recurrent leukemia.

## Decreased Intelligence Quotient

A preliminary analysis of 145 children studied immediately before and one or more years after TBI and BMT suggests that there is no significant impairment of fine-motor hand-eye coordination. Evaluation of full-scale, performance, and verbal-intelligence quotient (IQ) demonstrates a significant decrease in full-scale and performance IQ with increasing number of years after transplant.[250] Significant risk factors were age at time of initial cranial irradiation, total dose of cranial irradiation, and number of years after radiation. One practical implication of these observations is that children who performed well in grade school may begin to have difficulty in high school.

## Specific Learning Disability

Recognition that a child may develop learning disabilities after HCT is important to facilitate appropriate and timely psychological testing and placement of the child in special education classes if necessary. Deficits can be subtle learning difficulties or attention deficits. Parents should be told of this risk before the HCT, and inquiry regarding school performance should occur with each long-term follow-up visit. Neuropsychometric testing may be warranted and assessment by a multidisciplinary team is often helpful for the detection of specific learning disability.

## Leukoencephalopathy

Multifocal leukoencephalopathy after marrow transplantation is usually due to the same factors that influence its development in nontransplant settings.[251] After TBI and HCT for leukemia, a 7% incidence of leukoencephalopathy has been observed among patients who received pretransplant CNS treatment and posttransplant intrathecal therapy.[252] Symptoms often become evident four to six months after TBI. A cerebral MRI scan will be abnormal.

## Drug Induced Encephalopathy

Reversible neurotoxicity has occasionally been reported in patients treated with cyclosporine, tacrolimus, or high-dose acyclovir.[253]

## QUALITY OF LIFE

Two quality of life studies pertaining to pediatric bone marrow transplantation have focused on emotional well-being.[254,255] Both studies demonstrated overall improvement in quality of life by six months posttransplant and that family cohesion and the child's adaptive functioning were highly predictive of quality of life and behavioral adjustment. Neither study evaluated physical functioning, social functioning, or cognitive abilities. Sanders et al. used multidimensional validated instruments that were developed and tested in survivors of adult malignancies to evaluate cognitive difficulties, health care needs, and social adaptation of 234 adult survivors of childhood leukemia. The experimental groups comprised 114 patients treated with chemotherapy and 120 who underwent marrow transplant.[45] One hundred forty-nine control subjects were within five years of patient age and were selected by the patient from same sex siblings or friends. Sixty-five percent of the chemotherapy patients had received 1800 to 2400 cGy cranial irradiation, 645 of the marrow transplant patients had received 1000 to 1575 cGy of TBI, and 29% had received 1800 to 2400 cGy cranial irradiation plus TBI.

When compared to age- and sex-matched siblings or friends, survivors of childhood marrow transplant appear to have more health care needs as adults. Major illness was more often reported by marrow transplant survivors (21%) compared to chemotherapy patients (3.5%) and control subjects (4.7%; $P < 0.01$). During the past year, 66% of marrow transplant survivors reported more physician visits compared to 37% of chemotherapy patients and 41% of control subjects ($P < 0.01$). Diabetes, eye, hip, and joint problems each occurred more frequently in marrow transplant survivors compared to chemotherapy or control subjects. Second malignancies occurred in 8.4% of marrow transplant survivors compared to 2.6% of chemotherapy survivors and 1.4% of control subjects (0.009). Marrow transplant recipients perceived themselves as having more limited physical function, poorer general health, increased bodily pain, and a belief that their general health was worse than one year ago.

The Modified Memory Questionnaire (MMQ) and Neurobehavioral Rating Scale (NBRS) showed that marrow transplant survivors differed from chemotherapy survivors in that their memory and cognitive function was not impaired compared to control subjects. Among the chemotherapy survivors there was greater impairment of memory ($P = .013$) and learning ($P = .009$) in those who were six years of age or younger at the time of cranial irradiation compared to those who were seven years or older. Among the marrow transplant survivors, memory and cognitive function did not differ between those who received no irradiation, TBI, or TBI plus cranial irradiation ($P = .142$). Another study followed 47 children for up to six years after undergoing HCT without ever having received cranial irradiation.[256] The cognitive, behavioral, and social functioning of children three years and older was not detrimentally affected two years after HCT. Patients with more cognitive difficulties reported incomes of less than $30,000 per year ($P = .001$) and greater dependence on family or government disability for support ($P = .004$).[45]

Chemotherapy survivors perceived more difficulty with feelings of nervousness and depression than marrow transplant survivors ($P = .007$). No differences were noted in family relationships. Dating was infrequent or never for 68% of chemotherapy and 56% of marrow transplant survivors compared to 44% of control subjects ($P = 0.01$). Marital status did not differ between groups ($P = .149$). Insurance had been denied to 25% of chemotherapy and 33% of marrow transplant survivors compared to 3.4% of controls ($P < 0.01$). Future studies need to examine interventions aimed at improving quality of life in these patients.

# SECONDARY NEOPLASMS

Although many steps in the developmental pathway for malignant tumors remain elusive, etiologic factors have been identified from the study of genetic disorders such as Fanconi anemia, iatrogenic or inherited immunodeficiency, viral infections such as Epstein-Barr virus,[257] and epidemiological studies, for example, of the survivors of Hiroshima, Nagaski,[258] and Chernobyl nuclear disasters.[259,260] In addition, initial preclinical marrow transplant studies in dogs and monkeys demonstrated that malignancies occurred significantly more frequently in irradiated animals rescued with autologous or allogeneic marrow relative to controls.[261,262] Thus, it should not be surprising that new neoplasms occur in patients after HCT, when one or several of these potentially overlapping risk factors are present.

## Solid Tumors

Two very large studies have reported the incidence of solid tumors and posttransplant lymphoproliferative disease (PTLD) based on data collected from over 14,000 patients by the International Bone Marrow Transplant Registry (IBMTR) and over 4,000 patients by the Seattle group.[263,264] Using these combined data, Socié et al. recently reported the separate analysis of 3,182 children transplanted before age 17 years for acute leukemia.[48] Eighty-seven percent of the children received TBI-based preparative regimens and 10% received BU/CY. A 34-fold increased risk of solid tumors was demonstrated by the development of solid tumors in 25 children at a median of six years (range 0.3 to 14.3 years) posttransplant including: nine brain tumors, five thyroid papillary carcinomas, four melanomas, three squamous cell carcinomas of the tongue, two salivary gland mucoepidermoid carcinomas, two osteosarcomas, and one malignant fibrous histiocytoma. The actuarial probability of solid tumor development was 0.9%, 4.3%, and 11.0%, respectively, at 5, 10, and 15 years; however, 3,032 children died within ten years of transplant and were censored. Because death from other causes is a competing risk for solid tumor development the cumulative incidence method is preferred for estimating the risk of solid tumors at later times. Thus, the cumulative incidence for solid tumors was 1.7% and 3.9% at 10 and 15 years, respectively. Multivariate analyses showed an almost fourfold greater risk for the development of solid tumors in children aged zero to nine years compared to children aged 10 to 16 years ($P = .005$). Children who received high-dose TBI were approximately threefold more likely to develop solid tumors than children who received no or low-dose TBI ($P = .03$). Brain and thyroid tumors accounted for more than half of the solid tumors and 9 of these 14 children had received cranial irradiation in addition to TBI. The association of brain and thyroid tumors with age zero to nine years at transplantation ($P = .0009$) was even stronger than for solid tumors as a group, suggesting that brain and thyroid are highly sensitive to the effects of irradiation at very young ages.

It is noteworthy in the analysis of Socié et al. that no solid tumors developed in the 416 children who received non-radiation–based preparative regimens (315 received BU/CY).[48] The transplant teams at Seattle and Hopital St Louis in Paris, together with other European centers, had previously addressed the role of TBI in second malignancies by analyzing 700 patients who underwent marrow transplant for aplastic anemia.[265] This analysis indicated that irradiation, and especially total lymphoid or thoracoabdominal irradiation, significantly increased the risk for development of solid tumors compared to chemotherapy-only preparative regimens ($P = 0.0002$). Not surprisingly, the highest incidence of malignancy was observed among the subgroup of 79 patients in whom the etiology of marrow failure was Fanconi anemia. None of the Fanconi anemia patients developed hematologic malignancies and the five solid tumors (head and neck) all developed within six to eleven years posttransplant. If only the non-Fanconi patients were considered, in addition to irradiation (relative risk [RR] = 3.9, $P = .042$), treatment of chronic GVHD with azathioprine (RR = 7.5, $P = .0043$), and older age (RR = 1.1, $P = .025$) were significant.

## Posttransplant Lymphoproliferative Disease

The analysis by Socié et al. showed that 20 children developed B cell posttransplant lymphoproliferative disease (PTLD); 15 cases occurred within 12 months, four within 18 months, and one at 4.9 years posttransplant.[48] This represented a 182-fold increased risk compared to the expected risk among an age and sex-matched general population. The overall actuarial incidence of PTLD was 1.0% at five years posttransplant and the EBV genome was detected in all cases tested. This analysis of pediatric PTLD confirmed the risk factors that were identified by Curtis et al. in the much larger combined adult and pediatric analysis.[264] In descending order, the strongly associated ($P < .0001$) relative risks for early onset PTLD were anti-CD3 monoclonal antibody (RR = 43.2) for prophylaxis of acute GVHD, T cell depletion of the donor marrow (RR = 12.7), use of antithymocyte globulin (RR = 6.4), and unrelated or HLA-mismatched related donor (RR = 4.1). The only risk factor identified for late onset PTLD was extensive chronic GVHD (RR = 4.0, $P = .01$).[264]

The prognosis of PTLD in marrow transplant patients has been dismal.[266,267] This is partly because discontinuation of immunosuppression, which has helped to control PTLD after solid organ transplants, is usually not viable in marrow transplant recipients because of the potentially serious risk for flares of GVHD. All 20 of the children in the report by Socié died; in 16 cases, PTLD was the primary, and in two cases, the contributing cause of death. More recently, promising treatment approaches have included alpha-interferon,[268] anti-IL-6 antibody,[269] cellular therapy, and anti-B cell antibodies.[270] In 1994, infusions of unmodified donor leukocytes were first reported to have eradicated PTLD that developed in five patients who had undergone T-cell–depleted allogeneic marrow transplantation.[271] Because such therapy was complicated by subsequent development of chronic GVHD, EBV-specific CTL clones, or HSV-TK-transduced T lymphocytes have been used to control PTLD. In the latter case, subsequent development of GVHD can be treated with ganciclovir by way of activating the HSV-TK suicide gene.[272] The French initially reported that anti-B cell antibodies targeting CD21 and anti-CD24 were able to induce complete remissions in ten marrow transplant patients with PTLD and six survived at a median follow-up of 20 months.[270] More recently, a number of small case series have reported similar successful treatment of PTLD using the commercially available anti-CD20 antibody, rituximab.[273–275] An emerging strategy in patients at high risk for developing PTLD has been preemptive use of the anti-CD20, B cell monoclonal antibody, rituximab. Rituximab has been given based on early detection of rising plasma EBV DNA viral load using quantitative PCR techniques.[273,274,276,277] Recent studies that have reported serial plasma EBV viral loads after hematopoietic[273,277,278] and renal transplantation[279] have found that a plasma viral load of greater than 1000 genome equivalents per mL is helpful in predicting the development of PTLD. Emerging data also suggest that the absolute peripheral blood T cell count can be related to potential for development and control of PTLD. Gerritsen et al. found that children with T cell numbers below 50 per μL at one month post-HCT, and below 100 per μL at two months, were associated with an increased risk for developing PTLD.[280] In another study, 12 children had a median CD4 T cell count of 33 cells per μL (range 0 to 263 per μL) at the time of diagnosis of PTLD, and in the four children whose PTLD did not respond to rituximab the median CD4 count was only 4 per μL.[275]

## Myelodysplasia and Secondary Leukemia

Secondary myelodysplastic syndrome (MDS) or leukemia has infrequently been observed after allogeneic HCT, even in patients with Fanconi anemia in whom MDS developed frequently if not transplanted with normal cells.[281] It has been estimated that as many as 3% to 5% of leukemic recurrences may actually be derived from donor cells.[282]

Although secondary MDS and AML have occurred following conventional chemotherapy, several studies in the 1990s reported an unusually high incidence of secondary MDS and AML in patients who had undergone autologous transplantation for lymphoma.[283–285] The Minneapolis team reported ten who developed MDS and one who developed AML among 258 recipients of autologous transplants for Hodgkin's disease or non-Hodgkin's lymphoma for a cumulative probability of 13.5% ± 4.8% at six years.[286]

## Thyroid Neoplasms

Radiation to the thyroid is a well-established risk factor for the later development of benign and malignant thyroid neoplasms.[287,288] The latency of radiation-induced neoplasia has been as low as 1.5 to 6 years up to a peak incidence of 15 to 25 years after radiotherapy.[287,289] Two large studies each involving over 9000 childhood cancer survivors have reported the risks for development of thyroid cancers after thyroid irradiation in children. Ron et al. observed that children below five years of age were at greatest risk and that an estimated thyroid dose of 900 cGy was linked to a twofold increase in benign tumors, a fourfold increase in malignant tumors, and the radiation dose-response relationship was linear.[290] Tucker et al. were unable to separate the effects of age and dose on risk for thyroid cancer, but showed that radiation exposures of 200 to 999 cGy were associated with a 13-fold increased risk compared to doses below 200 cGy, and the risk after doses of 1000 to 2999 cGy was not significantly different.[287] The relative and absolute risks increased significantly with time since initial diagnosis ($P = .03$; $P < .001$, respectively). The cumulative probability ($\pm$ SE) that thyroid cancer would develop was 4.4 ± 2.0% at 26 years. In this regard, epidemiological studies pertaining to the 1986 Chernobyl accident indicated that among children under the age of 15 years the incidence rate of thyroid cancer progressively rose from 0.5 up to 97 per year per million children between 1991 and 1994.[259] More than 90% of these children were less than six years old at the time of the accident. In contrast, although 10.2% of 1984 male Chernobyl clean-up workers developed thyroid nodules, there were only two cases of papillary carcinoma.[260] At least six children at our Center[263] and two others reported in the literature[291] are known to have developed thyroid masses that occurred four or more years after TBI. These were determined to be papillary carcinoma (6), toxic goiter (1), and adenoma (1), so children should be examined annually. A history of thyroxine therapy appeared to reduce the risk of recurrent benign thyroid nodules but was not associated with reduced risk of thyroid carcinoma.[292]

## Monitoring and Surveillance

Anticipatory guidance and ongoing surveillance are likely to be crucial for early detection of secondary neoplasms to maximize potential to deliver effective treatments. Therefore, it is concerning that 635 consecutive survivors surveyed among the very large and well characterized Childhood Cancer Survivor Study Cohort[293] were observed to have important knowledge deficits in even the basic aspects of their initial cancer diagnoses and treatments.[194] Only 72% accurately reported their diagnosis, especially those who had CNS tumors or neuroblastoma. Among those who received radiotherapy, 70% recalled the site of radiotherapy. History of receiving a written medical summary, attending a long-term-follow-up clinic, and anxiety about late effects were not associated with greater knowledge. Thus, accurate treatment summaries need to be given to patients in a form that is accessible, even many years later, and whenever possible, medical records should be obtained from the treating institution prior to formulating long-term follow-up care.

The evaluation of the HCT survivor should include a thorough physical exam and a particularly detailed inspection of the skin, oral cavity, and thyroid gland for neoplastic growths. Benign melanocytic nevi have frequently been observed after chemoradiotherapy and may have an increased risk for melanoma.[294] Investigations should include periodic complete blood counts to monitor for myelodysplasia and secondary leukemias.

## CONCLUSIONS

The successful use of hematopoietic cell transplantation as a definitive therapy for childhood malignancies, bone marrow failure syndromes, and a variety of other inherited metabolic and immunodeficiency disorders has led to an increasing number of children who survive into adulthood. Many of these children develop normally, become healthy survivors, and return to a normal life. Some patients, however, continue to need long-term medical care and other assistance for chronic or delayed problems that arise because of pretransplant therapy, intensive preparative regimens, and chronic GVHD. Current new approaches are exploring the development of less toxic preparative regimens. Better preventive and therapeutic interventions are needed for acute and, particularly, chronic GVHD. In parallel, it will be important to improve patient knowledge, and transferability of treatment summaries of their prior cancer or preparative regiment therapy, so that future generations of their health professionals may have sufficiently detailed information to offer optimal long-term follow-up and to provide anticipatory guidance for secondary malignancies and the sequelae of chronic GVHD and disturbed endocrine, ophthalmological, skeletal, pulmonary, cardiac, and neuropsychological function.

# REFERENCES

1. Kubota C, Shinohara O, Hinohara T et al. Changes in hypothalamic-pituitary function following bone marrow transplantation in children. Acta Paediatr Jpn 1994;36:37–43.
2. Brauner R, Adan L, Souberbielle JC et al. Contribution of growth hormone deficiency to the growth failure that follows bone marrow transplantation. J Pediatr 1997;130:785–792.
3. Clement-De Boers A, Oostdijk W, Van Weel-Sipman MH et al. Final height and hormonal function after bone marrow transplantation in children. J Pediatr 1996;129:544–550.
4. Textbook of Pediatrics (15th ed). Philadelphia: W.B. Saunders Company, 1996.
5. Powell GF, Brasel JA, Blizzard RM. Emotional deprivation and growth retardation simulating idiopathic hypopituitarism. I. Clinical evaluation of the syndrome. N Engl J Med 1967;276:1271–1278.
6. Powell GF, Brasel JA, Raiti S et al. Emotional deprivation and growth retardation simulating idiopathic hypopituitarism. II. Endocrinologic evaluation of the syndrome. N Engl J Med 1967;276:1279–1283.
7. Albanese A, Hamill G, Jones J et al. Reversibility of physiological growth hormone secretion in children with psychosocial dwarfism. Clin Endocrinol 1994;40:687–692.
8. Sanders JE, Pritchard S, Mahoney P et al. Growth and development following marrow transplantation for leukemia. Blood 1986;68:1129–1135.
9. Leiper AD, Stanhope R, Lau T et al. The effect of total body irradiation and bone marrow transplantation during childhood and adolescence on growth and endocrine function. Br J Haematol 1987;67:419–426.
10. Thomas BC, Stanhope R, Plowman PN, Leiper AD. Growth following single fraction and fractionated total body irradiation for bone marrow transplantation. Eur J Pediatr 1993;152:888–892.
11. Brauner R, Fontoura M, Zucker JM et al. Growth and growth hormone secretion after bone marrow transplantation. Arch Dis Child 1993;68:458–463.
12. Giorgiani G, Bozzola M, Locatelli F et al. Role of busulfan and total body irradiation on growth of prepubertal children receiving bone marrow transplantation and results of treatment with recombinant human growth hormone. Blood 1995;86:825–831.
13. Holm K, Nysom K, Rasmussen MH et al. Growth, growth hormone and final height after BMT. Possible recovery of irradiation-induced growth hormone insufficiency. Bone Marrow Transplant 1996;18:163–170.
14. Cohen A, Rovelli A, Bakker B et al. Final height of patients who underwent bone marrow transplantation for hematological disorders during childhood: a study by the Working Party for Late Effects-EBMT. Blood 1999;93:4109–4115.
15. Sanders JE. Growth and development after hematopoietic cell transplantation. In: Hematopoietic Cell Transplantation (2nd ed.), Thomas ED, Blume KG, Forman SJ, (eds). Malden, MA: Blackwell Science, Inc 1999: 764–775.
16. Huma Z, Boulad F, Black P et al. Growth in children after bone marrow transplantation for acute leukemia. Blood 1995;86:819–824.
17. Papadimitriou A, Urena M, Hamill G et al. Growth hormone treatment of growth failure secondary to total body irradiation and bone marrow transplantation. Arch Dis Child 1991;66:689–692.
18. Borgström B, Bolme P. Growth and growth hormone in children after bone marrow transplantation. Horm Res 1988;30:98–100.
19. Ogilvy-Stuart AL, Clark DJ, Wallace WH et al. Endocrine deficit after fractionated total body irradiation. Arch Dis Child 1992;67:1107–1110.
20. Olshan JS, Willi SM, Gruccio D, Moshang T, Jr. Growth hormone function and treatment following bone marrow transplant for neuroblastoma. Bone Marrow Transplant 1993;12:381–385.
21. Hovi L, Rajantie J, Perkkiö M et al. Growth failure and growth hormone deficiency in children after bone marrow transplantation for leukemia. Bone Marrow Transplant 1990;5:183–186.
22. Harrison's Principles of Internal Medicine (15th ed.) New York: McGraw-Hill, 2001.
23. Shalet SM, Brennan BM. Growth and growth hormone status following treatment for childhood leukaemia (Review). Horm Res 1998;50:1–10.
24. Duffner PK, Cohen ME, Voorhess ML et al. Long-term effects of cranial irradiation on endocrine function in children with brain tumors. A prospective study. Cancer 1985;56:2189–2193.
25. Duffner PK, Cohen ME. Long-term consequences of CNS treatment for childhood cancer, Part II: Clinical consequences (Review). Pediatr Neurol 1991;7:237–242.
26. Shalet SM, Beardwell CG, Pearson D, Morris-Jones PH. The effect of varying doses of cerebral irradiation on growth hormone production in childhood. Clin Endocrinol 1976;5:287–290.
27. Brennan BM, Rahim A, Mackie EM et al. Growth hormone status in adults treated for acute lymphoblastic leukaemia in childhood. Clin Endocrinol 1998;48:777–783.
28. Sanders JE, Buckner CD, Sullivan KM et al. Growth and development in children after bone marrow transplantation. Horm Res 1988;30:92–97.
29. Michel G, Socié G, Gebhard F et al. Late effects of allogeneic bone marrow transplantation for children with acute myeloblastic leukemia in first complete remission: the impact of conditioning regimen without total-body irradiation—a report from the Société Française de Greffe de Moelle. J Clin Oncol 1997;15:2238–2246.

30. Afify Z, Shaw PJ, Clavano-Harding A, Cowell CT. Growth and endocrine function in children with acute myeloid leukaemia after bone marrow transplantation using busulfan/cyclophosphamide. Bone Marrow Transplant 2000;25:1087–1092.

31. Biller BMK, Samuels MH, Zagar A et al. Sensitivity and specificity of six tests for the diagnosis of adult GH deficiency. J Clin Endocrinol Metabol 2002;87:2067–2079.

32. Frasier SD. A preview of growth hormone stimulation tests in children. Pediatrics 1974;53:929–937.

33. Joss EE. Growth hormone deficiency in childhood. Evaluation of diagnostic procedures (Review). Monogr Paediatr 1975;5:1–83.

34. Hagenas L. Clinical tests as predictors of growth response in GH treatment of short normal children (Review). Acta Paediatr Scand 362(Suppl):36–43.

35. Ghigo E, Bellone J, Aimaretti G et al. Reliability of provocative tests to assess growth hormone secretory status. Study in 472 normally growing children. J Clin Endocrinol Metabol 1996;81:3323–3327.

36. Cohen A, Rovelli A, Van-Lint MT et al. Final height of patients who underwent bone marrow transplantation during childhood. Arch Dis Child 1996;74:437–440.

37. Bozzola M, Giorgiani G, Locatelli F et al. Growth in children after bone marrow transplantation. Horm Res 1993;39:122–126.

38. Ogilvy-Stuart AL, Shalet SM. Growth and puberty after growth hormone treatment after irradiation for brain tumours. Arch Dis Child 1995;73:141–146.

39. MacGillivray MH, Baptista J, Johanson A. Outcome of a four-year randomized study of daily versus three times weekly somatropin treatment in prepubertal naive growth hormone-deficient children. Genentech Study Group. J Clin Endocrinol Metabol 1996;81:1806–1809.

40. Rotnem D, Genel M, Hintz RL, Cohen DJ. Personality development in children with growth hormone deficiency. J Am Acad Child Psychiatry 1977;16:412–426.

41. de Boer H, Blok GJ, Van d V. Clinical aspects of growth hormone deficiency in adults (Review). Endocr Rev 1995;16:63–86.

42. Stabler B, Siegel PT, Clopper RR et al. Behavior change after growth hormone treatment of children with short stature. J Pediatr 1998;133:366–373.

43. Mauseth RS, Kelly BE, Sanders JE. Bone mineral density (BMD) in pediatric marrow transplant patients (Abstr #P1–488). Pediatr Res 2001;49(Part 2):82A.

44. Bhatia S, Ramsay NK, Weisdorf D et al. Bone mineral density in patients undergoing bone marrow transplantation for myeloid malignancies. Bone Marrow Transplant 1998;22:87–90.

45. Sanders JE, Syrjala KL, Hoffmeister PA, Foster LD. Quality of life (QOL) of adult survivors of childhood leukemia treated with chemotherapy (CT) or bone marrow transplant (BMT) (Abstr #3090). Blood 2001;98(Part 1):741a.

46. Swerdlow AJ, Reddingius RE, Higgins CD et al. Growth hormone treatment of children with brain tumors and risk of tumor recurrence. J Clin Endocrinol Metabol 2000;85:4444–4449.

47. Packer RJ, Boyett JM, Janss AJ et al. Growth hormone replacement therapy in children with medulloblastoma: use and effect on tumor control. J Clin Oncol 2001;19:480–487.

48. Socié G, Curtis RE, Deeg HJ et al. New malignant diseases after allogeneic marrow transplantation for childhood acute leukemia. J Clin Oncol 2000;18:348–357.

49. Wallace WH, Shalet SM, Hendry JH et al. Ovarian failure following abdominal irradiation in childhood: the radiosensitivity of the human oocyte. Br J Radiol 1989;62:995–998.

50. Mertens AC, Ramsay NK, Kouris S, Neglia JP. Patterns of gonadal dysfunction following bone marrow transplantation. Bone Marrow Transplant 1998;22:345–350.

51. Damewood MD, Grochow LB. Prospects for fertility after chemotherapy or radiation for neoplastic disease. Fertil Steril 1986;45:443–459.

52. Siris ES, Leventhal BG, Vaitukaitis TL. Effects of childhood leukemia and chemotherapy on puberty and reproductive function in girls. N Engl J Med 1976;294:1143–1146.

53. Marshall WA, Tanner JM. Variations in pattern of pubertal changes in girls. Arch Dis Child 1969;44:291–303.

54. Sarafoglou K, Boulad F, Gillio A, Sklar C. Gonadal function after bone marrow transplantation for acute leukemia during childhood. J Pediatr 1997;130:210–216.

55. Leiper AD, Stanhope R, Kitching P, Chessells JM. Precocious and premature puberty associated with treatment of acute lymphoblastic leukaemia. Arch Dis Child 1987;62:1107–1112.

56. Leiper AD, Stanhope R, Preece MA et al. Precocious or early puberty and growth failure in girls treated for acute lymphoblastic leukaemia. Horm Res 1988;30:72–76.

57. Sanders JE, Buckner CD, Amos D et al. Ovarian function following marrow transplantation for aplastic anemia or leukemia. J Clin Oncol 1988;6:813–818.

58. Sanders JE, Seattle Marrow Transplant Team. The impact of marrow transplant preparative regimens on subsequent growth and development. Semin Hematol 1991;28:244–249.

59. Ray H, Mattison D. How radiation and chemotherapy affect gonadal function. Contemp Ob Gyn 1985;109:106–115.

60. De Sanctis V, Galimberti M, Lucarelli G et al. Gonadal function after allogeneic bone marrow transplantation for thalassaemia. Arch Dis Child 1991;66:517–520.

61. Teinturier C, Hartmann O, Valteau-Couanet D et al. Ovarian function after autologous bone marrow transplantation in childhood: high-dose busulfan is a major cause of ovarian failure. Bone Marrow Transplant 1998;22:989–994.

62. Thibaud E, Rodriguez-Macias K, Trivin C et al. Ovarian function after bone marrow transplantation during childhood. Bone Marrow Transplant 1998;21:287–290.

63. Adan L, Sainte-Rose C, Souberbielle JC et al. Adult height after growth hormone (GH) treatment for GH deficiency due to cranial irradiation. Med Pediatr Oncol 2000;34:14–19.

64. Klein KO, Barnes KM, Jones JV et al. Increased final height in precocious puberty after long-term treatment with LHRH agonists: the National Institutes of Health experience. J Clin Endocrinol Metabol 2001;86:4711–4716.

65. Sklar C. Reproductive physiology and treatment-related loss of sex hormone production (Review). Med Pediatr Oncol 1999;33:2–8.

66. Sanders JE, Hawley J, Levy W et al. Pregnancies following high-dose cyclophosphamide with or without high-dose busulfan or total-body irradiation and bone marrow transplantation. Blood 1996;87:3045–3052.

67. Liesner, RJ, Leiper, AD, Hann et al. Late effects of intensive treatment for acute myeloid leukemia and myelodysplasia in childhood. J Clin Oncol 1994;12:916–924.

68. Lopez-Ibor B, Schwartz AD. Gonadal failure following busulfan therapy in an adolescent girl. Am J Pediatr Hematol Oncol 1986;8:85–87.

69. Giorgiani G, Bozzola M, Cisternino M et al. Gonadal function in adolescents receiving different conditioning regimens for bone marrow transplantation. Bone Marrow Transplant 1991;8(Suppl 1):53.

70. Grigg AP, McLachlan R, Zaja J, Szer J. Reproductive status in long-term bone marrow transplant survivors receiving busulfan-cyclophosphamide (120 mg/kg). Bone Marrow Transplant 2000;26:1089–1095.

71. Ash, P. The influence of radiation on fertility in man. Br J Radiol 1980;53:271–278.

72. Singhal S, Powles R, Treleaven J et al. Melphalan alone prior to allogeneic bone marrow transplantation from HLA-identical sibling donors for hematologic malignancies: alloengraftment with potential preservation of fertility in women. Bone Marrow Transplant 1996;18:1049–1055.

73. Borgna-Pignatti C, Marradi P, Rugolotto S, Marcolongo A. Successful pregnancy after bone marrow transplantation for thalassaemia. Bone Marrow Transplant 1996;18:235–236.

74. Jackson GH, Wood A, Taylor PR et al. Early high dose chemotherapy intensification with autologous bone marrow transplantation in lymphoma associated with retention of fertility and normal pregnancies in females. Scotland and Newcastle Lymphoma Group, UK. Leuk Lymphoma 1997;28:127–132.

75. Trounson A, Mohr L. Human pregnancy following cryopreservation, thawing and transfer of an eight-cell embryo. Nature 1983;305:707–709.

76. Fabbri R, Porcu E, Marsella T et al. Human oocyte cryopreservation: new perspectives regarding oocyte survival. Hum Reprod 2001;16:411–416.

77. Radford JA, Lieberman BA, Brison DR et al. Orthotopic reimplantation of cryopreserved ovarian cortical strips after high-dose chemotherapy for Hodgkin's lymphoma. Lancet 2001;357:1172–1175.

78. Sklar CA, Robison LL, Nesbit ME et al. Effects of radiation on testicular function in long-term survivors of childhood acute lymphoblastic leukemia: a report from the Children Cancer Study Group. J Clin Oncol 1990;8:1981–1987.

79. Shapiro E, Kinsella TJ, Makuch RW et al. Effects of fractionated irradiation on endocrine aspects of testicular function. J Clin Oncol 1985;3:1232–1239.

80. Brauner R, Caltabiano P, Rappaport R et al. Leydig cell insufficiency after testicular irradiation for acute lymphoblastic leukemia. Horm Res 1988;30:111–114.

81. Barton C, Waxman J. Effects of chemotherapy on fertility (Review). Blood Rev 1990;4:187–195.

82. Gianni AM, Bregni M, Siena S et al. High-dose chemotherapy and autologous bone marrow transplantation compared with MACOP-B in aggressive B-cell lymphoma. N Engl J Med 1997;336:1290–1297.

83. Tsatsoulis A, Shalet SM, Morris ID, de Kretser DM. Immunoactive inhibin as a marker of Sertoli cell function following cytotoxic damage to the human testis. Horm Res 1990;34:254–259.

84. Castillo LA, Craft AW, Kernahan J et al. Gonadal function after 12-Gy testicular irradiation in childhood acute lymphoblastic leukaemia. Med Pediatr Oncol 1990;18:185–189.

85. Leiper AD, Grant DB, Chessells JM. Gonadal function after testicular radiation for acute lymphoblastic leukaemia. Arch Dis Child 1986;61:53–56.

86. Sanders JE, Buckner CD, Leonard JM et al. Late effects on gonadal function of cyclophosphamide, total-body irradiation, and marrow transplantation. Transplantation 1983;36:252–255.

87. Bramsig JH, Heimes U, Heiermann E et al. The effects of different cumulative doses of chemotherapy on testicular function. Results in 75 patients treated for Hodgkin's disease during childhood or adolescence. Cancer 1990;65:1298–1302.

88. Kenney LB, Laufer MR, Grant FD et al. High risk of infertility and long term gonadal damage in males treated with high dose cyclophosphamide for sarcoma during childhood. Cancer 2001;91:613–621.

89. Sklar CA, Kim TH, Ramsay NKC. Testicular function following bone marrow transplantation performed during or after puberty. Cancer 1984;53:1498–1501.
90. Ortin TT, Shostak CA, Donaldson SS. Gonadal status and reproductive function following treatment for Hodgkin's disease in childhood: the Stanford experience. Int J Radiat Oncol Biol Phys 1990;19:873–880.
91. Relander T, Cavallin-Stahl E, Garwicz S et al. Gonadal and sexual function in men treated for childhood cancer. Med Pediatr Oncol 2000;35:52–63.
92. Mulvihill JJ. Sentinel and other mutational effects in offspring of cancer survivors. Progr Clin Biol Res 1990;340C:179–186.
93. Damani MN, Masters V, Meng MV et al. Postchemotherapy ejaculatory azoospermia: fatherhood with sperm from testis tissue with intracytoplasmic sperm injection. J Clin Oncol 2002;20:930–936.
94. Boulad F, Bromley M, Black P et al. Thyroid dysfunction following bone marrow transplantation using hyperfractionated radiation. Bone Marrow Transplant 1995;15:71–76.
95. Vexiau P, Perez-Castiglioni P, Socié G et al. The 'euthyroid sick syndrome': incidence, risk factors and prognostic value soon after allogeneic bone marrow transplantation. Br J Haematol 1993;85:778–782.
96. Katsanis E, Shapiro RS, Robison LL et al. Thyroid dysfunction following bone marrow transplantation: long-term follow-up of 80 pediatric patients. Bone Marrow Transplant 1990;5:335–340.
97. Ogilvy-Stuart AL, Shalet SM, Gattamaneni HR. Thyroid function after treatment of brain tumors in children. J Pediatr 1991;119:733–737.
98. Sklar C, Whitton J, Mertens A et al. Abnormalities of the thyroid in survivors of Hodgkin's disease: data from the Childhood Cancer Survivor Study. J Clin Endocrinol Metab 2000;85:3227–3232.
99. Wyatt DT, Lum LG, Casper J et al. Autoimmune thyroiditis after bone marrow transplantation. Bone Marrow Transplant 1990;5:357–361.
100. Glatstein E, McHardy-Young S, Brast N et al. Alterations in serum thyrotropin (TSH) and thyroid function following radiotherapy in patients with malignant lymphoma. J Clin Endocrinol Metab 1971;32:833–841.
101. Green DM, Brecher ML, Yakar D et al. Thyroid function in pediatric patients after neck irradiation for Hodgkin disease. Med Pediatr Oncol 1980;8:121–136.
102. Livesey EA, Brook CG. Thyroid dysfunction after radiotherapy and chemotherapy of brain tumours. Arch Dis Child 1989;64:593–595.
103. Hancock SL, McDougall IR, Constine LS. Thyroid abnormalities after therapeutic external radiation (Review). Int J Radiat Oncol Biol Phys 1995;31:1165–1170.
104. Hancock SL, Cox RS, McDougall R. Thyroid diseases after treatment of Hodgkin's disease. N Engl J Med 1991;325:599–606.
105. Sklar CA, Kim TH, Ramsay NKC. Thyroid dysfunction among long-term survivors of bone marrow transplantation. Am J Med 1982;73:688–694.
106. Sanders JE, the Long-Term Follow-Up Team. Endocrine problems in children after bone marrow transplant for hematologic malignancies. Bone Marrow Transplant 1991;8:2–4.
107. Thomas BC, Stanhope R, Plowman PN, Leiper AD. Endocrine function following single fraction and fractionated total body irradiation for bone marrow transplantation in childhood. Acta Endocrinol 1993;128:508–512.
108. Borgstrom B, Bolme P. Thyroid function in children after allogeneic bone marrow transplantation. Bone Marrow Transplant 1994;13:59–64.
109. Manenti F, Galimberti M, Lucarelli G et al. Growth and endocrine function after bone marrow transplantation for thalassemia major. Progr Clin Biol Res 1989;309:273–280.
110. Al-Fiar FZ, Colwill R, Lipton JH et al. Abnormal thyroid stimulating hormone (TSH) levels in adults following allogeneic bone marrow transplants. Bone Marrow Transplant 1997;19:1019–1022.
111. Franklyn JA, Betteridge J, Daykin J et al. Long-term thyroxine treatment and bone mineral density. Lancet 1992;340:9–13.
112. Greenspan SL, Greenspan FS. The effect of thyroid hormone on skeletal integrity (Review). Ann Intern Med 1999;130:750–758.
113. Hershman JM, Eriksen E, Kaufman N, Champlin RE. Thyroid function tests in patients undergoing bone marrow transplantation. Bone Marrow Transplant 1990;6:49–51.
114. Kami M, Tanaka Y, Chiba S et al. Thyroid function after bone marrow transplantation: possible association between immune-mediated thyrotoxicosis and hypothyroidism. Transplantation 2001;71:406–411.
115. Holland FJ, McConnon JK, Volpe R, Saunders EF. Concordant Graves' disease after bone marrow transplantation: implications for pathogenesis. J Clin Endocrinol Metab 1991;72:837–840.
116. Karthaus M, Gabrysiak T, Brabant G et al. Immune thyroiditis after transplantation of allogeneic CD34+ selected peripheral blood cells. Bone Marrow Transplant 1997;20:697–699.
117. Rocchini AP. Childhood obesity and a diabetes epidemic. N Engl J Med 2002;346:854–855.
118. Silink M. Childhood diabetes: a global perspective. Horm Res 2002;57(Suppl 1):1–5.
119. Strauss R. Perspectives on childhood obesity. Curr Gastroenterol Rep 2002;4:244–250.
120. Sklar CA, Mertens AC, Walter A et al. Changes in body mass index and prevalence of overweight in survivors of childhood acute lymphoblastic leukemia: role of cranial irradiation. Med Pediatr Oncol 2000;35:91–95.

121. Kamel A, Norgren S, Elimam A et al. Effects of growth hormone treatment in obese prepubertal boys. J Clin Endocrinol Metabol 2000;85:1412–1419.
122. Reilly JJ, Brougham M, Montgomery C et al. Effect of glucocorticoid therapy on energy intake in children treated for acute lymphoblastic leukemia. J Clin Endocrinol Metabol 2001;86:3742–3745.
123. Talvensaari KK, Lanning M, Tapanainen P, Knip M. Long-term survivors of childhood cancer have an increased risk of manifesting the metabolic syndrome. J Clin Endocrinol Metabol 1996;81:3051–3055.
124. Willman KY, Cox RS, Donaldson SS. Radiation induced height impairment in pediatric Hodgkin's disease. Int J Radiat Oncol Biol Phys 1994;28:85–92.
125. Dahllöf G, Heimdahl A, Bolme P et al. Oral condition in children treated with bone marrow transplantation. Bone Marrow Transplant 1988;3:43–51.
126. Dahllöf G, Barr M, Bolme P et al. Disturbances in dental development after total body irradiation in bone marrow transplant recipients. Oral Surg Oral Med Oral Pathol 1988;65:41–44.
127. Dahllöf G, Forsberg CM, Ringden O et al. Facial growth and morphology in long-term survivors after bone marrow transplantation. Eur J Orthod 1989;11:332–340.
128. Dahllöf G, Forsberg CM, Näsman M et al. Craniofacial growth in bone marrow transplant recipients treated with growth hormone after total body irradiation. Scand J Dent Res 1991;99:44–47.
129. Dahllöf G, Krekmanova L, Kopp S et al. Craniomandibular dysfunction in children treated with total-body irradiation and bone marrow transplantation. Acta Odontol Scand 1994;52:99–105.
130. Nasman M, Forsberg CM, Dahllöf G. Long-term dental development in children after treatment for malignant disease. Eur J Orthod 1997;19:151–159.
131. Nasman M, Bjork O, Soderhall S et al. Disturbances in the oral cavity in pediatric long-term survivors after different forms of antineoplastic therapy. Pediatr Dent 1994;16:217–223.
132. Shulman HM, Sullivan KM, Weiden PL et al. Chronic graft-versus-host syndrome in man. A long-term clinicopathologic study of 20 Seattle patients. Am J Med 1980;69:204–217.
133. Sullivan KM, Shulman HM, Storb R et al. Chronic graft-versus-host disease in 52 patients: adverse natural course and successful treatment with combination immunosuppression. Blood 1981;57:267–276.
134. Baker BW, Wilson CL, Davis AL et al. Busulphan/cyclophosphamide conditioning for bone marrow transplantation may lead to failure of hair regrowth. Bone Marrow Transplant 1991;7:43–47.
135. Socié G, Clift RA, Blaise D et al. Busulfan plus cyclophosphamide compared with total-body irradiation plus cyclophosphamide before marrow transplantation for myeloid leukemia: long-term follow-up of the 4 randomized studies. Blood 2001;98:3569–3574.
136. Vowels M, Chan LL, Giri N et al. Factors affecting hair regrowth after bone marrow transplantation. Bone Marrow Transplant 1993;12:347–350.
137. Ljungman P, Hassan M, Bekassy AN et al. Busulfan concentration in relation to permanent alopecia in recipients of bone marrow transplants. Bone Marrow Transplant 1995;15:869–871.
138. Slattery JT, Sanders JE, Buckner CD et al. Graft-rejection and toxicity following bone marrow transplantation in relation to busulfan pharmacokinetics. Bone Marrow Transplant 1995;16:31–42.
139. Palmas A, Tefferi A, Myers JL et al. Late-onset noninfectious pulmonary complications after allogeneic bone marrow transplantation. Br J Haematol 1998;100:680–687.
140. Freudenberger T, Madtes DK, Hackman RC. Characterization of bronchiolitis obliterans organizing pneumonia in a hematopoietic stem cell transplant population (Abstr). Am J Respir Crit Care Med 2000;161:A890.
141. Griese M, Rampf U, Hofmann D et al. Pulmonary complications after bone marrow transplantation in children: twenty-four years of experience in a single pediatric center. Pediatr Pulmonol 2000;30:393–401.
142. Hayes-Jordan A, Benaim E, Richardson S et al. Open lung biopsy in pediatric bone marrow transplant patients. J Pediatr Surg 2002;37:446–452.
143. Crawford SW, Hackman RC, Clark JG. Biopsy diagnosis and clinical outcome of focal pulmonary lesions after marrow transplantation. Transplantation 1989;48:266–271.
144. Crawford SW. Critical care and respiratory failure. In Hematopoietic Cell Transplantation (2nd ed.), Thomas ED, Blume KG, Forman SJ, (eds). Boston: Blackwell Science 1999;712–722.
145. Crawford SW, Pepe M, Lin D et al. Abnormalities of pulmonary function tests after marrow transplantation predict nonrelapse mortality. Am J Respir Crit Care Med 1995;152:690–695.
146. Sanders JE, Madtes D, Hoffmeister P, Storer B. The impact of pediatric marrow transplant (BMT) on late pulmonary function (Abstr #2392). Blood 2000;96(Part 1):557a.
147. Nysom K, Holm K, Hesse B et al. Lung function after allogeneic bone marrow transplantation for leukaemia or lymphoma. Arch Dis Child 1996;74:432–436.
148. Kaplan EB, Wodell RA, Wilmott RW et al. Late effects of bone marrow transplantation on pulmonary function in children. Bone Marrow Transplant 1994;14:613–621.
149. Tait RC, Burnett AK, Robertson AG et al. Subclinical pulmonary function defects following autologous and allogeneic bone marrow transplantation: relationship to total body irradiation and graft-versus-host disease. Int J Radiat Oncol Biol Phys 1991;20:1219–1227.
150. Thurlbeck WM. Postnatal growth and development of the lung. Am Rev Respir Dis 1975;111(6):803–844.

151. Calhoon JH, Levine S, Anzueto A et al. Lung transplantation in a patient with a prior bone marrow transplant. Chest 1992;102:948.
152. Clark JG, Schwartz DA, Flournoy N et al. Risk factors for airflow obstruction in recipients of bone marrow transplants. Ann Intern Med 1987;107:648–656.
153. Chan CK, Hyland RH, Hutcheon MA et al. Small-airways disease in recipients of allogeneic bone marrow transplants. An analysis of 11 cases and a review of the literature. Medicine 1987;66:327–340.
154. Paz HL, Crilley P, Patchefsky A et al. Bronchiolitis obliterans after autologous bone marrow transplantation. Chest 1992;101:775–778.
155. Schultz KR, Green GJ, Wensley D et al. Obstructive lung disease in children after allogeneic bone marrow transplantation. Blood 1994;84:3212–3220.
156. Worthy SA, Flint JD, Muller NL. Pulmonary complications after bone marrow transplantation: high-resolution CT and pathologic findings (Review). Radiographics 1997;17:1359–1371.
157. Urbanski SJ, Kossakowska AE, Curtis J et al. Idiopathic small airways pathology in patients with graft-versus-host disease following allogeneic bone marrow transplantation. Am J Surg Pathol 1987;11:965–971.
158. Ralph DD, Springmeyer SC, Sullivan KM et al. Rapidly progressive air-flow obstruction in marrow transplant recipients: Possible association between obliterative bronchiolitis and chronic graft-versus-host disease. Am Rev Respir Dis 1984;129:641–644.
159. Clark JG, Crawford SW, Madtes DK, Sullivan KM. Obstructive lung disease after allogeneic marrow transplantation. Ann Intern Med 1989;111:368–376.
160. McDonald GB, Sullivan KM, Schuffler MD et al. Esophageal abnormalities in chronic graft-versus-host disease in humans. Gastroenterology 1981;80:914–921.
161. Sullivan KM, Kopecky KJ, Jocom J et al. Immunomodulatory and antimicrobial efficacy of intravenous immunoglobulin in bone marrow transplantation. N Engl J Med 1990;323:705–712.
162. O'Hagan AR, Stillwell PC, Arroliga A, Koo A. Photopheresis in the treatment of refractory bronchiolitis obliterans complicating lung transplantation. Chest 1999;115:1459–1462.
163. Salerno CT, Park SJ, Kreykes NS et al. Adjuvant treatment of refractory lung transplant rejection with extracorporeal photopheresis. J Thorac Cardiovasc Surg 1999;117:1063–1069.
164. Villanueva J, Bhorade SM, Robinson JA et al. Extracorporeal photopheresis for the treatment of lung allograft rejection. Ann Transplant 2000;5:44–47.
165. Dall'Amico R, Rossetti F, Zulian F et al. Photopheresis in paediatric patients with drug-resistant chronic graft-versus-host disease. Br J Haematol 1997;97:848–854.
166. Klein AK, Wang H, Sprague K et al. Effective treatment of progressive post-transplant bronchiolitis obliterans with extracorporeal photopheresis (Abstr #5247). Blood 2001;98(Part 2):368b.
167. Salvaneschi L, Perotti C, Zecca M et al. Extracorporeal photochemotherapy for treatment of acute and chronic GVHD in childhood. Transfusion 2001;41:1299–1305.
168. Gascoigne A, Corris P. Lung transplants in patients with prior bone marrow transplants. Chest 1994;105:327.
169. Rabitsch W, Deviatko E, Keil F et al. Successful lung transplantation for bronchiolitis obliterans after allogeneic marrow transplantation. Transplantation 2001;71:1341–1343.
170. Heath JA, Kurland G, Spray TL et al. Lung transplantation after allogeneic marrow transplantation in pediatric patients: the Memorial Sloan-Kettering experience. Transplantation 2001;72:1986–1990.
171. Epler GR, Colby TV, McLoud TC et al. Bronchiolitis obliterans organizing pneumonia. N Engl J Med 1985;312:152–158.
172. Mathew P, Bozeman P, Krance RA et al. Bronchiolitis obliterans organizing pneumonia (BOOP) in children after allogeneic bone marrow transplantation. Bone Marrow Transplant 1994;13:221–223.
173. Thirman MJ, Devine SM, O'Toole K et al. Bronchiolitis obliterans organizing pneumonia as a complication of allogeneic bone marrow transplantation. Bone Marrow Transplant 1992;10:307–311.
174. Kleinau I, Perez-Canto A, Schmid HJ et al. Bronchiolitis obliterans organizing pneumonia and chronic graft-versus-host disease in a child after allogeneic bone marrow transplantation. Bone Marrow Transplant 1997; 19:841–844.
175. Yousem SA. The histological spectrum of pulmonary graft-versus-host disease in bone marrow transplant recipients. Hum Pathol 1995;26:668–675.
176. Clark JG, Hansen JA, Hertz MI et al. NHLBI workshop summary: idiopathic pneumonia syndrome after bone marrow transplantation (Review). Am Rev Respir Dis 1993;147:1601–1606.
177. Kantrow SP, Hackman RC, Boeckh M et al. Idiopathic pneumonia syndrome: changing spectrum of lung injury after marrow transplantation. Transplantation 1997;63:1079–1086.
178. Wingard JR, Santos GW, Saral R. Late-onset interstitial pneumonia following allogeneic bone marrow transplantation. Transplantation 1985;39:21–23.
179. Cooke KR, Kobzik L, Martin TR et al. An experimental model of idiopathic pneumonia syndrome after bone marrow transplantation: I. The roles of minor H antigens and endotoxin. Blood 1996;88:3230–3239.
180. Cooke KR, Krenger W, Hill G et al. Host reactive donor T cells are associated with lung injury after experimental allogeneic bone marrow transplantation. Blood 1998;92:2571–2580.

181. Clark JG, Madtes DK, Martin TR et al. Idiopathic pneumonia after bone marrow transplantation: cytokine activation and lipopolysaccharide amplification in the bronchoalveolar compartment. Crit Care Med 1999; 27:1800–1806.

182. Wingard JR, Sostrin MB, Vriesendorp HM et al. Interstitial pneumonitis following autologous bone marrow transplantation. Transplantation 1988;46:61–65.

183. Appelbaum FR, Sullivan KM, Buckner CD et al. Treatment of malignant lymphoma in 100 patients with chemotherapy, total body irradiation, and marrow transplantation. J Clin Oncol 1987;5:1340–1347.

184. Keane TJ, van Dyk J, Rider WD. Idiopathic interstitial pneumonia following marrow transplantation: the relationship with total body irradiation. Int J Radiat Oncol Biol Phys 1981;7:1365–1370.

185. Della Volpe A, Ferreri AJ, Annaloro C et al. Lethal pulmonary complications significantly correlate with individually assessed mean lung dose in patients with hematologic malignancies treated with total body irradiation. Int J Radiat Oncol Biol Phys 2002;52:483–488.

186. Crawford SW, Longton G, Storb R. Acute graft-versus-host disease and the risks for idiopathic pneumonia after marrow transplantation for severe aplastic anemia. Bone Marrow Transplant 1993;12:225–231.

187. Lipshultz SE, Sallan SE. Cardiovascular abnormalities in long-term survivors of childhood malignancy. J Clin Oncol 1993;11:1199–1203.

188. Pihkala J, Saarinen UM, Lundstrom U et al. Effects of bone marrow transplantation on myocardial function in children. Bone Marrow Transplant 1994;13:149–155.

189. Eames GM, Crosson J, Steinberger J et al. Cardiovascular function in children following bone marrow transplant: a cross-sectional study. Bone Marrow Transplant 1997;19:61–66.

190. Storb R, Buckner CD, Dillingham LA, Thomas ED. Cyclophosphamide regimens in rhesus monkeys with and without marrow infusion. Cancer Res 1970;30:2195–2203.

191. Lipshultz SE, Lipsitz SR, Mone SM et al. Female sex and drug dose as risk factors for late cardiotoxic effects of doxorubicin therapy for childhood cancer. N Engl J Med 1995;332:1738–1743.

192. Krischer JP, Epstein S, Cuthbertson DD et al. Clinical cardiotoxicity following anthracycline treatment for childhood cancer: the Pediatric Oncology Group experience. J Clin Oncol 1997;15:1544–1552.

193. Giantris A, Abdurrahman L, Hinkle A et al. Anthracycline-induced cardiotoxicity in children and young adults. Crit Rev Oncol Hematol 1998;27:53–68.

194. Kadan-Lottick NS, Robison LL, Gurney JG et al. Childhood cancer survivors' knowledge about their past diagnosis and treatment: Childhood Cancer Survivor Study. JAMA 2002;287:1832–1839.

195. Praga C, Beretta G, Vigo PL et al. Adriamycin cardiotoxicity: a survey of 1273 patients. Cancer Treat Rep 1979;63:827–834.

196. Gottdiener JS, Appelbaum FR, Ferrans VJ et al. Cardiotoxicity associated with high-dose cyclophosphamide therapy. Arch Intern Med 1981;141:758–763.

197. Aisenberg J, Hsieh K, Kalaitzoglou G et al. Bone mineral density in young adult survivors of childhood cancer. J Pediatr Hematol Oncol 1998;20:241–245.

198. Nysom K, Holm K, Michaelsen KF et al. Bone mass after allogeneic BMT for childhood leukaemia or lymphoma. Bone Marrow Transplant 2000;25:191–196.

199. Socié G, Cahn JY, Carmelo J et al. Avascular necrosis of bone after allogeneic bone marrow transplantation: analysis of risk factors for 4388 patients by the Société Française de Greffe de Moelle (SFGM). Br J Haematol 1997;97:865–870.

200. Enright H, Haake R, Weisdorf D. Avascular necrosis of bone: a common serious complication of allogeneic bone marrow transplantation. Am J Med 1990;89:733–738.

201. Jaffe N, Ried HL, Cohen M et al. Radiation induced osteochondroma in long-term survivors of childhood cancer. Int J Radiat Oncol Biol Phys 1983;9:665–670.

202. Harper GD, Dicks-Mireaux C, Leiper AD. Total body irradiation-induced osteochondromata. J Pediatr Orthop 1998;18:356–358.

203. Stern JM, Sullivan KM, Ott SM et al. Bone density loss after allogeneic hematopoietic stem cell transplantation: a prospective study. Biol Blood Marrow Transplant 2001;7:257–264.

204. Marshall D, Johnell O, Wedel H. Meta-analysis of how well measures of bone mineral density predict occurrence of osteoporotic fractures. BMJ 1996;312:1254–1259.

205. Hui SL, Slemenda CW, Johnston CC Jr. The contribution of bone loss to postmenopausal osteoporosis. Osteoporos Int 1990;1:30–34.

206. Wulff JC, Springmeyer SC, Deeg HJ, Storb R. Canine bronchoalveolar cells: antigen-presenting macrophages are Ia-positive, lymphocytes are of non-B lineage. Blut 1983;47:263–270.

207. Pearce G, Tabensky DA, Delmas PD et al. Corticosteroid-induced bone loss in men (Review). J Clin Endocrinol Metabol 1998;83:801–806.

208. Laan RF, van Riel PL, van de Putte LB et al. Low-dose prednisone induces rapid reversible axial bone loss in patients with rheumatoid arthritis. A randomized, controlled study. Ann Intern Med 1993;119:963–968.

209. Ebeling PR, Thomas DM, Erbas B et al. Mechanisms of bone loss following allogeneic and autologous hemopoietic stem cell transplantation. J Bone Miner Res 1999;14:342–350.

210. Gilsanz V, Carlson ME, Roe TF, Ortega JA. Osteoporosis after cranial irradiation for acute lymphoblastic leukemia. J Pediatr 1990;117:238–244.

211. Wüster C, Abs R, Bengtsson BA et al. The influence of growth hormone deficiency, growth hormone replacement therapy, and other aspects of hypopituitarism on fracture rate and bone mineral density. J Bone Miner Res 2001;16:398–405.

212. Anonymous. NIH Consensus Conference. Optimal calcium intake. NIH Consensus Development Panel on Optimal Calcium Intake (Review). JAMA 1994;272:1942–1948.

213. Anonymous. Recommendations for the prevention and treatment of glucocorticoid-induced osteoporosis. American College of Rheumatology Task Force on Osteoporosis Guidelines. Arthritis Rheum 1996; 39:1791–1801.

214. Stallings VA. Calcium and bone health in children: a review (Review). Am J Ther 1997;4:259–273.

215. Rossouw, JE, Anderson, GL, Prentice, RL et al. Risks and benefits of estrogen plus progestin in healthy postmenopausal women. JAMA 2002;288:321–333.

216. Lindsay R, Gallagher JC, Kleerekoper M, Pickar JH. Effect of lower doses of conjugated equine estrogens with and without medroxyprogesterone acetate on bone in early postmenopausal women. JAMA 2002;287:2668–2676.

217. Khosla S, Melton LJ, Riggs BL. Estrogens and bone health in men (Review). Calcif Tissue Int 2001;69:189–192.

218. Wiesmann A, Pereira P, Bohm P et al. Avascular necrosis of bone following allogeneic stem cell transplantation: MR screening and therapeutic options. Bone Marrow Transplant 1998;22:565–569.

219. Arlet J. Nontraumatic avascular necrosis of the femoral head. Past, present, and future (Review). Clin Orthop 1992;12–21.

220. Drescher W, Schneider T, Becker C et al. Selective reduction of bone blood flow by short-term treatment with high-dose methylprednisolone. An experimental study in pigs. J Bone Joint Surg British Volume 2001; 83:274–277.

221. Wang GJ, Dughman SS, Reger SI, Stamp WG. The effect of core decompression on femoral head blood flow in steroid-induced avascular necrosis of the femoral head. J Bone Joint Surg 1985;67:121–124.

222. Matsui M, Saito S, Ohzono K et al. Experimental steroid-induced osteonecrosis in adult rabbits with hypersensitivity vasculitis. Clin Orthop 1992;277:61–72.

223. Korompilias AV, Gilkeson GS, Seaber AV, Urbaniak JR. Hemorrhage and thrombus formation in early experimental osteonecrosis. Clin Orthop 2001;386:11–18.

224. Castro FPJ, Barrack RL. Core decompression and conservative treatment for avascular necrosis of the femoral head: a meta-analysis. Am J Orthop 2000;29:187–194.

225. Fink JC, Leisenring WM, Sullivan KM et al. Avascular necrosis following bone marrow transplantation: a case-control study. Bone 1998;22:67–71.

226. Koc S, Leisenring W, Flowers MED et al. Therapy for chronic graft-versus-host disease: a randomized trial comparing cyclosporine plus prednisone versus prednisone alone. Blood 2002;100:48–51.

227. Socié G, Selimi F, Sedel L et al. Avascular necrosis of bone after allogeneic bone marrow transplantation: clinical findings, incidence and risk factors. Br J Haematol 1994;86:624–628.

228. Ficat RP. Idiopathic bone necrosis of the femoral head. Early diagnosis and treatment. J Bone Joint Surg 1985;67:3–9.

229. Plakseychuk AY, Shah M, Varitimidis SE et al. Classification of osteonecrosis of the femoral head. Reliability, reproducibility, and prognostic value. Clin Orthop 2001; 386:34–41.

230. Koo KH, Kim R. Quantifying the extent of osteonecrosis of the femoral head. A new method using MRI. J Bone Joint Surg 1995;77:875–880.

231. Steinberg ME, Larcom PG, Strafford B et al. Core decompression with bone grafting for osteonecrosis of the femoral head. Clin Orthop 2001;386:71–78.

232. Mont MA, Carbone JJ, Fairbank AC. Core decompression versus nonoperative management for osteonecrosis of the hip (Review). Clin Orthop 1996;324:169–178.

233. Stulberg BN, Davis AW, Bauer TW et al. Osteonecrosis of the femoral head. A prospective randomized treatment protocol. Clin Orthop 268:1991;140–151.

234. Koo KH, Kim R, Ko GH et al. Preventing collapse in early osteonecrosis of the femoral head. A randomised clinical trial of core decompression. J Bone Joint Surg 1995;77:870–874.

235. Fraunfelder FT, Meyer SM. Ocular toxicity of antineoplastic agents. Ophthalmology 1983;90:1–3.

236. Merriam GRJ, Worgul BV. Experimental radiation cataract—its clinical relevance. Bull NY Acad Med 1983;59:372–392.

237. Axelrod L. Glucocorticoid therapy. Medicine 1976;55:39–65.

238. Urban RCJ, Cotlier E. Corticosteroid-induced cataracts (Review). Surv Ophthalmol 1986;31:102–110.

239. Benyunes MC, Sullivan KM, Deeg HJ et al. Cataracts after bone marrow transplantation: long-term follow-up of adults treated with fractionated total body irradiation. Int J Radiat Oncol Biol Phys 1995;32:661–670.

240. Belkacemi Y, Labopin M, Vernant JP et al. Cataracts after total body irradiation and bone marrow transplantation in patients with acute leukemia in complete remission: a study of the European Group for Blood and Marrow Transplantation. Int J Radiat Oncol Biol Phys 1998;41:659–668.

241. Belkacemi Y, Ozsahin M, Pene F et al. Cataractogenesis after total body irradiation. Int J Radiat Oncol Biol Phys 1996;35:53–60.
242. Fife K, Milan S, Westbrook K et al. Risk factors for requiring cataract surgery following total body irradiation. Radiother Oncol 1994;33:93–98.
243. Deeg HJ, Leisenring W, Storb R et al. Long-term outcome after marrow transplantation for severe aplastic anemia. Blood 1998;91:3637–3645.
244. Ridgway EW, Jaffe N, Walton DS. Leukemic ophthalmopathy in children. Cancer 1976;38:1744–1749.
245. Brown NP, Koretz JF, Bron AJ. The development and maintenance of emmetropia (Review). Eye 1999;13:83–92.
246. Dahan E, Drusedau MU. Choice of lens and dioptric power in pediatric pseudophakia. J Cataract Refractive Surg 1997;23(Suppl 1): 618–623.
247. Ellis FJ. Management of pediatric cataract and lens opacities (Review). Curr Opin Ophthalmol 2002;13:33–37.
248. Tichelli A, Duell T, Weiss M et al. Late-onset keratoconjunctivitis sicca syndrome after bone marrow transplantation: incidence and risk factors. European Group or Blood and Marrow Transplantation (EBMT) Working Party on Late Effects. Bone Marrow Transplant 1996;17:1105–1111.
249. Meadows AT, Massari D, Fergusson J et al. Declines in IQ scores and cognitive dysfunction in children with acute lymphocytic leukemia treated with cranial irradiation. Lancet 1981;2:1015–1018.
250. McGuire T, Sanders JE, Hill D et al. Neuropsychological function in children given total body irradiation for marrow transplantation (Abstr). Pediatr Res 1992;31:143A.
251. Bleyer WA. Neurologic sequelae of methotrexate and ionizing radiation: A new classification. Cancer Treat Rep 1981;65(Suppl 1):89–98.
252. Thompson CB, Sanders JE, Flournoy N et al. The risks of central nervous system relapse and leukoencephalopathy in patients receiving marrow transplants for acute leukemia. Blood 1986;67:195–199.
253. Wade JC, Meyers JD. Neurologic symptoms associated with parenteral acyclovir treatment after marrow transplantation. Ann Intern Med 1983;98:921–925.
254. Phipps S, Mulhern RK. Family cohesion and expressiveness promote resilience to the stress of pediatric bone marrow transplant: a preliminary report. Dev Behav Pediatr 1995;16:257–263.
255. Barrera M, Pringle LAB, Sumbler K, Saunders F. Quality of life and behavioral adjustment after pediatric bone marrow transplantation. Bone Marrow Transplant 2000;26:427–435.
256. Simms S, Kazak AE, Golomb V et al. Cognitive, behavioral, and social outcome in survivors of childhood stem cell transplantation. J Pediatr Hematol Oncol 2002;24:115–119.
257. Cohen JI. Epstein-Barr virus lymphoproliferative disease associated with acquired immunodeficiency (Review). Medicine 1991;70:137–160.
258. The Committee for the Compilation of Materials on Damage Caused by the Atomic Bombs in Hiroshima and Nagasaki. Hiroshima and Nagasaki: The Physical, Medical, and Social Effects of the Atomic Bombings. New York: Basic Books, Inc., 1981.
259. Antonelli A, Miccoli P, Derzhitski VE et al. Epidemiologic and clinical evaluation of thyroid cancer in children from the Gomel region (Belarus). World J Surg 1996;20:867–871.
260. Inskip PD, Hartshorne MF, Tekkel M et al. Thyroid nodularity and cancer among Chernobyl cleanup workers from Estonia. Radiat Res 1997;147:225–235.
261. Deeg HJ, Storb R, Prentice R et al. Increased cancer risk in canine radiation chimeras. Blood 1980;55:233–239.
262. Broerse JJ, Hollander CF, Van Zwieten MJ. Tumor induction in Rheesus monkeys after total body irradiation with X-rays and fission neutrons. Int J Radiat Biol 1981;40:671–676.
263. Curtis RE, Rowlings PA, Deeg HJ et al. Solid cancers after bone marrow transplantation. N Engl J Med 1997;336:897–904.
264. Curtis RE, Travis LB, Rowlings PA et al. Risk of lymphoproliferative disorders after bone marrow transplantation: a multi-institutional study. Blood 1999;94:2208–2216.
265. Deeg HJ, Socié G, Schoch G et al. Malignancies after marrow transplantation for aplastic anemia and Fanconi anemia: a joint Seattle and Paris analysis of results in 700 patients. Blood 1996;87:386–392.
266. Zutter MM, Martin PJ, Sale GE et al. Epstein-Barr virus lymphoproliferation after bone marrow transplantation. Blood 1988;72:520–529.
267. Shapiro RS, McClain K, Frizzera G et al. Epstein-Barr virus associated B cell lymphoproliferative disorders following bone marrow transplantation. Blood 1988;71:1234–1243.
268. Shapiro RS, Chauvenet A, McGuire W et al. Treatment of B-cell lymphoproliferative disorders with interferon alfa and intravenous gamma globulin. N Engl J Med 1988;318:1334.
269. Haddad E, Paczesny S, Leblond V et al. Treatment of B-lymphoproliferative disorder with a monoclonal anti-interleukin-6 antibody in 12 patients: a multicenter phase 1-2 clinical trial. Blood 2001;97:1590–1597.
270. Benkerrou M, Jais JP, Leblond V et al. Anti-B-cell monoclonal antibody treatment of severe posttransplant B-lymphoproliferative disorder: prognostic factors and long-term outcome. Blood 1998;92:3137–3147.
271. Papadopoulos EB, Ladanyi M, Emanuel D et al. Infusions of donor leukocytes to treat Epstein-Barr virus-associated lymphoproliferative disorders after allogeneic bone marrow transplantation. N Engl J Med 1994;330:1185–1191.

272. Bonini C, Ferrari G, Verzeletti S et al. HSV-TK gene transfer into donor lymphocytes for control of allogeneic graft-versus-leukemia. Science 1997;276:1719–1724.

273. Kuehnle I, Huls MH, Liu Z et al. CD20 monoclonal antibody (rituximab) for therapy of Epstein-Barr virus lymphoma after hemopoietic stem-cell transplantation. Blood 2000;95:1502–1505.

274. Carpenter PA, Appelbaum FR, Corey L et al. A humanized non-FcR-binding anti-CD3 antibody, visilizumab, for treatment of steroid-refractory acute graft-versus-host disease. Blood 2002;99:2712–2719.

275. Faye A, Quartier P, Reguerre Y et al. Chimaeric anti-CD20 monoclonal antibody (rituximab) in posttransplant B-lymphoproliferative disorder following stem cell transplantation in children. Br J Haematol 2001; 115:112–118.

276. van Esser JW, Niesters HG, Thijsen SF et al. Molecular quantification of viral load in plasma allows for fast and accurate prediction of response to therapy of Epstein-Barr virus-associated lymphoproliferative disease after allogeneic stem cell transplantation. Br J Haematol 2001;113:814–821.

277. van Esser JW, Niesters HG, van der Holt B et al. Prevention of Epstein-Barr virus-lymphoproliferative disease by molecular monitoring and preemptive rituximab in high-risk patients after allogeneic stem cell transplantation. Blood 2002;99:4364–4369.

278. van Esser JW, van der Holt B, Meijer E et al. Epstein-Barr virus (EBV) reactivation is a frequent event after allogeneic stem cell transplantation (SCT) and quantitatively predicts EBV-lymphoproliferative disease following T cell–depleted SCT. Blood 2001;98:972–978.

279. Wagner HJ, Wessel M, Jabs W et al. Patients at risk for development of posttransplant lymphoproliferative disorder: plasma versus peripheral blood mononuclear cells as material for quantification of Epstein-Barr viral load by using real-time quantitative polymerase chain reaction. Transplantation 2001;72:1012–1019.

280. Gerritsen EJ, Stam ED, Hermans J et al. Risk factors for developing EBV-related B cell lymphoproliferative disorders (BLPD) after non-HLA-identical BMT in children. Bone Marrow Transplant 1996;18:377–382.

281. Fefer A. Immunotherapy and chemotherapy of Moloney sarcoma virus induced tumors in mice. Cancer Res 1969;29:2177–2183.

282. Boyd CN, Ramberg RE, Thomas ED. The incidence of recurrence of leukemia in donor cells after allogeneic bone marrow transplantation. Leuk Res 1982;6:833–837.

283. Stone RM, Neuberg D, Soiffer R et al. Myelodysplastic syndrome as a late complication following autologous bone marrow transplantation for non-Hodgkin's lymphoma. J Clin Oncol 1994;12:2535–2542.

284. Kumar L. Secondary leukaemia after autologous bone marrow transplantation. Lancet 1995;345:810.

285. Socié G. Secondary malignancies. Curr Opin Hematol 1996;3:468–470.

286. Bhatia S, Ramsay NK, Steinbuch M et al. Malignant neoplasms following bone marrow transplantation. Blood 1996;87:3633–3639.

287. Tucker MA, Jones PH, Boice JD et al. Therapeutic radiation at a young age is linked to secondary thyroid cancer. The Late Effects Study Group. Cancer Res 1991;51:2885–2888.

288. Ron E, Lubin JH, Shore RE et al. Thyroid cancer after exposure to external radiation: a pooled analysis of seven studies. Radiat Res 1995;141:259–277.

289. Shore RE, Woodard E, Hildreth N et al. Thyroid tumors following thymus irradiation. J Natl Cancer Inst 1985;74:1177–1184.

290. Ron E, Modan B, Preston D et al. Thyroid neoplasia following low-dose radiation in childhood. Radiat Res 1989;120:516–531.

291. Uderzo C, Van Lint MT, Rovelli A et al. Papillary thyroid carcinoma after total body irradiation. Arch Dis Child 1994;71:256–258.

292. Fogelfeld L, Wiviott MBT, Shore-Freedman E et al. Recurrence of thyroid nodules after surgical removal in patients irradiated in childhood for benign conditions. N Engl J Med 1989;320:835–840.

293. Robison LL, Mertens AC, Boice JD et al. Study design and cohort characteristics of the Childhood Cancer Survivor Study: a multi-institutional collaborative project. Med Pediatr Oncol 2002;38:229–239.

294. Hughes BR, Cunliffe WJ, Bailey CC. Excess benign melanocytic naevi after chemotherapy for malignancy in childhood. BMJ 1989;299:88–91.

# Drugs Commonly Used in Pediatric Stem Cell Transplantation

PAULETTE MEHTA

Most of the drugs used in pediatric stem cell transplantation have other uses. This Appendix describes the uses of these drugs in pediatric stem cell transplantation. It is likely that new drugs will be introduced and that old drugs will continue to find new applications and novel ways of administration.

## DRUGS FOR GRAFT-VERSUS-HOST DISEASE

### Cyclosporine

Cyclosporine is a cyclic polypeptide immunosuppressive used for prophylaxis against graft-versus-host disease (GVHD). It has been used since the mid 1980s and is currently the standard against which all new drugs are compared.[1] New drugs such as tacrolimus are now increasingly being used instead of cyclosporine in many protocols, although none of these regimens has proven to be more efficacious than the other. Cyclosporine is usually used in combination with methotrexate, and sometimes in combination with methotrexate and methylprednisone, although the latter triple-drug regimen has not been proven to be better than the dual regimen alone.[2] The combination of cyclosporine plus prednisone appears to be superior to the drug alone in the setting of chronic GVHD,[2,3] however, some investigators have found that prophylaxis with cyclosporine and prednisone is associated with increased risk of chronic GVHD.[4,5] Once chronic GVHD sets in, the combination of cyclosporine plus prednisone seems to be more effective than prednisone alone as therapy.[3]

Two forms of cyclosporine are available: conventional preparation (Sandimmune™) and a microemulsion (Neoral™). Neoral has greater absorption and bioavailability compared to Sandimmune,[6-8] although there is great inter-patient variability. A topical form of cyclosporine is available also, although it has not yet been fully evaluated for skin-only GVHD to date.

Cyclosporine doses must be higher for children than adults because of increased clearance in the very young. It should be used intravenously during the time of chemotherapy condition until the gastrointestinal tract is completely healed; subsequently it should be substituted by the oral preparation. The usual oral dose is 6.25 mg every hour, and the drug is usually used in combination with low dose methotrexate. Lower doses of cyclosporine have been suggested in some protocols in order to maximize graft-versus-leukemia (GVL) effects through lowering of GVHD prophylaxis.

Blood levels of parent or of total cyclosporine levels are needed to prevent renal toxicity and to assure adequate amounts. Trough concentrations are usually used, although areas under the curve (AUCs) are used in some centers.[7,9,10] Cyclosporine levels must be taken from a lumen of a line in which the drug had not been previously infused, otherwise falsely high levels are obtained.[11,12]

The major adverse effects of cyclosporine are anemia, thrombocytopenia, erythrocytosis, and thromboembolism. Hypertension as a result of renal compromise is also common, and usually begins within a few days of starting the medicine; it may result in seizures, tremors, confusion, and paresthesia. Other neurological abnormalities may include lethargy, tinnitus, speech disorders, coma, and hemiplegia. Encephalopathy with impaired consciousness, convulsions, and visual disturbances including cortical blindness have been reported.[13,14] These manifestations are usually reversible after discontinuation from cyclosporine and they are more likely to occur in patients who have concomitant hypertension who are being treated with high dose steroids, and who have low cholesterol and/or magnesium levels. Some cases show a diffuse white hypodensity on their computed tomography (CT) scan.[13] Other neurological problems that have been reported are seizures, and pseudotumor cerebri. Other side effects include hyperglycemia, gynecomastia, adrenal suppression, fever, and hyperkalemia. Cyclosporine also causes hyperlipidemia with high cholesterol and low high-density lipoproteins and a markedly increased ratio of low density to high density lipoproteins. The long-term ramifications of these findings are not known.

Gastrointestinal side effects are common and include gum hyperplasia, diarrhea, nausea, vomiting, abdominal discomfort, hyperbilirubinemia, and cholestasis. Gingival hyperplasia has been reported in 10 to 70% of patients and is related to dose and usually begins after three months from starting therapy.[15] It may be related to salivary concentration and these side effects may be worse in young patients and in those patients on higher doses. It is more common in patients undergoing solid organ transplantation compared to stem cell transplantation.

Cyclosporine rarely causes thrombotic thrombocytopenia purpura; this resolves upon interruption of cyclosporine, but some patients have required more extensive therapy including plasma infusions and/or exchange transfusions.

Patients also commonly develop gynecomastia, alopecia, brittle fingernails, and myopathy. This can result in dysmorphic features over the long run, including coarse features, cheek puffiness, mandibular prognastism, and thickening of the ears.

Absorption of cyclosporine involves cytochrome p450 enzymes and therefore can be altered when used in combination with many different drugs including acetazolamide, acyclovir, angiotensin-converting enzyme (ACE) inhibitors, allopurinol, amikacin, and rifampin. Nifedipine accentuates gingival hyperplasia,[15] although the mechanism for this is not clear. Absorption is also decreased in patients who have diarrhea and in African-American compared to white patients. There are also different pharmacokinetics in Latino and Caucasian pediatric renal transplantation recipients, suggesting that absorption patterns are genetically determined.[16] Foods affect cyclosporine absorption; milk, grapefruit, and grapefruit juice all increase absorption. Grapefruit and grapefruit juice also decrease metabolism of cyclosporine, and some investigators have suggested that the combination could result in higher cyclosporine levels for lower cost.

An interesting paradoxical effect of cyclosporine is that in addition to its protective effect against GVHD, it can actually cause GVHD in the patient undergoing chemotherapy or undergoing autologous bone marrow transplantation. This observation has given rise to protocols in which GVHD has been induced in patients undergoing autologous stem cell transplantation in an attempt to increase GVHD, and therefore harness the GVL (tumor) effect.[17] This concept needs further testing before it can be validated and/or recommended as a treatment plan.

## Tacrolimus

Tacrolimus is a macrolide compound also used to prevent GVHD. Increasingly it is being used as front line therapy instead of cyclosporine, and is continuing to be used as salvage therapy for patients who either fail to respond to cyclosporine or who develop intolerable side effects. The advantages of tacrolimus over cyclosporine are (a) the absorption is independent of bile; (b) therapeutic blood levels are achieved with oral preparation early on; and (c) it does not cause hirsutism or gingival hyperplasia, common disfiguring effects of cyclosporine.[18-20] Yanik et al. have recently described the role of tacrolimus in 41 patients who were receiving tacrolimus as prophylaxis for GVHD.[21] Twenty patients were undergoing related donor transplants and 20 undergoing unrelated donor transplants. For patients who had received related donor stem cells, grade II–IV GVHD was 33% and for grades III–IV it was 19%. Similarly, for patients undergoing unrelated donor stem cell transplantation the incidence of grade IV GVHD was 55%.[21]

Przepiorka et al. also found tacrolimus to be effective in preventing GVHD in children undergoing cord blood transplantation.[25] In their study, 10 children underwent cord blood stem cell transplantation from unrelated donors. The actuarial risk of grade II GVHD was 77% and no patient had grades III–IV GVHD. Two patients had chronic GVHD. Some but not all of the patients had also received methotrexate.

Another use of tacrolimus is as salvage therapy if there is suboptimal response to cyclosporine or intolerable side effects from cyclosporine. In one study in which 39 patients had been changed from cyclosporine-prednisone to treatment with tacrolimus, 29% were able to stop all immunosuppressives by three years posttransplantation.[22] Resolution of the GVHD was sometimes related to relapse of malignancy, and death. Other investigators have shown that patients resistant to cyclosporine could respond to tacrolimus, but in a small percentage only.[23] In one study, the investigators described the outcome in 53 patients who were changed from cyclosporine treatment to tacrolimus either because of resistance to the drug or because of serious complications including either hemolytic uremic syndrome or neurotoxicity. Nine patients (17%) responded and remained alive, including six who had therapy changed for neurotoxicity. Only one patient who was changed because of resistance to the drug subsequently responded to tacrolimus. Thus, the change from cyclosporine to tacrolimus can be successful, but usually only when it is done for tolerability rather than for effectiveness.

Children have higher clearance rates of tacrolimus than do adults.[24,25] We studied tacrolimus administration in seven patients (8 to 17 years of age) undergoing allogeneic stem cell transplantation, of whom four had received unrelated donor transplant, one matched-related transplant and one other  unrelated umbilical cord transplant. All patients received tacrolimus by continuous infusion at 0.03 to 0.04 mg/k/d on the day prior to transplant and levels of tacrolimus were adjusted to stay within blood levels of 10 to 20 μg/mL. Once patients tolerated the oral medications, the intravenous form was changed to the oral form in a 4:1 conversion. Mean clearance for achieving a therapeutic level was 108 mL/h/kg (range 79 to 142), greater than that in adult patients (71 mL/h/k). The average dose required to achieve a therapeutic range was 0.035. Over the entire course of intravenous tacrolimus, mean clearance was 97 mL/h/kg. Sharp drops in clearance occurred with changes in liver function tests. Patients with the higher clearance had a greater chance of dying of severe acute GVHD. Thus, we recommended that children needed higher starting doses of tacrolimus and needed to begin therapy earlier than adults in order to achieve these levels by the time of donor stem cell infusion. Przepiorka et al. also found that tacrolimus clearance was age-dependent, and that children under six years of age required markedly higher doses than children over six or compared to adults.[25]

A consensus panel published recommendations of tacrolimus use in adults and in children incorporating this information.[26] The panel recommended administering tacrolimus at 0.03 mg/k/d by lean body weight intravenously by continuous infusion from one to two days prior to the start of the transplant. Our own experience, however, suggests that higher doses (0.035 mg/k/d) are better for the child less than six years of age. Therapeutic drug monitoring is essential to keep target range for whole blood levels between 10 and 20 ng/mL. Tacrolimus should be discontinued for intolerable tremor, hemolytic uremic syndrome, leukoencephalopathy, or other serious toxicity. It is usually used in combination with methotrexate or mini-methotrexate (10 or 5 mg/m$^2$ IV on days 1, 3, 6, and 11, respectively), and tapered.[21,26]

The intravenous form should be used if there is gastrointestinal distress as occurs after bone marrow transplantation.[6,27] However, the intravenous form contains a castor oil derivative that has been associated in some patients with anaphylaxis. As soon as the patient's intestinal condition improves, he or she should be treated with the oral form. With either preparation, frequent monitoring of blood levels is required.[7-12,16,28-31] Once the oral dose is begun, it should be used 8 to 12 hours after stopping the intravenous infusion.

Whole blood tacrolimus concentration should be measured and used to guide therapy. Levels between 5 and 10 ng/mL are usually used for pediatric patients.[26,32,33] There is also a topical form of tacrolimus as therapy for skin-only GVHD.

Other side effects of tacrolimus include hypersensitivity to the drug or to the castor oil in which the drug is prepared. This is a particular problem in patients with Netherton syndrome. The drug should be used with caution in patients with renal or hepatic insufficiency, diabetes mellitus, hyperkalemia, and hypertension.

The major side effects reported have been anemia, leukocytosis, thrombocytopenia, leukopenia, and microangiopathic hemolytic anemia. Cardiovascular side effects include hypertension secondary to renal complications and concentric hypertrophic cardiomyopathy in very young pediatric patients. A constant side effect is immunosuppression, which predisposes to cause an increased risk of infection as well as posttransplant lymphoproliferative diseases, especially for patients who have had prior Epstein-Barr virus infections and/or those who undergo T cell-depleted stem cell transplantation. Posttransplant lymphoproliferative disease usually resolves after withdrawal or dose reduction in the dose. As for patients who are taking cyclosporine, leukoencephalopathy can occur and usually responds to withdrawal of the drug.[13,14] The mechanism is not known, but it is common to immunosuppression used during transplantation and is associated with white matter changes on CT scan and/or magnetic resonance imaging (MRI) scans. Other side effects include hyperkalemia, hyperuricemica, nausea, vomiting, anorexia, constipation, and diarrhea. Gingival hyerplasia is very rare, as is pancreatitis. Skin abnormalities reported include itching, rash, and Stevens-Johnson syndrome. Anaphylaxis has also been reported.

There are important drug interactions with amikacin, caspofungin, cimetidine, cisapride, clotrimazole, diltiazm, fluconazole, erythromycin, nonsteroidal antiinflammatory drugs, rifampin, St. John's wort, theophylline, and many others.[34]

## Methotrexate

Methotrexate is an antimetabolite that reversibly inhibits dihydrofolate reductase, which then reduces folic acid to tetrahydrofolic acid and therefore interferes with DNA synthesis, repair, and replication.[21,34-37] It is most commonly used for treatment of pediatric malignancies such as acute lymphocytic leukemia and osteogenic sarcoma, but also it is used as an adjunct to the treatment of GVHD along with other stronger immunosuppressives. It cannot be used alone as an immunosuppressive and protective agent, since it suppresses engraftment of new stem cells at higher doses.

Methotrexate most often is used in combination with either cyclosporine or tacrolimus, usually at doses of 10 mg/m$^2$ four times during the conditioning regimen. Recently minimethotrexate (5 mg/m$^2$, four times during the conditioning regimen on days 1, 3, 6, and 11[37] has been suggested. Major toxicities include pancytopenia and liver function abnormalities. These side effects are usually reversible with leucovorin (folinic acid) and are usually transient. A Stevens-Johnson–like syndrome has occurred with low doses of methotrexate and can be fatal. Gastrointestinal side effects include mucositis, diarrhea, stomatitis, nausea vomiting, diarrhea; these coexist and overlap with similar effects from drugs in the conditioning regimen. Nephrotoxicity is low at such low doses. Photosensitivity occurs after methotrexate and there can be radiation recall dermatitis in some patients.

## Daclizumab

Daclizumab was used for many years in solid organ transplantation before it was introduced into the bone marrow transplantation armamentarium for prophylaxis and for treatment of GVHD.[36,38-42] It is a genetically engineered human IgG1 monoclonal antibody that binds specifically to the alpha chain of the interleukin-2 (IL-2) receptor and thus may reduce the risk of GVHD after stem cell transplantation. It has been used effectively in patients undergoing renal transplants to prevent rejection. Early studies in humans shows that it is safe and that it has efficacy in preventing and treating GVHD in patients undergoing stem cell transplantation.[19,35,36,39,42,43]

In studies on renal transplant patients, Vincenti et al. showed that the drug was safe.[40,41] They evaluated 126 patients who received daclizumab, administered intravenously before transplantation and once every other week afterward for a total of five doses, and compared results of these patients to 134 other patients who received placebo. Rates of solid organ rejection were significantly lower in patients who received daclizumab compared to those receiving placebo. Patients given daclizumab did not have adverse reactions to the drug, nor any increased risk of infections. The serum half-life of daclizumab was 20 days.

Since that time, there have been increasing numbers of reports of daclizumab in patients undergoing stem cell transplantation.[19,35,36,38,39,42,43] In a phase I study of 24 patients with steroid-resistant acute GVHD, patients were treated with single doses of 0.5, 1, or 1.5 mg/k of daclizumab.[2] Responses were seen at all dose levels and in all three organ systems: skin, liver, and gut. Overall improvement was seen in 42% of patients. Anasetti et al. reported on one or two doses of daclizumab in 20 patients who developed acute GVHD after stem cell transplants.[44] These patients were all refractory to cyclosporine and to steroids. Clinical improvement of GVHD was documented in 40% of these patients.

Adverse events of daclizumab in patients undergoing renal transplantation did not differ from those seen in placebo subjects.[1,2] In Phase I studies in 24 patients in whom safety and pharmacokinetics were evaluated, the drug was safe and well tolerated. The only daclizumab-related adverse events were mild shivering in one patient and sweating in another patient. Fifteen of these 24 patients had a total of 24 serious adverse events and 12 patients died from these events; however, none of these events were considered related to the drug, but rather to the patients' underlying disease and to concomitant therapy.

Safety also was shown in the Roche-sponsored phase II/III randomized, double-blind, placebo-controlled trial for prevention of acute GVHD in 260 recipients of matched unrelated donor transplants.[3] Almost all patients experienced adverse events involving the gastrointestinal system (including inflammation of the mucosa, epigastric pain, oral hemorrhage, abdominal pain, buccal mucosal ulceration); however, these events occurred with similar incidence in the daclizumab and placebo groups. Adverse events affecting the autonomic nervous system, respiratory system, metabolic and nutritional systems were also similar in both daclizumab- and placebo-treated groups. Commonly reported adverse events that occurred in a slightly higher frequency in daclizumab-treated patients than placebo-treated patients were hypertension, leg pain, tremor, and pulmonary hypostasis; however, these differences were not statistically significant and patients also were receiving cyclosporine. Willenbacher et al. also showed that daclizumab was beneficial in the treatment of graft-versus-host disease.[42] Sixteen patients with steroid refractory GVHD received daclizumab 1 mg/kg body weight on days 1, 2, –5, 7, 14 and 21. Twelve patients suffered grade III–IV acute GVHD and four patients suffered extensive chronic GVHD. Responses were observed in nine patients (6 with acute and 3 with chronic GVHD). Infections were present in 14 of 16 patients and three deaths were infection related in this series. Thus, daclizumab is effective in some patients with GVHD but an increased incidence of infection may occur.

Przepiorka et al. showed that daclizumab ameliorated GVHD in 43 patients with advanced or steroid refractory graft-versus-host disease. Two separate regimens were tried: (1) daclizumab 1 mg/kg on days 1, 8, 10, 15, 22, and 29; and (2) daclizumab 1 mg/kg on days 1, 4, 8, 15, and 22. The second regimen yielded better results than the first regimen (complete response rates on day 120: 53% vs. 29%).[39]

## Campath-1H

Campath-1H (alemtuzumab) is named for the place where it was discovered, Cambridge-Pathology in England. The H connotes that the molecule has been humanized. It is a recombinant DNA-derived humanized monoclonal antibody against the cell surface glycoprotein CD52 and has been used in many settings including autoimmune neutropenia, non-Hodgkin's lymphoma, rheumatoid arthritis, vasculitis, and B cell chronic lymphocytic leukemia.[45–50] It has a long history as a preventive agent for GVHD after stem cell transplantation, especially in the most high risk situations (i.e., unrelated and/or mismatched transplantation).

Campath is one of the few agents that can be used to protect against GVHD in the very high risk situation in which posttransplant lymphoproliferative disease does not occur. The lack of occurrence of posttransplant lymphoproliferative disease is due to combined inactivation of both T and B cell antigens; thus, the B cell-mediated lymphoproliferation after other forms of T cell-depleted bone marrow transplants does not occur.

Campath-1H is primarily used as an in vitro treatment to purge bone marrow harvests of T cells in order to reduce the amount of GVHD.[45,47,49–54] This procedure is especially important when the risk for GVHD is particularly high and dangerous, as when unrelated and/or mismatched donors are used. Many groups have shown that T cell depletion (through Campath-1H or through other means) decreases GVHD in very high risk patients. T cell depletion through Campath-1H treatment may be particularly advantageous because the antibody is potent and since B-cells are also depleted, thus avoiding the potential complication of posttransplant B-cell–driven lymphoproliferative disease.[49]

Similarly, Hale et al. studied 2,828 patients with leukemia treated by transplantation from human leukocyte antigen (HLA) matched-siblings using Campath-1H depletion.[50] Graft-versus-host disease grades II–IV was 12%. Naparstek et al. studied 146 patients with acute leukemia (81 with acute nonlymphocytic leukemia and 65 with acute lymphocytic leukemia) who received matched sibling transplants.[53] Of these patients, 121 underwent T cell depletion with campath-1H. Rejection of marrow occurred in 6.8% of T cell-depleted transplants, and these patients also received posttransplant donor lymphocyte infusions to include graft versus leukemia; this was associated with clinically significant GVHD and with a decreased relapse rate.

Gennery studied Campath-1M in patients with severe combined immunodeficiency.[46] They reported on 30 patients with who were treated with Campath-1M treated bone marrow as a method of T cell depletion. Survival was 63%. Eleven children died, but this was presumably in most cases due to preexisting infections. Seventeen of 19 long-term survivors had normal immune function, good quality of life, and full remission of disease.[46]

It is associated with infusional toxicity and therefore should be used with premedication to modulate cytokine-associated inflammatory side effects. Campath is also intensely immunosuppressive, and the risk for serious life-threatening infections is very high. Therefore, patients should receive prophylactic treatment to ward off infection as well as preemptive therapy at the first sign of infection. An additional precaution is harvesting and storage of stem cells so that if recovery does not occur after campath administration, infusion of stored stem cells could help to restore an otherwise aplastic and immunoincompetent patient.

Patients who have systemic infections and/or proven hypersensitivity to the drug should not be given Campath-1H. Adverse reactions include prolonged and profound pancytopenia and marrow dysplasia. Cardiovascular effects include hypotension as an infusional related adverse event secondary to cytokine activation. Central nervous system toxicity includes headaches, dysesthesias, dizziness and tremors. Gastrointestinal side effects such as nausea, vomiting, and diarrhea are common as are rash and urticaria. The most serious problem by far is opportunistic infection.

# MOST COMMONLY USED DRUGS IN CONDITIONING REGIMENS FOR STEM CELL TRANSPLANTATION

## Cyclophosphamide

Cyclophosphamide is an alkylating agent that is similar to nitrogen mustard—in that it cross links tumor cell DNA, thereby preventing replication of cells.[55-63] It was the first drug to be used in conditioning regimens for stem cell transplantation and remains the gold standard to which other drugs are compared for conditioning. Despite definite toxicity, cyclophosphamide does not destroy stem cell compartments and therefore patients do not die of pancytopenia if the graft fails to take. Cyclophosphamide is used in very high doses in stem cell transplantation, although not truly ablative doses since the stem cell is not injured. At these high doses, however, toxicities rarely seen at lower doses may occur. The most serious of these are hemorrhagic cystitis and hemorrhagic myocarditis.

Hemorrhagic cystitis can be devastating; risk factors include prior episode of hemorrhagic cystitis, pelvic radiation, total body irradiation, or total lymphoid radiation and concurrent viral infection.[64-69] Infections that can cause hemorrhagic cystitis and aggravate chemotherapy-mediated cystitis are adenovirus, papillomavirus, cytomegalovirus, and bacterial infections.[68] In one study, Efros and colleagues reviewed the records of 217 consecutive patients undergoing bone marrow transplantation.[64] Cystitis developed in 27% and was severe in 6% of patients. Severe cystitis manifested as gross hematuria, clot retention, and drop in hematocrit necessitating blood transplantation. Treatments range from increased hydration, correction of coagulation abnormalities, continuous bladder irrigation, and alum irrigation and intravesical formalin installation. In their study, formalin was the single best treatment for severe, refractory hemorrhagic cystitis. Another treatment that has been recommended is prostaglandin $F_{2\alpha}$.[66] Prophylactic treatment with abundant hyperhydration prior to administration of cyclophosphamide, and treatment with MESNA (2-mercaptoethane sulfonate)[69] are important in preventing the complication. Imaging studies can be very helpful in diagnosing and in following patients with hemorrhagic cystitis.[70] Findings on two-dimensional sonography, color Doppler, power Doppler sonography, CT, MRI, antegrade pyelography, and cystography are also sometimes helpful.[70]

Another major complication, albeit rare, is hemorrhagic myocarditis.[60,61,71-78] This has been only infrequently described and usually in patients who have risk factors for cardiomyopathy such as prior full doses of adriamycin.[69] Murdych and Weisdorf studied serious cardiac complications in patients being treated at the University of Minnesota and found that the overall incidence of serious cardiac events within 100 days of bone marrow transplantation was <1%.[72] The low frequency is mostly attributable to appropriate pretransplant clinical evaluation with exclusion of patients with preexisting serious cardiac disease from treatment with high dose cyclophosphamide and irradiation. Fortunately, nonmyeloablative regimens are now available, allowing such patients to be transplanted on less cardiac toxic regimens. Mori et al. described left ventricular diastolic dysfunction due to cyclophosphamide in blood stem cell transplantation.[71] This group studied 27 consecutive patients, those who received cyclophosphamide in a median dose of 120 mg/k, range 100 to 200 mg/k, and another group that did not, which served as a control group. Ultrasound cardiograms and signaled averaged electrocardiograms (SAECG) were recorded before and after blood stem cell transplantation. Significant posttransplant increases in interventricular septal wall thickness and in Ap/Ep ratio were noted in the first group, as was the QRS duration time, and summated left ventricle (LV) voltage which were reduced in this group. Thus, the cardiotoxicity was characterized by left ventricular diastolic rather than systolic dysfunction. The best way to follow cyclophosphamide-induced cardiac toxicity is through echocardiograms, MUGA scans, as well as noninvasive blood monitoring for natriuretic atrial peptide and for troponin.[73]

Cyclophosphamide causes reproductive defects. The younger the child, the less toxic and long lasting is this effect. Thus, very young girls and boys usually recover their reproductive potential, whereas older teenaged children often do not, and adults usually do not recover.

Cyclophosphamide is metabolized in the liver to 4-hydroxycyclophosphamide, which then breaks down to its activated metabolite. It is the metabolite, 4-hydroxycyclophosphamide, which causes hemorrhagic cystitis.

During stem cell transplantation, it is used in intravenous form because of the high doses that are required. It is associated with hematological toxicity in all patients, increased risk of infection in most patients, and with hemorrhagic cystitis and myocarditis in some patients. Unfortunately, these patients cannot be predicted before they are given their doses of cyclophosphamide. The mechanism of the cardiomyopathology is myocardial necrosis with interstitial myocardial edema and intramyocardial extravasation of blood. Echocardiogram (ECG) analysis with emphasis on QT dispersion can sometimes be useful to predict who will develop cardiotoxicity. Also, infusion of cyclophosphamide is sometimes associated with immediate ECG changes.

Other problems include transient and mild hepatic function abnormalities, blurred vision, and interstitial pneumonitis.[80] The syndrome of interstitial pneumonitis can relate to the drug as well as other insults to the lungs including effects of other drugs, GVHD, infections, and others.

Inappropriate antidiuretic hormone (ADH) secretion can occur resulting in water in toxicity, seizures, and death. As with most chemotherapy drugs, alopecia occurs but the hair returns. As with other immunosuppressive drugs, there is an increased risk of infections after bone marrow transplantation and there is a greater risk of secondary malignancies. Drug-to-drug interactions occur when cyclophosphamide is used in combination with busulfan, allopurinol, ondansetron, and others.

## Fludarabine

Fludarabine, the 2-fluoro, 5-6 phosphate derivative of vidarabine, has been newly introduced into the armamentarium of conditioning regimens, especially for the so-called "mini transplant" conditioning regimens.[81–85] The advantage of fludarabine is that it is immunoabative, not myeloablative, and thus provides the backbone for nonmyeloablative regimens. Levels must be monitored as either area under the curve or as total level.

Fludarabine is available in oral, subcutaneous, or intravenous form. The oral bioavailability is ~55% and therefore the subcutaneous and intravenous forms are preferred for conditioning. Side effects include pancytopenia and autoimmune hemolytic anemia, sometimes with cross-reacting antibodies affecting platelets (i.e., Evans syndrome). Neutropenia and thrombocytopenia are common and are dose limiting. Some patients have experienced neurotoxicity including dysarthria, paresthesia, weakness, seizures, cortical blindness, confusion, and coma. This is similar to the neurotoxicity syndromes seen with cyclosporine and tacrolimus. Visual disturbances also are not uncommon especially when high doses are used. Gastrointestinal side effects are common and usually consist of nausea, vomiting, and diarrhea, although stomatitis and gastrointestinal bleeding have been reported. Dermatological symptoms with skin rashes also occur.

Initial reports indicate that mini-transplantation regimens using fludarabine are effective in allowing engraftment of allogeneic cells. For example, in one study ten patients (5 adults, 5 children) with chronic granulomatosis disease underwent allogeneic stem cell transplantation with a nonmyeloablative regimen consisting of fludarabine 25 mg/m$^2$ on days −5 to −1, cyclophosphamide 60 mg/k on days −7 and −6 and antithymocyte globulin (ATG).[85] All children engrafted and all were alive and well from the time of engraftment, from 16 to 26 months of follow up.[86] In another study, seven children (4 to 17 years of age) who had leukemia or thalassemia major received a fludarabine-based conditioning regimen on an outpatient basis. Of these patients, six engrafted and of these, two relapsed and died at 120 and 360 days, while the rest were alive and in complete remission for 30 to 600 days. In still another study, total body irradiation, fludarabine 30 mg/m$^2$ × 4 d followed by Melphalan 140 mg/m$^2$ on the day prior to stem cell transplantation, resulted in successful engraftment in three children. All received unrelated umbilical cord blood stem cells that were mismatched by one or two HLA antigens. Two of the three patients had a full recovery. The other one developed GVHD and infections; he died on day +96 from respiratory failure.[83]

## Busulfan

Busulfan is often used in pediatric stem cell transplantation to replace the need for radiation therapy at least in very young children. It is a bifunctional alkylating agent, non-cell cycle specific analogue of the nitrogen mustards. Side effects include myelosuppression, seizures, venoocclusive disease, interstitial pneumonia, hemorrhagic cystitis, and alopecia when used in high doses. The complications such as venoocclusive disease have been the most difficult clinically, and can be avoided with accurate drug levels. Drug monitoring is required because the absorption from the oral form is erratic. Moreover, younger children do not tolerate the drug. Low doses predispose to nonengraftment and high doses predispose to venoocclusive disease. Doses must be absolutely in the right range to prevent either of these complications. Yet, monitoring of doses is not available in most centers. When blood is sent out for monitoring of levels, monitoring becomes very difficult because results need to be returned within sufficient time to adjust subsequent doses occurring only hours after the prior dose.

Thus, the advent of intravenous busulfan was a boon to pediatric stem cell transplanters. Nevertheless, this also was problematic because the intravenous drug is expensive, and because monitoring is still required. Even though absorption is not a problem with intravenous administration, drug metabolism is highly variable from one person to another. Younger patients need much higher doses of the drug than older patients because of their higher metabolism of the drug. Moreover, they need more frequent doses because they clear the drug more quickly. There is probably a genetic basis for differences in drug metabolism and drug clearance, although it is not yet possible to screen patients for differences in metabolism and to adjust accordingly.

The usual dose of busulfan in conditioning regimen is 1 mg/k orally four times a day for a total of 16 days. It is usually combined with cyclophosphamide, either before or after, and it replaces the need for radiation therapy as an immunosuppressant allowing engraftment of allogeneic cells.

Major toxicities include myelosuppression, bronchopulmonary dysplasia, cellular dysplasia in organs other than the lungs, mutagenic and carcinogenic changes, ovarian suppression, amenorrhea, hepatic venoocclusive disease, cardiac tamponade, and seizure.

## Melphalan

Melphalan is an alkylating agent that cross links with DNA and is cell cycle nonspecific. It is widely used as treatment for multiple myeloma, Hodgkin's lymphoma, and other diseases. In pediatric patients, however, the major use has been for neuroblastoma, although its use has decreased recently. The major problems have been gastrointestinal toxicity, which can lead to catastrophic results (including typhilitis) and can be fatal.

It is available in oral and intravenous form. When used as an intravenous dose, it should be given as a single infusion over 20 minutes. There is no required adjustment for renal disease, although some investigators recommend reduction if the blood urea nitrogen (BUN) is over 30, especially in children or if the serum creatinine is greater than 1.5 mg/mL. No adjustment is needed in liver failure, since it is not metabolized in the liver, but rather undergoes spontaneous degradation.

The major toxicity of melphalan is bone marrow suppression, and secondary malignancy. Bone marrow suppression is usual and there is permanent damage to the stem cells. Thus, high dose melphalan must only be used in the setting in which stem cells are to be given thereafter and in the setting in which additional stem cells are stored so that the bone marrow can be restored in case of irreversible suppression or myelodysplasia.

Cardiovascular complications can occur and consist of atrial fibrillation. Seizures have been described. Inappropriate ADH secretion can occur also. Gastrointestinal problems include nausea, vomiting, diarrhea, and stomatitis. Sterility and menstrual disorders may occur. Renal failure also may occur, as can liver insufficiency. Pulmonary fibrosis with interstitial pneumonitis is a catastrophic complication that may occur, although it may reverse after withdrawal of the drug. These complications have not been described in children yet. The major drug interactions are with buthionine, cimetidine, and cyclosporine.

Food should be taken in the fasting state since food inhibits the bioavailability of the drug. The drug is often used in combination with either busulfan or radiation therapy.

# MOST COMMONLY USED GROWTH FACTORS FOR CHILDREN UNDERGOING BONE MARROW TRANSPLANTATION

## Erythropoietin

Erythropoietin can be used after bone marrow transplantation to reduce the need for blood transfusions, although it is not routinely used after stem cell transplantation in children.[87] It is, however, used in pediatric patients undergoing cancer chemotherapy and has been used in doses of 25 to 300 units/kg intravenously or subcutaneously three to seven times per week. The major significant side effect has been hypertension. A new major complication has become recognized after use of erythropoietin: pure red cell aplasia, which develops after 3 to 657 months of treatment, is related to neutralizing antierythropoietin antibodies, and may persist even after withdrawal of patient from the medication.[88–92] Some patients develop a functional iron deficiency probably because the demand for hemoglobulin synthesis exceeds ability of the reticuloendothelial system to release iron to transferring.[93–97] There is also risk of myocardial infarction, cerebrovascular accidents, transient ischemic attacks, and other manifestations of clotting, especially in patients who are also receiving hemodialysis and in whom there are central lines. Polycythemia and thrombocytosis can occur after treatment with erythropoietin. Hypertension can occur and is associated with an increase in erythrocyte mass and hematocrit, and also may be due to an increase in vasoconstrictor responses to catecholamines. Central nervous system effects can occur including seizures, aphasia, and confusion. Gastrointestinal effects can occur including nausea, vomiting, and diarrhea.

## Filgastim (Neupogen™)

Granulocyte colony-stimulating factors (G-CSF) are widely used for the mobilization of peripheral blood cells for collection in patients who will receive myeloablative therapy.[98–102] It is also used for the use of neutropenia in patients who are neutropenic as a result of chemotherapy, whether or not it is associated with bone marrow transplant conditioning.

It is an orphan drug with the orphan indication of mobilization of blood progenitor cells; treatment of patients with severe chronic neutropenia; treatment of myelodysplastic syndrome; reduction in the duration of neutropenic; fever; to reduce antibiotic use and hospitalization following therapy for acute myeloid leukemia; and for treatment of neutropenia associated with bone marrow transplantation.

A new form of granulocyte colony-stimulating factor has become available, neulasta, which is the pegylated form of filgastim that can be used once per chemotherapy cycle to decrease the risk of infection and febrile neutropenia.[103–105] It has not been used for peripheral blood progenitor cell mobilization, however, and has not been studied for neutropenia after bone marrow transplantation.

# REFERENCES

1. Kennedy MS, Deeg HJ, Storb R et al. Treatment of acute graft-versus-host disease after allogeneic marrow transplantation. Randomized study comparing corticosteroids and cyclosporine. Am J Med 1985;78(6 Pt 1):978–983.
2. Deeg HJ, Flowers ME, Leisenring W et al. Cyclosporine (CSP) or CSP plus methylprednisolone for graft-versus-host disease prophylaxis in patients with high-risk lymphohemopoietic malignancies: long-term follow-up of a randomized trial. Blood 2000;96:1194–1195.
3. Koc S, Leisenring W, Flowers ME et al. Therapy for chronic graft-versus-host disease: a randomized trial comparing cyclosporine plus prednisone versus prednisone alone. Blood 2002;100:48–51.
4. Arnold AN, Wombolt DG, Whelan TV et al. Mycophenolate mofetil, with cyclosporine and prednisone, reduces early rejection while allowing the use of less antilymphocytic agent induction and cyclosporine in renal recipients with delayed graft function. Clin Transplant 2000;14(4 Pt 2): 421–426.
5. Kumar S, Chen MG, Gastineau DA et al. Prophylaxis of graft-versus-host disease with cyclosporine-prednisone is associated with increased risk of chronic graft-versus-host disease. Bone Marrow Transplant 2001;27:1133–1140.
6. Bokenkamp A, Offner G, Hoyer PF et al. Improved absorption of cyclosporin A from a new microemulsion formulation: implications for dosage and monitoring. Pediatr Nephrol 1995;9:196–198.
7. Kelles A, Herman J, Tjandra-Maga TB et al. Sandimmune to Neoral conversion and value of abbreviated AUC monitoring in stable pediatric kidney transplant recipients. Pediatr Transplant 1999;3:282–287.
8. van Mourik ID, Thomson M, Kelly DA. Comparison of pharmacokinetics of Neoral and Sandimmune in stable pediatric liver transplant recipients. Liver Transplant Surg 1999;5:107–111.
9. Hoyer PF. Therapeutic drug monitoring of cyclosporin A: should we use the area under the concentration-time curve and forget trough levels? Pediatr Transplant 2000;4:2–5.
10. Meier-Kriesche HU, Kaplan B, Brannan P et al. A limited sampling strategy for the estimation of eight-hour neoral areas under the curve in renal transplantation. Ther Drug Monit 1998;20:401–407.
11. Shulman RJ, Ou C, Reed T, Gardner P. Central venous catheters versus peripheral veins for sampling blood levels of commonly used drugs. JPEN J Parenter Enteral Nutr 1998;22:234–237.
12. Busca A, Miniero R, Vassallo E et al. Monitoring of cyclosporine blood levels from central venous lines: a misleading assay? Ther Drug Monit 1994;16:71–74.
13. Jeruss J, Braun SV, Reese JC, Guillot A. Cyclosporine-induced white and grey matter central nervous system lesions in a pediatric renal transplant patient. Pediatr Transplant 1998;2:45–50.
14. Rodriguez E, Delucchi A, Cano F. [Neurotoxicity caused by cyclosporin A in renal transplantation in children.] (Spanish) Rev Med Chil 1992;120:300–303.
15. David-Neto E, Lemos FB, Furusawa EA et al. Impact of cyclosporin A pharmacokinetics on the presence of side effects in pediatric renal transplantation. J Am Soc Nephrol 2000;11:343–349.
16. Lemire J, Capparelli EV, Benador N et al. Neoral pharmacokinetics in Latino and Caucasian pediatric renal transplant recipients. Pediatr Nephrol 2001;16:311–314.
17. Baron F, Gothot A, Salmon JP et al. Clinical course and predictive factors for cyclosporin-induced autologous graft-versus-host disease after autologous haematopoietic stem cell transplantation. Br J Haematol 2000;111:745–753.
18. Cox KL, Freese DK. Tacrolimus (FK506): the pros and cons of its use as an immunosuppressant in pediatric liver transplantation. Clin Invest Med 1996;19:389–392.
19. Jacobsohn DA, Vogelsang GB. Novel pharmacotherapeutic approaches to prevention and treatment of GVHD. Drugs 2002;62:879–889.
20. McDiarmid SV, Busuttil RW, Ascher NL et al. FK506 (tacrolimus) compared with cyclosporine for primary immunosuppression after pediatric liver transplantation. Results from the U.S. Multicenter Trial. Transplantation 1995;59:530–536.
21. Yanik G, Levine JE, Ratanatharathorn V et al. Tacrolimus (FK506) and methotrexate as prophylaxis for acute graft-versus-host disease in pediatric allogeneic stem cell transplantation. Bone Marrow Transplant 2000;26:161–167.
22. Carnevale-Schianca F, Martin P, Sullivan K et al. Changing from cyclosporine to tacrolimus as salvage therapy for chronic graft-versus-host disease. Biol Blood Marrow Transplant 2000;6:613–620.
23. Furlong T, Storb R, Anasetti C et al. Clinical outcome after conversion to FK 506 (tacrolimus) therapy for acute graft-versus-host disease resistant to cyclosporine or for cyclosporine-associated toxicities. Bone Marrow Transplant 2000;26:985–991.
24. Mehta P, Beltz S, Kedar A et al. Increased clearance of tacrolimus in children: need for higher doses and earlier initiation prior to bone marrow transplantation. Bone Marrow Transplant 1999;24:1323–1327.
25. Przepiorka D, Blamble D, Hilsenbeck S et al. Tacrolimus clearance is age-dependent within the pediatric population. Bone Marrow Transplant 2000;26:601–605.

26. Przepiorka D, Devine S, Fay J et al. Practical considerations in the use of tacrolimus for allogeneic marrow transplantation. Bone Marrow Transplant 1999;24:1053–1056.
27. Novelli M, Muiesan P, Mieli-Vergani G et al. Oral absorption of tacrolimus in children with intestinal failure due to short or absent small bowel. Transplant Int 1999;12:463–465.
28. David OJ, Johnston A. Limited sampling strategies for estimating cyclosporin area under the concentration-time curve: review of current algorithms. Ther Drug Monit 2001;23:100–114.
29. de Lima M, van Besien K, Gajewski J et al. High-dose melphalan and allogeneic peripheral blood stem cell transplantation for treatment of early relapse after allogeneic transplant. Bone Marrow Transplant 2000;26:333–338.
30. Yuhki Y, Tadano K, Takahashi Y et al. [Cyclosporine level in blood as monitored by area-under-the-curve (AUC). III. The influence of absorption phase after orally dosing.] (Japanese) Yakugaku Zasshi 1994;114:589–596.
31. Pettersen MD, Driscoll DJ, Moyer TP et al. Measurement of blood serum cyclosporine levels using capillary "fingerstick" sampling: a validation study. Transplant Int 1999;12:429–432.
32. Asante-Korang A, Boyle GJ, Webber SA et al. Experience of FK506 immune suppression in pediatric heart transplantation: a study of long-term adverse effects. J Heart Lung Transplant 1996;15:415–422.
33. Moreno M, Manzanares C, Castellano F et al. Monitoring of tacrolimus as rescue therapy in pediatric liver transplantation. Ther Drug Monit 1998;20:376–379.
34. Chao NJ, Schmidt GM, Niland JC et al. Cyclosporine, methotrexate, and prednisone compared with cyclosporine and prednisone for prophylaxis of acute graft-versus-host disease. N Engl J Med 1993;329:1225–1230.
35. Simpson D. Drug therapy for acute graft-versus-host disease prophylaxis. J Hematother Stem Cell Res 2000;9:317–325.
36. Simpson D. New developments in the prophylaxis and treatment of graft versus host disease. Expert Opin Pharmacother 2001;2:1109–1117.
37. Vettenranta K, Hovi L, Parto K, Saarinen-Pihkala UM. Very low-dose methotrexate in the treatment of GVHD in children. Bone Marrow Transplant 1997;20:75–77.
38. Bumgardner GL, Ramos E, Lin A, Vincenti F. Daclizumab (humanized anti-IL-2R alpha mAb) prophylaxis for prevention of acute rejection in renal transplant recipients with delayed graft function. Transplantation 2001;72:642–647.
39. Przepiorka D, Kernan NA, Ippoliti C et al. Daclizumab, a humanized anti-interleukin-2 receptor alpha chain antibody, for treatment of acute graft-versus-host disease. Blood 2000;95:83–89.
40. Vincenti F, Nashan B, Light S. Daclizumab: outcome of phase III trials and mechanism of action. Double Therapy and the Triple Therapy Study Groups. Transplant Proc 1998;30:2155–2158.
41. Vincenti F, Kirkman R, Light S et al. Interleukin-2-receptor blockade with daclizumab to prevent acute rejection in renal transplantation. Daclizumab Triple Therapy Study Group. N Engl J Med 1998;338:161–165.
42. Willenbacher W, Basara N, Blau IW et al. Treatment of steroid refractory acute and chronic graft-versus-host disease with daclizumab. Br J Haematol 2001;112:820–823.
43. Jacobsohn DA. Novel therapeutics for the treatment of graft-versus-host disease. Expert Opin Investig Drugs 2002;11:1271–1280.
44. Anasetti C, Hansen JA, Waldmann TA et al. Treatment of acute graft-versus-host disease with humanized anti-Tac: an antibody that binds to the interleukin-2 receptor. Blood 1994;84:1320–1327.
45. Hamblin M, Marsh JC, Lawler M et al. Campath-1G in vivo confers a low incidence of graft-versus-host disease associated with a high incidence of mixed chimaerism after bone marrow transplantation for severe aplastic anaemia using HLA-identical sibling donors. Bone Marrow Transplant 1996;17:819–824.
46. Gennery AR, Dickinson AM, Brigham K et al. CAMPATH-1M T-cell depleted BMT for SCID: long-term follow-up of 19 children treated 1987–98 in a single center. Cytotherapy 2001;3:221–232.
47. Dickinson AM, Reid MM, Abinun M et al. In vitro T cell depletion using Campath 1M for mismatched BMT for severe combined immunodeficiency (SCID). Bone Marrow Transplant 1997;19:323–329.
48. Fischer A, Friedrich W, Fasth A et al. Reduction of graft failure by a monoclonal antibody (anti-LFA-1 CD11a) after HLA nonidentical bone marrow transplantation in children with immunodeficiencies, osteopetrosis, and Fanconi's anemia: a European Group for Immunodeficiency/European Group for Bone Marrow Transplantation report. Blood 1991;77:249–256.
49. Jacobs P, Wood L, Fullard L et al. T cell depletion by exposure to Campath-1G in vitro prevents graft-versus-host disease. Bone Marrow Transplant 1994;13:763–769.
50. Hale G, Cobbold S, Waldmann H. T cell depletion with CAMPATH-1 in allogeneic bone marrow transplantation. Transplantation 1988;45:753–759.
51. Marks DI, Bird JM, Vettenranta K et al. T cell-depleted unrelated donor bone marrow transplantation for acute myeloid leukemia. Biol Blood Marrow Transplant 2000;6:646–653.
52. Champlin RE, Passweg JR, Zhang MJ et al. T-cell depletion of bone marrow transplants for leukemia from donors other than HLA-identical siblings: advantage of T-cell antibodies with narrow specificities. Blood 2000;95:3996–4003.

53. Champlin RE, Passweg JR, Zhang MJ et al. T-cell-depleted allogeneic bone marrow transplantation for acute leukaemia using Campath-1 antibodies and post-transplant administration of donor's peripheral blood lymphocytes for prevention of relapse. Br J Haematol 1995;89:506–515.

54. Ringden O, Potter MN, Oakhill A et al. Transplantation of peripheral blood progenitor cells from unrelated donors. Bone Marrow Transplant 1996;17(Suppl 2):S62–S64.

55. Deeg HJ, Storer B, Slattery JT et al. Conditioning with targeted busulfan and cyclophosphamide for hemopoietic stem cell transplantation from related and unrelated donors in patients with myelodysplastic syndrome. Blood 2002;100:1201–1207.

56. Hamilton VM, Norris C, Bunin N et al. Cyclophosphamide-based, seven-drug hybrid and low-dose involved field radiation for the treatment of childhood and adolescent Hodgkin disease. J Pediatr Hematol Oncol 2001;23:84–88.

57. Leung CK. Fifteen years' review of advanced childhood neuroblastoma from a single institution in Hong Kong. Chin Med J (English) 1998;111:466–469.

58. Stoppa AM, Hirn J, Blaise D et al. Autologous bone marrow transplantation for B cell malignancies after in vitro purging with floating immunobeads. Bone Marrow Transplant 1990;6:301–307.

59. Vossen JM, Brinkman DM, Bakker B et al. Rationale for high-dose cyclophosphamide and medium-dose total body irradiation in the conditioning of children with progressive systemic and polyarticular juvenile chronic arthritis before autologous stem cell transplantation. Rheumatology (Oxford) 1999;38:762–763.

60. Weigel BJ, Breitfeld PP, Hawkins D et al. Role of high-dose chemotherapy with hematopoietic stem cell rescue in the treatment of metastatic or recurrent rhabdomyosarcoma. J Pediatr Hematol Oncol 2001;23:272–276.

61. Yule SM, Foreman NK, Mitchell C et al. High-dose cyclophosphamide for poor prognosis and recurrent pediatric brain tumors: a dose-escalation study. J Clin Oncol 1997;15:3258–3265.

62. Zecca M, Pession A, Messina C et al. Total body irradiation, thiotepa, and cyclophosphamide as a conditioning regimen for children with acute lymphoblastic leukemia in first or second remission undergoing bone marrow transplantation with HLA-identical siblings. J Clin Oncol 1999;17:1838–1846.

63. Zoubek A, Holzinger B, Mann G et al. High-dose cyclophosphamide, adriamycin, and vincristine (HD-CAV) in children with recurrent solid tumor. Pediatr Hematol Oncol 1994;11:613–623.

64. Efros MD, Ahmed T, Coombe N et al. Urologic complications of high-dose chemotherapy and bone marrow transplantation. Urology 1994;43:355–360.

65. Erer B, Angelucci E, Baronciani D et al. Hemorrhagic cystitis after allogeneic bone marrow transplantation for thalassemia. Bone Marrow Transplant 1993;12(Suppl 1):93–95.

66. Levine LA, Jarrard DF. Treatment of cyclophosphamide-induced hemorrhagic cystitis with intravesical carboprost tromethamine. J Urol 1993;149:719–723.

67. Lou FD, Liu HC, Yao SQ. [Hemorrhagic cystitis in the course of hematopoietic stem cell transplantation.] (Chinese) Zhonghua Nei Ke Za Zhi 1993;32:250–252.

68. Russell SJ, Vowels MR, Vale T. Haemorrhagic cystitis in paediatric bone marrow transplant patients: an association with infective agents, GVHD and prior cyclophosphamide. Bone Marrow Transplant 1994;13:533–539.

69. Sencer SF, Haake RJ, Weisdorf DJ. Hemorrhagic cystitis after bone marrow transplantation. Risk factors and complications. Transplantation 1993;56:875–879.

70. McCarville MB, Hoffer FA, Gingrich JR et al. Imaging findings of hemorrhagic cystitis in pediatric oncology patients. Pediatr Radiol 2000;30:131–138.

71. Mori T, Yanagi N, Maruyama T et al. Left ventricular diastolic dysfunction induced by cyclophosphamide in blood stem cell transplantation. Jpn Heart J 2002;43:249–261.

72. Murdych T, Weisdorf DJ. Serious cardiac complications during bone marrow transplantation at the University of Minnesota, 1977–1997. Bone Marrow Transplant 2001;28:283–287.

73. Snowden JA, Hill GR, Hunt P et al. Assessment of cardiotoxicity during haemopoietic stem cell transplantation with plasma brain natriuretic peptide. Bone Marrow Transplant 2000;26:309–313.

74. von Herbay A, Dorken B, Mall G, Korbling M. Cardiac damage in autologous bone marrow transplant patients: an autopsy study. Cardiotoxic pretreatment as a major risk factor. Klin Wochenschr 1988;66:1175–1181.

75. Abe T, Takaue Y, Okamoto Y et al. Syndrome of inappropriate antidiuretic hormone secretion (SIADH) in children undergoing high-dose chemotherapy and autologous peripheral blood stem cell transplantation. Pediatr Hematol Oncol 1995;12:363–369.

76. Galotto M, Berisso G, Delfino L et al. Stromal damage as consequence of high-dose chemo/radiotherapy in bone marrow transplant recipients. Exp Hematol 1999;27:1460–1466.

77. Kimby E, Brandt L, Nygren P, Glimelius B; SBU-group. Swedish Council of Technology Assessment in Health Care. A systematic overview of chemotherapy effects in B-cell chronic lymphocytic leukaemia. Acta Oncol 2001;40:224–230.

78. Schlegel PG, Haber HP, Beck J et al. Hepatic veno-occlusive disease in pediatric stem cell recipients: successful treatment with continuous infusion of prostaglandin E1 and low-dose heparin. Ann Hematol 1998;76:37–41.

79. Stillwell TJ, Bernson RC Jr, and Burgert EO. Cyclophosphamide-induced hemorrhagic cystitis in Ewing's sarcoma. J Clin Oncol 1988;6:76–82.
80. Kushner BH, O'Reilly RJ, LaQuaglia M, Cheung NK. Dose-intensive use of cyclophosphamide in ablation of neuroblastoma. Cancer 1990;66:1095–1100.
81. Aker M, Varadi G, Slavin S, Nagler A. Fludarabine-based protocol for human umbilical cord blood transplantation in children with Fanconi anemia. J Pediatr Hematol Oncol 1999;21:237–239.
82. Boulad F, Gillio A, Small TN et al. Stem cell transplantation for the treatment of Fanconi anaemia using a fludarabine-based cytoreductive regimen and T-cell-depleted related HLA-mismatched peripheral blood stem cell grafts. Br J Haematol 2000;111:1153–1157.
83. Chan KW, Bekassy AN, Ha CS et al. Fludarabine-based preparative protocol for unrelated donor cord blood transplantation in children: successful engraftment with minimal toxicity. Bone Marrow Transplant 1999;23:849–851.
84. Chan KW, Li CK, Worth LL et al. A fludarabine-based conditioning regimen for severe aplastic anemia. Bone Marrow Transplant 2001;27:125–128.
85. Pedrazzoli P, Da Prada GA, Giorgiani G et al. Allogeneic blood stem cell transplantation after a reduced-intensity, preparative regimen: a pilot study in patients with refractory malignancies. Cancer 2002;94: 2409–2415.
86. Horwitz ME, Barrett AJ, Brown MR et al. Treatment of chronic granulomatous disease with nonmyeloablative conditioning and a T-cell-depleted hematopoietic allograft. N Engl J Med 2001;344:881–888.
87. Baron F, Sautois B, Baudoux E et al. Optimization of recombinant human erythropoietin therapy after allogeneic hematopoietic stem cell transplantation. Exp Hematol 2002;30:546–554.
88. Casadevall N. Antibodies against rHuEPO: native and recombinant. Nephrol Dial Transplant 2002;17(Suppl 5):42–47.
89. Gershon SK, Luksenburg H, Cote TR, Braun MM. Pure red-cell aplasia and recombinant erythropoietin. N Engl J Med 2002;346:1584–1586, 2002; discussion 1584–1586.
90. Mercadal L, Sutton L, Casadevall N, Bagnis C. Immunological reaction against erythropoietin causing red-cell aplasia. Nephrol Dial Transplant 2002;17:943.
91. Okoshi Y, Imagawa S, Higuchi M et al. A patient with acquired pure red cell aplasia showing a positive antiglobulin test and the presence of inhibitor against erythroid precursors. Intern Med 2002;41:589–592.
92. Sokol L, Prchal JT. Pure red-cell aplasia and recombinant erythropoietin. N Engl J Med 2002;346:1584–1586; discussion 1584–1586.
93. Deeg HJ, Storer B, Slattery JT et al. Conditioning with targeted busulfan and cyclophosphamide for hemopoietic stem cell transplantation from related and unrelated donors in patients with myelodysplastic syndrome. Blood 2002;100:1201–1207.
94. Hawkins D, Barnett T, Bensinger W et al. Busulfan, melphalan, and thiotepa with or without total marrow irradiation with hematopoietic stem cell rescue for poor-risk Ewing-Sarcoma-Family tumors. Med Pediatr Oncol 2000;34:328–337.
95. Carli M, Colombatti R, Oberlin O et al. High-dose melphalan with autologous stem-cell rescue in metastatic rhabdomyosarcoma. J Clin Oncol 1999;17:2796–2803.
96. Diaz MA, Vicent MG, Madero L. High-dose busulfan/melphalan as conditioning for autologous PBPC transplantation in pediatric patients with solid tumors. Bone Marrow Transplant 1999;24:1157–1159.
97. Hassan M. The role of busulfan in bone marrow transplantation. Med Oncol 1999;16:166–176.
98. Cairo MS. Myelopoietic growth factors after stem cell transplantation: does it pay? J Pediatr Hematol Oncol 2001;23:2–6.
99. Frenck RW Jr, Shannon KM. Hematopoietic growth factors in pediatrics. Curr Opin Pediatr 1993;5:94–102.
100. Hann IM. Haemopoietic growth factors and childhood cancer. Eur J Cancer 1995;31A:1476–1478.
101. Levine JE, Boxer LA. Clinical applications of hematopoietic growth factors in pediatric oncology. Curr Opin Hematol 2002;9:222–227.
102. Madero L, Villa M, Benito A et al. Peripheral blood progenitor cells for autologous transplant in children. Bone Marrow Transplant 1998;21(Suppl 2):S8–S10.
103. Pegfilgrastim (Neulasta) for prevention of febrile neutropenia. Med Lett Drugs Ther 2002;44:44–45.
104. Bence AK, Adams VR. Pegfilgrastim: a new therapy to prevent neutropenic fever. J Am Pharm Assoc (Wash) 2002;42:806–808.
105. Curran MP, Goa KL. Pegfilgrastim. Drugs 2002;62:1207–1213; discussion 1214–1215.

Fatty acid
 Essential fatty acid deficiency, 79
Female puberty and fertility, after HSCT,
  419–422
Fertility, after HSCT, 418–425
Filgastim (Neupogen™), for BMT
  patients, 468
Final adult height, and growth hormone
  deficiency, after HSCT, 413–418
First phase, after HSCT, 391–393
Fludarabine, for conditioning regimens
  for HSCT, 465–466
Follow-up, after HSCT, 61
Fucosidosis, 249–250
Full-myeloablation approach, 34–35
Fungal infections, after HSCT, 397–398

# G

Gaucher disease, 248
GCT. *See* Germ cell tumors (GCT)
Genes, polymorphism of, 51
Genetic diseases, donor testing for,
  121–123
Germ cell tumors (GCT), 179–181
Germ cells, after HSCT, 424–425
Gliomas, 176–178
Globoid cell leukodystrophy, 245–246
Glutamine, for HSCT patients, 83–84
$G_{M2}$ activator deficiency disease, 250
$G_{M2}$ gangliosidoses, 250
Gonadal function, puberty, and fertility,
  after HSCT, 418–425
Graft-versus-host disease (GVHD), 6–7,
  401–410
 acute, 71–72, 401–407, 402t
 chronic, 74–75, 401, 407–410
 cytokine secretion in, 403
 drugs for, 457–463
 of the gut, 71
 hyperacute, 403
 treatment of, 7
 in umbilical cord blood
   transplantations, 345, 346t
Graft-versus-leukemia (GVL), 346–347

Growth and development, delayed, in
  HSCT patient, 75
Growth and direct tissue effects, after
  HSCT, 427–428
Growth factors, most commonly used, for
  bone marrow transplantation
  patients, 467–468
Growth hormone deficiency, after HSCT,
  413–418
Gut, graft-versus-host disease of the, 71
GVHD. *See* Graft-versus-host disease
  (GVHD)
GVL. *See* Graft-versus-leukemia (GVL)

# H

Haplotype-disparate transplants,
  noninherited maternal, 345
Haplotypes, frequency of HLA, 52, 53t
HCT. *See* Hematopoietic stem cell
  transplantation (HSCT)
The heart, after HSCT, effects on, 434–435
Height, final adult, and growth hormone
  deficiency after HSCT, 413–418
Height standard deviation, after HSCT,
  414f–416f
Hematologic/metabolic disorders,
  undetected, 348–349
Hematopoiesis, mouse models of, 360
Hematopoietic cell expansion, ex vivo,
  363–365, 365t
Hematopoietic cell transplantation
  (HCT). *See* Hematopoietic stem
  cell transplantation (HSCT)
Hematopoietic content, in cord blood
  units, 339
Hematopoietic precursors, 338–339
Hematopoietic stem cell transplantation
  (HSCT). *See also* Specific diseases
 after
  deficits in host defenses, 389–391,
    390t
  infectious complications, 389–398
  late effects, 413–445
 allogeneic *versus* autologous, 142–143